Clinical Atlas of Canine and Feline Dermatology

Clinical Atlas of Canine and Feline Dermatology

Edited by

Kimberly S. Coyner, DVM, DACVD

Dermatology Clinic for Animals
Lacey, WA, USA

WILEY Blackwell

This edition first published 2020

Registered Office
John Wiley & Sons, Inc., 111 River Street, Hoboken, NJ 07030, USA

Editorial Office
111 River Street, Hoboken, NJ 07030, USA

For details of our global editorial offices, customer services, and more information about Wiley products visit us at www.wiley.com.

Wiley also publishes its books in a variety of electronic formats and by print-on-demand. Some content that appears in standard print versions of this book may not be available in other formats.

Library of Congress Cataloging-in-Publication Data

Names: Coyner, Kimberly S., editor.
Title: Clinical atlas of canine and feline dermatology / edited by Kimberly S. Coyner.
Description: Hoboken, NJ : Wiley-Blackwell, 2020. | Includes bibliographical references and index. |
Identifiers: LCCN 2019003283 (print) | LCCN 2019004616 (ebook) | ISBN 9781119226321 (Adobe PDF) | ISBN 9781119226314 (ePub) | ISBN 9781119226307 (hardback)
Subjects: LCSH: Dogs–Disease. | Cats–Disease. | Veterinary dermatology. | MESH: Skin Diseases–veterinary | Dog Diseases–diagnosis | Dog Diseases–drug therapy | Cat Diseases–diagnosis | Cat Diseases–drug therapy | Atlas
Classification: LCC SF992.S55 (ebook) | LCC SF992.S55 C55 2019 (print) | NLM SF 992.S55 | DDC 636.7/08965–dc23
LC record available at https://lccn.loc.gov/2019003283

Cover Design: Wiley
Cover Image: © Kimberly S. Coyner

Set in 10/12pt Warnock by SPi Global, Pondicherry, India

10 9 8 7 6 5 4 3 2 1

For Marc, my best friend, my support, my love.

Contents

List of contributors

Patricia Ashley, DVM, DACVD
Veterinary Allergy and Dermatology Services
Springfield, OR, USA

Jacquelyn Campbell, DVM, DACVD
Animal Allergy and Dermatology of Colorado
Colorado Springs, CO, USA

Kimberly S. Coyner, DVM, DACVD
Dermatology Clinic for Animals
Lacey, WA, USA

Alexandra Gould, DVM
Dermatology Clinic for Animals, Lacey, WA, USA
Animal Allergy and Dermatology, Las Vegas, NV, USA

Heide Newton, DVM, DACVD
Dermatology for Animals
Tucson, AZ, USA

Anthea Schick, DVM, DACVD
Dermatology for Animals, Gilbert, AZ, USA
Dermatology for Animals, Scottsdale, AZ, USA

Amy Shumaker, DVM, DACVD
VCA Southshore (Weymouth) Animal Hospital
South Weymouth, MA, USA

Preface

Veterinary dermatology can be, at once, inspiring, interesting, and frustrating. When I first became a general practice veterinarian I disliked dermatology cases, as they all seemed to have similar symptoms with a huge laundry list of possible causes and I had no idea where to start diagnostically. The dermatology books I had access to were excellent, but discussed dermatology diagnosis and treatment disease by disease, and the animals that entered my exam room did not walk in with their diseases labelled on their charts. After a frustrating time in general practice, I had the fortunate and life-changing experience of working with Dr. Linda Medleau, the brilliant veterinary dermatologist at the University of Georgia, who taught me the joy and ease of veterinary dermatology. I learned that with consideration of species, breed, clinical signs, and recognizing pattern and type of lesions, as well as using a simple and methodical workup of every case, dermatology became an intuitive and enjoyable specialty. When I was asked to design a new veterinary dermatology atlas, I envisioned a book which did not only present cases disease by disease, but by how the animals present to veterinarians, as itchy, crusty, and/or alopecic, then guided readers how to accurately recognize specific lesions and patterns of lesions to formulate a reasonable list of differential diagnoses, and utilize and interpret appropriate diagnostics to make the correct diagnosis. I asked for input from six other experienced private practice veterinary dermatologists to obtain a wide range of practical knowledge. We present efficient algorithms for diagnosis and treatment of the most common clinical presentations of dermatologic disorders in companion animals, including pruritus, alopecia, otitis, atopy, pyoderma, dermatophytosis, and pemphigus foliaceus. We tried to include many pictures in our descriptions of diagnostic techniques, lesions, and diseases, as dermatology is the most visual specialty. Once the diagnosis is achieved, then treatment options are presented in simple tables easily referenced in a busy practice. Treatment options are presented not as an exhaustive or dogmatic list, but as I and my collaborators would choose to ideally treat our patients; when appropriate, first-line, second-line, and third-line treatments are offered. A dermatology formulary gives more detail of specific drugs and topical therapies which were available at the time of publication. This Atlas is not intended to replace a veterinary dermatology reference book such as *Small Animal Dermatology*, but to help busy private practitioners treat dermatology patients efficiently and accurately.

Acknowledgments

I am indebted to all my friends and amazing dermatologists who contributed their knowledge and images to this book, to the VINers who very helpfully donated many great images, and to all my dermatology patients and their dedicated owners who make veterinary dermatology such a fulfilling specialty.

About the companion website

This book is accompanied by a companion website:

www.wiley.com/go/coyner/dermatology

The website features video clips, demonstrating dermatologic diagnostic techniques, including skin scrapings and cytology, aspiration of skin masses for cytology, and biopsy.

1

Dermatology diagnostics

Kimberly S. Coyner, DVM, DACVD

Dermatology Clinic for Animals, Lacey, WA, USA

Indications:

- All cases with hair loss, scaling, crusting, papules, pustules, lichenification, or otitis should be screened for infectious organisms with skin scrapings and surface skin cytology; flea combing to screen for fleas and flea feces as well as for lice is also necessary, even in indoor pets.
- These quick and easy in-house tests will not only allow for the accurate diagnosis of the dermatitis and guide appropriate therapy, but are also revenue generators.
- Additionally, with the emerging problem of antibiotic-resistant bacterial skin infections, cytology to monitor response to antimicrobial therapy is important and can guide decisions about culture submission.
- The first important consideration is to buy a good microscope! There are numerous affordable, high quality microscopes available; I use the Swift M10 series biological lab microscope, but there are many other options.
- It is important to teach our veterinary technicians and assistants how to appropriately take care of microscopes, and there are numerous online resources including http://micro.magnet.fsu.edu/primer/anatomy/cleaning.html.

1.1 Skin scrapings (*See video on companion website*)

- Skin scrapings are used to diagnose mites such as scabies, *Demodex*, and *Cheyletiella*.
- A dulled #10 scalpel blade or medical curette/spatula and mineral oil are used to collect skin debris (Figures 1.1–1.4), which is then mixed with more mineral oil on a microscope slide and observed under 4–10×, with the condenser down for maximum contrast.
- For scabies, multiple wide superficial scrapings of crusted, papular, or alopecic lesions on elbows, pinnal margins, and ventral trunk should be obtained (Figures 1.5 and 1.6).
  - The mites live in the stratum corneum and are often few in number, and consequently false negative scrapings are common, so any animal with pruritus consistent with scabies should be trial-treated with appropriate acaricidal therapy.
- For surface living *Cheyletiella* mites, wide superficial scrapings of scaly lesions are obtained; these large surface-dwelling mites are quite visible on 4× magnification (Figure 1.7).
  - Mites can also be low in number, and as for scabies empiric acaricidal therapy is often prescribed in suspect cases.
  - In some cases, *Cheyletiella* mites can be found using multiple applications of clear acetate tape onto scaly areas; after sample collection the tape is applied to a microscope slide (no oil or stain is used) and observed under 4×.
- *Demodex* mites live in hair follicles and so require deeper skin scrapings.
  - The dulled blade is scraped briskly in one direction on the skin (be careful not to press down on the blade which could cause cutting of the skin) until capillary oozing is observed on the skin as well as on the blade (Figure 1.8). Intermittently squeezing the sampled skin area between scrapings can be helpful to express mites and increase scraping yield (Figures 1.9 and 1.10A–1.10C).
  - *Demodex* mites can also be obtained using hair plucks placed into mineral oil, then observe the roots to look for mites (especially helpful for hard to scrape areas such as paws, eyelids, and lips, or in very thickened, scarred areas of skin; Figure 1.11).

Clinical Atlas of Canine and Feline Dermatology, First Edition. Edited by Kimberly S. Coyner.

Companion website: www.wiley.com/go/coyner/dermatology

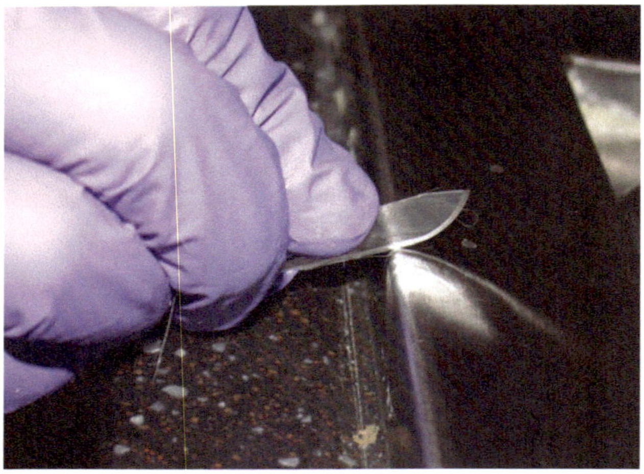

Figure 1.1 The scalpel blade is dulled by repeatedly scraping the edge on a hard surface.

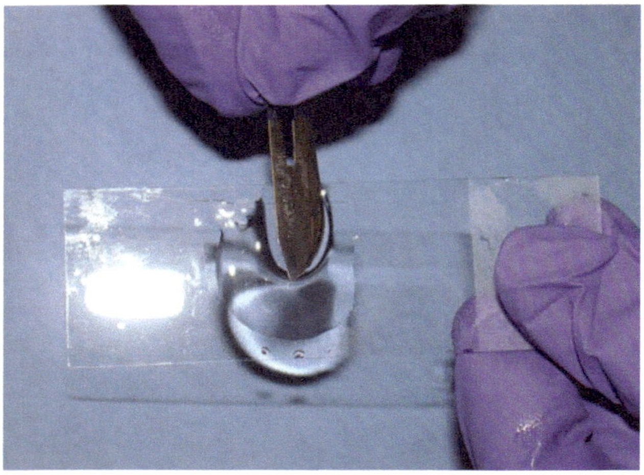

Figure 1.2 Mineral oil is applied to the dulled blade and the microscope slide.

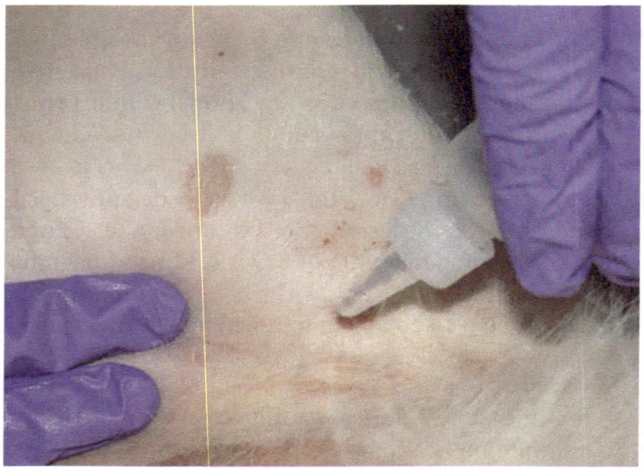

Figure 1.3 Mineral oil is applied to the lesion to be scraped.

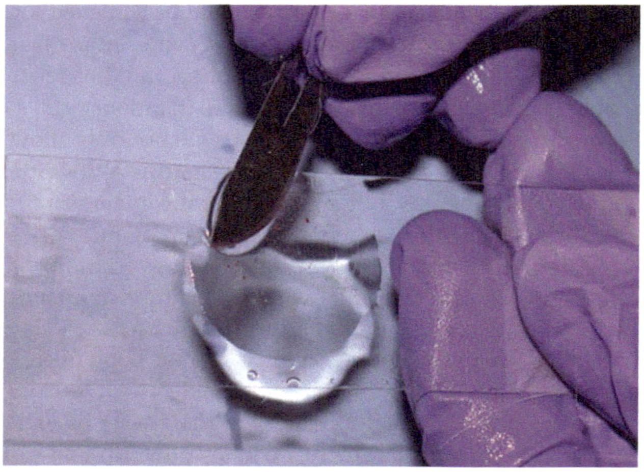

Figure 1.4 Accumulated debris on the blade is mixed into the mineral oil on the microscope slide.

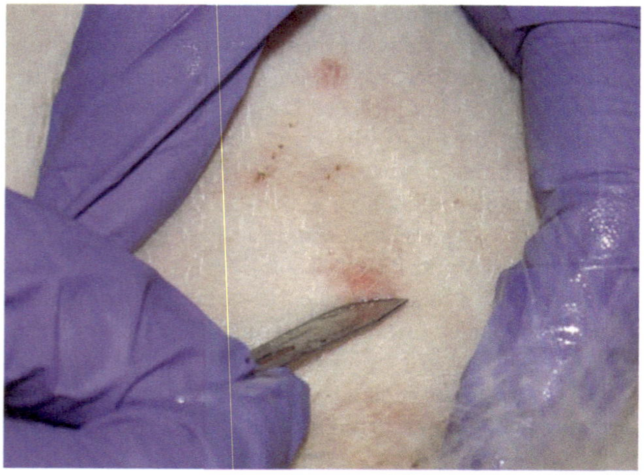

Figure 1.5 Superficial skin scraping.

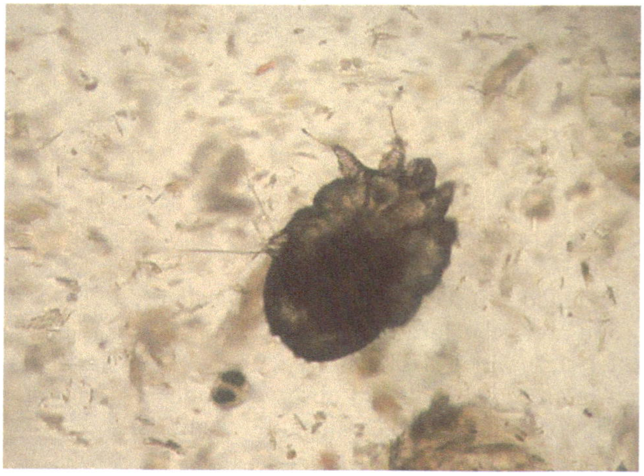

Figure 1.6 Scabies mite (10× with digital zoom).

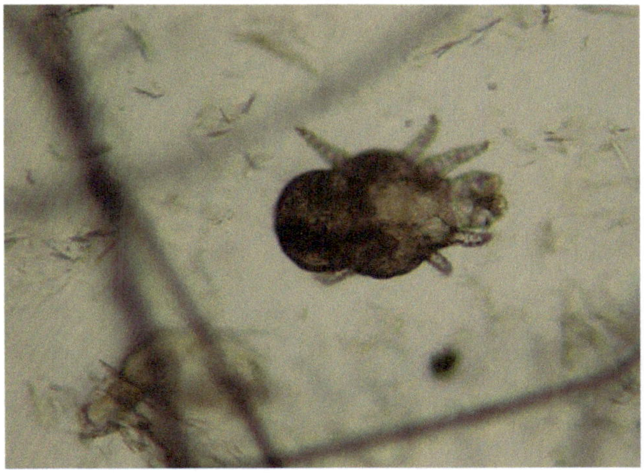

Figure 1.7 *Cheyletiella* mite (10×).

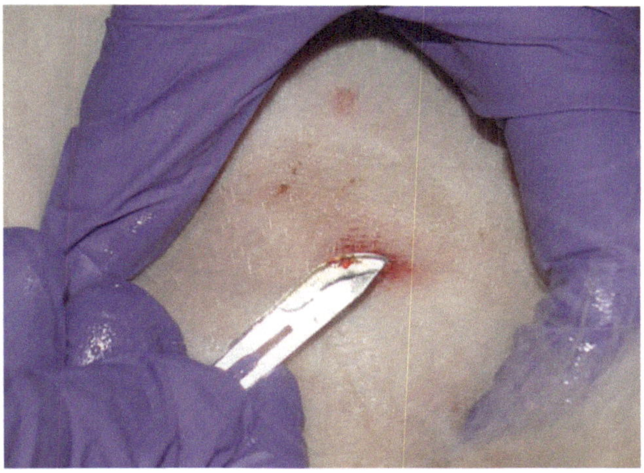

Figure 1.8 For *Demodex*, scrape until capillary oozing is observed.

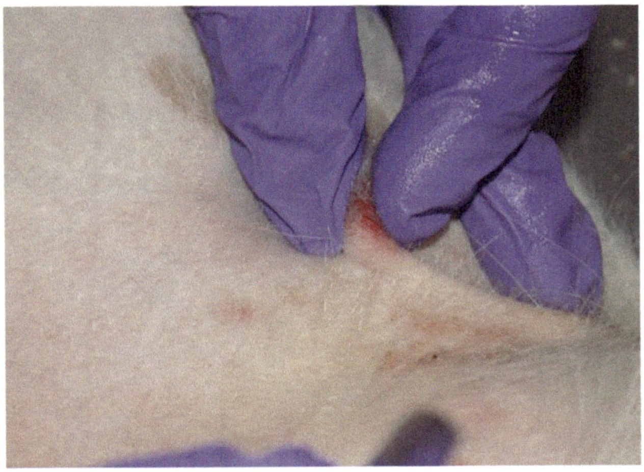

Figure 1.9 Squeeze the scraped area to increase mite yield.

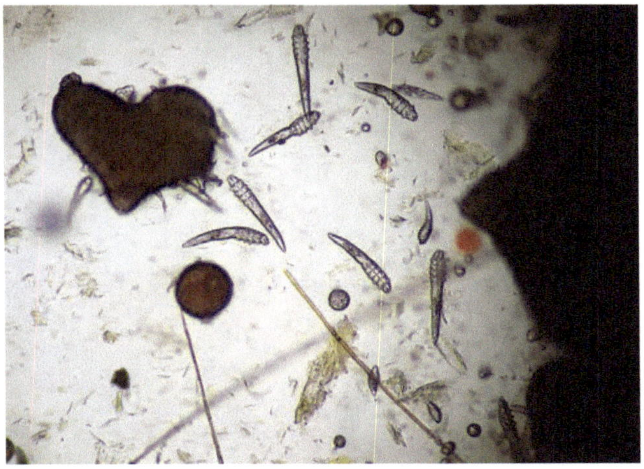

Figure 1.10A *Demodex canis* mites (4× with digital zoom).

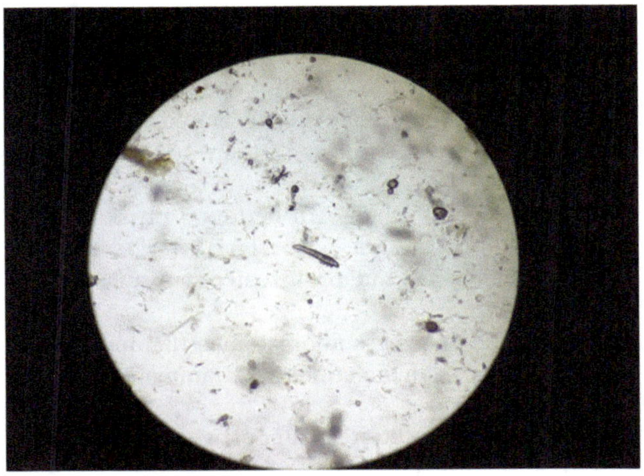

Figure 1.10B A *Demodex* mite at 4× with the microscope condenser down.

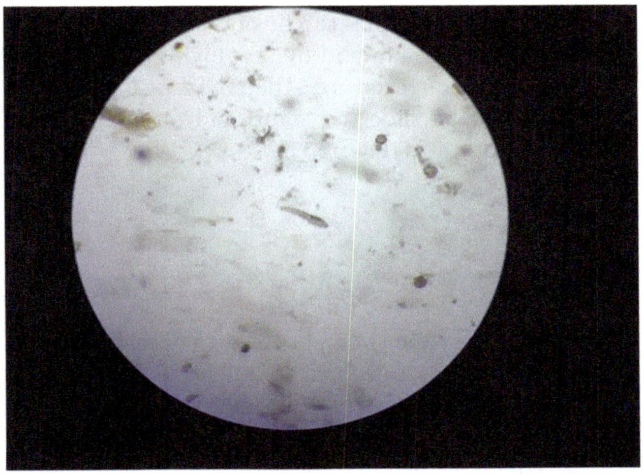

Figure 1.10C The same mite with the microscope condenser up; the mite is washed out and less visible.

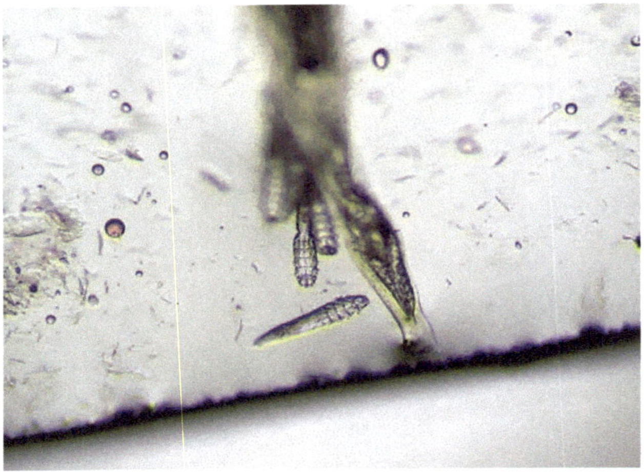

Figure 1.11 *Demodex* mites from a hair pluck, encased in keratin around a hair root (4× with digital zoom).

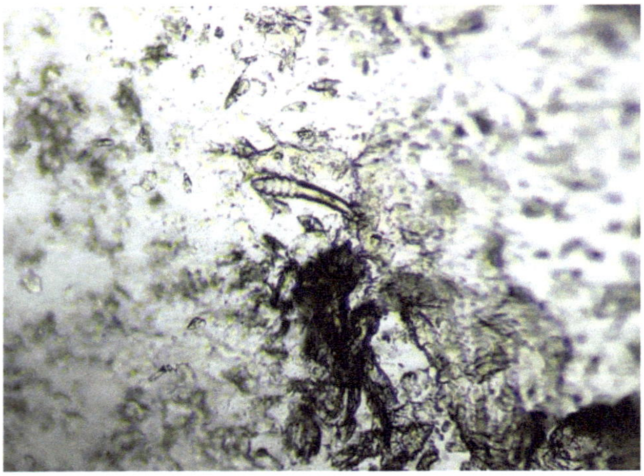

Figure 1.12 *Demodex* mite on a tape prep (4×).

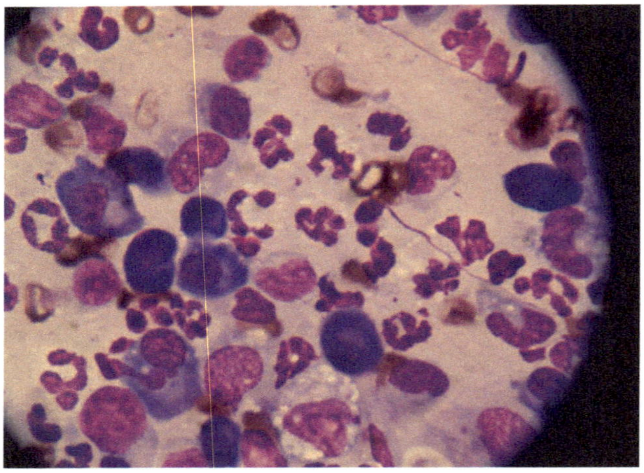

Figure 1.13 Mixed (neutrophils, macrophages, plasma cells) inflammation due to deep interdigital pyoderma (100×).

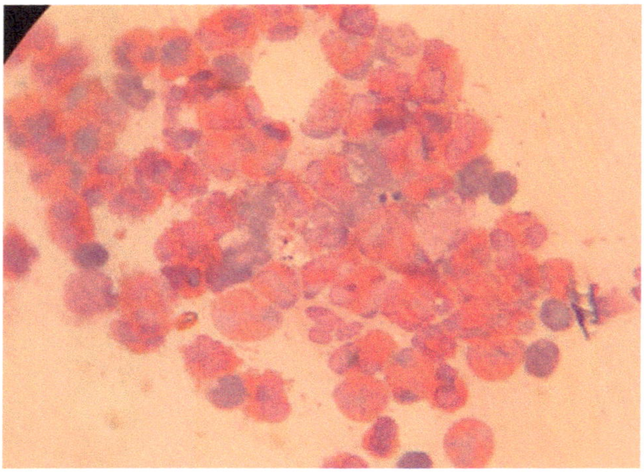

Figure 1.14 Eosinophilic inflammation found on impression smear from a feline eosinophilic plaque (100×).

- Additionally, samples can be obtained by repeatedly squeezing the skin and then applying clear acetate tape to the squeezed area, then the tape is applied to a microscope slide (no stain) and observed under 4–10× for mites (Figure 1.12).

1.2 Cytology – Skin and ear (*See videos on companion website*)

- Skin and ear cytology can be used to obtain information on bacterial or *Malassezia* infection, as well as to characterize inflammatory infiltrate.
- Skin cytology.
  - Less than one of each type of organism (yeast, cocci, or rod) per oil-immersion field (OIF) is seen in normal skin.
  - Inflammatory cells are not found on normal skin cytology.
- Samples are applied to a microscope slide and stained with Diff-Quik or similar stain, scanned under 10× to identify an area of interest, then observed under 40–100×.
- Infectious agents which can be found on skin cytology include cocci and rod bacteria, *Malassezia* and fungal organisms, and protozoal organisms such as *Leishmania*.
- Neutrophilic or pyogranulomatous inflammation can be supportive of an infectious or inflammatory process (Figure 1.13).
- An eosinophilic infiltrate is supportive of a hypersensitivity dermatitis (Figure 1.14).
- Acantholytic cells can suggest pemphigus complex (but can also be seen with chronic bacterial or dermatophyte

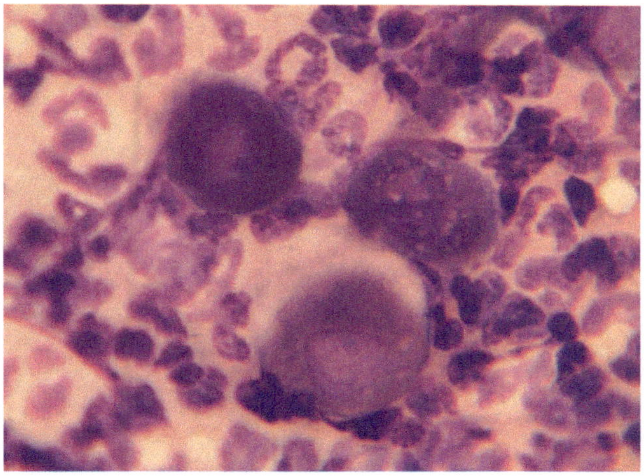

Figure 1.15 Acantholytic cells and neutrophils in a case of canine pemphigus foliaceus (100×).

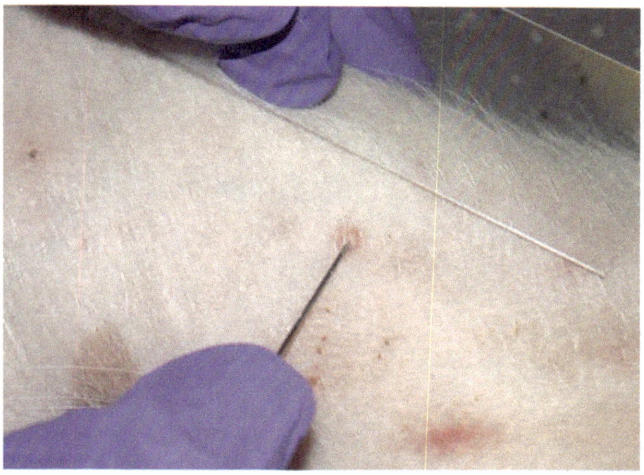

Figure 1.16A To sample a pustule, a needle is used to rupture the pustule and the contents are smeared onto a microscope slide.

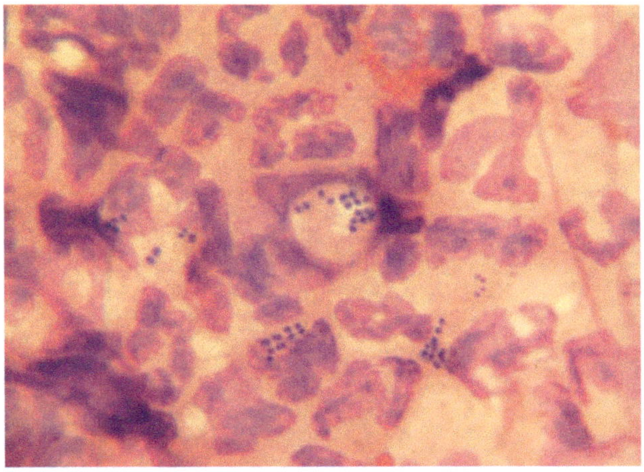

Figure 1.16B Cytologic evaluation of pustule contents reveals neutrophils and intracellular cocci (100×).

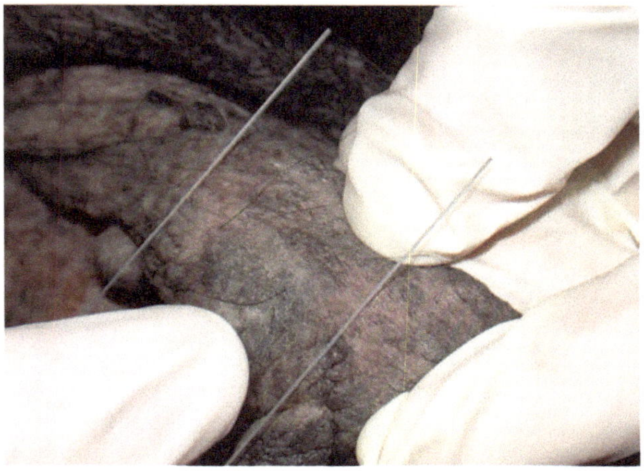

Figure 1.17 Impression smear: Lichenified skin is firmly pressed onto the microscope slide. Clinically, the lichenification and hyperpigmentation are suspicious for *Malassezia* dermatitis.

infection) and support the need for biopsy and histologic diagnosis (Figure 1.15).

- Skin cytology can be obtained in a variety of ways:
  - If a pustule is present, it can be ruptured with a needle and the contents smeared onto a slide (Figures 1.16A and 1.16B).
  - If a moist or greasy lesion is present, it can be sampled by firmly pressing a microscope slide on the surface of the lesion (Figure 1.17).
  - For dry scaling or diffuse crusting lesions, use of a dulled scalpel blade without mineral oil can be helpful to collect surface debris which is then smeared like a spatula onto the microscope slide (Figures 1.18A–1.18D). If larger crusts are present, use the blade or microscope slide edge to raise the edge of the crust and then obtain an impression smear of the exudate or debris under the crust.
  - For interdigital lesions, samples can be obtained via direct impression of the interdigital web onto a slide, cotton tipped swab of interdigital debris which is then rolled onto a slide, or by acetate tape impression (see acetate tape impressions below). In cases of paronychia, nailbed debris can be collected with a dull blade or the wooden end of a cotton swab, then smeared onto a microscope slide.
  - Acetate tape impressions can be used to sample dry, lichenified, and interdigital areas. A piece of clear (not frosted) acetate tape is firmly pressed to the lesion, then applied onto a microscope slide over a few drops of blue Diff-Quik stain (or stained using routine Diff-Quik stain omitting methanol) and observed under 40–100× (Figures 1.19A–1.19F).

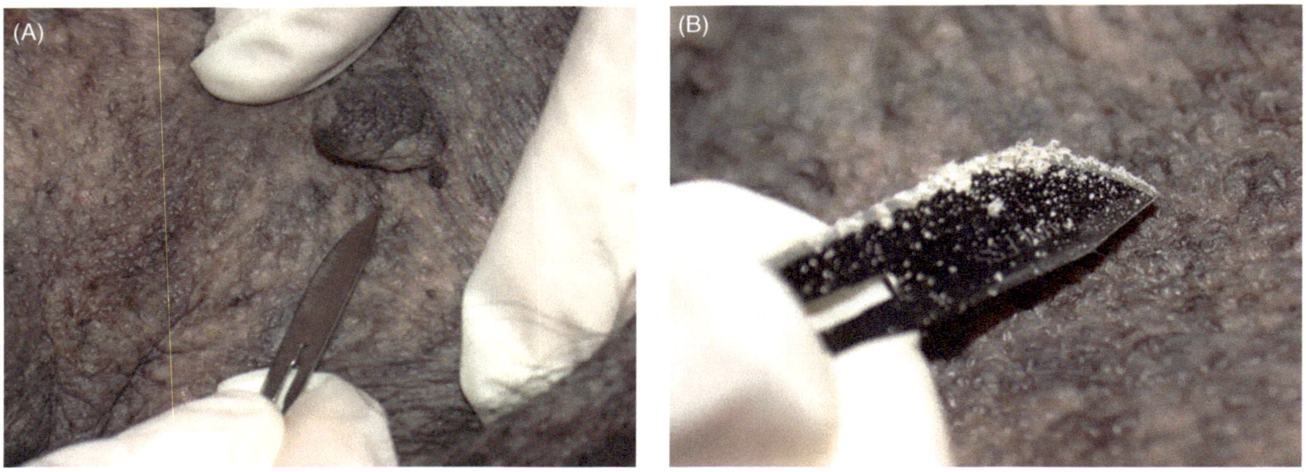

Figures 1.18A and B The lichenified skin is scraped with a dry, dull scalpel blade.

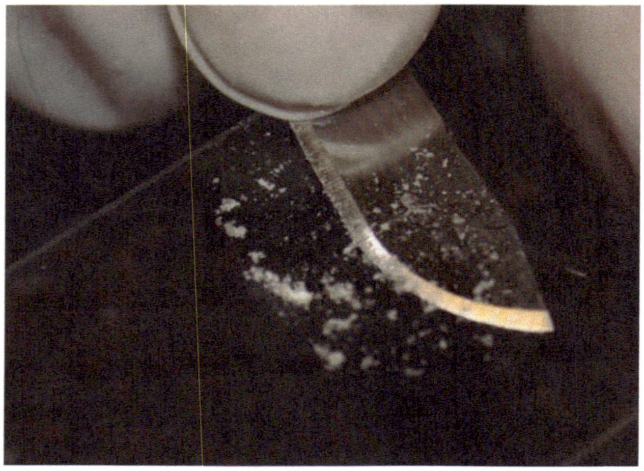

Figure 1.18C The accumulated debris is smeared onto the microscope slide.

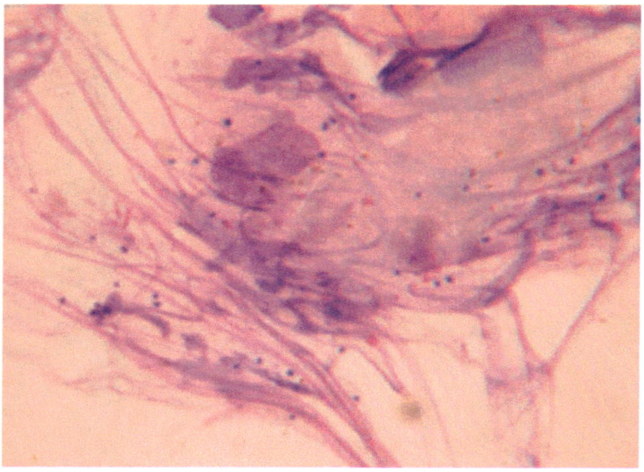

Figure 1.18D Cytology reveals streaming neutrophilic debris and bacterial cocci, but no *Malassezia* are found (100×).

- For otic cytology, gently obtain a swab of external ear debris (insert the swab into the canal no further than the proximal vertical canal, Figure 1.20), then roll the swab onto a microscope slide; both ear samples can be placed onto one slide with each side labeled (Figure 1.21A and 1.21B).
  - Otic cytology:
    a) >3 yeast/OIF in dogs and >1 yeast organism/OIF in cats may be considered abnormal (Figure 1.22).
    b) >5 cocci/OIF and >1 rod/OIF is considered abnormal (Figures 1.23 and 1.24).
    c) Presence of inflammatory cells is also abnormal.
- Red herrings: Non-significant cytology findings which can mimic infectious organisms include:
  - Melanin granules (Figures 1.25A and 1.25B).
  - Keratohyalin granules (Figure 1.26).
  - *Simonsiella* oral bacteria, huge rod bacteria, often found on the lips and paws (Figure 1.27).
  - Pollen (Figures 1.28A–1.28C).
  - Saprophytic fungal spores (Figure 1.29).
  - Stain precipitate (Figure 1.30; to avoid this, stain solutions should ideally be changed weekly).

1.3 Cytology – Mass aspirates (*See videos on companion website*)

- Ideally, every new mass should be evaluated. Dermal or subcutaneous masses can be aspirated for in-house cytology in order to determine:
  - If the mass is inflammatory vs. cyst vs. potential neoplasia.
  - Potential need for biopsy or tissue cultures (if neoplastic cells or inflammatory cells are seen).
  - If sample submission to a reference laboratory for pathology evaluation will be needed or diagnostic (if suspected neoplastic cells are found).

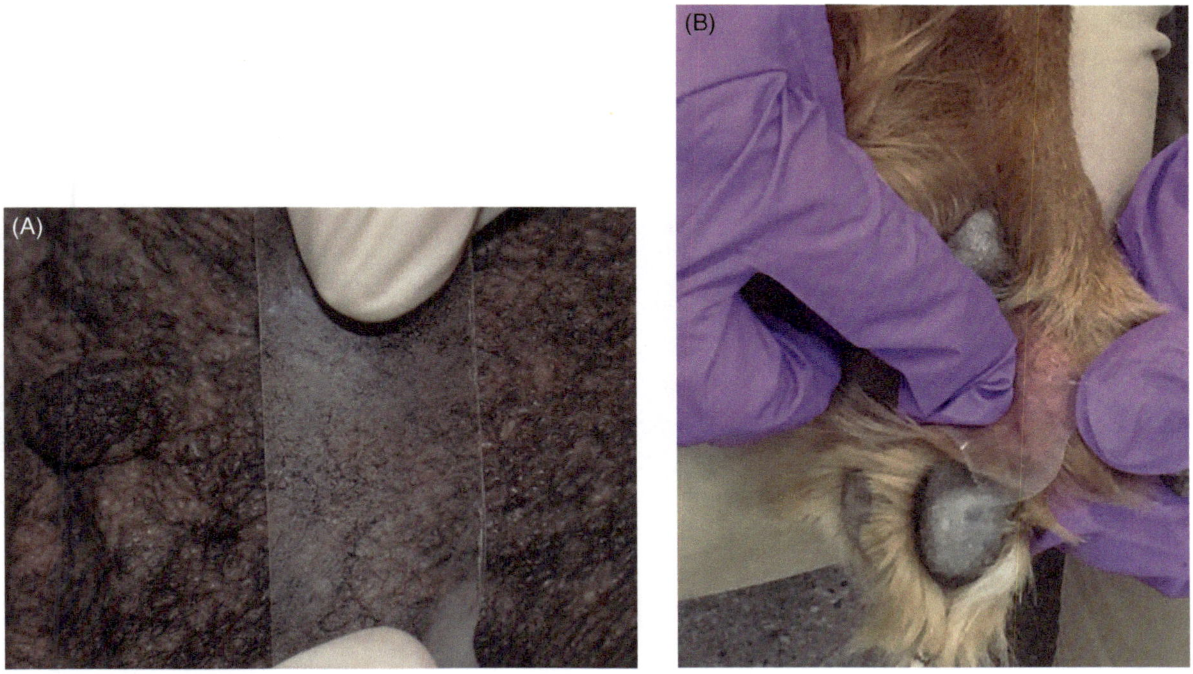

Figures 1.19A and B For a tape prep, the clear acetate tape is repeatedly impressed onto the lichenified skin; to sample interdigital areas, the web is pressed up onto the tape.

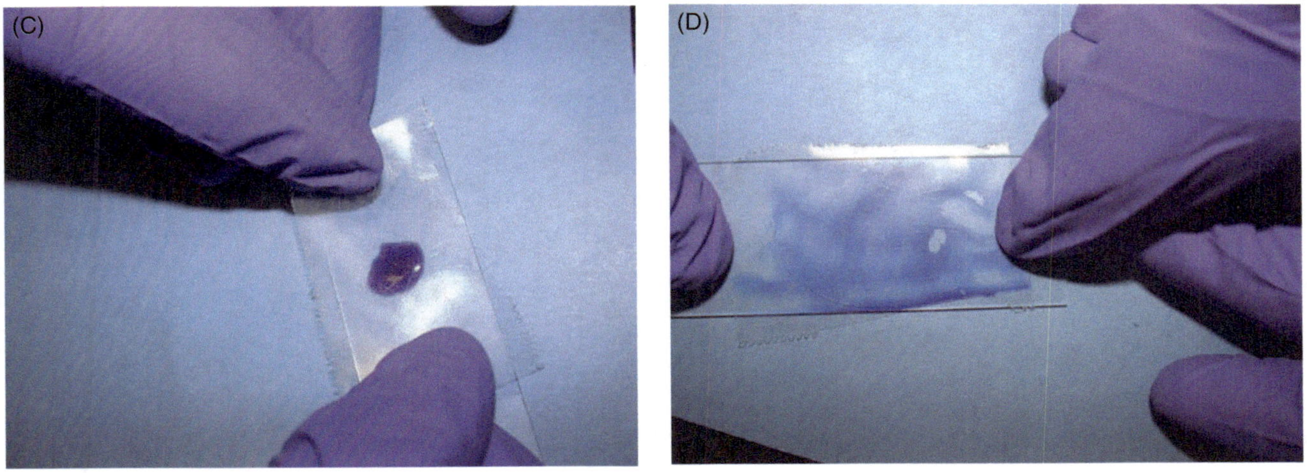

Figures 1.19C and D The tape is then applied onto the microscope slide on top of a drop of blue Diff-Quik stain.

- Procedure:
  a) Use a 25–22 g needle and a 3–6 cc syringe.
  b) Insert needle into lesion, aspirate, redirect, and aspirate again (Figure 1.31A; if lesion is vascular, then only insert needle in once then withdraw to avoid blood dilution).
  c) Take needle off syringe, draw air into syringe, replace needle and expel needle contents onto slide (Figure 1.31B).
  d) Use a second slide for gentle squash prep to form monolayer of cells (Figure 1.31C).
  e) Stain with Diff-Quick, observe under 10× to find a diagnostic area, then observe under 40–100×.
- Appropriate action based on findings:
  a) Potential “wait and see” nodules: Follicular cysts (Figure 1.32), lipoma (Figure 1.33), histiocytoma (Figure 1.34).

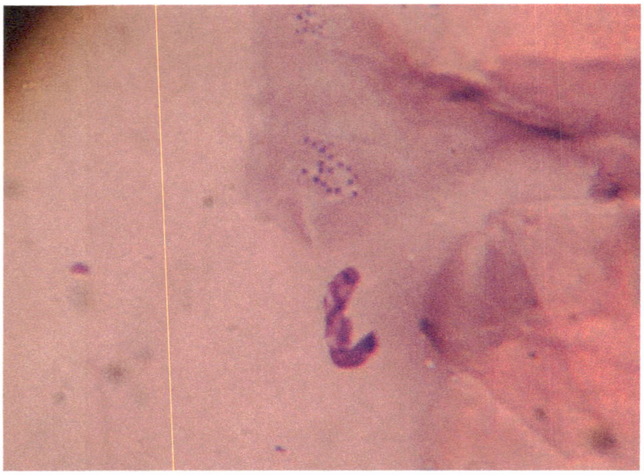

Figure 1.19E Cytological analysis reveals keratinocytes with scattered neutrophils and cocci (100×).

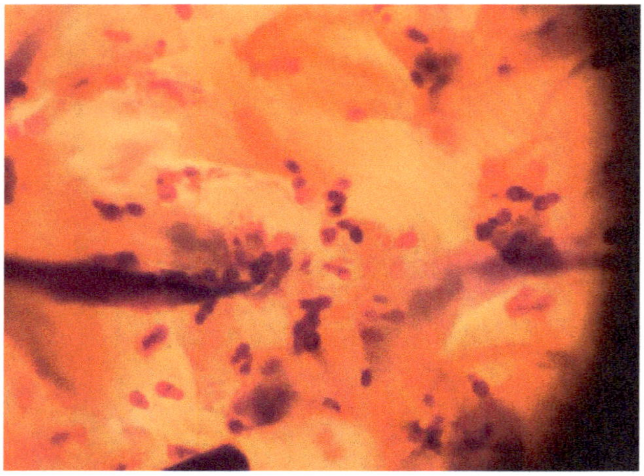

Figure 1.19F In a different case, numerous *Malassezia* are found on tape prep (100×).

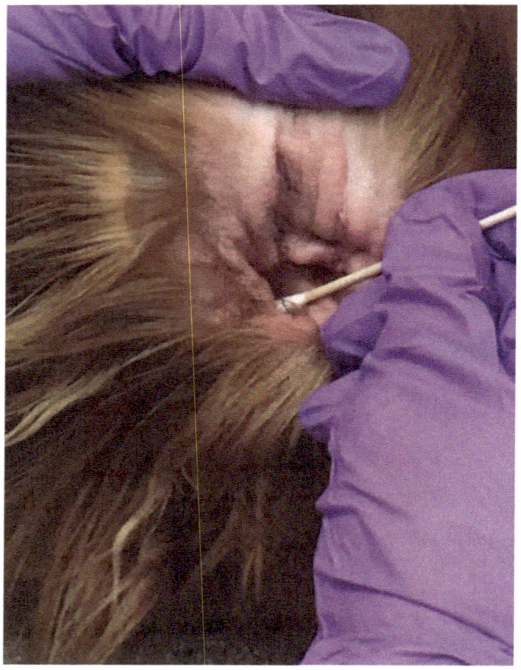

Figure 1.20 To obtain otic cytology, the cotton swab is inserted into the ear canal, no further than the vertical canal.

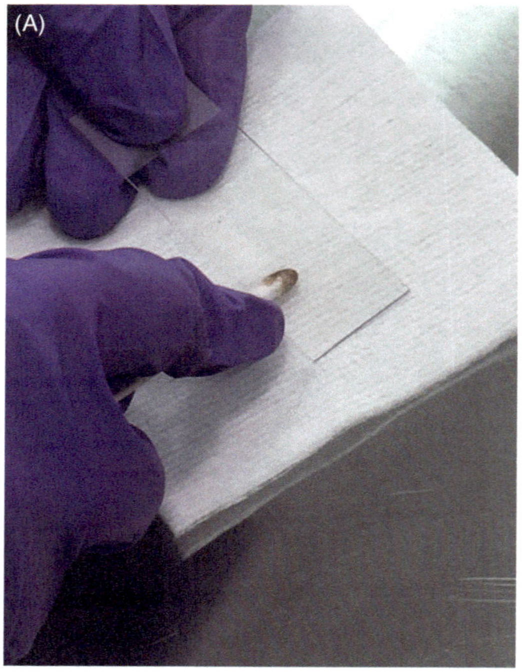

Figure 1.21A and B The swabs are then rolled onto one slide, left and right ears are labeled.

b) We need biopsy +/− staging lesions: mast cell tumor (Figure 1.35), lymphoma (Figure 1.36), plasmacytoma, melanoma (Figure 1.37).
c) We need biopsy/special stains/tissue cultures: Pyogranulomatous inflammation (Figure 1.13).
d) We need biopsy: everything else.

1.4 Trichograms

- Indications for trichogram/microscopic hair shaft evaluation when faced with cases of localized or generalized alopecia include:
  - To evaluate anagen/telogen ratio (Figures 1.38 and 1.39):
    a) Anagen: Growing stage of the hair follicle, during which the follicle is actively producing hair.

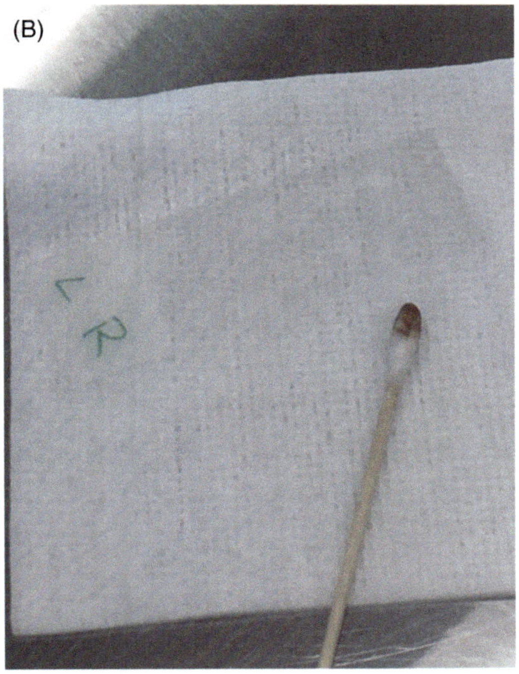

Figure 1.21A and B (Continued)

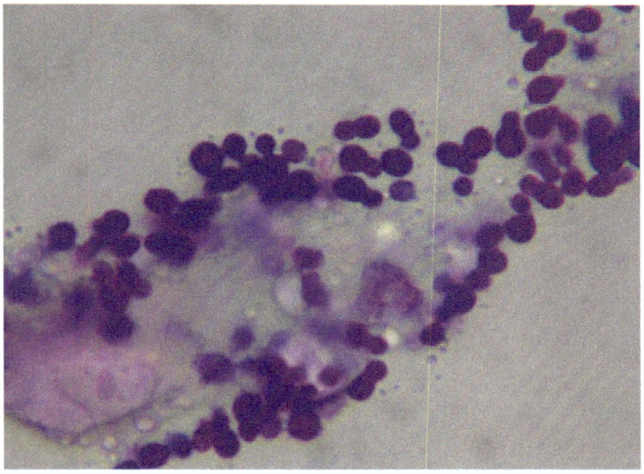

Figure 1.22 Cytology of yeast otitis (100×).

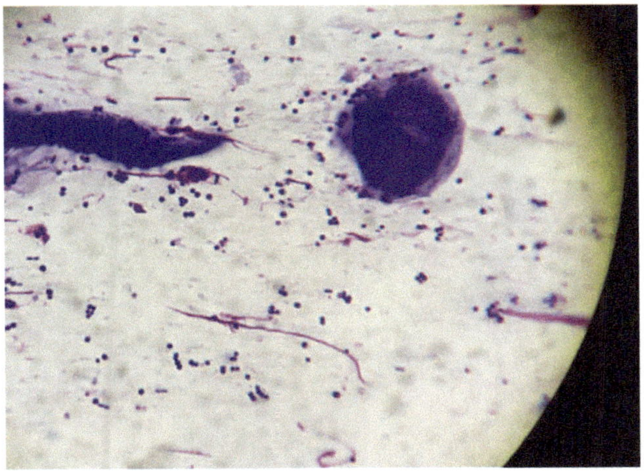

Figure 1.23 Cytology of bacterial otitis caused by cocci bacteria (100×).

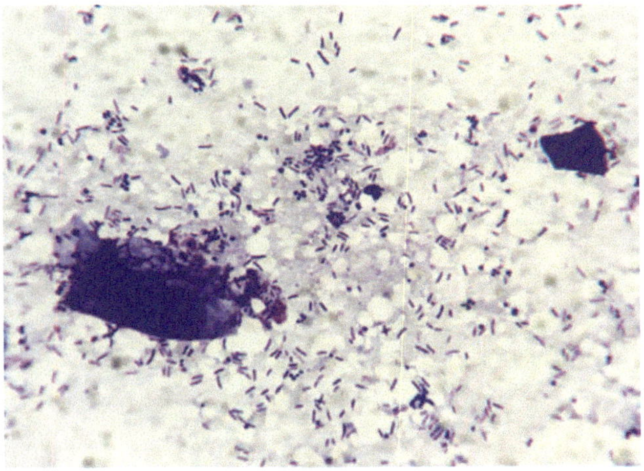

Figure 1.24 Cytology of a mixed bacterial otitis (100×).

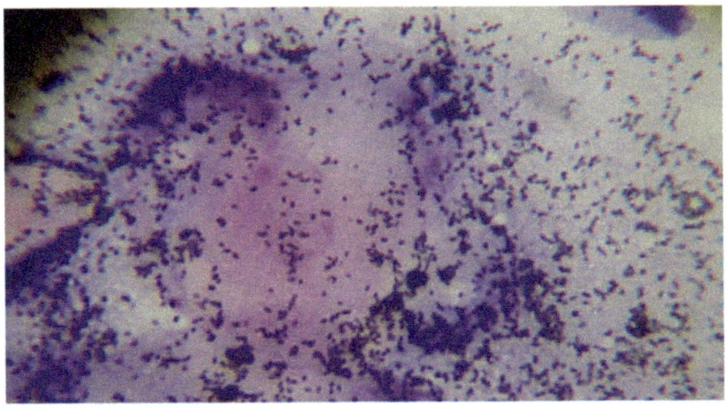

Figure 1.25A Melanin pigment granules found on cytology of a dry skin scraping of a black dog (100×).

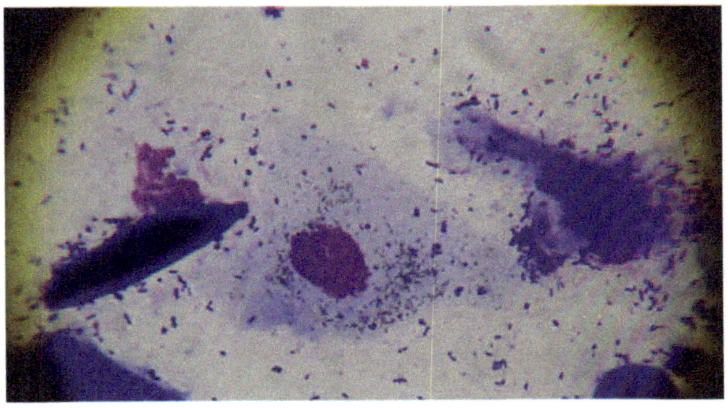

Figure 1.25B Cytology demonstrating melanin granules on an epithelial cell, surrounded by cocci and rod bacteria (100×).

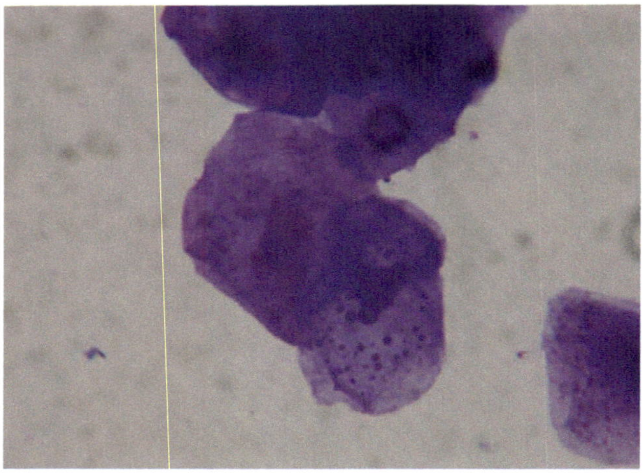

Figure 1.26 Cytology of an epithelial cell with large pink intracellular keratohyaline granules which vary in shape and size (100×).

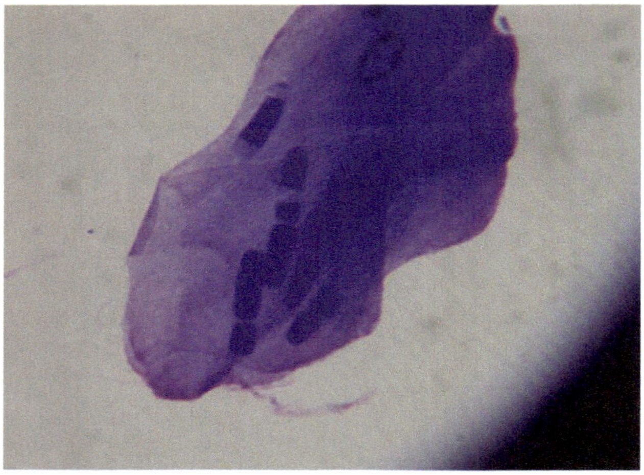

Figure 1.27 An epithelial cell from a lip fold impression, colonized by very large *Simonsiella* oral bacteria (100×).

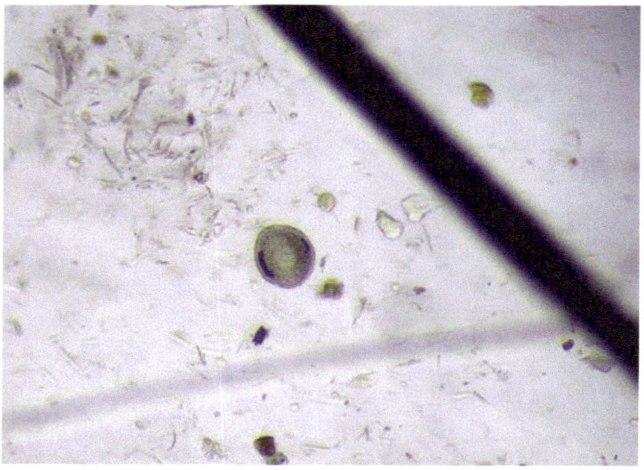

Figure 1.28A Pollen on a skin scraping (10×), which could potentially be mistaken for a parasite egg.

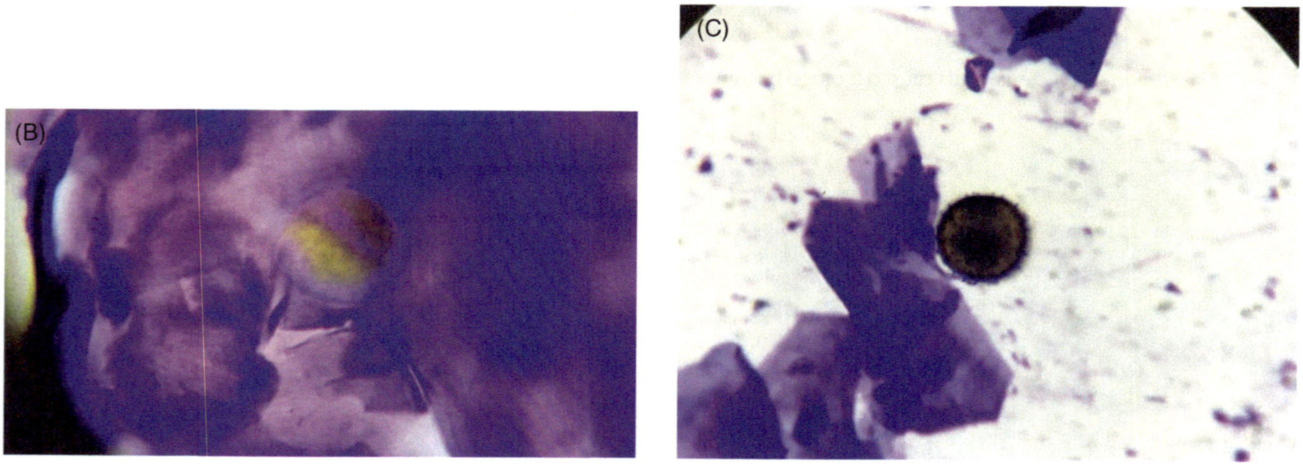

Figures 1.28B and C Pollen on skin cytology obtained by tape prep (100×).

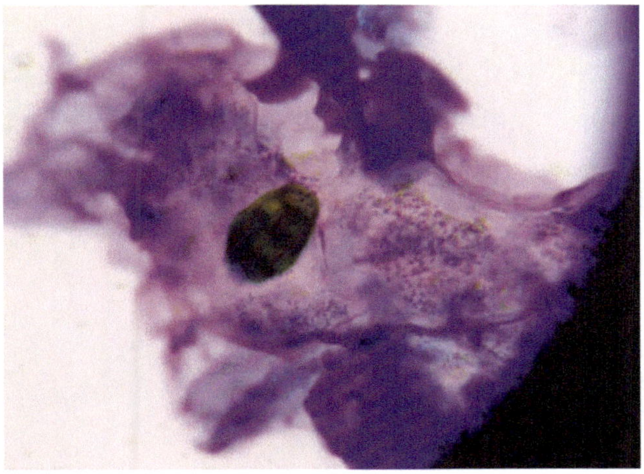

Figure 1.29 In this skin cytology, lightly pigmented epithelial cells are seen as well as a pigmented environmental mold spore, likely *Alternaria* (100×).

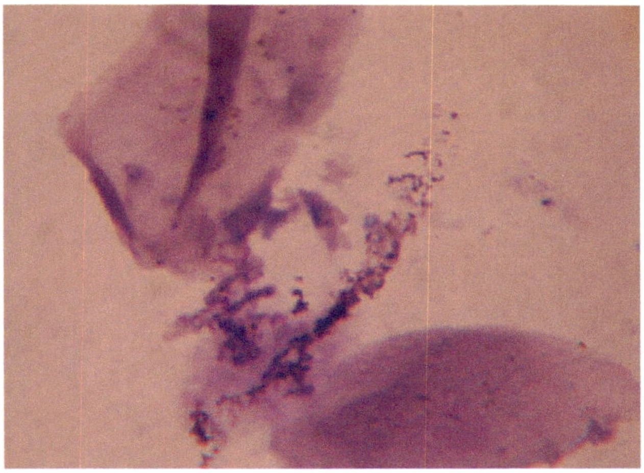

Figure 1.30 This skin cytology shows epithelial cells and amorphous purple debris which is stain precipitate (100×).

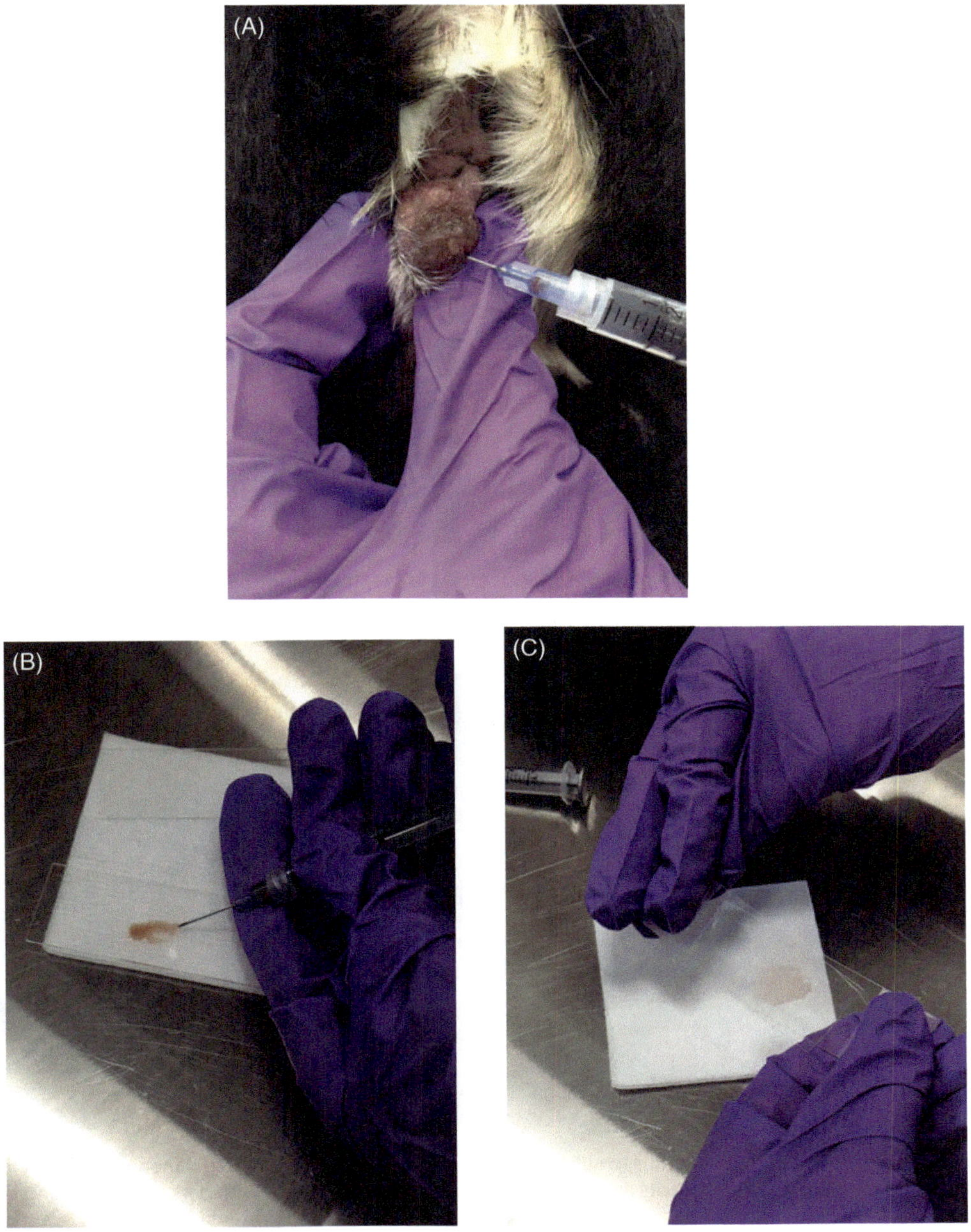

Figure 1.31A–C Aspiration of a dermal mass for cytology.

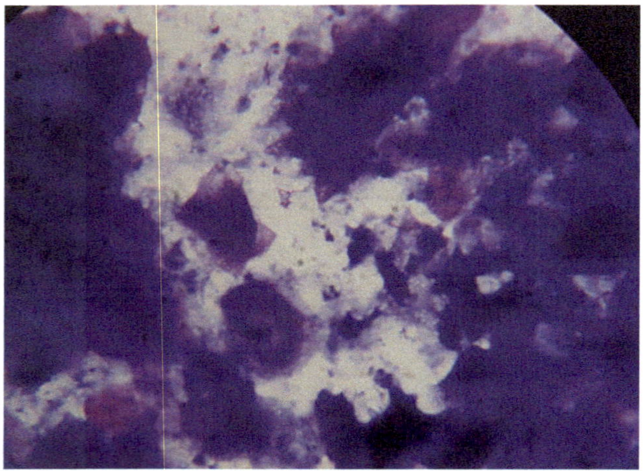

Figure 1.32 This skin mass aspirate cytology shows amorphous keratinaceous debris consistent with a benign follicular cyst/tumor (100×).

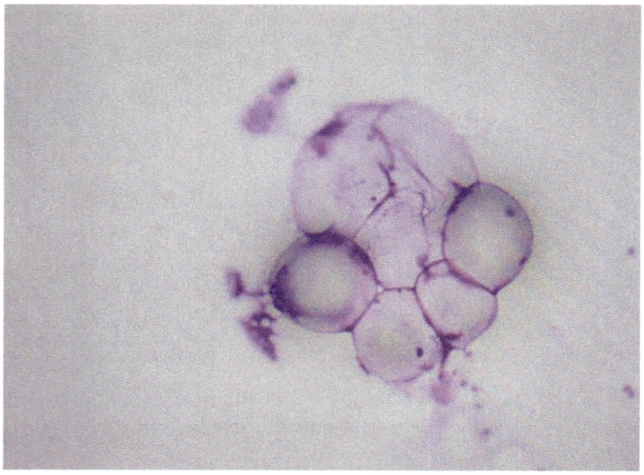

Figure 1.33 Most cells and lipid from lipoma aspirates will dissolve in the methanol stain, but sometimes the delicate adipocyte cells can be found (100×).

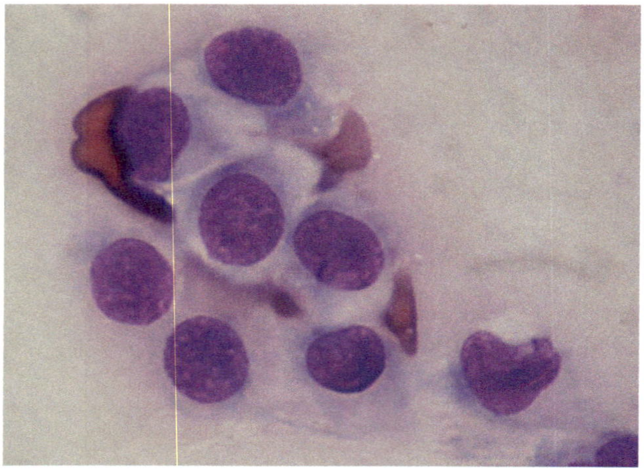

Figure 1.34 Cytology of a histiocytoma shows round cells with moderate light blue, wispy cytoplasm, occasional small vacuoles, and some nuclei can be indented in a "kidney bean" shape (100×).

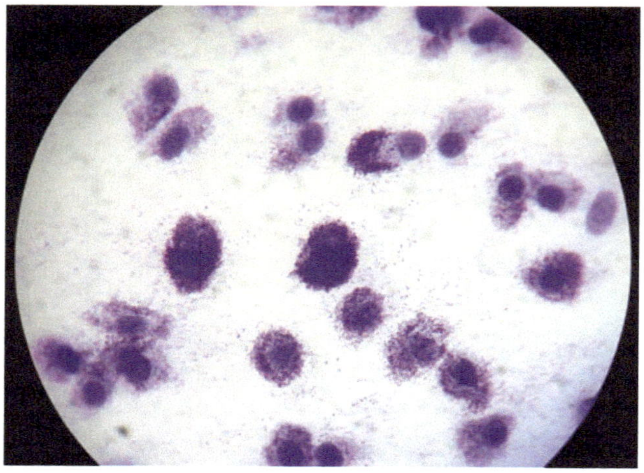

Figure 1.35 Cytology of a mast cell tumor demonstrating round cells with purple granules (100×).

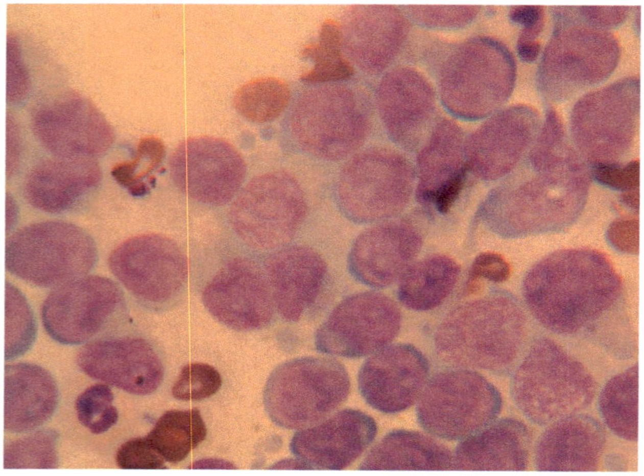

Figure 1.36 Impression smear cytology of cutaneous lymphoma showing round cells (lymphoblasts) with large nuclei and scant dark blue cytoplasm (100×).

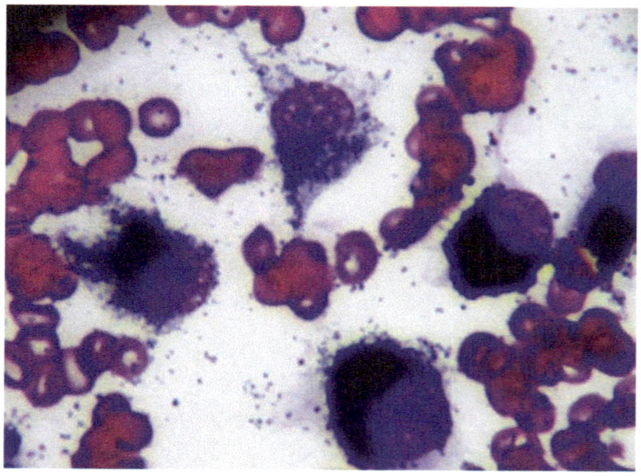

Figure 1.37 Cytology of a cutaneous melanocytoma, showing round to stellate cells with dark pigment granules; numerous red blood cells are also present (100×).

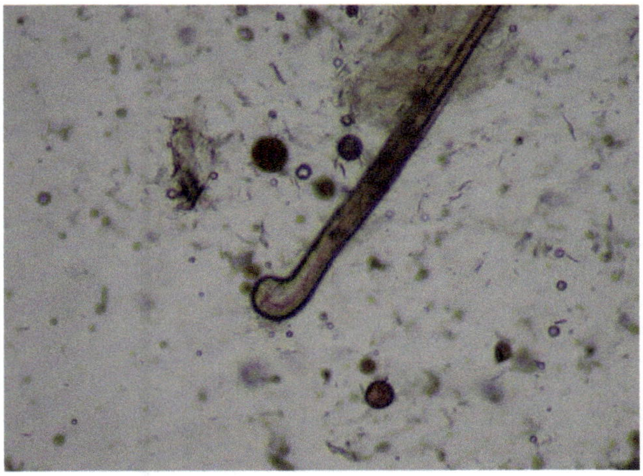

Figure 1.38 A typical club shaped anagen hair root (10×).

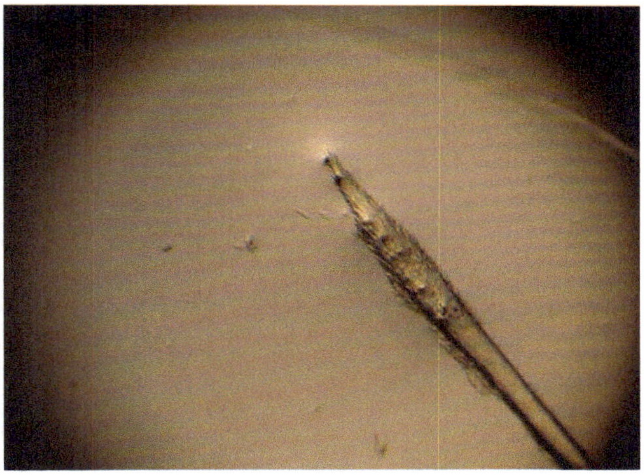

Figure 1.39 The telogen hair root has a spear shape (10×).

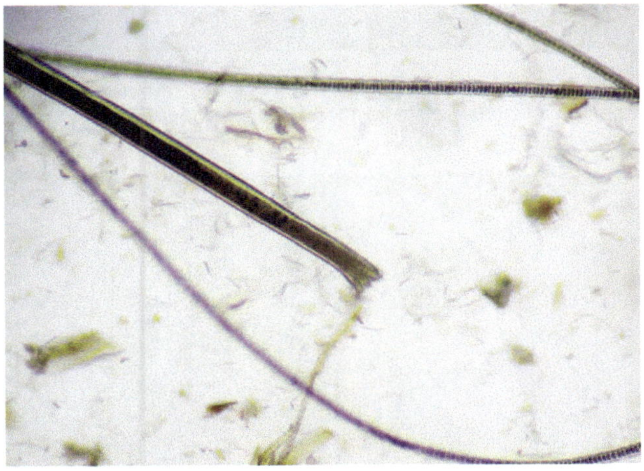

Figure 1.40 Trichogram of an overgrooming cat shows hairs sheared off mid-shaft (10×).

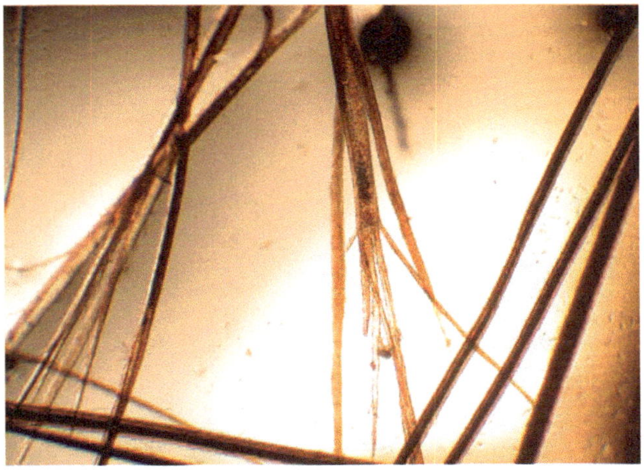

Figure 1.41 This trichogram demonstrates hair damage due to aggressive brushing (4×).

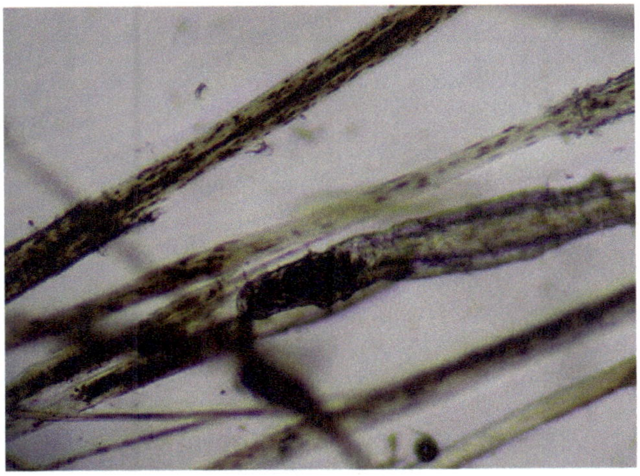

Figure 1.42 Trichogram of a dog with color dilution alopecia; note the clumps of pigment causing distortion of the hair cuticles as well as the hair root (10×).

b) Telogen: Resting stage of the hair follicle, in which the non-growing hair is retained in the follicle and subsequently lost.

- To investigate barbering potential in cases in which the animal is not witnessed to be licking or chewing at the fur (Figure 1.40).
- To evaluate hair shaft integrity in cases of suspected chemical or physical injury to the fur such as aggressive brushing (Figure 1.41).
- To evaluate hair shaft pigment distribution, in suspected cases of color dilution alopecia (Figure 1.42).
- To evaluate potential hair shaft infection such as dermatophytosis (Figure 1.43).

• The hair cycle can vary with breed, age, gender, season, and health status:
  - Beagles were reported to have approx. 50 : 50 anagen : telogen ratio in one study (Al-Bagdadi, Titkemeyer, and Lovell, 1977), though another reference states 20 : 80.

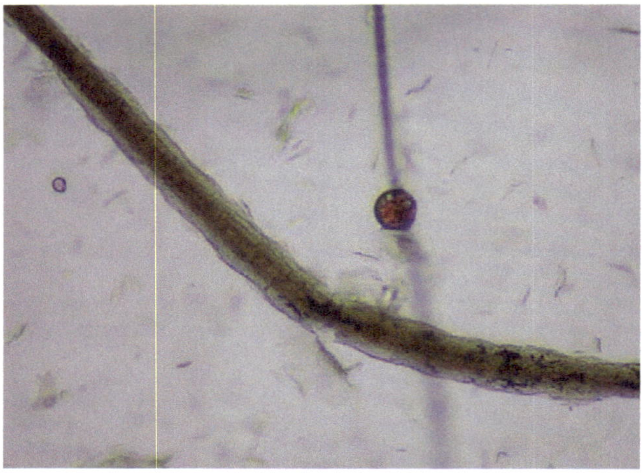

Figure 1.43 Trichogram of a cat with dermatophytosis showing the dermatophyte organisms invading the walls of the hair shaft, creating a "rotten log" appearance. The hair was obtained in this case via skin scrapings, causing the micelle of red blood cells within mineral oil above the affected hair (10×).

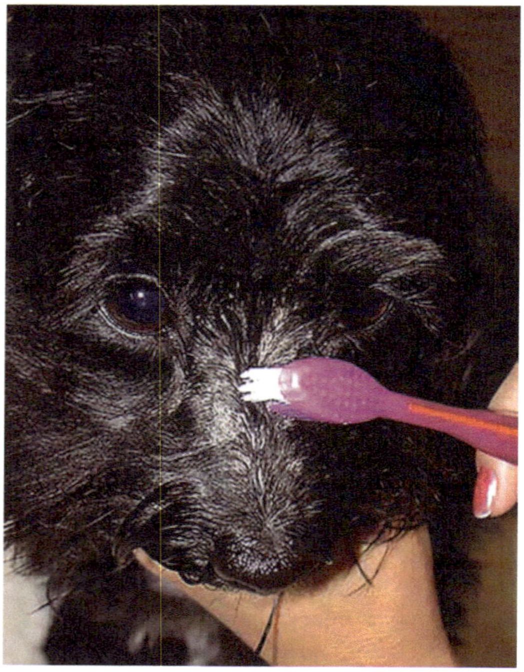

Figure 1.45A Toothbrush samples are obtained with a new toothbrush vigorously brushed across affected areas.

- Nordic breeds are thought to have a telogen predominant cycle (10 : 90) (Dunstan et al. 2001); Welle and Wiener, 2016), though one study on normal Huskies showed a 50 : 50 anagen/telogen ratio (Diaz et al. 2006).
- There is no exact "normal ratio" but observing trends in anagen and telogen hairs can be helpful.

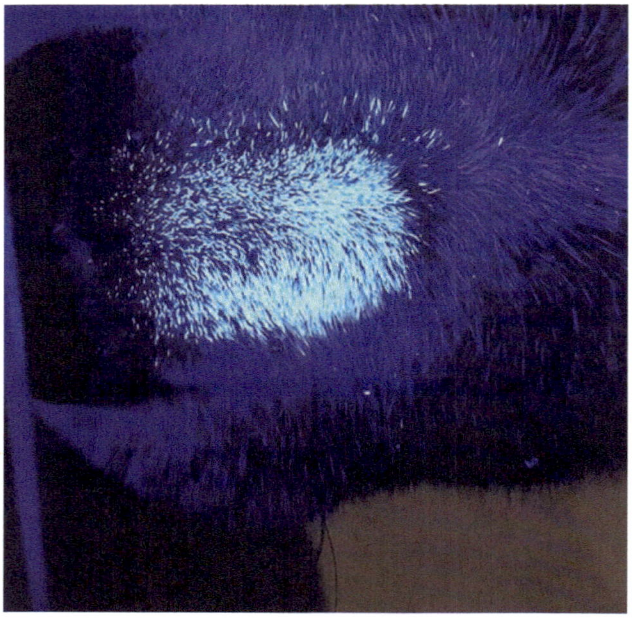

Figure 1.44 Wood's lamp examination of a dog with *Microsporum canis*; the infected hair shafts fluoresce apple green.

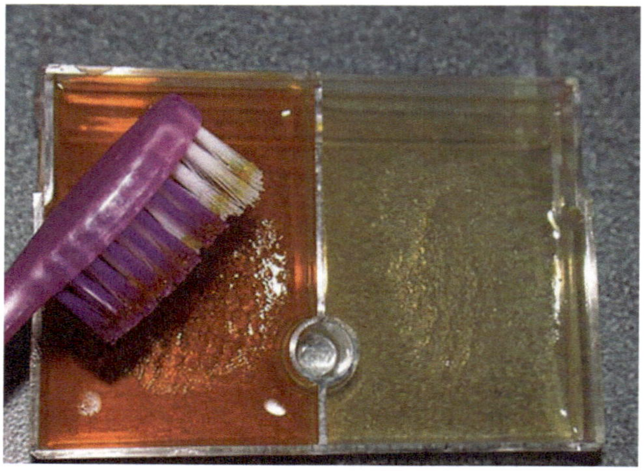

Figure 1.45B The toothbrush bristles are then gently and partially embedded into the dermatophyte culture media.

- In a study of Boxers and Labradors, more telogen hairs were found during the hottest months of the year, and an increase in anagen hairs during the coldest months (Favarato and Conceição, 2008).
- The mean percentage of telogen hairs was 93, 90, and 55.3% for Boxer, Labrador, and Schnauzer.
- Adult Labradors housed indoors had >80% telogen hairs in all seasons.
- Dogs with continuously growing haircoats (i.e. Poodles) have approx. 90% anagen hair bulbs (similar to humans).
  - Trichogram of a Poodle with only 50% anagen roots may increase suspicion for possible endocrinopathy.

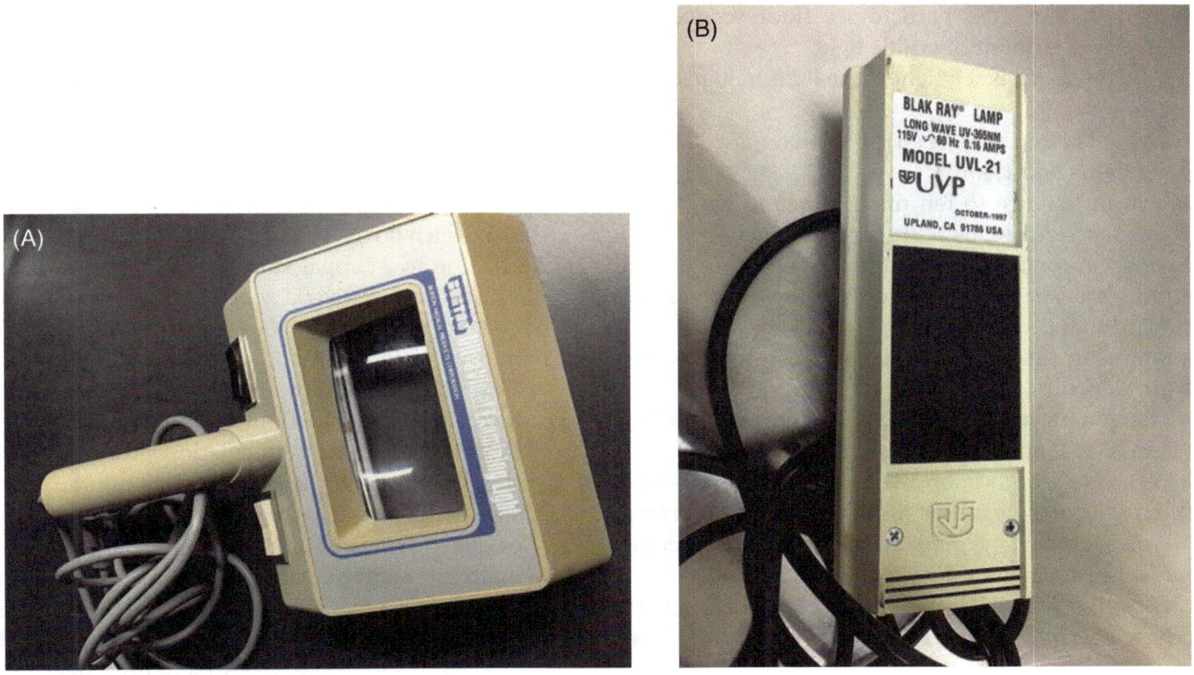

Figure 1.46A and B Use a high-quality Wood's lamps ideally with magnification.

1.5 Dermatophyte culture technique

- To obtain samples for dermatophyte culture, use sterile hemostats to pluck hairs from around the periphery of a newly formed or expanding skin lesion, and avoid areas which may have been recently medicated.
- Ideal hairs to select are those in areas of active crusting, and hairs which appear damaged or misshapen and/or fluoresce under a Wood's lamp (Figure 1.44).
- In addition to hair plucks (which can potentially miss infected hairs and may not sample infected epithelium adequately), it is ideal to also obtain samples using the MacKenzie toothbrush technique:
  - In this technique, a new toothbrush is removed from its packaging and the toothbrush is rubbed gently over the suspect area, including the skin and haired margins of alopecic or scaly lesions (Figure 1.45A).
  - If culturing a suspected asymptomatic dermatophyte carrier, use the toothbrush to sample the fur over the entire body, ending on the face and paws.
  - The toothbrush bristles are then gently embedded into the fungal culture media, taking care not to embed the bristles too deeply (which risks displacement of culture media when the bristles are removed (Figure 1.45B).
  - Hair and debris which are caught within the bristles can be removed with sterile hemostats and then placed on the fungal culture surface.
  - Toothbrushes can be obtained inexpensively in bulk from dollar stores or from online distributors.
  - The MacKenzie toothbrush technique is helpful to screen asymptomatic carriers, and to obtain samples from animals undergoing antifungal treatment in which skin lesions have clinically resolved. In these cases, the toothbrush is stroked over the entire body, concentrating especially in areas with prior lesions and, in cats, on the face, ears, and paws.
  - In cases of suspected onychomycosis, the toothbrush can be used on the affected nail bed; additionally, samples of nail bed fur can be obtained with sterile hemostats, and the proximal affected nail can be sampled using a scalpel blade to shave off small pieces of keratin (precleaning of the nail with alcohol is recommended to help reduce accumulated saprophytic or environmental fungal organisms). If an avulsed toenail is considered for fungal culture, the distal part of the nail should be discarded, and ideally samples for culture obtained by scraping the proximal concave aspect of the claw.

1.6 Wood's lamp examination

- Wood's lamps and black lights are different!
  - A Wood's lamp is a UV light which emits wavelength 320–450 nm (peak 365 nm), filtered through a cobalt or nickel filter.
  - A black light is composed of a clear glass that filters medium and short-wave UV light and emits a large amount of blue visible light along with long

wave UV light; It is hard to see fluorescence due to the large amount of visible light.
  - An example of a black light is the light bulb in a bug catcher.
- Use a Wood's lamp with electric plug and magnification (Figure 1.46A and 1.46B):
  - Warm up for five to ten minutes before use, light's wavelength and intensity are temperature dependent.
  - Expose fur for three to five minutes, some ringworm strains may be slow to fluoresce (or our eyes are slow to adapt to darkness).
  - Examine in dark room, hold lamp a few inches away from skin/fur.
- Pluck fluorescing hairs (Figure 1.44) for dermatophyte test medium (DTM) and direct microscopic examination.
- False negative Wood's lamp results can occur in 20–50% of *Microsporum canis* cases (usually due to user error), in all *Microsporum gypseum* and *Trichophyton mentagrophytes* cases, and after use of topical iodine.
- False positive Wood's lamp reactions can occur due to pyoderma, *Demodex*, keratin, soap, topical medications, and carpet fibers.
- The fluorescent metabolic product is a pigment that is incorporated into the hairs and will remain even when the fungus is dead.
- As infection resolves, fluorescence is lost in the proximal hairs and glowing tips may remain yet be culture negative.

1.7 Dermatophyte culture medium selection and incubation

- DTM contains Sabouraud's dextrose agar with cycloheximide, gentamycin, and chlortetracycline as antifungal and antibacterial agents to retard growth of contaminant organisms. Additionally, the pH indicator phenol red is added.
  - Dermatophytes preferentially metabolize protein in the culture medium, causing alkaline metabolites and turning the yellow fungal culture medium to a red color at exactly the same time as the dermatophyte colony appears.
  - Most other fungi initially utilize carbohydrates with resultant acidic metabolites; these saprophytic fungi can eventually consume protein and cause media color change, but this usually happens several days after fungal growth occurs.
- Daily observation and logging of fungal growth correlated with media color change is thus very important in correctly interpreting DTM culture results.
- Additionally, since some non-dermatophyte fungal organisms can cause positive media color change concurrent with colony growth and mimic dermatophytes, microscopic examination of all suspect colonies is very important to avoid misidentification.
- Microscopic examination can be done in the clinic, or the entire culture plate can be sent to a reference laboratory for fungal identification (usually at a reduced cost compared to fungal culture).
- To facilitate fungal sporulation and identification, it is helpful to use a DTM plate which also has a separate area of plain Sabouraud's agar or rapid sporulation medium (RSM) which do not contain inhibiting agents.
- According to a fungal culture manufacturer's recommendations (www.vetlab.com), culture media should be stored at 2–25°C (36–77°F) and protected from light prior to inoculation.
  - Plates should be allowed to warm to room temperature prior to inoculation.
  - Prior to and during inoculation procedures, plates should be handled in a manner that minimizes exposure of the media to the environment. Expired plates or plates that exhibit drying, cracking, discoloration, microbial contamination, or other signs of deterioration should not be used. The presence of excessive condensation may appear in plates that have been damaged by exposure to temperature extremes.
- Fungal cultures should be incubated at room temperature (25–30°C) with 30% humidity.
- Most organisms will appear within 7–10 days, however plates should be kept for 14–21 days, especially when no growth is seen initially, or when the sample has been obtained from a pet currently under therapy with antifungal medications.
  - According to one DTM manufacturer (www.vetlab.com), dermatophyte culture plates may be incubated in full light, although some recommend incubation in the dark to avoid UV light-induced inhibition of fungal growth.
  - In dry climates, culture plates should be placed in plastic bags or containers to prevent dehydration of the media which can inhibit growth of organisms.
- After 48–72 hours, begin examining the plates daily for characteristic media color changes and fungal growth.
- If optimal dermatophyte culture storage conditions, daily observation of fungal colony growth and media color change, and subsequent microscopic identification of suspect fungal organisms are not feasible in the individual clinic situation, then submission of skin and hair samples (placed in a sterile red top tube) from suspect cases to a veterinary reference laboratory for fungal culture is recommended to avoid misdiagnosis. Even some veterinary dermatologists elect this option to minimize the chance of false negative or false positive dermatophyte cultures.

1.8 Identification of dermatophytes

- Macroscopic fungal colony morphology is an important first step in determining if a dermatophyte is present.

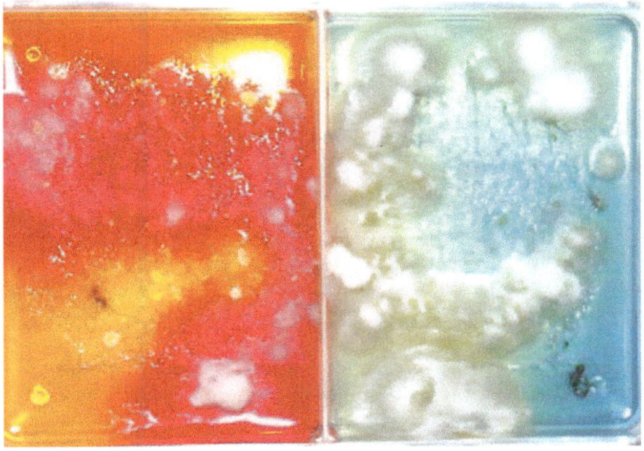

Figure 1.47 A dermatophyte culture plate growing *Microsporum canis*; white to cream cottony colonies with concurrent media color change.

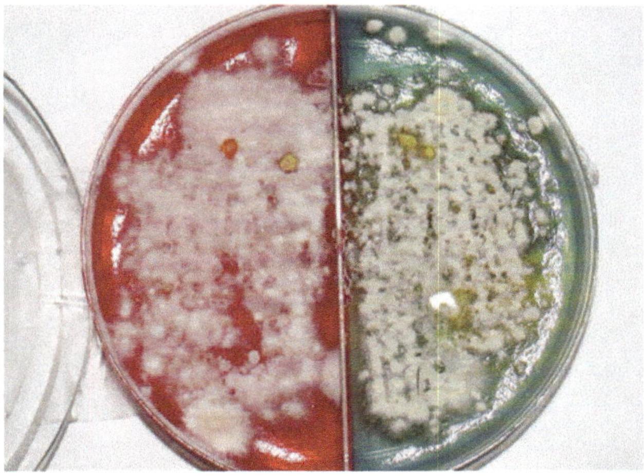

Figure 1.48 *Microsporum gypseum* has a white to buff-colored, slightly powdery appearance.

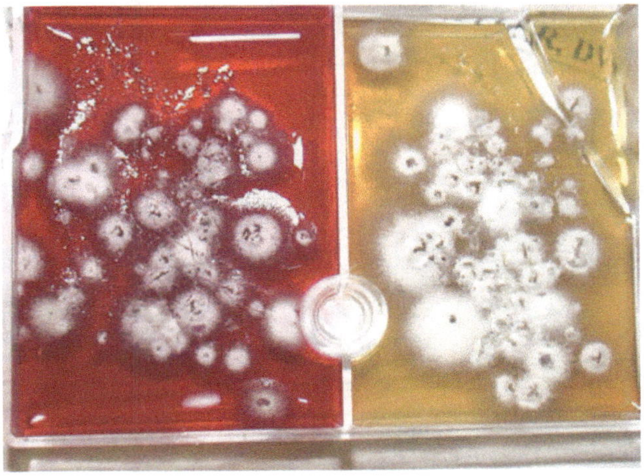

Figure 1.49 *Trichophyton mentagrophytes* colonies are white to cream in color with a powdery to granular texture.

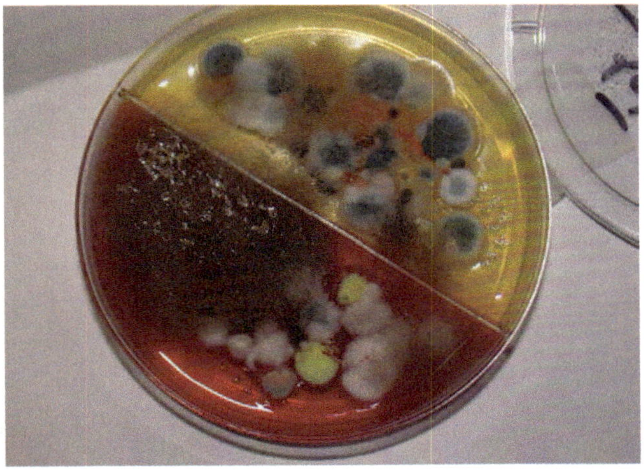

Figure 1.50 Dermatophytes are never black, green, or gray; this dermatophyte culture has numerous contaminant colonies, and any colonies of interest should be recultured onto a new plate. Contaminant fungi can also cause media color change usually after several days of incubation.

- *Microsporum* and *Trichophyton*, the most important dermatophytes in dogs and cats, appear as white, light yellow, tan, or buff-colored, cottony to powdery appearing colonies (Figures 1.47–1.49).
- Dermatophytes are never black, green, or gray (Figure 1.50).
- Microscopic evaluation of suspect fungal growth is also important, since some environmental fungi can mimic dermatophytes in gross colony morphology and ability to turn the media red.
- Gloves should be worn to avoid transmission of dermatophyte spores to the hands. A small piece of clear acetate tape is gently touched to the surface of the fungal colony and then the tape is applied to a glass slide over a drop of blue stain such as methylene blue, or the blue Diff-Quik solution (basophilic thiazine dye).
- The slide is examined under 10–40× for the characteristic dermatophyte macroconidia.
- In early cultures, only fungal hyphae with no macroconidia may be seen (especially in cases of *Trichophyton*), and these cultures should be incubated longer to allow for spore development.
- *M. canis* has numerous large spindle-shaped, thick-walled spores with a terminal knob and six or more internal cells (Figure 1.51).
- *M. gypseum* produces numerous large spindle-shaped spores with thin walls, no terminal knob, and six or less internal cells (Figure 1.52).

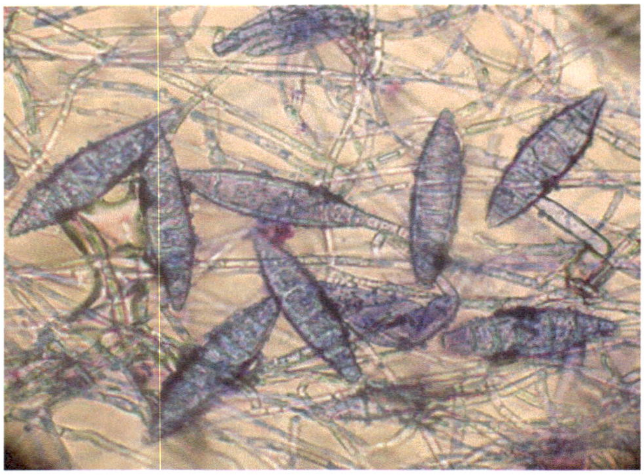

Figure 1.51 *Microsporum canis* has numerous large spindle-shaped, thick-walled spores with a terminal knob and six or more internal cells (40×).

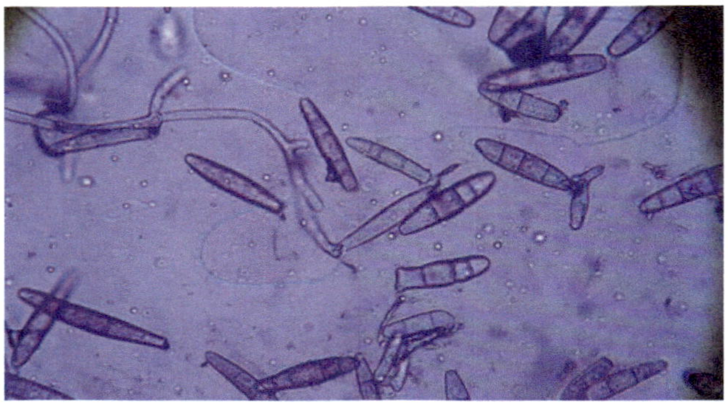

Figure 1.52 *Microsporum gypseum* produces numerous large spindle-shaped spores with thin walls, no terminal knob, and six or less internal cells (40×).

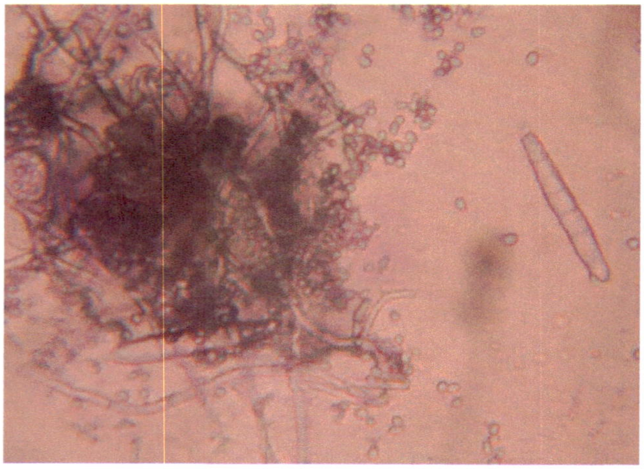

Figure 1.53 *Trichophyton mentagrophytes* produces sparse, cigar-shaped spores with thin walls; there are numerous round microconidia (40×).

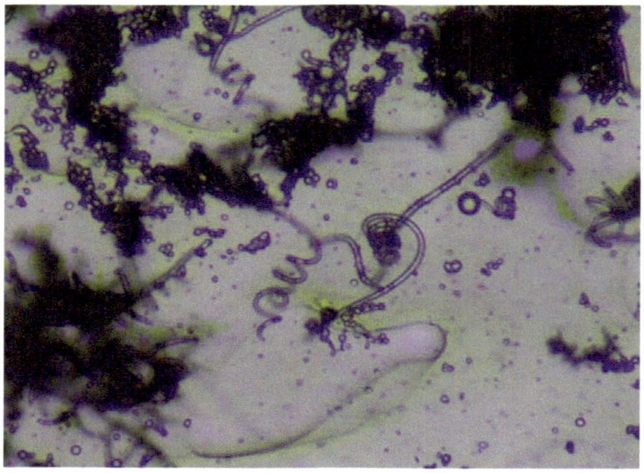

Figure 1.54 Spiral hyphae are also suggestive of *Trichophyton mentagrophytes* (40×).

- *T. mentagrophytes* produces long cigar-shaped macroconidia with thin walls; spores may be few in number; spiral-shaped hyphae are also characteristic of *Trichophyton* (Figures 1.53 and 1.54).
- In cases in which the fungal species cannot be easily identified in the clinic, then the dermatophyte culture should be submitted to a veterinary reference laboratory for fungal identification.

1.9 Dermatophyte PCR

- In recent years, dermatophyte PCR (polymerase chain reaction) has become an available screening test for dermatophyte infections in dogs and cats.
- Samples for PCR should be obtained from lesions using a toothbrush and by collecting scales and crusts.
  - If toothbrushes are submitted, wrap the head of the sample in a plastic bag (do not tape shut) and then place this into a second bag.
  - If crusts or scales are submitted, use a sterile red top tube. Dry skin scraping samples can be collected using a skin scraping spatula or forceps.
- Because dermatophyte PCR is very sensitive, false negative results are rare, but can occur if not enough material is submitted for analysis; it is important to submit adequate hairs with intact roots.
- Because PCR testing accurately identifies fungal DNA but does not discriminate between viable and nonviable fungal DNA, discordant test results between PCR and dermatophyte culture can occur when dead dermatophyte DNA is detected by PCR in successfully treated animals in which the dermatophyte culture is negative.
  - Rarely, a positive PCR may be misinterpreted as clinical infection if a single environmental dermatophyte spore such as *M. gypseum* or *Trichophyton* is coincidentally picked up.

- Fungal PCR is reported as positive or negative. Unlike follow-up dermatophyte cultures in which decreasing colony counts can be assessed as a measure of treatment efficacy, PCR cannot accurately determine number of dermatophyte spores present.
- Ideally, both dermatophyte PCR and dermatophyte culture should be used concurrently for optimal diagnosis of dermatophytosis, then follow-up dermatophyte cultures are obtained by toothbrush technique every one to two weeks to determine when treatment may be discontinued (after two negative cultures).

1.10 Bacterial culture

- Culture is indicated if there is poor response to empiric antibiotics, deep pyoderma, or rod bacteria on skin cytology.
- In superficial infections, aerobic bacterial culture is the only culture needed.
- In animals with draining tracts or nodules, samples may also be needed for anaerobic culture, fungal culture, or mycobacterial culture.
  - In these cases, a deep tissue biopsy rather than a swab is the best sample.
- Prior to culture, stop topical and systemic antimicrobials for 48 hours if possible (however, if numerous bacteria are found on cytology despite antibiotic treatment, culture delay may not be necessary).
- To obtain the culture sample, options include using a sterile culturette to swab a freshly ruptured pustule (Figure 1.55) or lift a crust and use the swab to sample the exudate under crust. In dry lesions, use a saline moistened swab to rub under rim of epidermal collarette or to vigorously rub several scaly areas (Figure 1.56).

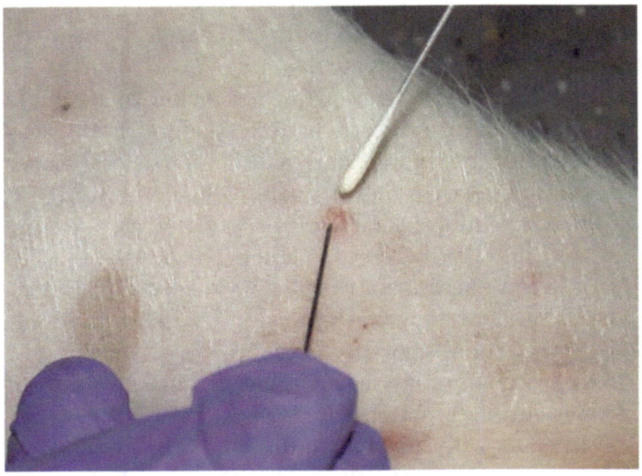

Figure 1.55 A sterile culturette for aerobic culture is used to sample a pustule ruptured by a sterile needle.

- Alternatively, bacterial skin cultures can be performed by obtaining a 4–6 mm punch biopsy of papule, pustule, or crusted lesion, which is then placed in a sterile red top tube (+/− with 0.25–0.5 cc sterile/not bacteriostatic saline to keep it moist; contact the laboratory you are using to determine their preferred submission protocol), then submit for macerated tissue culture.
  - Lidocaine has antibacterial properties, so ideally use sedation to obtain biopsies for culture.
- It is important to always perform skin (or ear) cytology at the time of culture in order to be able to interpret culture results, for example, if cocci bacteria were seen on cytology, but only rods were cultured, this indicates that the culture should be rechecked by the lab or resubmitted. Or if only yeast are found on cytology of skin or ears, then this would mean bacterial culture is not indicated.

1.11 Skin biopsies (*See videos on companion website*)

- Skin biopsies should be performed in cases of suspected neoplasia, vesicular or ulcerative diseases, unusual or atypical cases, and in cases which have not responded to conventional trial therapy.

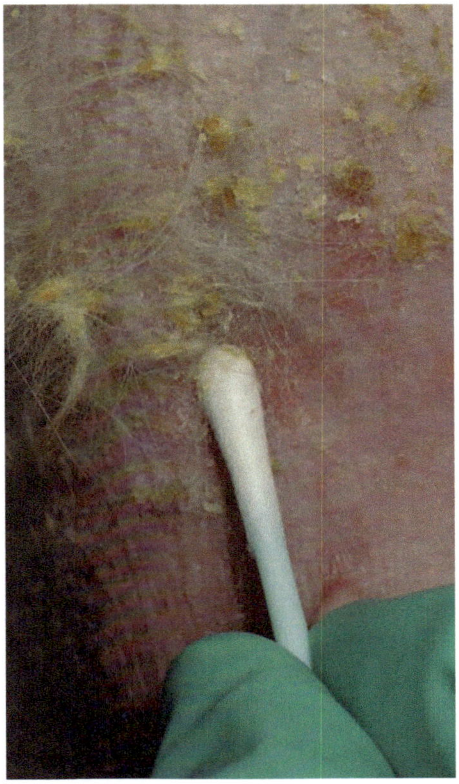

Figure 1.56 When pustules are not present, use a saline moistened culturette to sample under multiple crusts and submit for aerobic culture.

- In general, skin biopsies should be performed within three to four weeks of the onset of the disease, since more chronic lesions can be difficult to interpret due to changes secondary to infection, scarring, or steroid therapy.
- Check cytology of superficial or crusty lesions prior to biopsy; since secondary infection can alter histopathologic findings (e.g. discoid lupus and mucocutaneous pyoderma appear very similar histologically), pretreatment with antibiotics for two to three weeks may be necessary.
- Steroid therapy can also change biopsy results, and ideally patients should not receive oral or topical steroids within two to three weeks and injectable long-acting steroids within six to eight weeks of performing the biopsy procedure (severe, life-threatening cases would obviously be an exception to this rule).
- If possible, choose primary lesions such as papules, pustules, vesicles, macules, or nodules. In suspected cases of discoid lupus erythematosus, select early depigmented lesions (before erosion or scarring occurs).
  - Even if primary lesions are not present, diagnostic information can be obtained from crusts, which should be carefully preserved with the skin biopsies. Lesions which are less likely to be diagnostic include excoriations, ulcers, or chronically scarred areas.
- More information is gained by performing multiple (three to five) samples, obtained from a variety of lesions.
- To obtain biopsy samples, local anesthetic (0.5–1 cc of 1–2% lidocaine injected with a 25G needle subcutaneously under the lesion) and/or mild sedation will be needed (Figure 1.57).
  - Hair overlying the lesion may be gently clipped, but the clipper blades should not touch the skin.

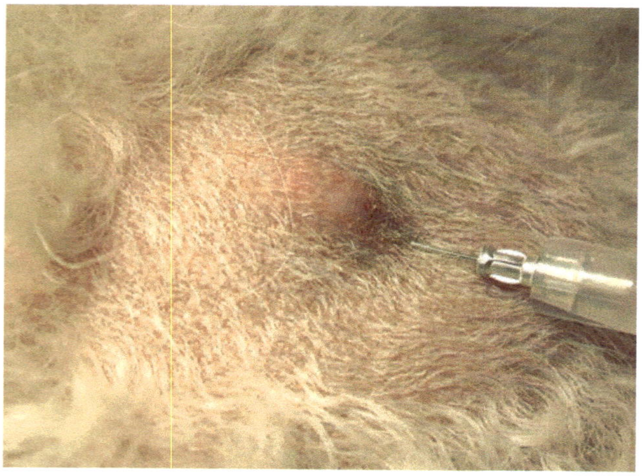

Figure 1.57 Lidocaine is injected using a 25G needle subcutaneously under the lesion to be sampled.

  - Do not surgically prep or disinfect the areas, as important skin debris will be lost.
  - Do not exceed a total lidocaine dose of 5 mg/kg for dogs or 2.5 mg/kg for cats (2% lidocaine = 20 mg/ml); lidocaine may be diluted 1 : 1 with saline if needed for small patients.
- 6 mm punch biopsies are preferred for most cases; 4 mm punches may be necessary for difficult areas such as near the eye, on the ear, and on the nasal planum or footpads of smaller patients.
  - Use new, sharp biopsy punches, as older used ones tend to shear and distort tissue and create artifact.
- Excisional biopsy with a scalpel may be indicated for larger or nodular lesions or for diseases of the subcutaneous fat.
- Place the area of interest in the center of the biopsy punch and do not include a significant amount of normal skin with the biopsy (Figure 1.58A and 1.58B); the only time a lesion should be biopsied on the margin is in the case of an ulcerative skin disease.
  - If a large lesion appears different in the center and leading edges, biopsy both areas.
- Push the biopsy punch down gently in a rotational motion in one direction to avoid shearing artifact until the epidermis and dermis are penetrated and the biopsy punch rotates freely.
  - When handling the skin biopsy, avoid crush artifact by grasping only the subcutaneous tissue with thumb forceps (Figure 1.59).
  - Prior to fixation, skin biopsies can be placed fat side down on pieces of wooden tongue depressor to prevent tissue folding and aid in orientation when samples are processed.
- Biopsies from radically different lesions or nodules should be tagged with a suture or placed in individually labeled containers for differentiation.
- Within five minutes of obtaining the specimens, skin biopsies should be fixed in 10% neutral phosphate buffered formalin (minimum 10 parts formalin to 1 part tissue for adequate fixation).
- Close skin biopsy sites with 3-0 Nylon in a simple interrupted or cruciate pattern (Figure 1.60A and 1.60B). To close biopsy sites in difficult to access places for future suture removal, use absorbable suture.
- When obtaining a sample for tissue cultures, place the biopsy in a sterile red top tube (+/− with 0.25–0.5 cc sterile/not bacteriostatic saline to keep it moist; contact the laboratory you are using to determine their preferred submission protocol).
- Skin histopathology results are optimized by utilizing experienced dermatopathologists.
  - In cases with histologic inflammation suspected to be related to infectious disease, special stains to highlight organisms are indicated, and many

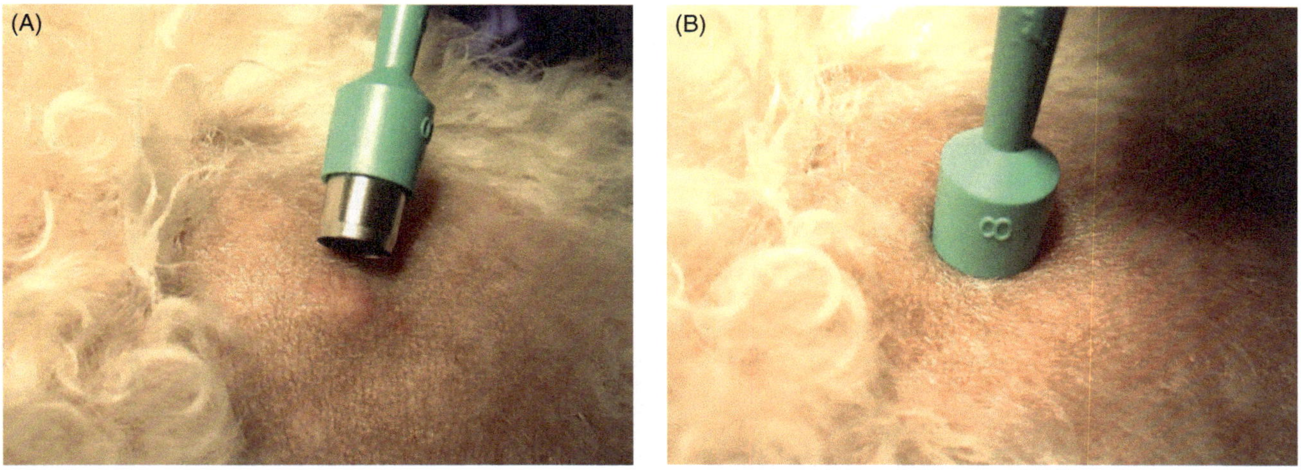

Figures 1.58A and B Place the biopsy punch in the center of the area of interest, then push down gently in a rotational motion in one direction to avoid shearing artifact until the biopsy punch rotates freely.

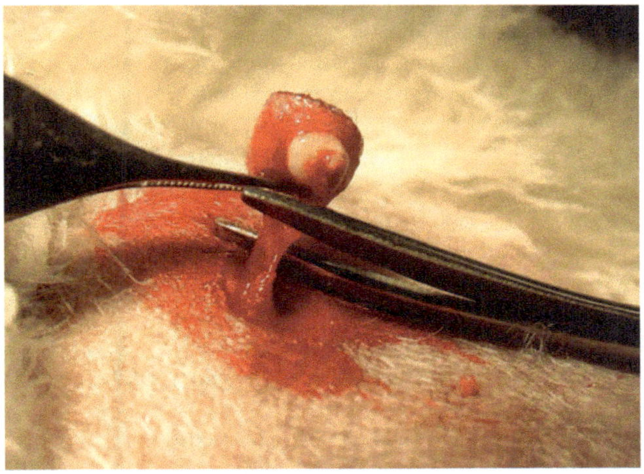

Figure 1.59 Avoid crush artifact by grasping the subcutaneous tissue/fat with the forceps.

dermatopathologists will add these stains on at no extra cost.
- Special stains which may be needed include Gram stain for bacteria, GMS (Gomori methenamine silver)and/or PAS Periodic acid–Schiff) stains for fungal organisms and Zygomycetes such as pythiosis, and acid-fast stains for mycobacteria and filamentous bacteria.

- It is also essential to give a complete signalment and history, including description and distribution of lesions, other symptoms and results of pertinent diagnostic tests, current or past therapy/response to therapy, and the clinician's differential diagnoses. Many pathologists will accept and appreciate digital patient photographs. These elements are important to allow the pathologist to formulate an accurate diagnosis, and if there are questions, most pathologists are happy to discuss their findings with the clinician.

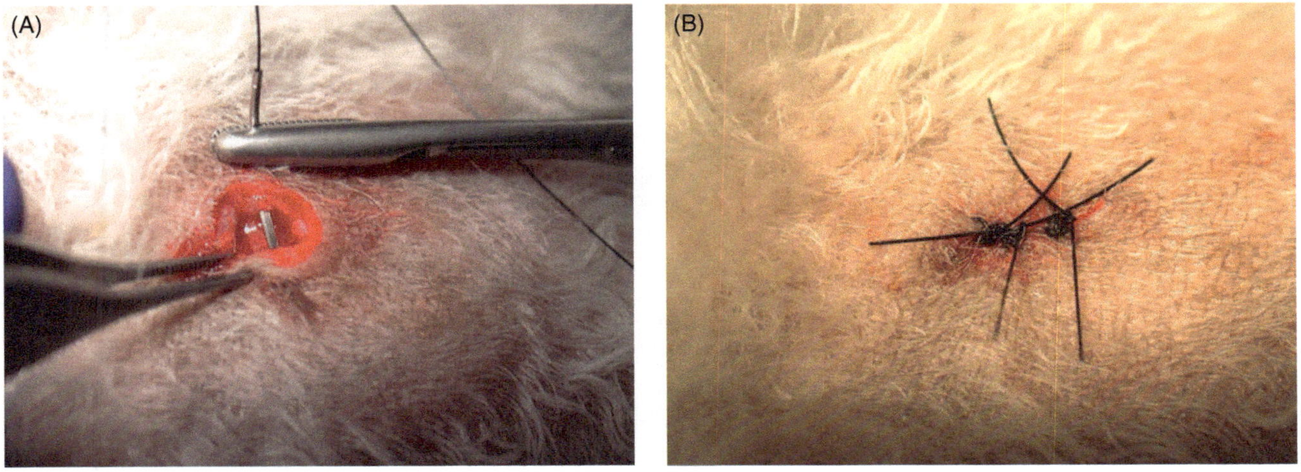

Figures 1.60A and B Close the biopsy site with two to three simple interrupted, or one or two cruciate sutures.

1.12 Allergy testing

- It is important to emphasize that allergy testing is not a first line screening test in the work up of dogs and cats with dermatologic disease.
- Allergy testing for environmental allergens, whether by serology or intradermal testing, is only performed when the clinical diagnosis of atopic dermatitis has been made by first ruling out all other causes of pruritus/dermatitis.
  - Rule out parasites with skin scrapings and trial treatment for parasites such as fleas and mites.
  - Rule out infection with cytology/culture and treatment of infectious organisms.
  - Rule out adverse food reaction with a carefully performed prescription or home cooked hypoallergenic diet trial for six to eight weeks with no other treats, table scraps, rawhides, milkbones, pill pockets, fish oil, chewable flavored medications, or supplements.
  - Serology for food allergy is not accurate and cannot be used as an alternative to a hypoallergenic diet trial.
- The purpose of allergy testing is to determine which allergens will be selected for a hyposensitization vaccine.
- Please see Chapter 10 for more information about allergy testing and allergen selection.

References/Further reading

Albanese, F. (2017). *Canine and Feline Skin Cytology: A Comprehensive and Illustrated Guide to the Interpretation of Skin Lesions via Cytological Examination.* Cham, Switzerland: Springer International Publishing.

Al-Bagdadi, F.A., Titkemeyer, C.W., and Lovell, J.E. (1977). Hair follicle cycle and shedding in male beagle dogs. *Am. J. Vet. Res.* 38 (5): 611–616.

Beco, L., Guagere, E., Lorente Mendez, C. et al. (2013). Suggested guidelines for using systemic antimicrobials in bacterial skin infections (1): diagnosis based on clinical presentation, cytology and culture. *Vet. Rec.* 172 (3): 72–78.

Bowman, D. (2014). *Georgis' Parasitology for Veterinarians*, 10e. St. Louis, MO: Elsevier Saunders.

Coyner, K. (2010). How to perform and interpret dermatophyte cultures. *Vet. Med.* 105 (7): 304–307.

Coyner, K. (2011). Skills laboratory: how to perform skin scraping and skin surface cytology. *Vet. Med.* 106 (11): 554–563.

Coyner, K. (2011). Skills laboratory: skin biopsy. *Vet. Med.* 106 (10): 505–507.

Diaz, S.F1., Torres, S.M., Nogueira, S.A. et al. (2006). The impact of body site, topical melatonin and brushing on hair regrowth after clipping normal Siberian Husky dogs. *Vet. Dermatol.* 17 (1): 45–50.

Dunstan, R.W., Credille, K.M., Mansell, J. et al. A common sense approach to the morphology of alopecia: Addressing 10 points of follicular confusion. In: Proceedings of the 16th Annual Meeting of American Academy of Veterinary Dermatology and American College of Veterinary Dermatology. Norfolk, USA, 2001

Favarato, E.S. and Conceição, L.G. (2008). Hair cycle in dogs with different hair types in a tropical region of Brazil. *Vet. Dermatol.* 19 (1): 15–20. https://doi.org/10.1111/j.1365-3164.2007.00642.x.

Miller, W.H., Griffen, C.E., and Campbell, K.L. (2013). *Muller and Kirk's Small Animal Dermatology*, 7e. St Louis, MO: Elsevier Mosby.

Moriello, K.A. (2014). Feline dermatophytosis. Aspects pertinent to disease management in single and multiple cat situations. *J. Feline Med. Surg.* 16 (5): 419–431.

Moriello, K.A. and Leutenegger, C.M. (2018). Use of a commercial qPCR assay in 52 high risk shelter cats for disease identification of dermatophytosis and mycological cure. *Vet. Dermatol.* 29: 66–e26.

Welle, M.M. and Wiener, D.J. (2016). The Hair follicle: a comparative review of canine hair follicle anatomy and physiology. *Toxicol. Pathol.* 44 (4): 564–574.

2

Dermatology lesions and differential diagnoses

Kimberly S. Coyner, DVM, DACVD

Dermatology Clinic for Animals, Lacey, WA, USA

One of the most important skills to master when approaching a dermatology case is to correctly identify skin lesions and to know what diseases are associated with what type of skin lesions. We tend to define lesions as primary lesions (those that develop spontaneously as a direct manifestation of an underlying disease, such as a papule or pustule due to folliculitis), and secondary lesions (which evolve from a primary lesion, such as an epidermal collarette evolving from a pustule, or excoriations induced by pruritus/scratching of a popular dermatitis). In some cases, lesions can be both primary or secondary in character, such as alopecia which can be a primary issue in an alopecic breed, but in a different patient may be secondary to many other diseases including folliculitis, endocrinopathy, or self-induced barbering due to pruritus. Being able to correctly identify primary lesions, or recognize that a secondary lesion evolved from a prior primary lesion, can help narrow down a list of differentials and guide further diagnostics.

2.1 Primary lesions

2.1.1 Macule/Patch

Definition:

1) Macule – a circumscribed flat area of color change <1 cm diameter.
2) Patch – a circumscribed flat area of color change >1 cm diameter.

Common causes:

1) Pigment change (increased or decreased melanin) in the skin cells due to inflammation, immune mediated disease (vitiligo), viral infection of epidermal cells, or aging changes, or as a normal finding on nasal and lip/eyelid mucosae of orange cats (lentigo). Less commonly, cutaneous lymphoma can cause patches of skin and fur depigmentation.
2) Increased red blood cells in the skin due to hemorrhage or vascular dilation/inflammation.

Differentials based on lesion distribution/location:

1) Post-inflammatory hyperpigmented or depigmented lesions are located in prior areas of inflammation/infection.
2) Pigmented viral macules are often found on the ventral trunk and may eventually become slightly raised/scaly (Figure 2.1).
3) Senile pigmented macules can occur anywhere.
4) Lentigo in orange cats causes dark macules on nasal planum, lips, and eyelids (Figure 2.2).
5) Vitiligo often affects face/nose/paws (Figure 2.3).
6) Atopic patches often occur on the lateral axillary and inguinal areas (Figure 2.4).
7) Thrombocytopenic ecchymoses are most visible in thinly furred areas (Figure 2.5).
8) Cutaneous lymphoma often causes depigmentation on the lips, nasal planum, and eyelids and may also involve paw pads and trunk.

Diagnostics:

1) Cytology of lesions which are inflamed or scaly to evaluate for type of inflammatory cells and bacteria.
2) Complete blood count/platelet count/coagulation panel/tick titers in cases of hemorrhagic skin lesions.
3) Biopsy in cases of suspected viral infection, immune mediated disease, or neoplasia.

2.1.2 Papule/pustule

Definition:

1) Papule – a solid elevated lesion <1 cm diameter; a small, raised, solid bump usually originating from an underlying infected hair follicle, and typically

Clinical Atlas of Canine and Feline Dermatology, First Edition. Edited by Kimberly S. Coyner.

Companion website: www.wiley.com/go/coyner/dermatology

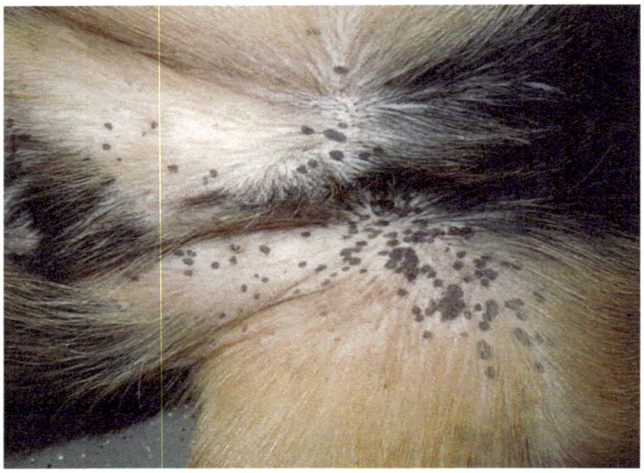

Figure 2.1 A dog with pigmented macules due to papilloma infection.

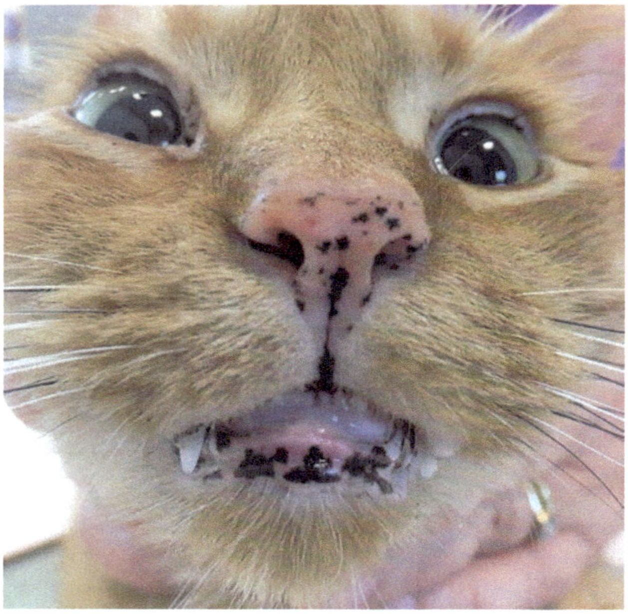

Figure 2.2 A cat with lentigo, a normal pigment variation in orange cats.

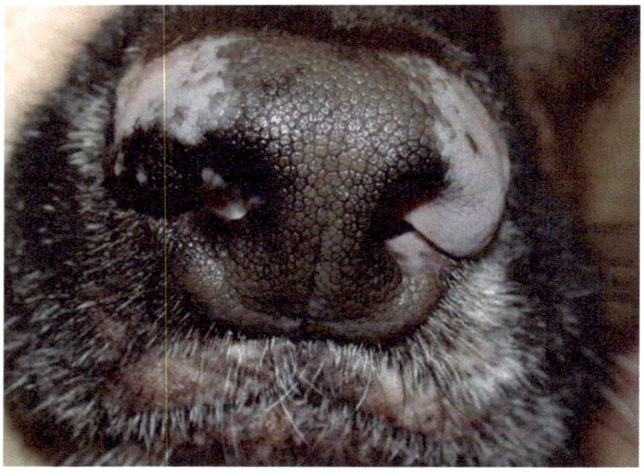

Figure 2.3 A dog with depigmented macules and patches due to vitiligo; the normal nasal reticular pattern is preserved.

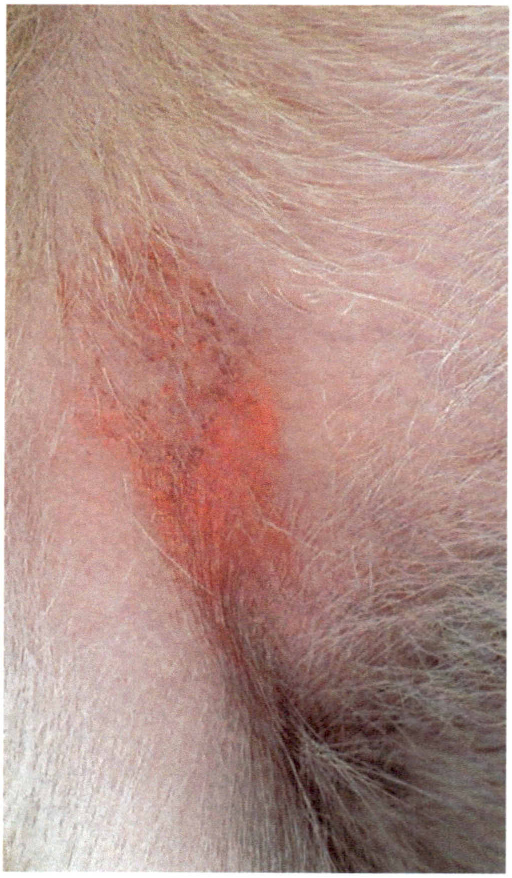

Figure 2.4 A dog with an erythematous axillary patch due to atopic dermatitis.

inflamed and may have slight surface crusting but not producing pus (Figure 2.6A and 2.6B); may be part of a more generalized rash on the skin.

2) Pustule – a small circumscribed elevation of the skin (epidermis or hair follicle) containing pus and having an inflamed base. It often evolves from a papule in cases of bacterial, demodectic, or dermatophyte induced folliculitis (Figure 2.6A and 2.6B).

Common causes:

1) Folliculitis/infection of hair follicles due to bacteria, *Demodex* mites, or dermatophytosis.
2) Other skin parasites such as fleas, scabies, *Cheyletiella*, and lice can also cause papules/pustules due to direct damage to the skin by biting, or by inducing a secondary infection.
3) Papules can also be seen with chronic sun damage (solar dermatosis, Figure 2.7).
4) Tiny papules in non-haired areas such as the groin can be a primary lesion of atopic dermatitis.

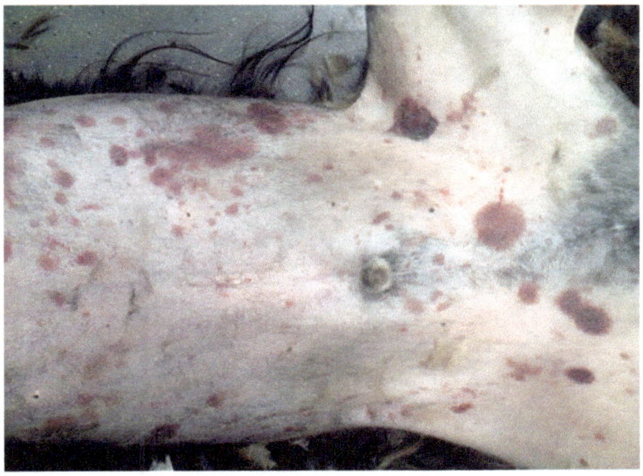

Figure 2.5 A dog with hemorrhagic macules and patches due to thrombocytopenia.

5) Pemphigus foliaceus causes pustules which span multiple hair follicles (Figure 2.8) and rupture quickly, leaving crusts.

Differentials based on lesion distribution/location:

1) Bacterial pyoderma most commonly occurs on the trunk, groin, and axillary areas and can sometimes involve the neck and perineum; lesions can be localized or generalized and can be symmetric or asymmetric. Bacterial pyoderma less commonly involves the legs or face, including ear pinnae.
2) *Demodex* and dermatophytosis commonly affect the face and paws but can occur anywhere on the body and can be localized/asymmetric or generalized.
3) Solar dermatitis most commonly occurs on nonpigmented skin on the groin, axillary areas, trunk, and face.
4) Pemphigus foliaceus commonly affects the face, ear pinnae, trunk, neck, legs; footpads and nasal planum can also be affected. Pustules are transient/rupture quickly, and often only residual crusting is seen clinically.

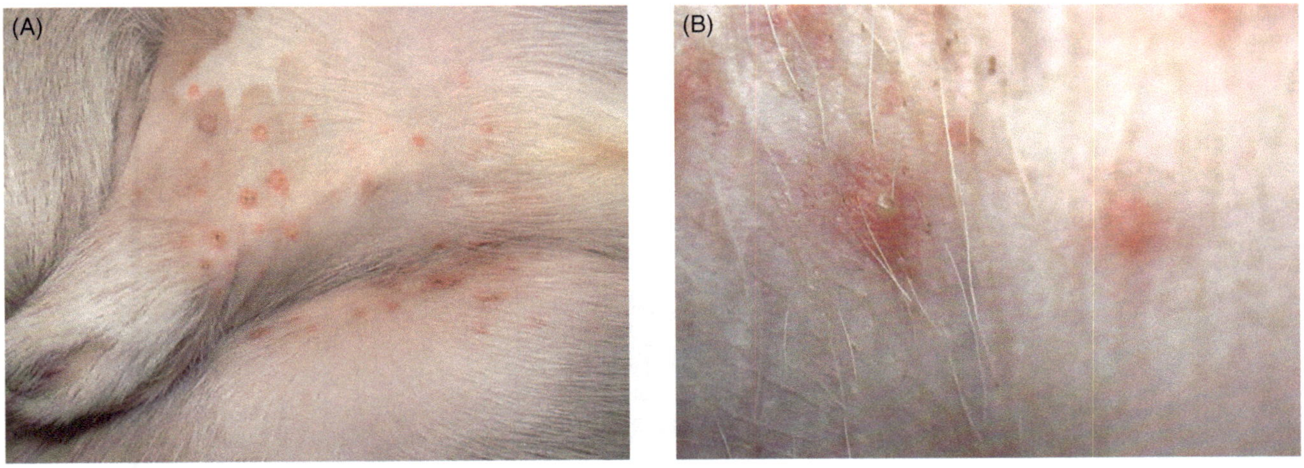

Figures 2.6A and B Inguinal papules and pustules due to bacterial folliculitis in an atopic dog.

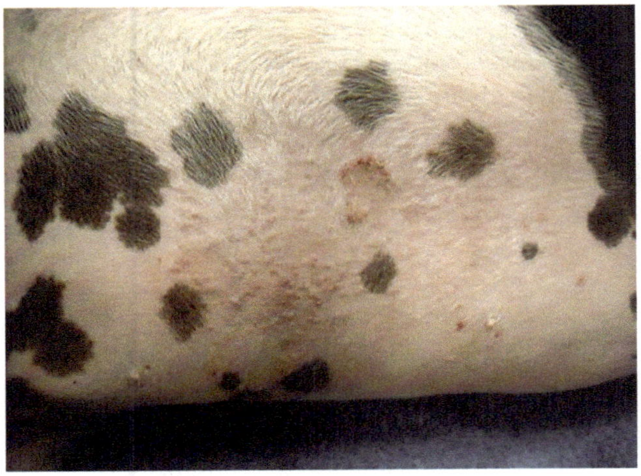

Figure 2.7 Papules caused by solar dermatitis.

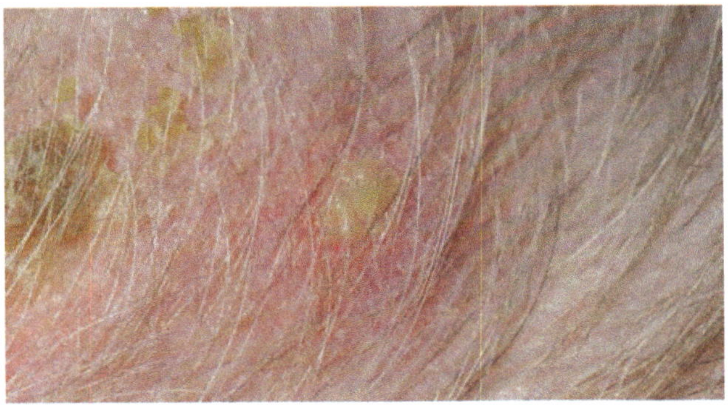

Figure 2.8 A dog with pustules due to pemphigus foliaceus.

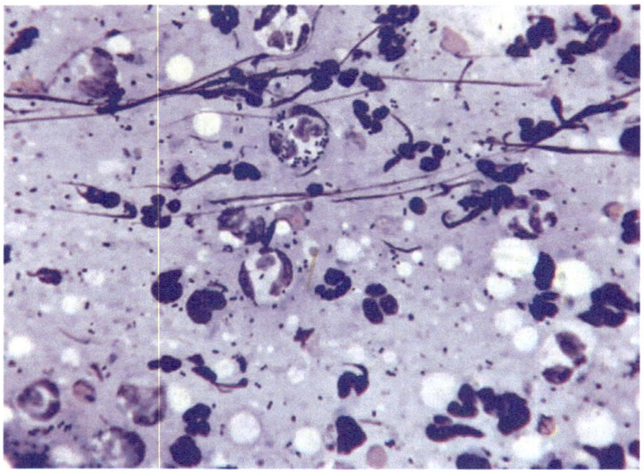

Figure 2.9 Cytology of pustules reveal neutrophils with numerous intracellular and extracellular cocci bacteria.

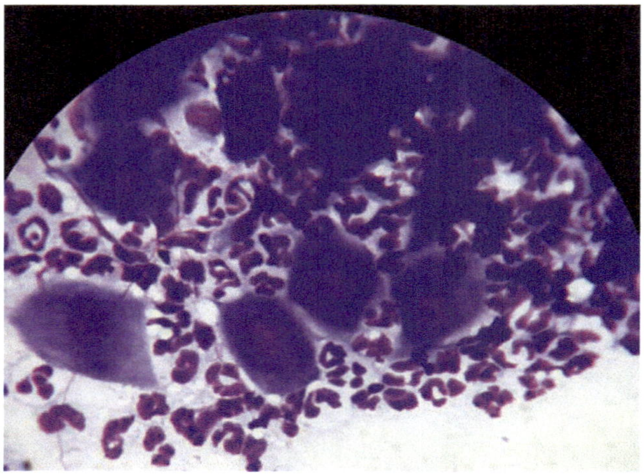

Figure 2.10 Cytology of pemphigus pustule contents reveal neutrophils and large acantholytic cells.

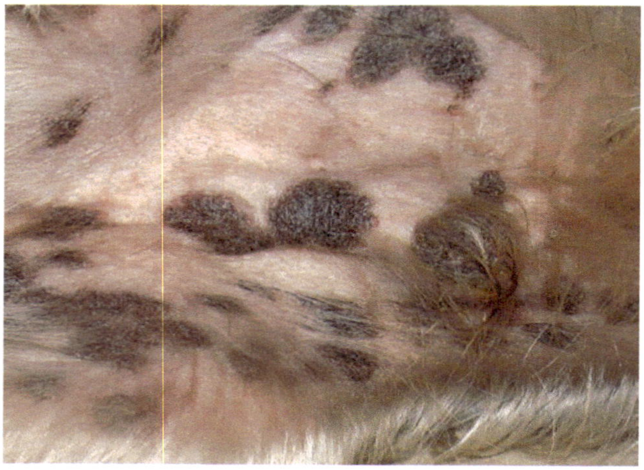

Figure 2.11 A dog with scaly hyperpigmented inguinal plaques due to bacterial infection; viral pigmented plaques can appear similar.

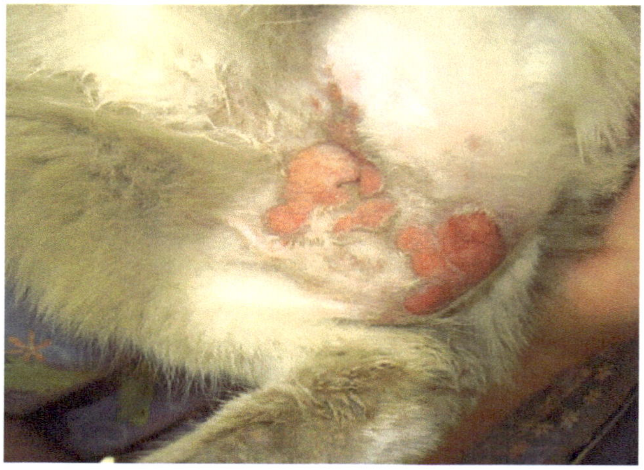

Figure 2.12 A cat with raised erythematous moist inguinal plaques secondary to atopy and flea bite hypersensitivity.

Diagnostics:

1) Superficial and deep skin scrapings for parasites.
2) Cytology to evaluate for type of inflammatory cells and bacteria (Figure 2.9), as well as to screen for acantholytic cells on suspected cases of pemphigus foliaceus (Figure 2.10).
3) Culture (aerobic) if bacteria are seen despite prior empiric antibiotics, or infection is recurrent.
4) Biopsy and dermatophyte culture if papules/pustules persist despite treatment of any secondary infection, or if no organisms are found on cytology and scrapings.

2.1.3 Plaque

Definition:

1) A flat-topped, firm, raised skin lesion >1 cm diameter.

Common causes:

1) Chronic inflammation due to skin infection (bacterial, *Demodex*, dermatophyte, *Malassezia*, viral), allergic inflammation, solar dermatitis, calcinosis cutis, cutaneous lymphoma.

Differentials based on lesion distribution/location:

1) Infectious/inflammatory lesions can occur anywhere but are more common on the inguinal area (Figure 2.11).
2) Feline eosinophilic plaques occur more commonly on the trunk, axilla, and groin (Figure 2.12).
3) Solar dermatitis occurs in white-coated, short-haired dogs in areas of thinly haired skin (Figure 2.13).
4) Calcinosis cutis most commonly occurs on the dorsal shoulders/trunk, axillae, and groin (Figure 2.14).

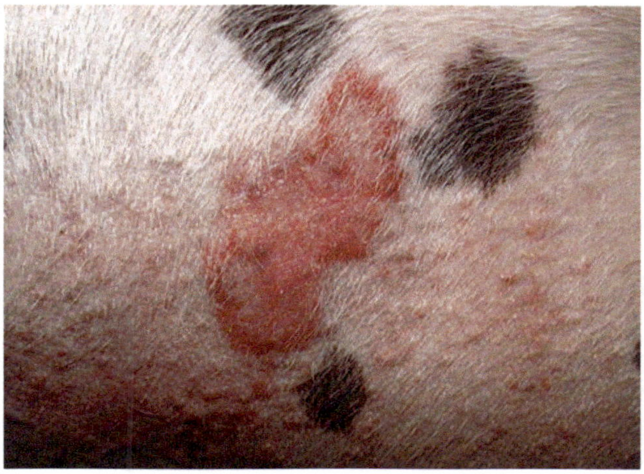

Figure 2.13 A raised erythematous plaque due to solar dermatitis.

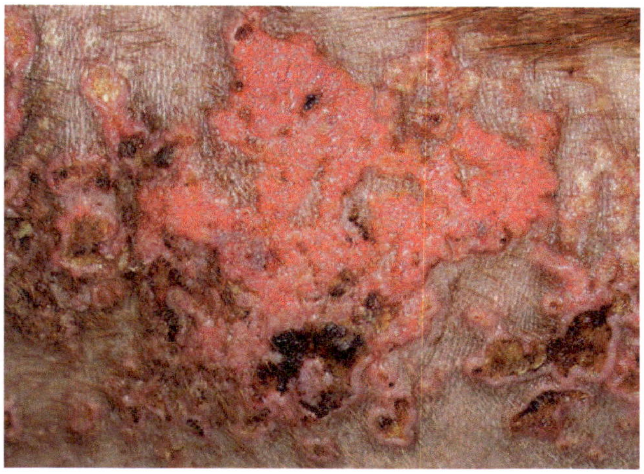

Figure 2.14 A dog with gritty raised plaques due to calcinosis cutis induced by chronic prednisone treatment.

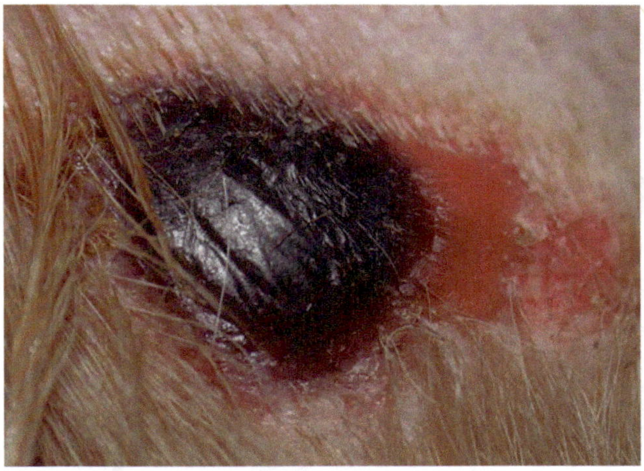

Figure 2.15 A blood filled bulla on the dorsal trunk of a dog due to solar thermal damage after a long walk.

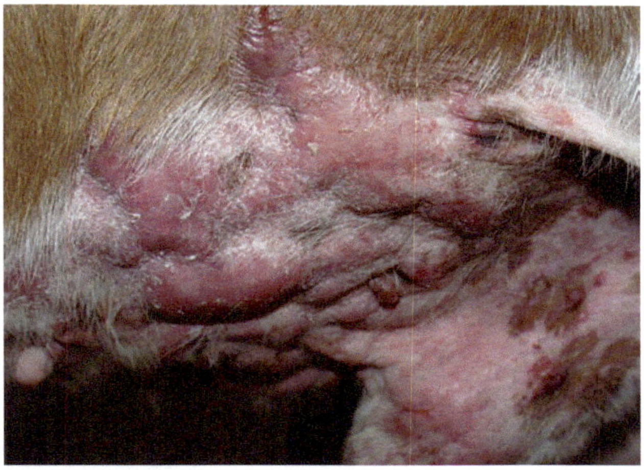

Figure 2.16 Inguinal bullae due to severe solar dermatitis.

Diagnostics:

1) Superficial and deep skin scrapings for parasites.
2) Cytology to evaluate for type of inflammatory cells and bacteria.
3) Culture (aerobic) if bacteria are seen despite prior empiric antibiotics, or infection is recurrent.
4) Biopsy and dermatophyte culture if plaques persist despite treatment of any secondary infection, or if no organisms are found on cytology and scrapings.

2.1.4 Vesicle/bulla

Definition:

1) Thin-walled, fluid-filled sac <1 cm diameter (vesicle) or >1 cm (bulla) containing clear to blood-tinged fluid. In most cases lesions are very fragile and rupture easily, leaving an ulceration which may crust.

Common causes:

1) Immune mediated diseases (i.e. pemphigus vulgaris, bullous pemphigoid, erythema multiforme, toxic epidermal necrolysis, systemic and cutaneous lupus, epidermolysis bullosa (Figure 11.8A), dermatomyositis).
2) Viral diseases (herpes virus, calicivirus, pox virus).
3) Acute epithelial damage caused by irritants/caustic chemicals/burn (Figures 2.15 and 2.16).
4) Mucinosis in Shar-Pei dogs.

Differentials based on lesion distribution/location:

1) Immune-mediated diseases often affect the face, pinnae, oral cavity, nasal planum, and paw pads.
2) Herpes and calicivirus often affect the face and oral cavity.
3) Mucinosis occurs in Shar-Pei dogs and often affects trunk and limbs (Figure 2.17).

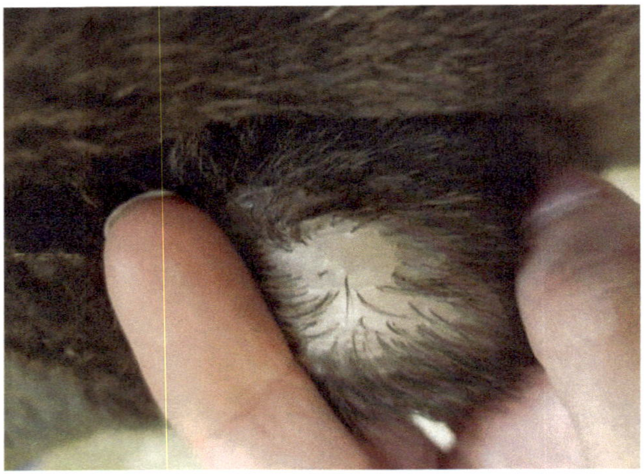

Figure 2.17 Mucin filled vesicles in a Shar-Pei dog. *Source:* Photo courtesy of Dr. Amy Shumaker, DACVD.

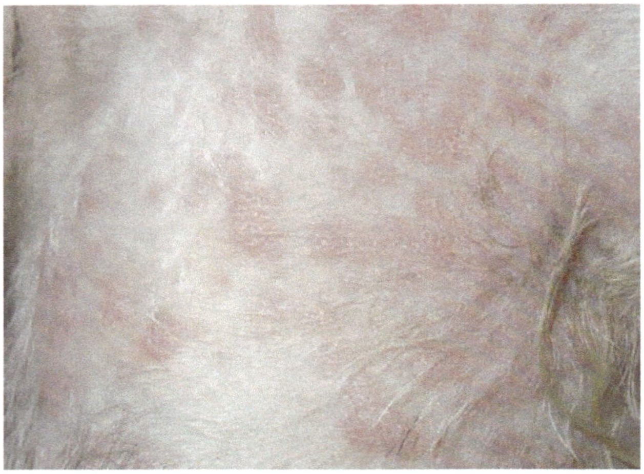

Figure 2.18 Acute urticarial reaction to a shampoo in an atopic dog.

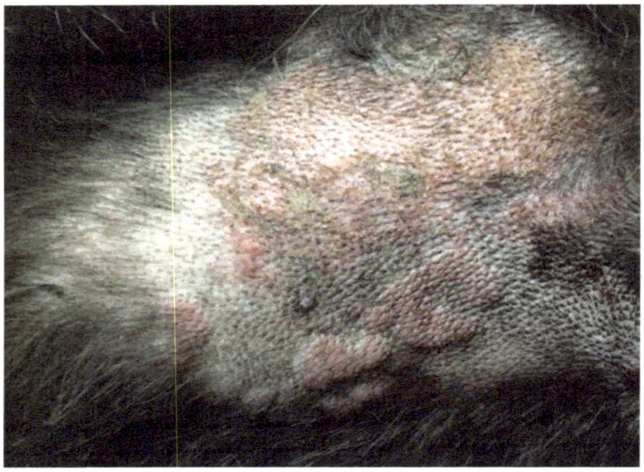

Figure 2.19 Urticarial wheals in a dog due to food allergy, with surrounding crusted excoriations due to scratching/self-trauma.

Diagnostics:

1) Cytology to evaluate for any inflammatory cells or bacteria.
2) Biopsy of intact vesicle, if present, or margin of erosion/ulceration.

2.1.5 Wheal

Definition:

1) An acute, flat-topped, firm, raised, edematous lesion which can range in size from 4 mm–1 cm; also known as hives (Figures 2.18 and 2.19). Large coalescing wheals involving the lips/eyelids is termed angioedema.

Common causes:

1) An acute allergic reaction to an insect bite or sting, drug or vaccine, or in chronic cases, to food or an environmental allergen.

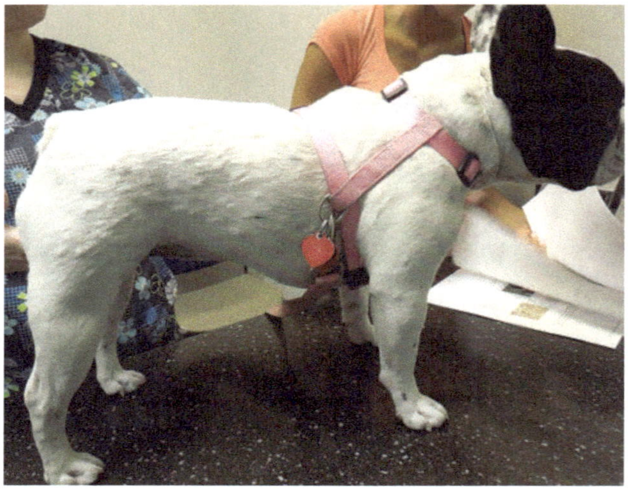

Figure 2.20 This French Bulldog has a bacterial folliculitis which can mimic hives; careful examination of the skin under the raised tufts of fur reveals slightly crusty papules.

Differentials based on lesion distribution/location:

1) Lesions may begin on the face or nose of dogs which have been stung by an insect, then hives can generalize and are usually pruritic.
2) In haired areas, wheals cause the fur to raise up slightly into tufts.
3) Wheals/hives are flat topped and come and go, never losing fur or becoming crusted; this differentiates them from a bacterial folliculitis which can also cause raised tufts of fur on the trunk that can be mistaken for hives, however they will eventually crust and lose fur (Figure 2.20).

Diagnostics:

1) Cytology to evaluate for any inflammatory cells or bacteria.

2) Biopsy shows eosinophilic inflammation and edema.
3) Obtain a thorough history including onset of lesions, possible insect exposure, and drug history including shampoos, vaccines, and oral drugs, and discontinue anything that is new. In chronic cases, begin a hypoallergenic diet trial for possible food allergy.

2.1.6 Nodule

Definition:

1) A solid mass >1 cm diameter.

Common causes:

1) Nodules can be caused by tumors (benign or malignant, Figures 2.21–2.23), infectious or sterile granulomas (Figure 2.24), histiocytic disorders (Figure 2.25), or miscellaneous disorders such as calcinosis circumscripta.

Differentials based on lesion distribution/location:

1) Tumors can occur anyplace on the body and are usually single in number, though sebaceous adenomas can be multiple in older dogs.
2) Histiocytic disorders and sterile granulomas can cause multiple nodules on multiple areas of the body and can occur rapidly.
3) Calcinosis circumscripta usually occurs in areas of trauma such as elbows, tongue, paw pads, or on pinnal margins after ear crop.

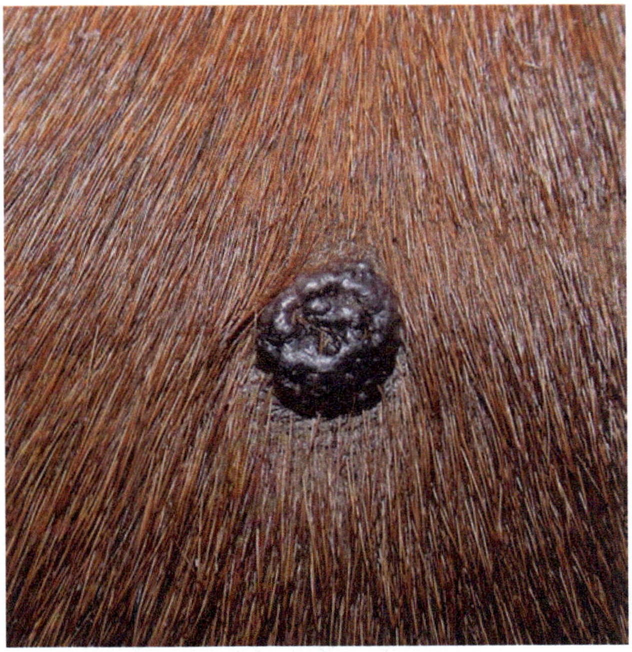

Figure 2.21 A sebaceous epithelioma.

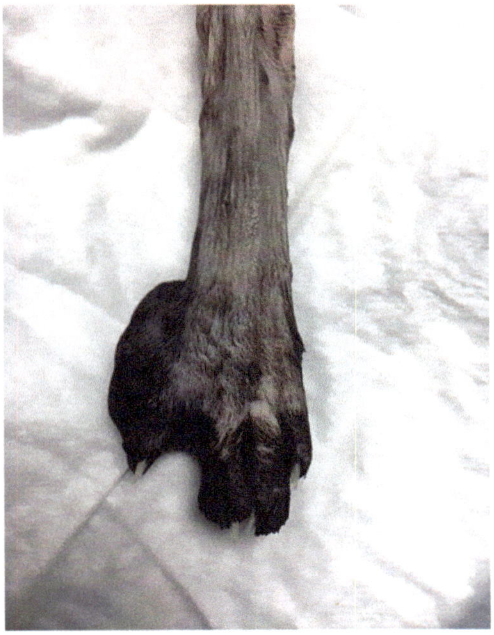

Figure 2.22 A cat with a distal limb subcutaneous hemangiosarcoma. *Source:* Photo courtesy of Dr. Eric Hoots, DACVS.

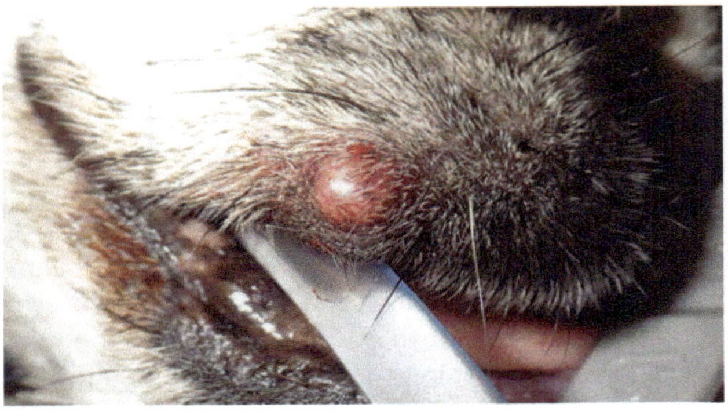

Figure 2.23 A mast cell tumor on the lip of a Pug.

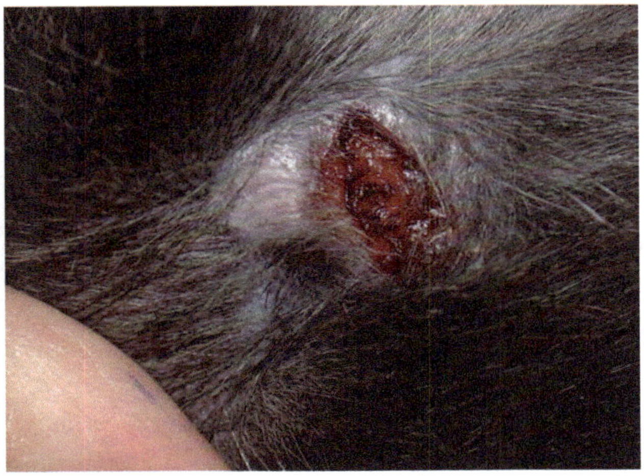

Figure 2.24 An ulcerated granulomatous mass on a cat caused by a mycobacterial infection.

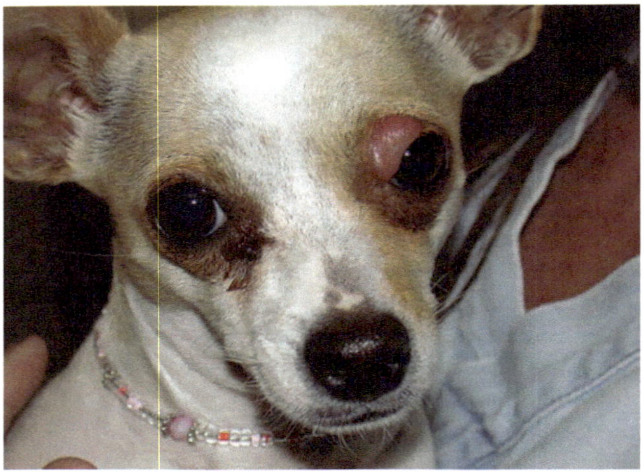

Figure 2.25 A dog with a histiocytoma on the eyelid; this resolved spontaneously in six weeks.

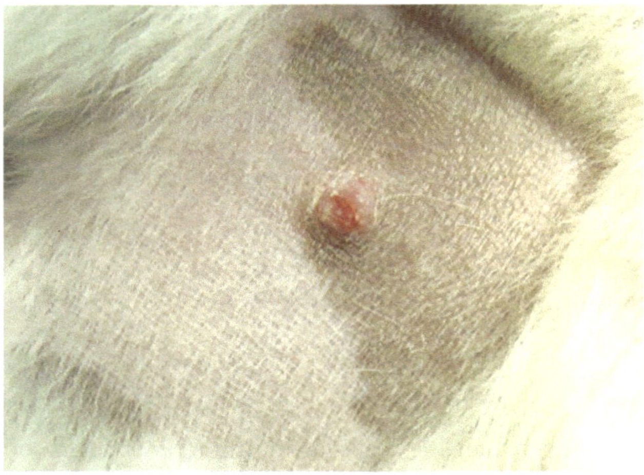

Figure 2.26A A follicular cyst.

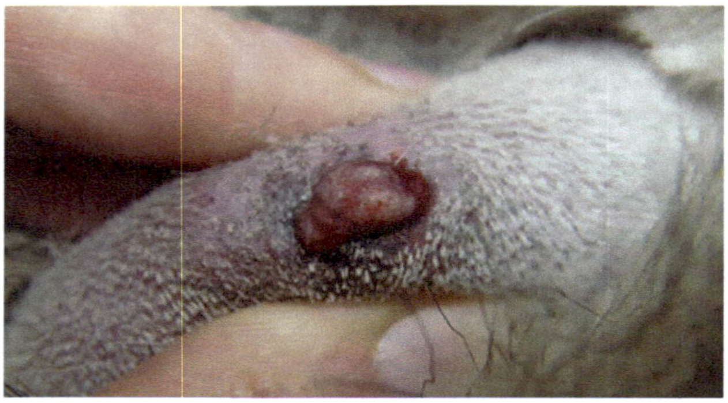

Figure 2.26B This Norwegian Elkhound had multiple intracornifying epitheliomas, which would often open and drain flocculent material.

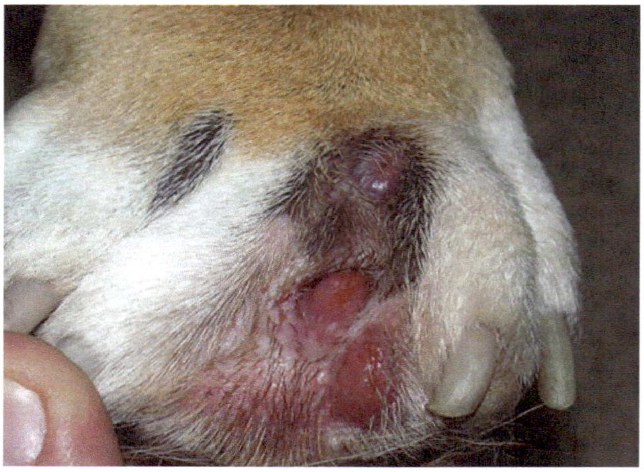

Figure 2.26C The atopic Bulldog had multiple interdigital follicular cysts which would become inflamed, rupture, and drain.

Diagnostics:

1) Fine needle aspirate for cytology to evaluate for any inflammatory or neoplastic cells or organisms.
2) Biopsy; if initial cytology shows inflammatory cells, then tissue cultures may be needed.

2.1.7 Cyst

Definition:

1) Epithelial lined cavity containing fluid or cellular and/or sebaceous debris.

Common causes:

1) Usually originate from hair follicles or glands.

Differentials based on lesion distribution/location:

1) Cysts can occur anyplace on the body and are usually single, though can be multiple especially in predisposed breeds (Figures 2.26A and 2.26B).
2) Interdigital cysts are distended inflamed obstructed hair follicles which occur secondarily to underlying atopy, food allergy, conformational abnormalities +/− obesity, and then rupture and cause infected granulomas (Figure 2.26C).

Diagnostics:

1) Fine needle aspirate of non-inflammatory sebaceous or follicular cysts for cytology usually shows amorphous keratinaceous debris (Figure 2.27A); aspirate of apocrine cyst typically shows clear to light yellow acellular to poorly cellular fluid, or sometimes brown turbid fluid due to melanin content (i.e. apocrine cystomatosis); aspirates of ruptured and inflamed interdigital cysts shows pyogranulomatous inflammation which may include eosinophils, keratin, and hair

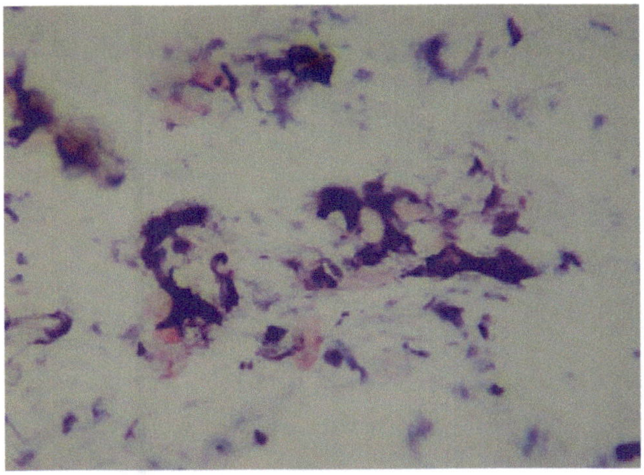

Figure 2.27A Cytology of a fine needle aspirate of the follicular cyst reveals amorphous keratinaceous and/or sebaceous material and may also contain melanin granules.

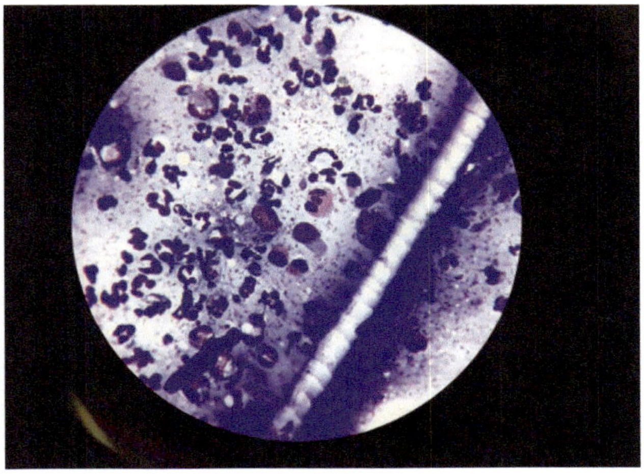

Figure 2.27B Cytology of a draining interdigital cyst/granuloma often shows neutrophils and macrophages; eosinophils, keratin, and fragments of degenerating hair shafts may also be found. Bacteria may be few in number and difficult to find due to severity of inflammation (100×).

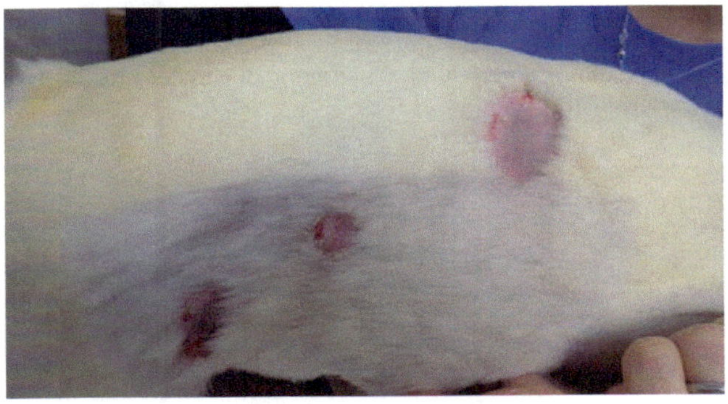

Figure 2.28 A dog with multifocal alopecia due to bacterial folliculitis; *Demodex* or dermatophyte infections can appear identical, and skin scrapings and cytology are indicated ± dermatophyte culture if definitive organisms are not found on screening tests.

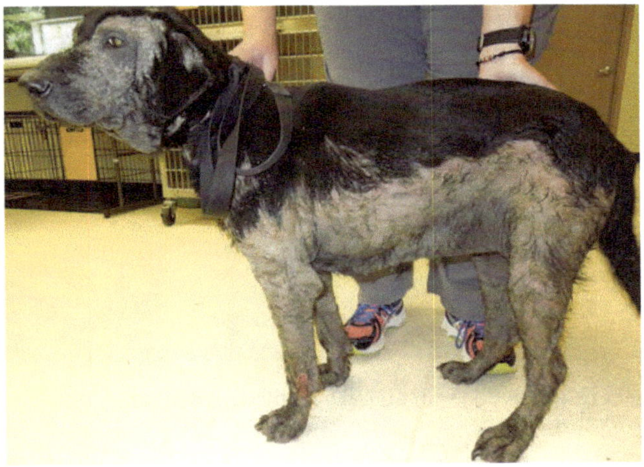

Figure 2.29 A dog with alopecia due to pruritus and severe bacterial and *Malassezia* skin infections secondary to atopy and food allergy.

fragments; bacteria may be present in low numbers or obscured by inflammatory infiltrate (Figure 2.27B).
2) Biopsy.
3) Culture interdigital cysts to guide antibiotic treatment while the underlying cause is addressed.

2.2 Primary or secondary lesions

2.2.1 Alopecia (Also see chapters 12 and 13)

Definition:

1) Localized, multifocal, or generalized loss of hair.

Common causes:

1) Folliculitis (bacterial [Figures 2.28 and 2.29], *Demodex*, dermatophyte).
2) Pruritus/barbering (Figures 2.30A and 2.30B).
3) Endocrinopathies.
   a) Hypothyroidism (Figure 2.31).
   b) Hyperadrenocorticism.
   c) Excess sex hormone (endogenous vs. exogenous).
4) Follicular dysplasia/Hair cycle disorder.
   a) Breed related, i.e. Doberman, Irish water spaniel, Curly coated retriever.
   b) Alopecia X.
   c) Canine recurrent flank alopecia (Figure 2.32A).
   d) Pattern baldness (Figure 2.32B).
5) Immune-mediated disorders.
   a) Alopecia areata (Figure 2.33A), mural folliculitis, dermatomyositis (Figure 2.33B).
   b) Vaccine reaction.

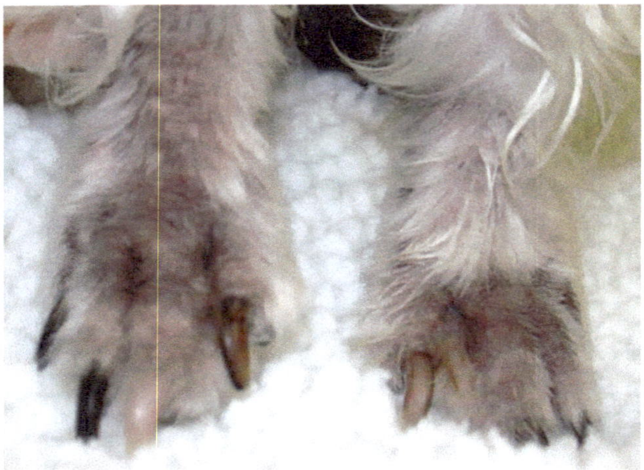

Figure 2.30A A dog with pedal barbering due to atopy.

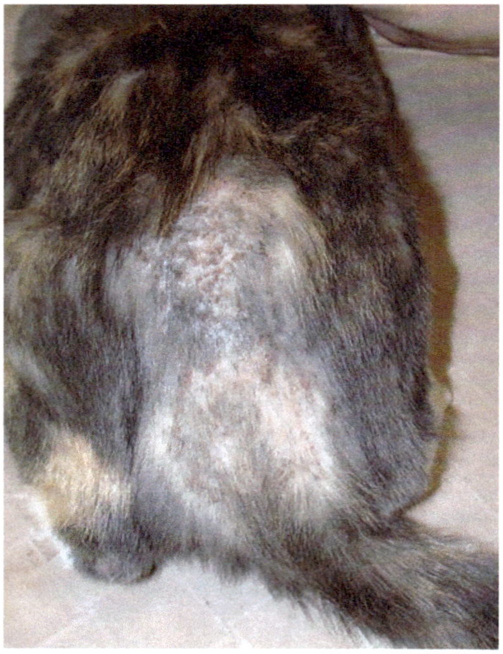

Figure 2.30B A cat with lumbar barbering due to flea bite hypersensitivity.

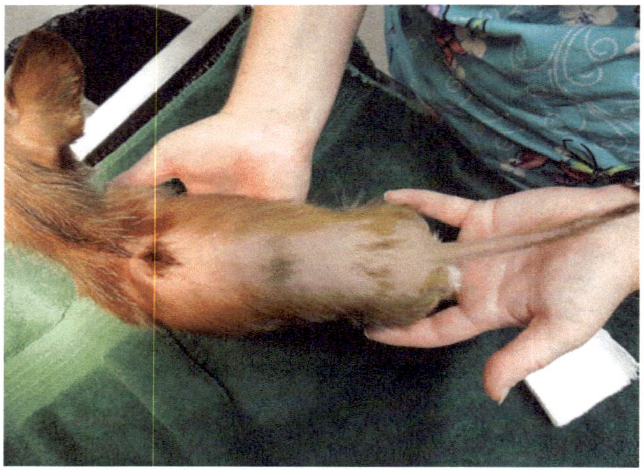

Figure 2.31 A dog with truncal hypotrichosis due to hypothyroidism.

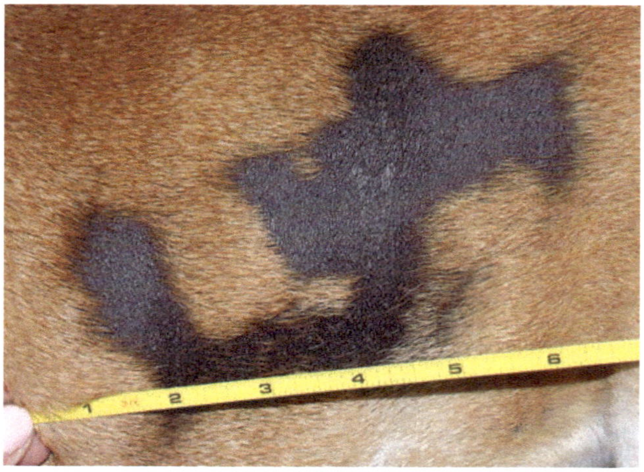

Figure 2.32A A dog with regional alopecia and hyperpigmentation due to seasonal flank alopecia.

6) Keratinization disorders.
   a) Color dilution alopecia (Figure 2.34), black hair follicular dysplasia.
   b) Sebaceous adenitis.
7) Congenital or breed related alopecia (Figure 2.35).
8) Scarring due to prior injury (trauma, burn) or prior severe infection or inflammatory disease causing follicular destruction.

Differentials based on lesion distribution/location:

1) Folliculitis usually causes patchy, multifocal hair loss often associated with scaling/crusting/papules +/− pruritus.
2) Barbering occurs in areas the pet can reach with paws or mouth or by rubbing.
3) Endocrinopathies cause non-pruritic (unless secondarily infected) symmetrical truncal, neck, and tail alopecia that spares the head and distal limbs, usually occur in older animals (unless iatrogenic Cushing's or exposure to human transdermal hormone replacements).
4) Follicular dysplasia is non-pruritic, symmetrical, and often affects lumbar area/trunk.
5) Immune-mediated alopecic diseases are usually non-pruritic and cause multifocal alopecia that can mimic folliculitis but papules/crusting are not present.
6) Vaccine-induced alopecia usually occurs a few weeks to months post vaccination (especially rabies).
7) Color dilution alopecia and black hair follicular dysplasia affect 6mo–18mo, affect blue, fawn, or black fur, and is non-pruritic (unless secondary infection occurs).

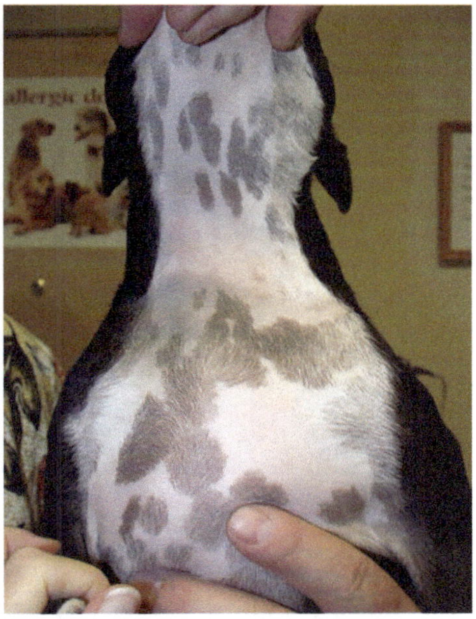

Figure 2.32B A young Boston Terrier with non-inflammatory ventral neck alopecia due to pattern baldness.

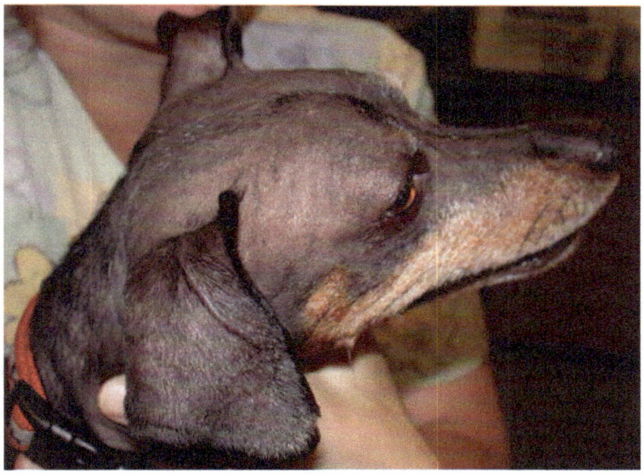

Figure 2.33A A Miniature Pinscher with facial and pinnal alopecia due to alopecia areata.

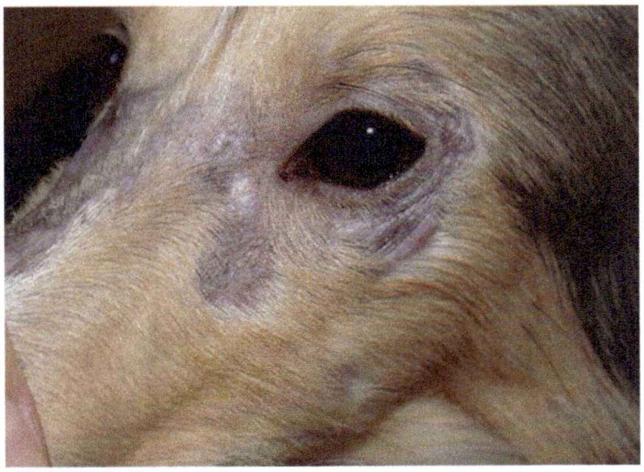

Figure 2.33B Patchy facial scarring alopecia in a Sheltie with dermatomyositis

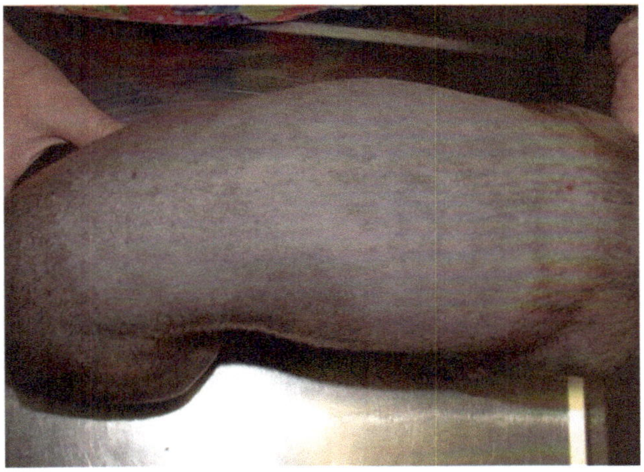

Figure 2.34 A dog with generalized non-inflammatory alopecia due to color dilution alopecia.

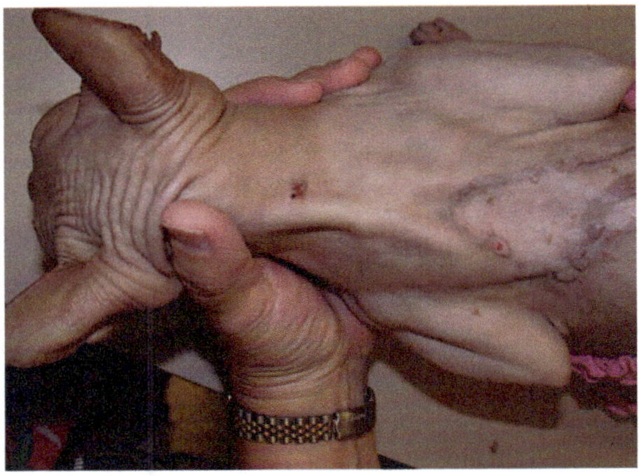

Figure 2.35 Congenital alopecia in a Sphynx cat.

8) Sebaceous adenitis often occurs in Standard poodles, Akitas, Vizslas, and Havanese, but can occur in any breed, causes follicular casting in most affected dogs, and may or may not be pruritic.
9) Congenital/breed related alopecias are present at birth or soon after.

Diagnostics:

1) Skin scrapings for mites.
2) Skin cytology for bacteria.
3) Dermatophyte culture.

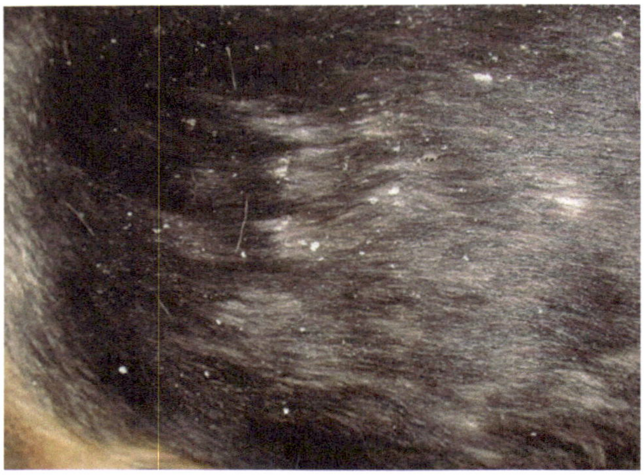

Figure 2.36A Scaling caused by a superficial pyoderma in an atopic dog.

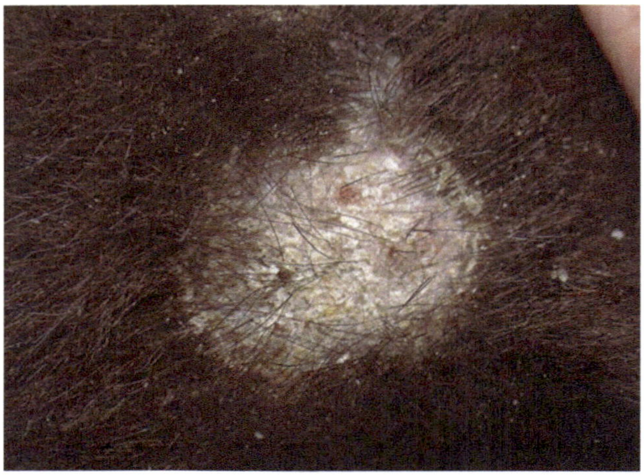

Figure 2.36B Scaling due to *Cheyletiella* infection.

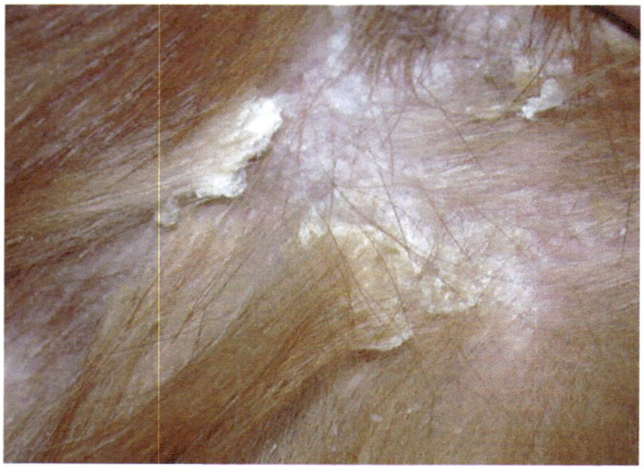

Figure 2.36C Scaling due to cutaneous lymphoma.

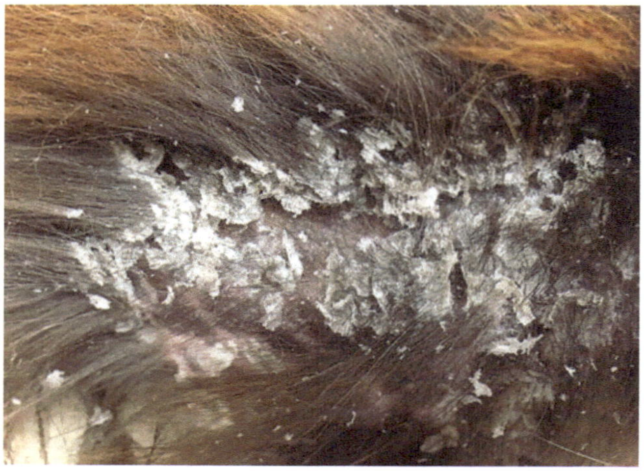

Figure 2.36D A cat with thymoma-associated exfoliative dermatitis.

4) Trichogram to screen for color dilution alopecia if appropriate, or to evaluate hairs for evidence of barbering/self-induced alopecia.
5) CBC/Chemistry panel/urinalysis/thyroid panel +/− adrenal testing if endocrinopathy suspected.
6) Skin biopsies if no infectious agents are found.

2.2.2 Scale

Definition:

1) Accumulation of fragments of surface epithelium which can be adherent or exfoliative, small to large flakes of keratin varying in color from white/tan/gray.

Common causes:

1) Secondary (more common): Inflammation due to any cause (infection (Figure 2.36A)/allergy/parasite (Figure 2.36B), xerosis of the skin due to underlying endocrinopathy, fatty acid or other nutritional imbalance, harsh shampoos; sebaceous adenitis, cutaneous epitheliotropic lymphoma (Figure 2.36C), feline thymoma-associated exfoliative dermatitis (Figure 2.36D).
2) Primary (rare): Keratinization disorders such as ichthyosis (Figure 2.37), primary seborrhea.

Differentials based on lesion distribution/location:

1) Scaling on the periphery of an alopecic lesion can suggest folliculitis.

Diagnostics:

1) Skin scrapings for mites.
2) Skin cytology for infection.
3) Dermatophyte culture.
4) Biopsy.

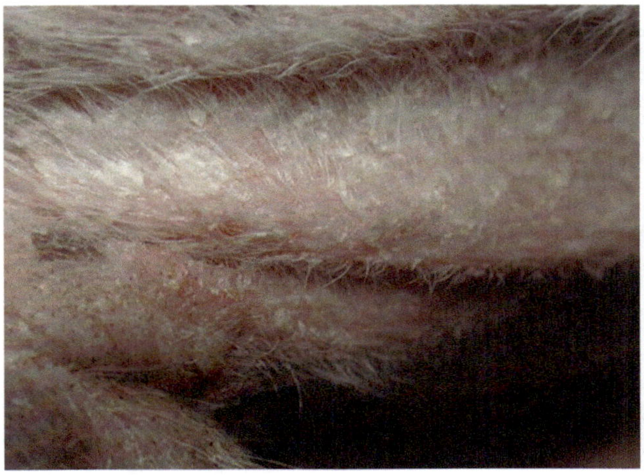

Figure 2.37 Adherent scaling in an American Bulldog due to ichthyosis.

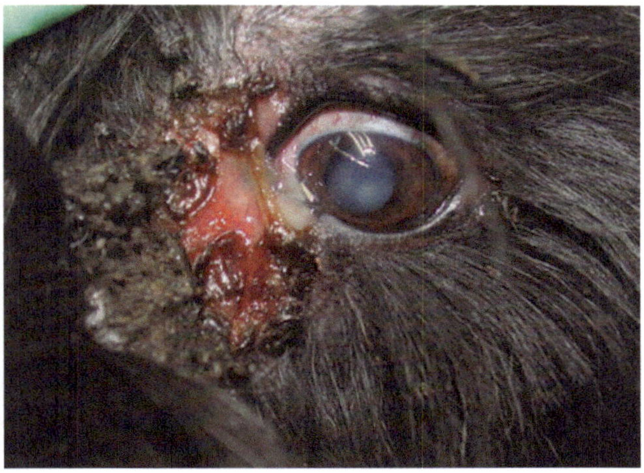

Figure 2.38 Crusting caused by deep pyoderma.

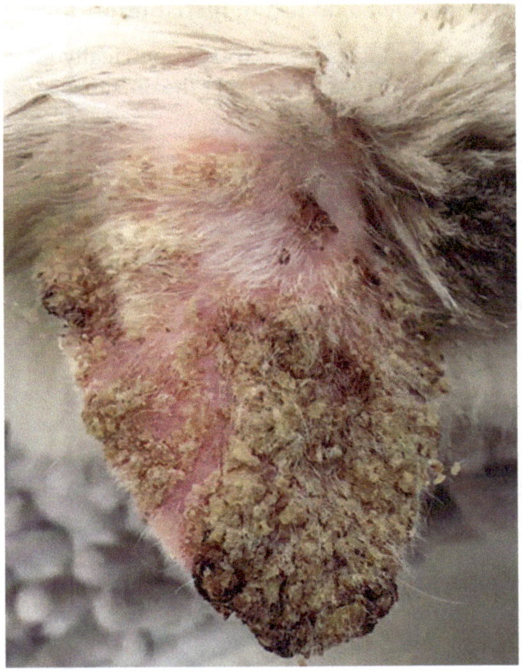

Figure 2.39 Pinnal crusting in a cat due to pemphigus foliaceus.

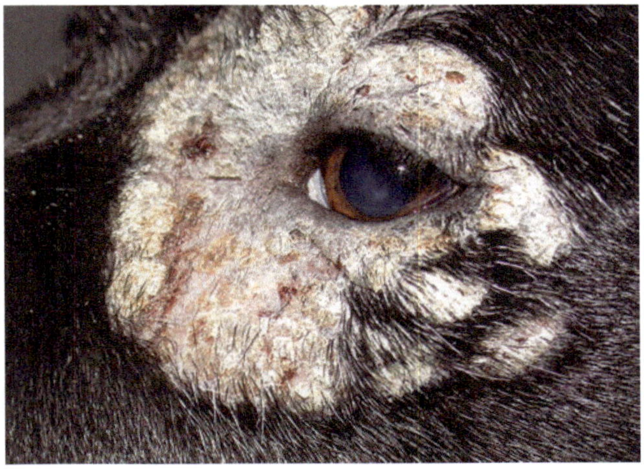

Figure 2.40 Periocular crusting due to zinc responsive dermatosis.

2.2.3 Crust

Definition:

1) Accumulation of dried exudate which may include pus, blood, and skin cells.

Common causes:

1) Secondary (more common): Pruritus/self-trauma, inflammation due to any cause (infection (Figure 2.38)/allergy/parasite/immune-mediated disease (Figure 2.39).
2) Primary (less common): Zinc responsive dermatosis (Figure 2.40), hepatocutaneous syndrome (superficial necrolytic dermatitis).

Differentials based on lesion distribution/location:

1) Pruritic crusts occur in areas the animal can reach to scratch, chew, or rub.
2) Crusts due to pyoderma are often (but not always) on the trunk.
3) Crusts due to scabies are often on pinnal margins and pressure points.
4) Crusts due to immune-mediated disease are often (but not always) on the face/muzzle, pinnae, and paw pads.
5) Crusts due to hepatocutaneous syndrome are often on the paw pads and pressure points, +/− face or perineum.
6) Crusts due to zinc responsive dermatosis are often on the lips, eyelids, pressure points, +/− paw pads and inner pinnae.

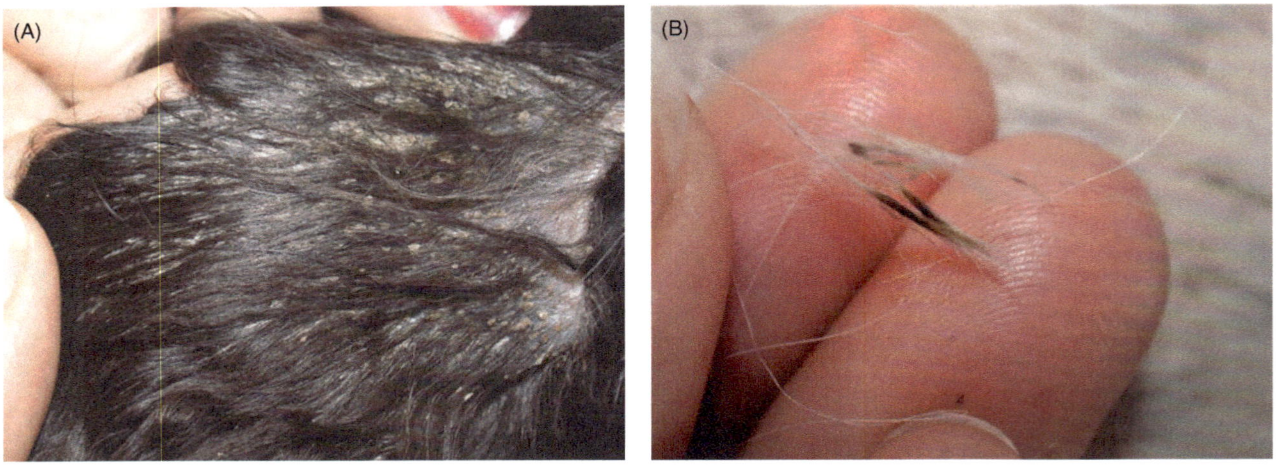

Figures 2.41A and B Follicular casting due to sebaceous adenitis.

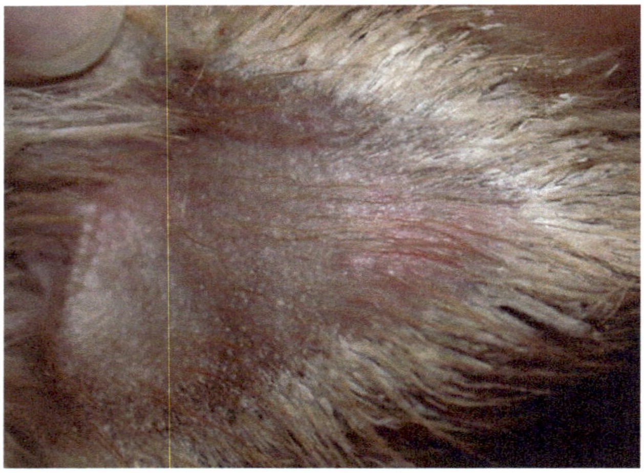

Figure 2.42 Follicular casts on the pinnae due to generalized demodicosis.

Diagnostics:

1) Skin scrapings for mites.
2) Skin cytology for infection and to evaluate inflammatory cells/screen for acantholysis.
3) Bacterial culture if bacteria are found on cytology despite prior empiric antibiotics.
4) Dermatophyte culture.
5) Biopsy.

2.2.4 Follicular cast

Definition:

1) Keratinaceous debris wrapped around proximal hair shafts (Figures 2.41A and 2.41B).

Common causes:

1) Secondary (more common): Demodicosis (Figure 2.42), dermatophytosis, bacterial folliculitis.
2) Primary: Sebaceous adenitis most common, rarely primary seborrhea, vitamin A responsive dermatosis.

Differentials based on lesion distribution/location:

1) Sebaceous adenitis tends to symmetrically affect the dorsal trunk, and also can affect the dorsal head/muzzle and outer pinnae.

Diagnostics:

1) Skin scrapings for mites.
2) Skin cytology for infection.
3) Dermatophyte culture.
4) Biopsy.

2.2.5 Comedo (Comedones)

Definition:

1) Dilated plugged hair follicle which may be closed at the surface ("whitehead") or open ("black head").

Common causes:

1) Secondary (more common): Demodicosis (Figure 2.43), dermatophytosis (Figure 2.44), bacterial folliculitis, endocrinopathy (Figure 2.45), overuse of topical or systemic steroids (Figure 2.46), solar dermatosis, friction/callus sites.
2) Primary: Schnauzer comedo syndrome (Figure 2.47), feline acne, alopecic breed related (Chinese crested), vitamin A responsive dermatosis (rare).

Differentials based on lesion distribution/location:

1) Schnauzer comedones occur on the dorsal midline.
2) Comedones due to endocrinopathy and overuse of systemic steroids occur on the dorsal trunk and groin.
3) Comedones due to overuse of topical steroid products occur at the site of application.
4) Comedones due to solar dermatosis occur in thinly haired, non-pigmented skin.

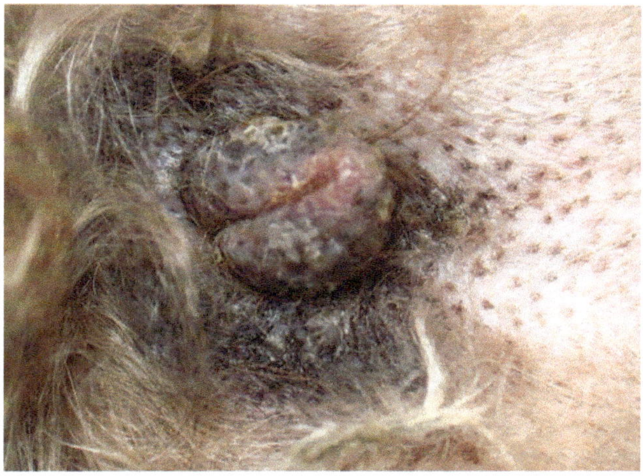

Figure 2.43 Perivulvar comedones due to demodicosis in the same dog.

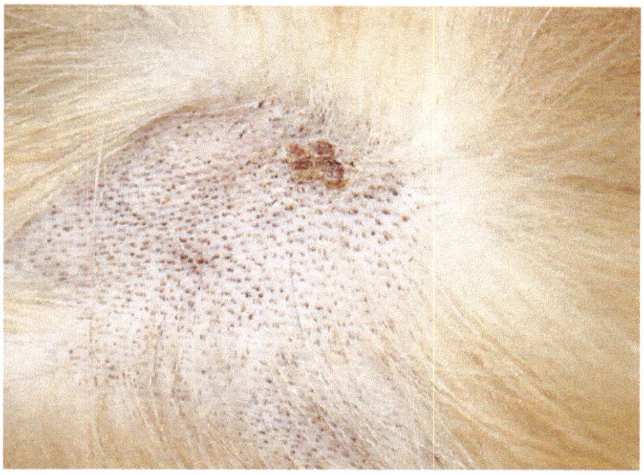

Figure 2.44 Comedones in a cat due to dermatophytosis.

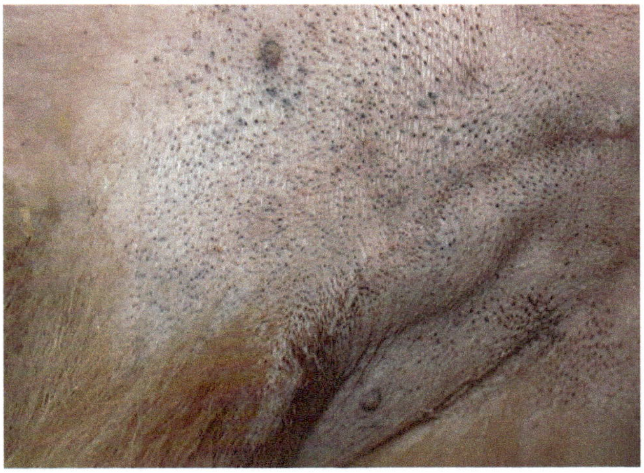

Figure 2.45 Comedones in a dog due to endocrine disease.

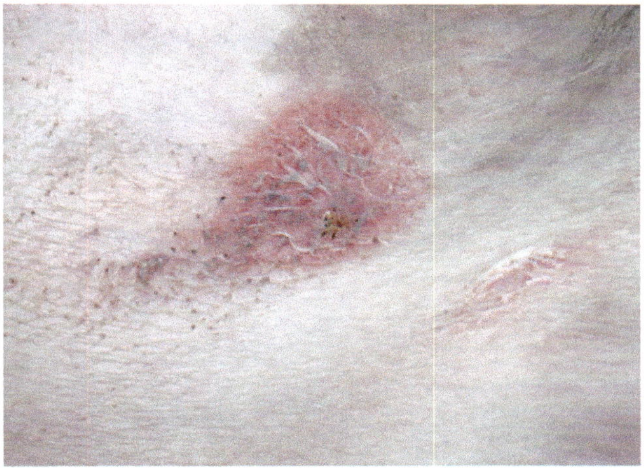

Figure 2.46 Comedones and milia on the groin of an atopic dog overtreated with topical steroid sprays and ointments.

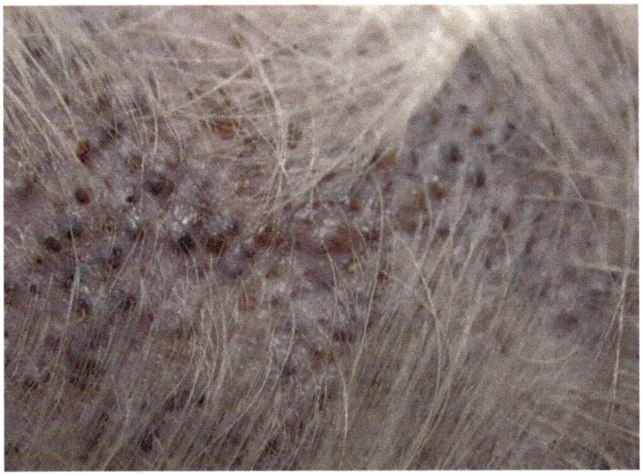

Figure 2.47 Comedones on the dorsal midline of a Miniature Schnauzer.

5) Comedones due to friction occur on pressure points such as elbows and ventral chest (Figure 2.48).

Diagnostics:

1) Skin scrapings for mites.
2) Skin cytology for infection.
3) Lab work/endocrine testing if appropriate based on age and location of comedones.
4) Biopsy.

2.2.6 Pigment change

Definition:

1) Hypopigmentation/hypomelanosis: loss of epidermal melanin. Hyperpigmentation/hypermelanosis: increased epidermal melanin.
2) Leukoderma: white skin. Leukotrichia: White fur.
3) Melanoderma: dark skin. Melanotrichia: Dark fur.

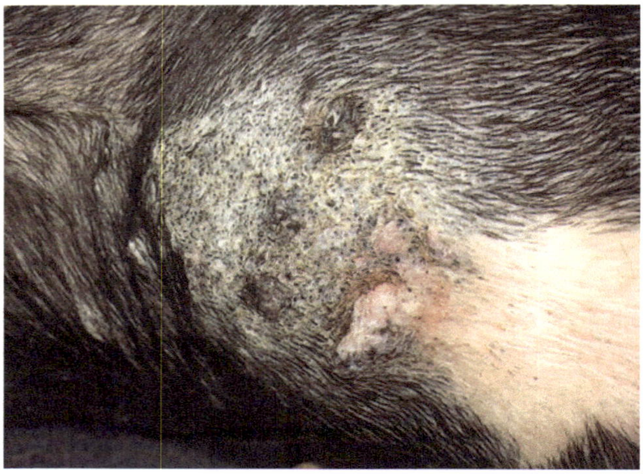

Figure 2.48 Comedones on the ventral sternum of a Miniature Dachshund due to chronic friction/pressure.

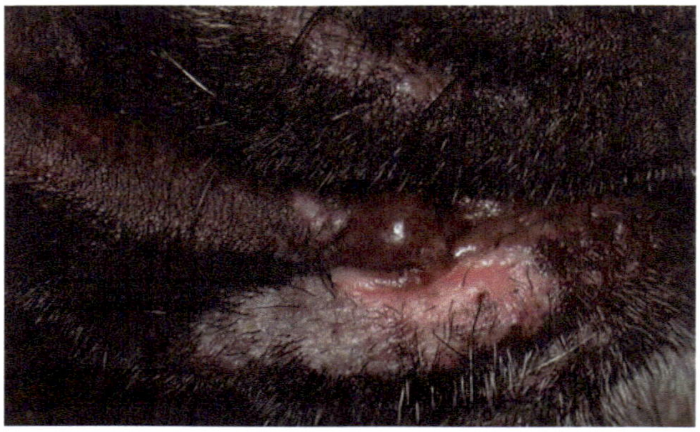

Figure 2.49A Post inflammatory depigmentation due to mucocutaneous pyoderma.

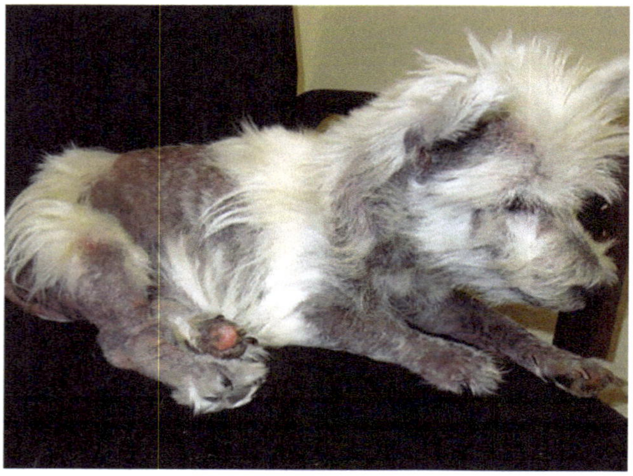

Figure 2.49B Generalized hyperpigmentation secondary to demodicosis and *Malassezia* dermatitis.

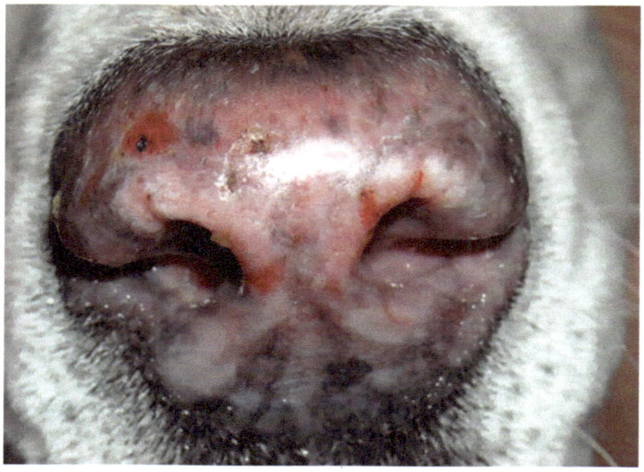

Figure 2.50 Nasal depigmentation due to discoid lupus, note the nasal reticular pattern is lost.

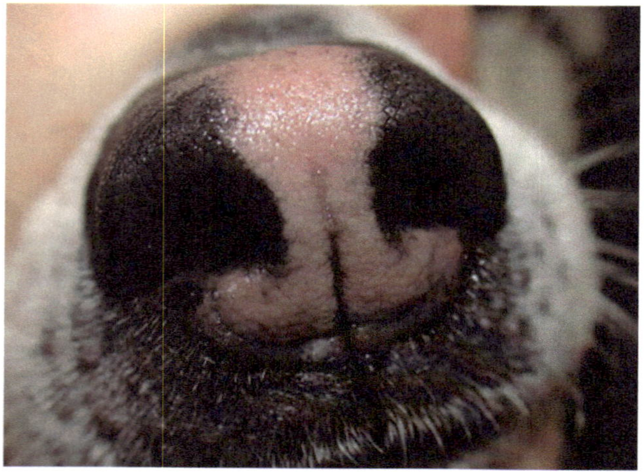

Figure 2.51 Nasal pigment loss with retention of normal reticular nasal pattern, due to Dudley nose.

Common causes:

1) Both hypo and hyperpigmentation of skin and fur can occur after an inflammatory event (infection due to bacterial, fungal, or parasitic causes [Figures 2.49A and 2.49B], trauma, allergy, immune-mediated skin diseases).
2) Hypopigmentation of skin and fur on the eyelids and nose is characteristic of uveodermatologic syndrome.
3) Nasal planum hypopigmentation also commonly occurs in discoid lupus (Figure 2.50), pemphigus foliaceus, vitiligo, and Dudley or Snow nose (Figure 2.51).
4) Cutaneous epitheliotropic lymphoma commonly causes hypopigmentation of nasal planum, lips, eyelids +/− paw pads (Figures 2.52 and 2.53).
5) Post inflammatory hyperpigmentation (reticulated/latticework appearance) of the inguinal and axillary skin and inner pinnae is common in canine atopic dermatitis (Figure 2.54).

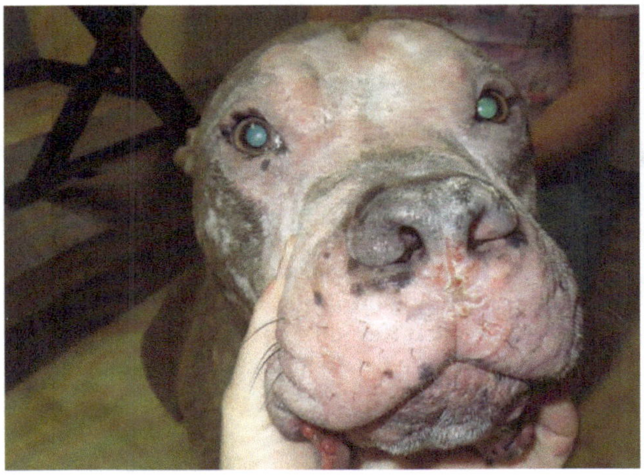

Figure 2.52 Depigmentation of nasal planum and facial skin and fur due to epitheliotropic lymphoma.

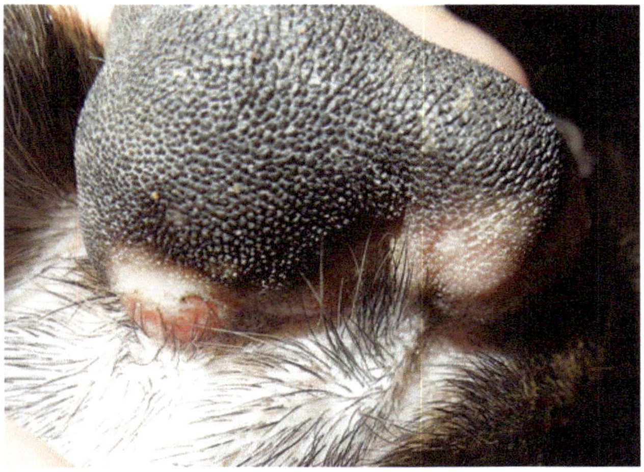

Figure 2.53 Paw pad depigmentation due to epitheliotropic lymphoma.

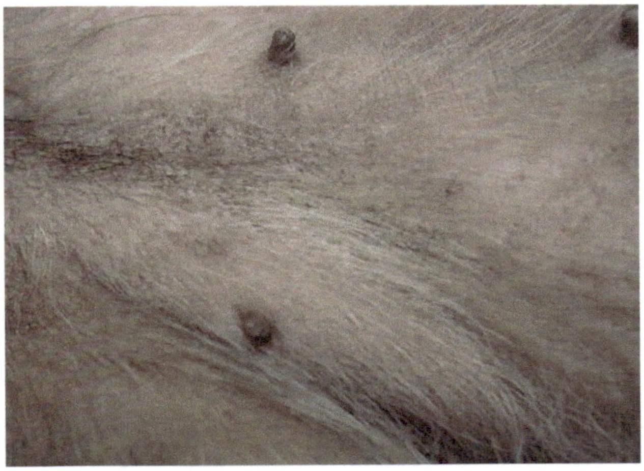

Figure 2.54 Post inflammatory inguinal hyperpigmentation due to atopy.

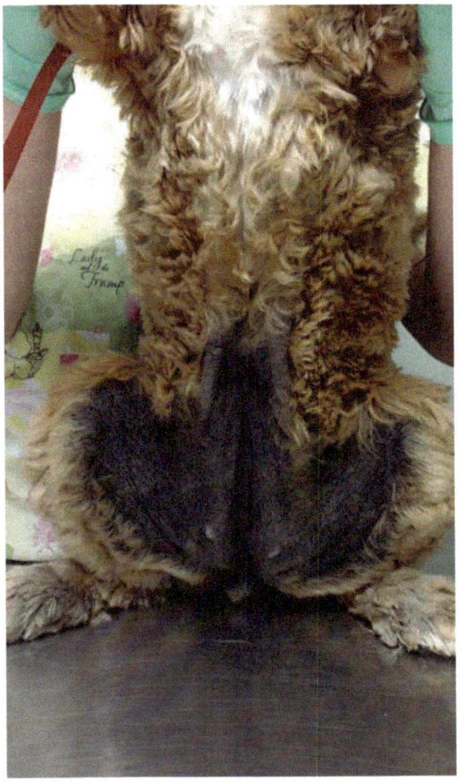

Figure 2.55 Inguinal hyperpigmentation due to hypothyroidism.

6) Diffuse hyperpigmentation of the skin is common in canine endocrine dermatoses (Figure 2.55).
7) Vitiligo is an immunologic disease targeting melanocytes and can cause both leukoderma and leukotrichia.

Differentials based on lesion distribution/location:

1) Facial, nasal, and/or paw pad hypopigmentation suggests immune-mediated disease or cutaneous lymphoma.
2) Inguinal and axillary reticulated hyperpigmentation suggests atopic dermatitis.
3) Diffuse truncal hyperpigmentation with hair loss suggests endocrinopathy.
4) Hyperpigmentation in the centers of circular areas of alopecia with peripheral scaling (epidermal collarettes) is commonly seen with canine bacterial pyoderma.
5) Hyperpigmentation around ulcerated or eroded lesions on the groin/axillae/perianal/perivulvar areas suggest immune-mediated disease, especially erythema multiforme and cutaneous or mucocutaneous lupus erythematosus (Figure 3.77).
6) Hyperpigmented macules on the nasal planum and lips of orange cats is a common benign change called lentigo (Figures 17.2A and B).
7) Hyperpigmented macules and scaly raised plaques in cats are commonly due to papillomavirus induced squamous cell carcinoma in situ (Bowen's disease).

Diagnostics:

1) Skin scrapings for mites.
2) Skin cytology for infection and to evaluate inflammatory cells.
3) Bacterial culture if bacteria are found on cytology despite prior empiric antibiotics.
4) Dermatophyte culture.
5) Biopsy.

2.3 Secondary lesions (lesions which occur as sequelae or progression of primary lesions)

2.3.1 Epidermal collarette

Definition:

1) Circular rim of scaling around an alopecic lesion, which originated initially from a prior pustule or bulla then expanded outward.

Common causes:

1) Dogs: Most commonly due to bacterial pyoderma (Figures 2.56 and 2.57), less commonly to dermatophytosis, insect bites, and immune-mediated diseases.
2) Cats: Most commonly due to dermatophytosis (Figure 8.24E) but can also occur with bacterial pyoderma and immune-mediated diseases.

Differentials based on lesion distribution/location:

1) Truncal and inguinal epidermal collarettes are typical for canine bacterial folliculitis.
2) Epidermal collarettes due to dermatophytosis tend to be few in number and asymmetrical and can occur anyplace, including the limbs, face, and ears.
3) Epidermal collarettes due to pemphigus foliaceus tend to involve the trunk, limbs, and head equally.

Diagnostics:

1) Skin scrapings for mites.
2) Skin cytology for infection and to evaluate inflammatory cells/screen for acantholysis.
3) Bacterial culture if bacteria are found on cytology despite prior empiric antibiotics.
4) Dermatophyte culture.
5) Biopsy.

2.3.2 Scar

Definition:

1) Fibrous tissue which has replaced damaged dermis +/− subcutis.

Common causes:

1) Prior severe skin trauma such as very deep chronic infection, chronic ulcerative immune-mediated diseases such as vasculitis (Figure 2.58), sterile panniculitis (Figure 2.59), burns, or trauma.

Differentials based on lesion distribution/location:

1) Facial scarring can occur after severe juvenile cellulitis.
2) Focal to patchy truncal scarring can occur after severe panniculitis.
3) Serpiginous truncal scars can occur after thermal solar injury.

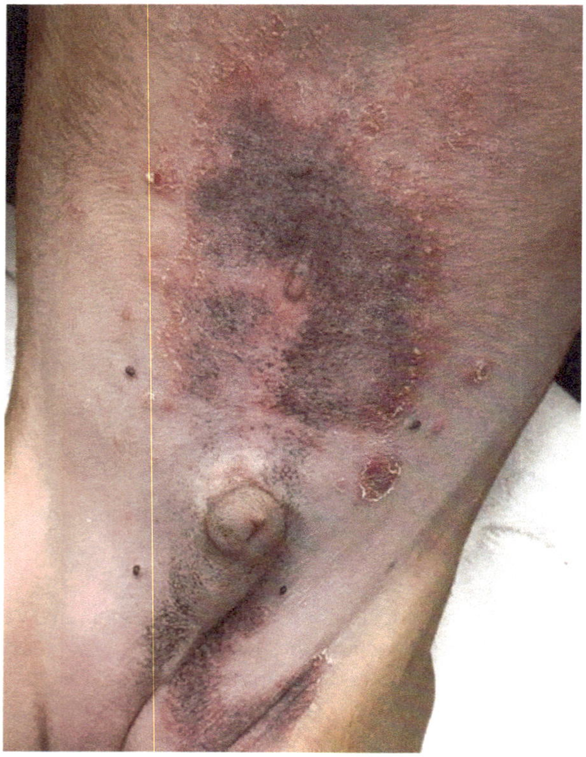

Figure 2.56 An atopic dachshund with inguinal epidermal collarettes.

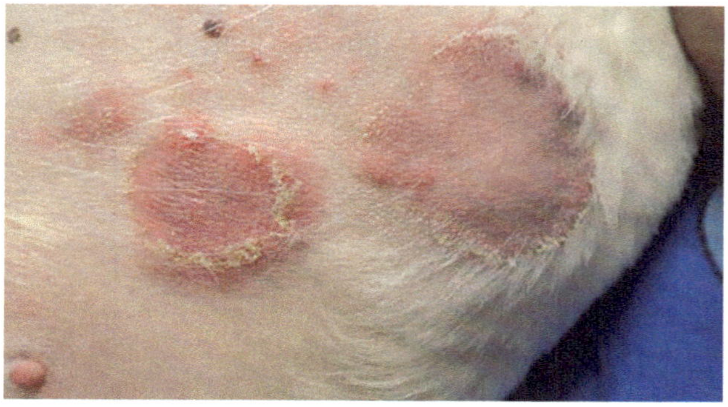

Figure 2.57 An atopic French Bulldog with truncal epidermal collarettes due to bacterial pyoderma.

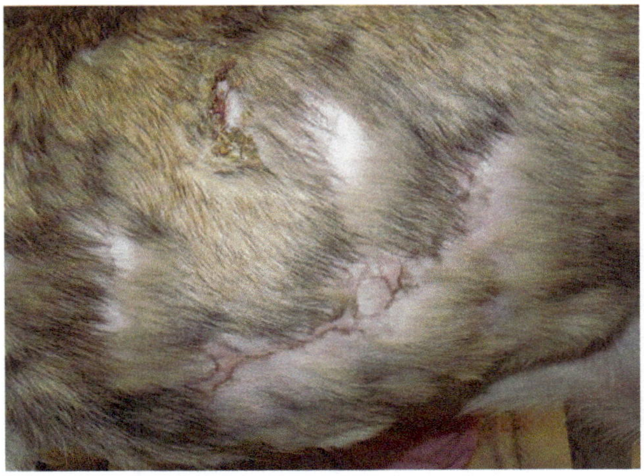

Figure 2.58 Scarring due to vasculitis.

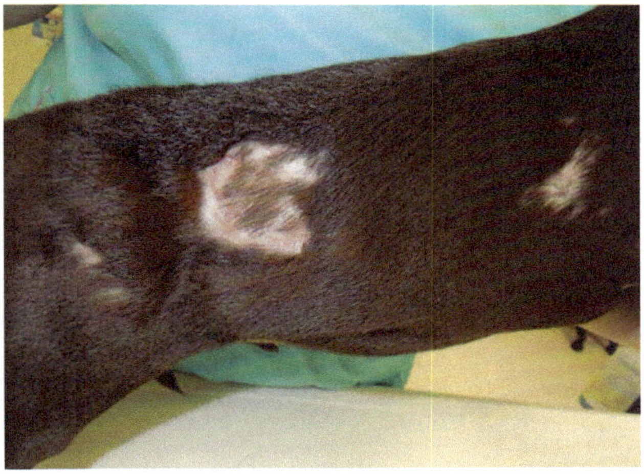

Figure 2.59 Scarring post treatment of sterile panniculitis.

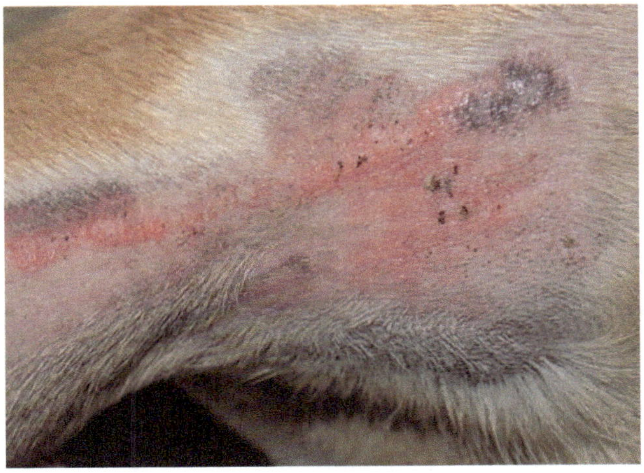

Figure 2.60 Excoriations due to self-trauma in a pruritic dog.

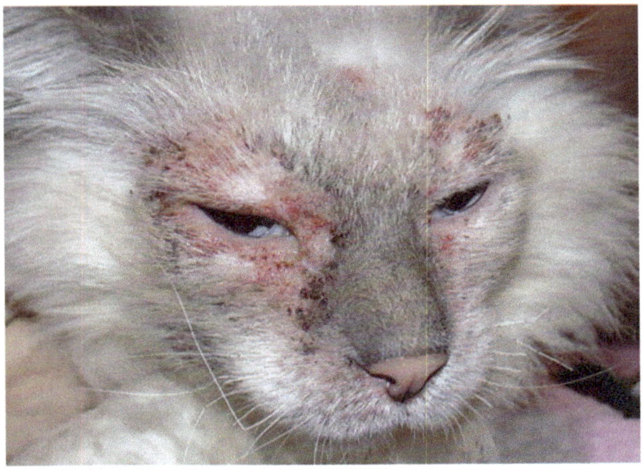

Figure 2.61 Facial excoriations in an atopic cat.

4) Rabies vaccine-induced localized vasculitis can induce follicular atrophy and scar formation at the prior injection site.

Diagnostics:

1) Biopsies demonstrate fibrosis but usually cannot elucidate prior cause of the scarring.

2.3.3 Excoriation

Definition:

1) Erosion or ulceration caused by chewing/scratching/self-trauma (Figure 2.60).

Common causes:

1) Ectoparasites.
2) Hypersensitivity dermatitis (atopy, food allergy, contact hypersensitivity).
3) Secondary bacterial or yeast infections.

Differentials based on lesion distribution/location:

1) Lumbar excoriations/barbering often signify flea bite hypersensitivity.
2) Axillary, facial, and pedal excoriations are common in canine atopic dermatitis and adverse food reaction.
3) Facial and truncal excoriations are common with feline atopic dermatitis and adverse food reaction (Figure 2.61).

Diagnostics:

1) Skin scrapings for mites, trial treatment for ectoparasites.
2) Skin cytology for infection and to evaluate inflammatory cells.
3) Bacterial culture if bacteria are found on cytology despite prior empiric antibiotics.
4) Dermatophyte culture.
5) Biopsy is usually not helpful but may support underlying hypersensitivity.

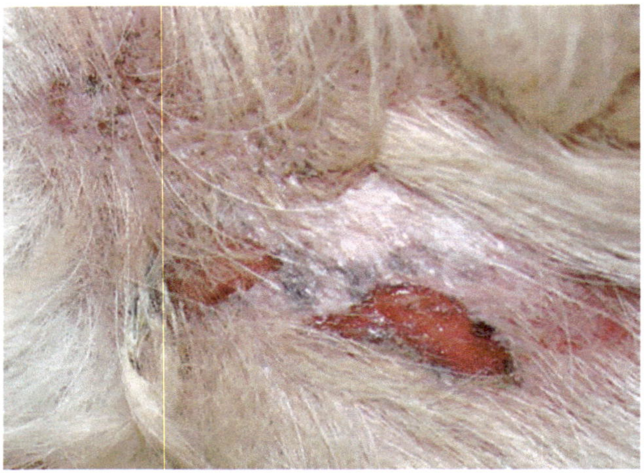

Figure 2.62 Erosion due to vasculitis.

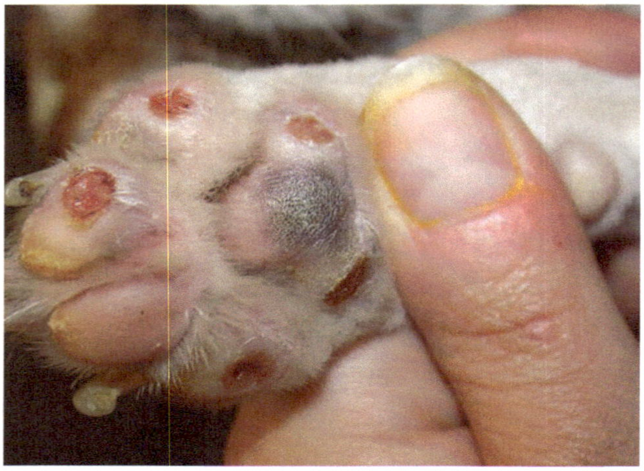

Figure 2.64 Paw pad ulcers due to vasculitis.

2.3.4 Erosion

Definition:

1) Shallow epidermal defect that does not expose dermis (Figure 2.62).

Common causes:

1) Self-trauma due to the same causes as excoriation, see 2.3.3 Excoriation.
2) Rupture of a vesicle caused by an immune-mediated disease.

Differentials based on lesion distribution/location:

1) See 2.3.3 Excoriation for distribution of excoriations due to self-trauma.
2) Erosions due to immune-mediated disease are not usually pruritic and often involve the face, pinnae, and mucocutaneous junctions.

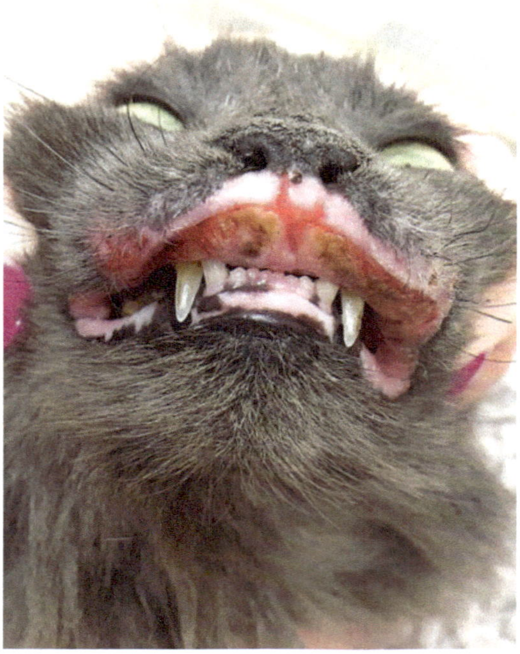

Figure 2.63 Thickening and ulceration of the lip in an atopic cat (indolent ulcer) which was poorly steroid responsive due to untreated secondary bacterial infection.

Diagnostics:

1) Skin scrapings for mites, trial treatment for ectoparasites.
2) Skin cytology for infection and to evaluate inflammatory cells.
3) Bacterial culture if bacteria are found on cytology despite prior empiric antibiotics.
4) Biopsy on the margin of the lesion to include intact epidermis.

2.3.5 Ulcer

Definition:

1) Epidermal defect with exposure of dermis.

Common causes:

1) Deep infection due to bacterial or fungal organisms, such as canine deep pyoderma, feline mycobacteriosis.
2) Feline indolent ulcer (Figure 2.63).
3) A physical cause such as trauma or thermal/chemical burn.
4) Immune-mediated disease such as vasculitis (Figure 2.64), sterile panniculitis (Figure 2.65), systemic lupus erythematosus (SLE), nasal arteritis (Figure 2.66), severe discoid lupus erythematosus (DLE), epidermolysis bullosa, pemphigus vulgaris.
5) If located over a mass, underlying granuloma (induced by a foreign body or deep infection) or neoplasia (Figure 2.67).

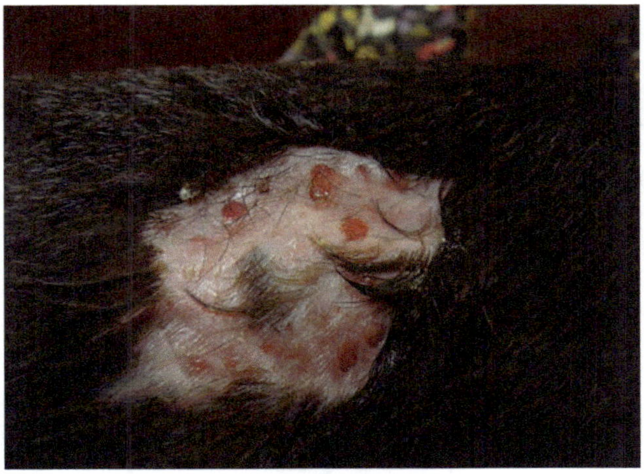

Figure 2.65 Truncal ulcerations and draining tract due to sterile panniculitis.

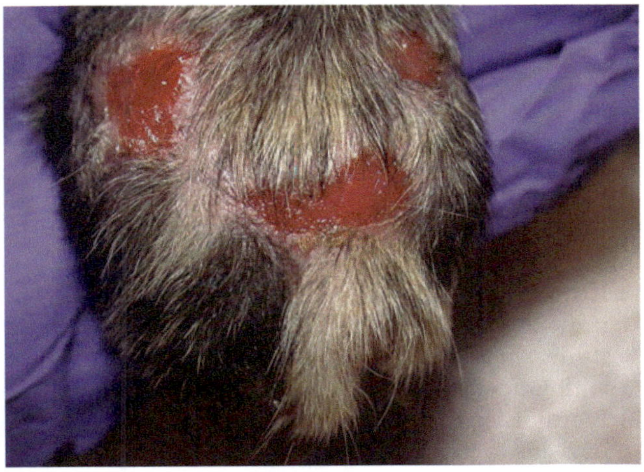

Figure 2.67 Ulcerations on the paws of a cat with lymphoma.

Differentials based on lesion distribution/location:

1) Canine deep pyoderma commonly occurs on the dorsal and lateral trunk.
2) Feline mycobacteriosis can occur anywhere but commonly occurs on the inguinal and lumbar areas.
3) Feline indolent ulcer occurs on the lip mucocutaneous junction.
4) Immune-mediated diseases commonly affect the face, nasal planum, oral cavity, pinnae, and paw pads.

Diagnostics:

1) Cytology for infection.
2) Bacterial +/− fungal cultures, ideally deep tissue culture.
3) Biopsy for pathology and special stains for organisms if deep infection suspected.
4) If immune-mediated disease is suspected, it's important to biopsy on the margin of the ulcerated lesion to include intact epidermis, and to sample several areas.

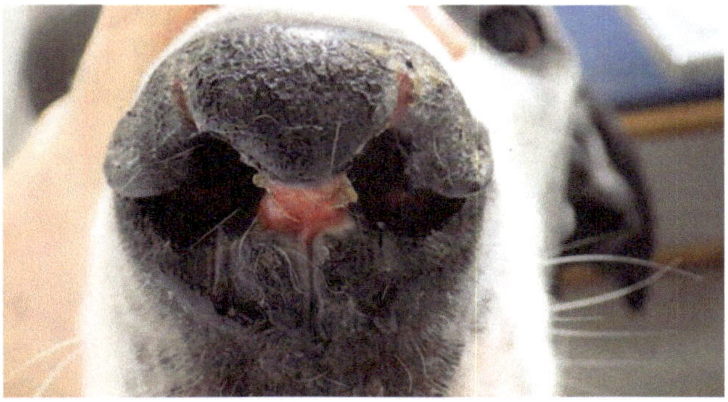

Figure 2.66 Nasal ulceration due to nasal arteritis.

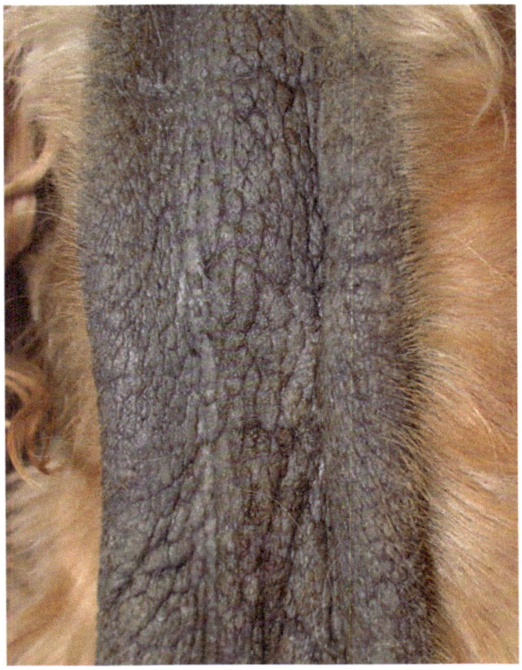

Figure 2.68 Chronic bacterial pyoderma can create lichenification.

2.3.6 Lichenification

Definition:

1) Thickened, elephant-like skin which is also often, but not always, hyperpigmented.

Common causes:

1) Signifies chronic inflammation due to friction or chronic bacterial (Figure 2.68) or *Malassezia* infection (Figure 2.69), secondary to an underlying primary hypersensitivity dermatitis (parasite, atopy, food allergy), endocrinopathy or keratinization disorder.

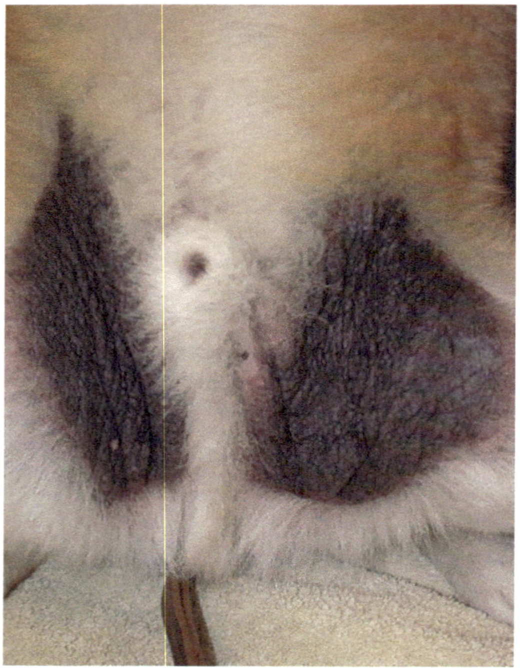

Figure 2.69 Lichenification due to *Malassezia* dermatitis caused by hypothyroidism.

Differentials based on lesion distribution/location:

1) Commonly seen on the ventral neck, inguinal, and axillary areas of atopic dogs with secondary infections.

Diagnostics:

1) Skin scrapings for mites, trial treatment for ectoparasites.
2) Skin cytology for infection.
3) Bacterial culture if bacteria are found on cytology despite prior empiric antibiotics.
4) Dermatophyte culture.
5) Biopsy is usually not helpful but may support underlying hypersensitivity.

2.3.7 Callus

Definition:

1) A noninflammatory hyperplastic response of the skin causing thickening and hair loss, most commonly on pressure points such as elbows and hocks; can become secondarily infected.

Common causes:

1) Chronic pressure/friction.

Differentials based on lesion distribution/location:

1) Most commonly occurs on lateral elbows (Figure 2.70), hocks, ventral sternum, and hips.

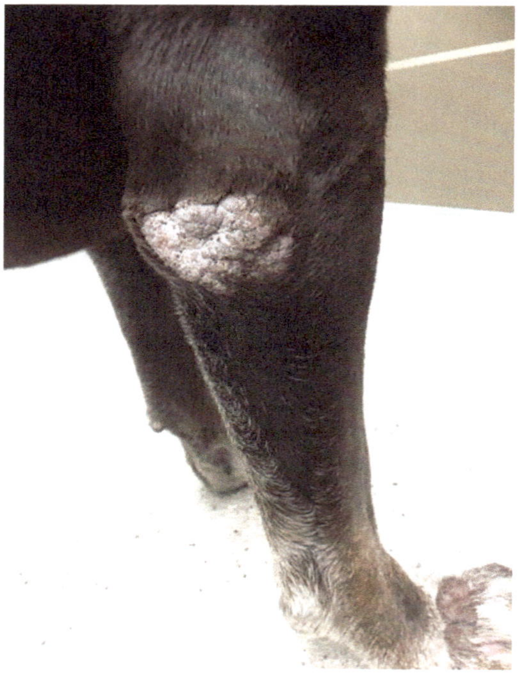

Figure 2.70 An elbow callus in a large breed dog.

Diagnostics:

1) If crusting, inflammation, and/or drainage are present, perform cytology for infection +/− culture if organisms are present despite prior empiric antibiotics.
2) Biopsy is not usually helpful and can be difficult to heal due to location.

2.3.8 Fissure

Definition:

1) Linear cleavage through epidermis +/− into dermis.

Common causes:

1) Thickened, inelastic, or crusted skin or paws subjected to inflammation or friction/trauma.
2) Often occurs on paw pads, nasal planum, pinnal margins, oral, and anal mucocutaneous borders.

Differentials based on lesion distribution/location:

1) Hyperkeratotic fissured paw pads can be caused by immune-mediated diseases (pemphigus foliaceus), zinc responsive dermatosis, hepatocutaneous syndrome (Figure 2.71), severe chronic sarcoptic mange (Figure 2.72), and canine distemper.
2) Hyperkeratotic fissured nasal planum can be due to idiopathic nasodigital hyperkeratosis (Figure 2.73), severe nasal pyoderma (Figure 2.74) pemphigus foliaceus, hepatocutaneous syndrome.

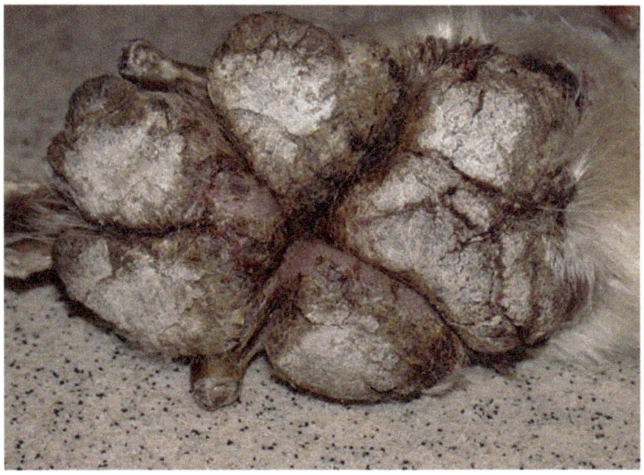

Figure 2.71 Fissured, hyperkeratotic paw pads due to hepatocutaneous syndrome.

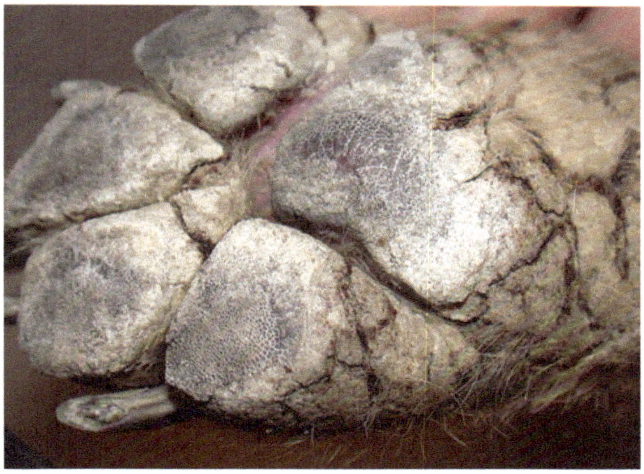

Figure 2.72 Fissured, hyperkeratotic paw pads due to chronic untreated sarcoptic mange; this is a rare finding.

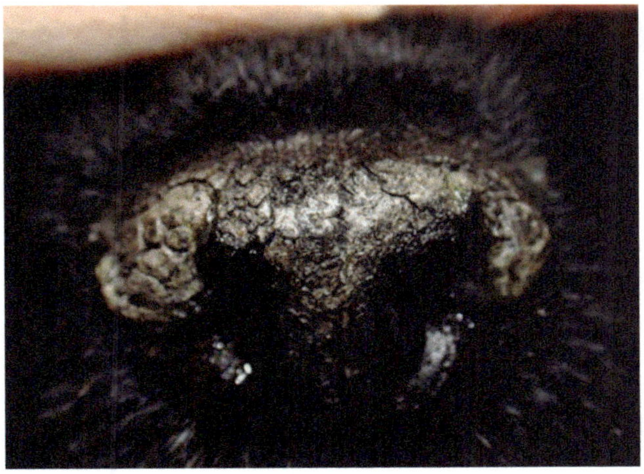

Figure 2.73 Crusting and fissuring of the dorsal nasal planum due to idiopathic nasodigital hyperkeratosis. Mucocutaneous nasal pyoderma can appear identical but no bacteria were found on cytology.

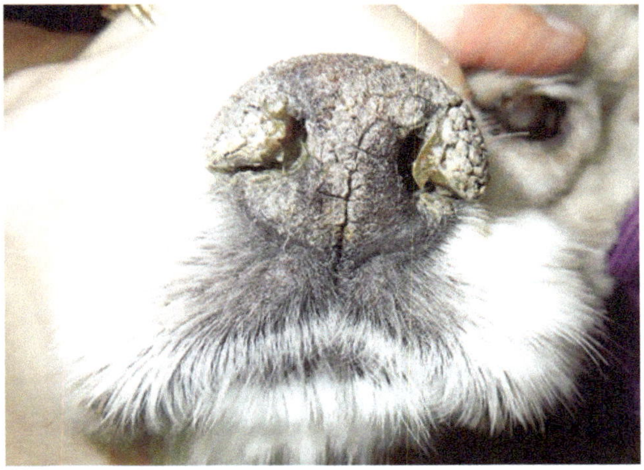

Figure 2.74 Nasal planum crusting and fissuring due to nasal mucocutaneous pyoderma secondary to atopic dermatitis.

3) Fissured lip and anal mucocutaneous junction lesions can be due to mucocutaneous pyoderma or immune-mediated disease (vasculitis, mucocutaneous lupus erythematosus).
4) Fissured ear margins can be due to pinnal vasculitis or chronic repetitive trauma due to head/ear flapping secondary to otitis and/or hypersensitivity (parasite, atopy, food).

Diagnostics

1) Skin scrapings for mites, trial treatment for ectoparasites.
2) Skin cytology for infection.
3) Bacterial culture if bacteria are found on cytology despite prior empiric antibiotics.
4) Dermatophyte culture.
5) Biopsy.

Further reading

Albanese, F. (2017). *Canine and Feline Skin Cytology: A Comprehensive and Illustrated Guide to the Interpretation of Skin Lesions via Cytological Examination*. Cham, Switzerland: Springer International Publishing.

Beco, L., Guagere, E., Lorente Mendez, C. et al. (2013). Suggested guidelines for using systemic antimicrobials in bacterial skin infections (1): diagnosis based on clinical presentation, cytology and culture. *Vet. Rec.* 172 (3): 72–78.

Coyner, K. (2011). Skills laboratory: how to perform skin scraping and skin surface cytology. *Vet. Med.* 106 (11): 554–563.

Coyner, K. (2011). Skills laboratory: skin biopsy. *Vet. Med.* 106 (10): 505–507.

Meckenburg, L., Linke, M., and Tobin, D. (2009). *Hair Loss Disorders in Domestic Animals.* Ames, IA: Wiley Blackwell.

Miller, W.H., Griffen, C.E., and Campbell, K.L. (2013). *Muller and Kirk's Small Animal Dermatology*, 7e. St Louis, MO: Elsevier Mosby.

3

Lesion location and differentials

Kimberly S. Coyner, DVM, DACVD

Dermatology Clinic for Animals, Lacey, WA, USA

Although any disease can potentially affect any part of the body, some diseases occur more commonly in certain parts of the body, and certain parts of the body are more prone to certain diseases, so consider the lesion location as well as the lesion to formulate your differential diagnosis. This chapter lists the most common diseases by location and type of lesion; the diagnosis of all these diseases is, as always, obtained by first performing baseline dermatologic diagnostics of skin cytology (+/− culture if bacteria are found despite empiric antibiotics), skin scrapings and plucks for mites in haired areas, +/− dermatophyte culture or PCR and/or biopsies depending on initial test results. Symmetry of lesions is also helpful to consider: infections and neoplasia tend to be asymmetrical, while immune-mediated diseases and endocrinopathies tend to be symmetrical.

3.1 Face

3.1.1 Nasal planum

a) Crusty
   - Nasal pyoderma (Figure 3.1)
   - Idiopathic nasodigital hyperkeratosis (Figure 3.2)
   - Immune-mediated disease (i.e. pemphigus foliaceus/PF, Figure 3.3)
   - Metabolic disease (hypothyroidism, hepatocutaneous syndrome, Figure 3.4)
   - Parasympathetic nose (chronic unilateral demarcated crusting, Figure 3.5)

b) Depigmented/loss of reticular pattern
   - Nasal pyoderma
   - Immune-mediated disease (i.e. PF, discoid lupus erythematosus/DLE, Figure 3.6)
   - Cutaneous lymphoma (Figure 3.7)

c) Depigmented, normal nasal reticular pattern
   - Vitiligo (Figure 3.8)
   - Snow nose/Dudley nose (Figure 3.9)

d) Ulcerated
   - Immune-mediated disease (PF, DLE, systemic lupus erythematosus/SLE, erythema multiforme/EM, vasculitis, histiocytosis, sterile granuloma; Figure 3.10).
   - Deep fungal infection (i.e. cryptococcosis, blastomycosis, histoplasmosis, aspergillosis, coccidioidomycosis; Figure 3.11A).
   - Viral (i.e. feline herpesvirus, Figure 3.11B).
   - Neoplasia (i.e. cutaneous lymphoma, squamous cell carcinoma).

3.1.2 Lips/Eyelids

a) Alopecic
   - Infection (bacterial, yeast, *Demodex*, or dermatophyte; Figures 3.12A and 3.12B).
   - Barbering due to rubbing/pruritus due to hypersensitivity dermatitis (Figure 3.13).
   - Immune-mediated disease (dermatomyositis/DM, vasculitis, Figure 3.14).

b) Crusty
   - Self-trauma/pruritus due to hypersensitivity dermatitis (Figures 3.15A and 3.15B).
   - Infection: Mucocutaneous and/or lipfold pyoderma (Figure 3.16A); *Malassezia* dermatitis (Figure 3.16B), feline herpesvirus dermatitis.
   - Demodicosis (Figure 3.17).
   - Juvenile cellulitis (Figure 3.18).
   - Immune-mediated disease (i.e. PF, vasculitis [Figure 3.19], mucocutaneous lupus erythematosus/MCLE, DM).
   - Metabolic disease (i.e. zinc responsive dermatosis [Figure 3.20], hepatocutaneous syndrome [Figure 3.21]).

c) Depigmented
   - Mucocutaneous pyoderma
   - Immune-mediated disease (PF/EM/vasculitis/DM/SLE)
   - Cutaneous lymphoma (Figure 3.22)
   - Vitiligo (if non-ulcerated, Figure 3.23)

Clinical Atlas of Canine and Feline Dermatology, First Edition. Edited by Kimberly S. Coyner.

Companion website: www.wiley.com/go/coyner/dermatology

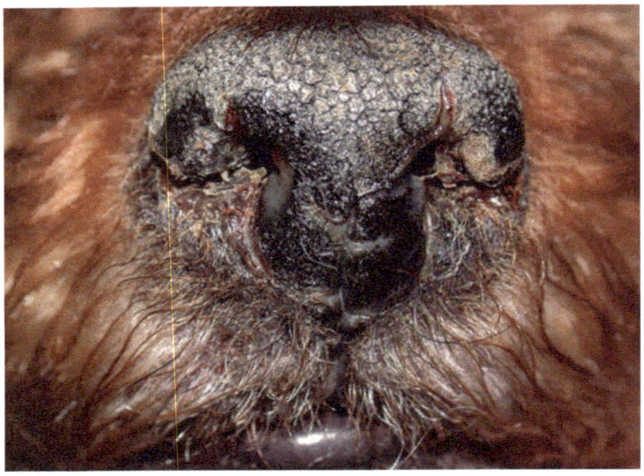

Figure 3.1 Nasal crusting caused by a bacterial infection, secondary to atopy.

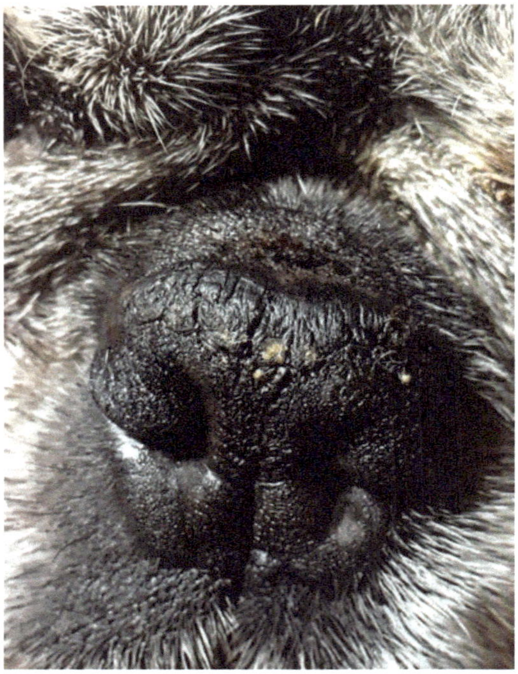

Figure 3.2 Chronic non-pruritic hyperkeratosis of the dorsal nasal planum is typical canine idiopathic nasodigital hyperkeratosis.

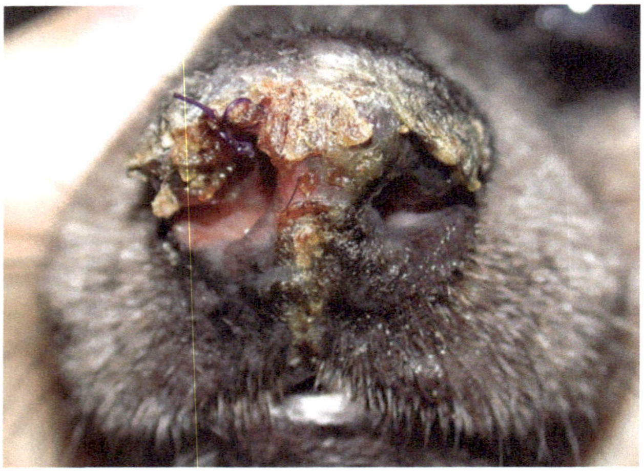

Figure 3.3 A dog with pemphigus foliaceus with associated nasal planum depigmentation, erosion, and crusting.

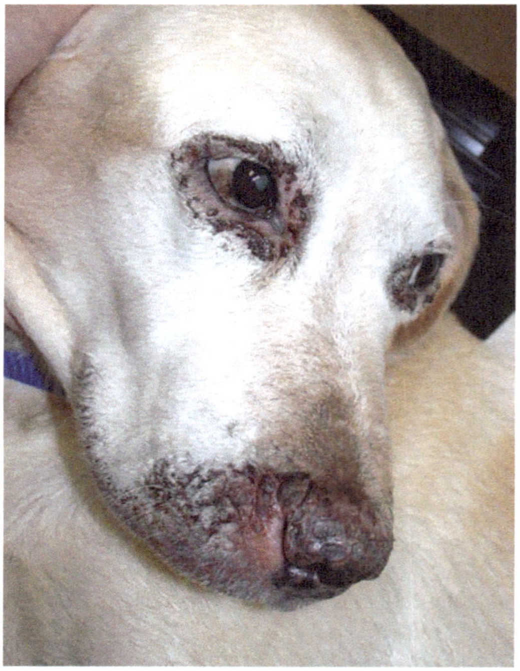

Figure 3.4 In this dog with hepatocutaneous syndrome, crusting moist dermatitis is present on the nasal planum as well lips and eyelids.

Lips/Eyelids (cont.)

d) Ulcerated
  - Deep bacterial or fungal infection.
  - Feline rodent ulcer secondary to allergic dermatitis (Figure 3.24).
  - Immune-mediated disease (PF/pemphigus vulgaris (PV)/DLE/SLE/EM/vasculitis/MCLE, drug eruption Figure 3.25).
  - Neoplasia (cutaneous lymphoma [Figure 3.26A], squamous cell carcinoma [Figure 3.26B]).

e) Mass
  - Oral papilloma (Figure 3.26C)
  - Infectious granuloma (fungal, mycobacterial)
  - Neoplasia

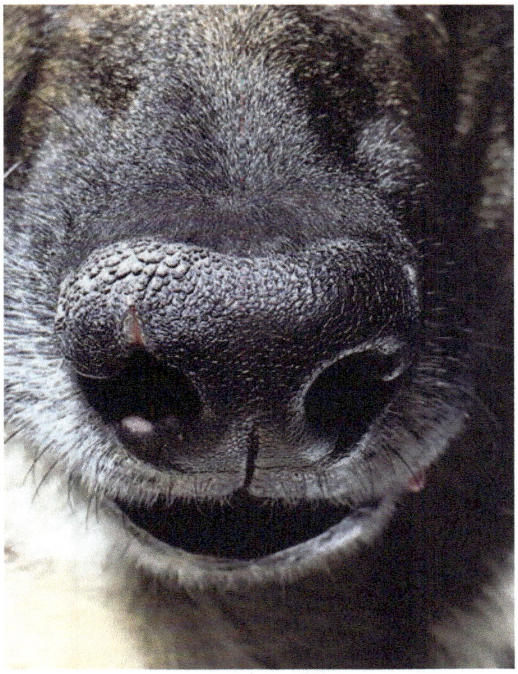

Figure 3.5 Parasympathetic nose is characterized by chronic unilateral nasal hyperkeratosis; no bacteria were found on cytology.

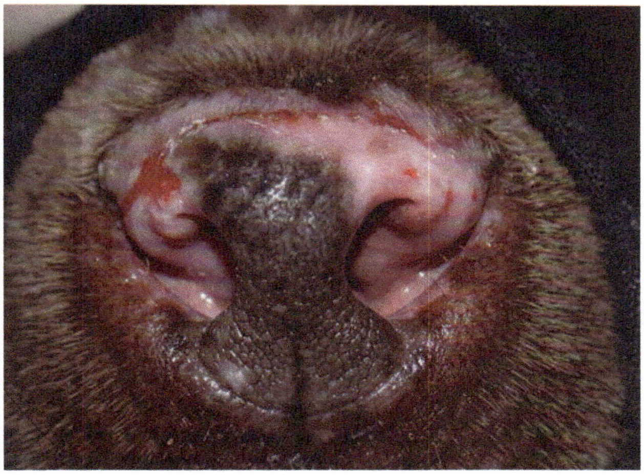

Figure 3.6 In this dog with discoid lupus there is loss of nasal planum pigment, as well as cartilage.

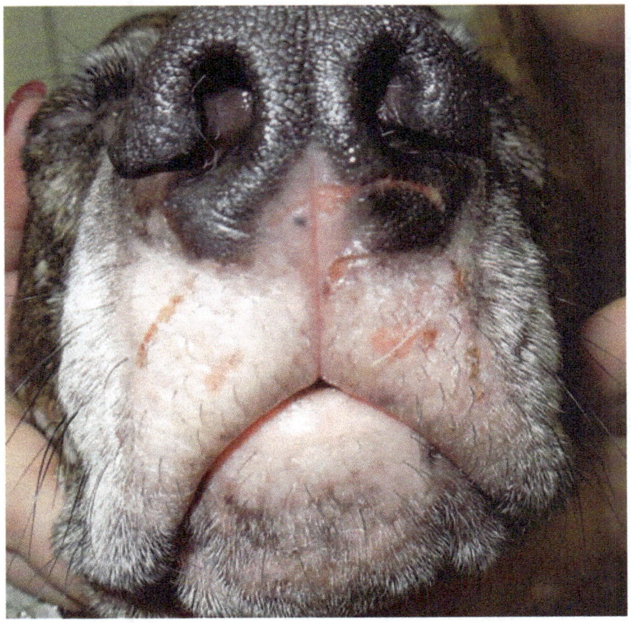

Figure 3.7 Cutaneous lymphoma often causes nasal planum depigmentation which starts on the ventral aspect.

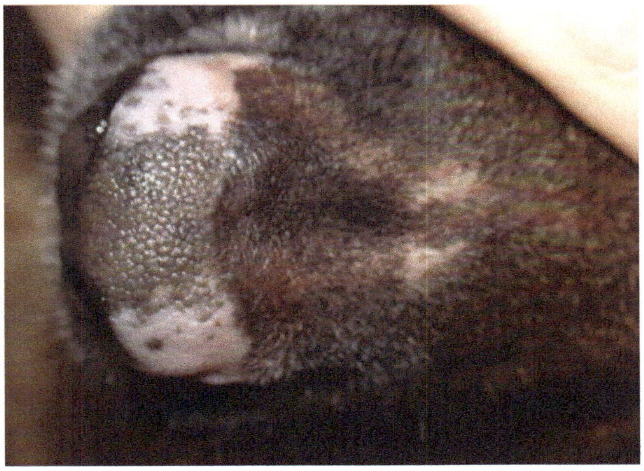

Figure 3.8 A dog with vitiligo; note the retention of the normal reticular nose print pattern.

3.1.3 Muzzle

a) Alopecic
   - Infection (bacterial, *Demodex*, or dermatophyte, Figure 3.27A)
   - Barbering due to rubbing/pruritus due to hypersensitivity dermatitis (Figure 3.27B)
   - Hypothyroidism (Figure 3.28)
   - Canine recurrent (flank) alopecia
   - Immune-mediated disease (i.e. vasculitis, DM, Figure 3.29)

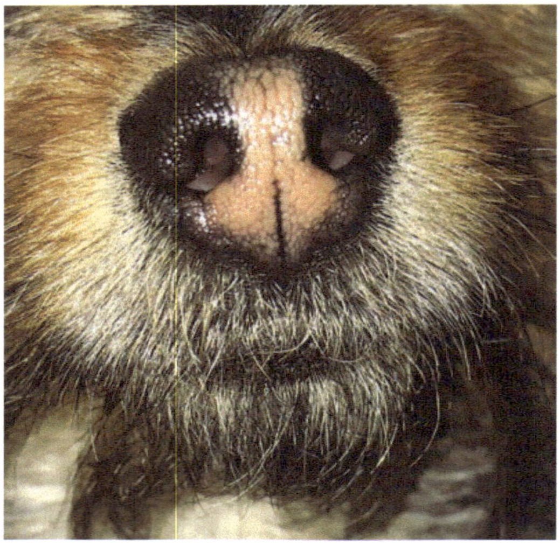

Figure 3.9 Dudley nose is characterized by a strip of central planum hypopigmentation which may wax and wane and never becomes eroded or crusted.

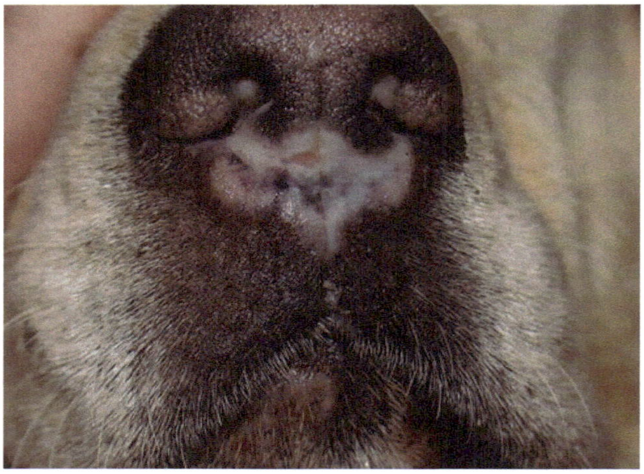

Figure 3.10 In this dog nasal depigmentation was shown on biopsy to be due to sterile granuloma syndrome.

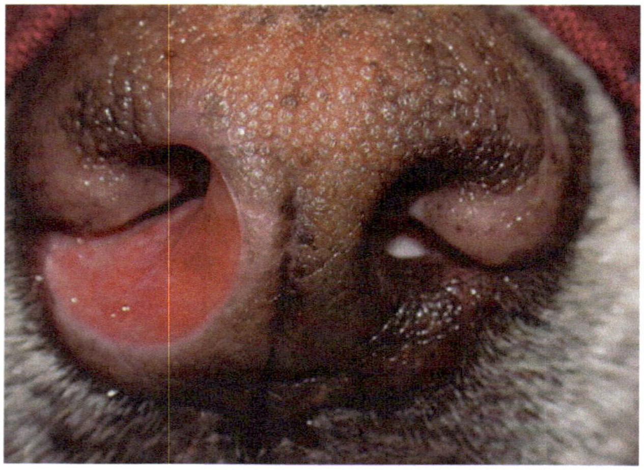

Figure 3.11A Unilateral nasal swelling and ulceration which was determined to be due to coccidioidomycosis.

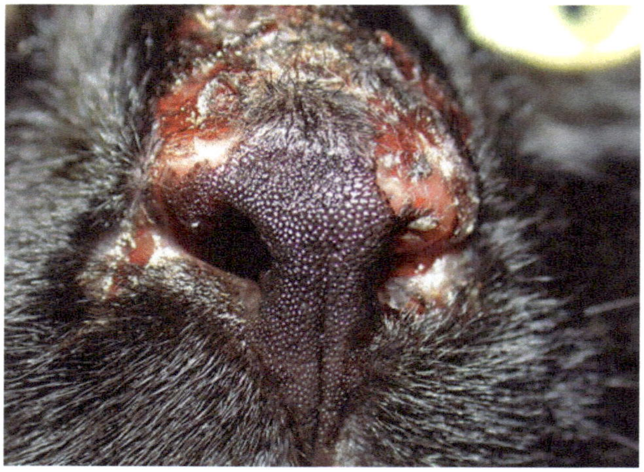

Figure 3.11B Crusting, erythema and erosion on the nasal planum and dorsal nose of a cat with herpesvirus dermatitis.

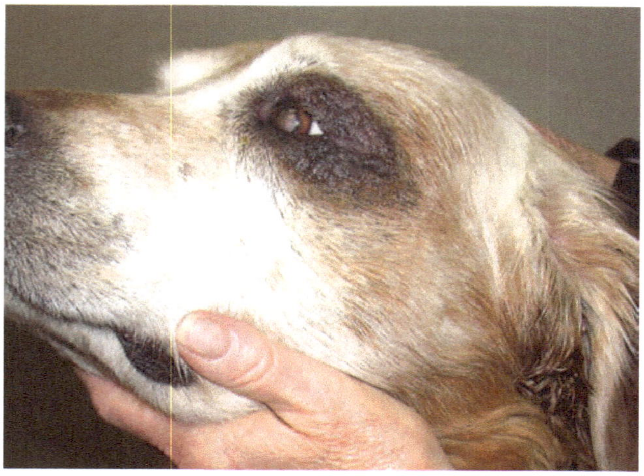

Figure 3.12A Alopecia and lichenification due to bacterial and yeast blepharitis in an atopic dog.

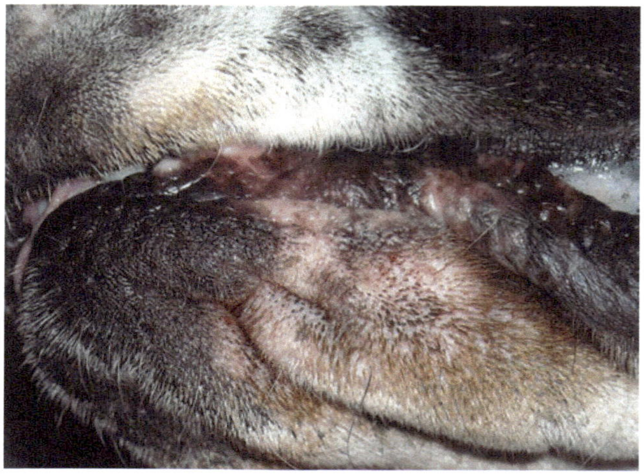

Figure 3.12B Alopecia caused by barbering/pruritus due to atopy and secondary yeast cheilitis.

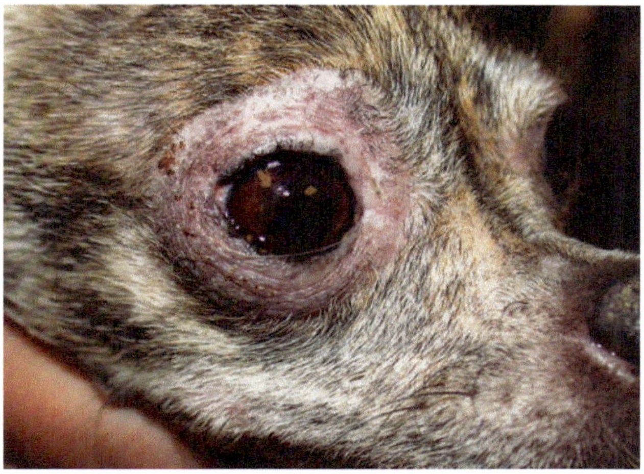

Figure 3.13 An atopic chihuahua with periocular barbering.

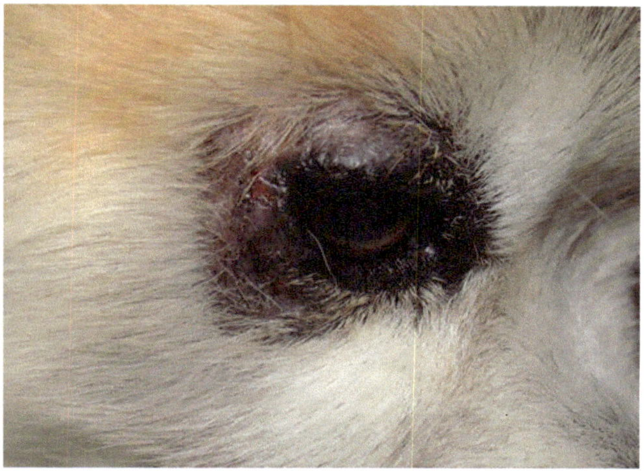

Figure 3.14 Non-pruritic scarring alopecia of the eyelids caused by vasculitis.

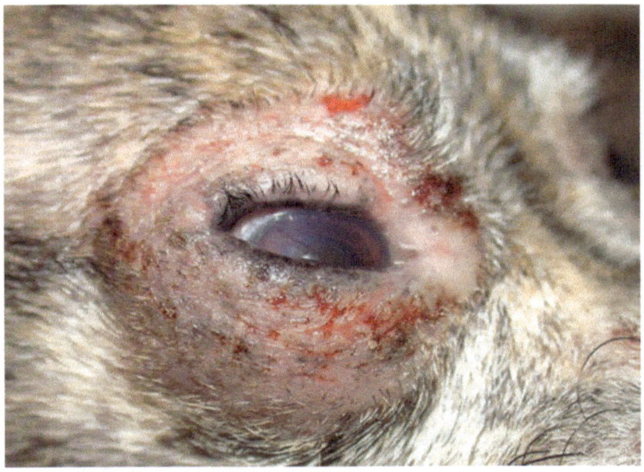

Figure 3.15A Periocular barbering, erythema, and crusting due to atopic dermatitis and secondary bacterial blepharitis.

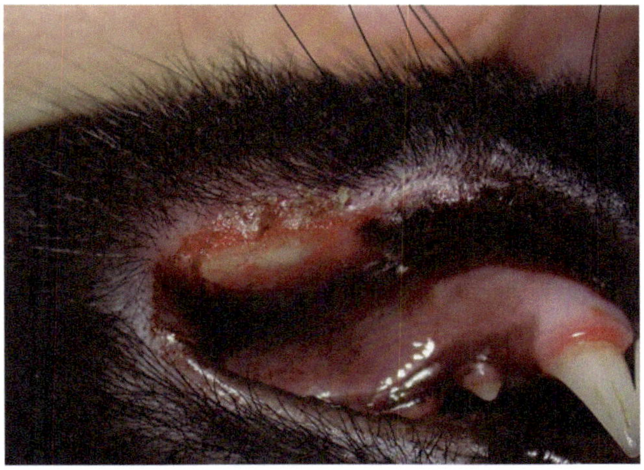

Figure 3.15B Crusting and erythema on the lip of an atopic cat with an eosinophilic granuloma complicated by bacterial mucocutaneous pyoderma.

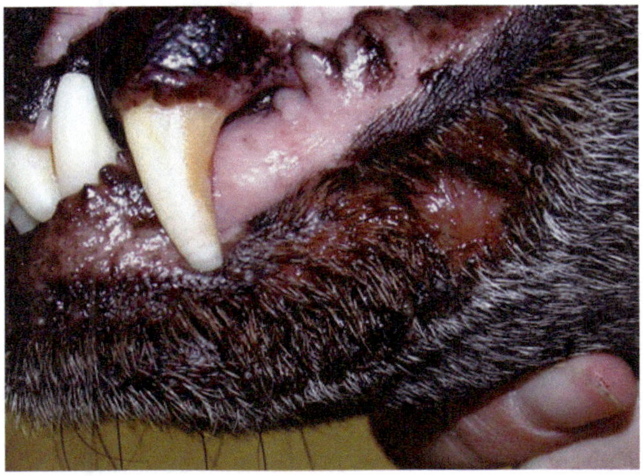

Figure 3.16A Mucocutaneous and lipfold pyoderma in an atopic dog.

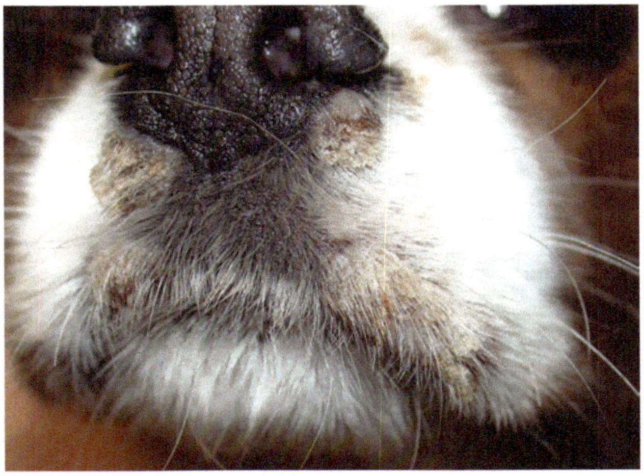

Figure 3.16B Focal crusts on the lips of this allergic spaniel showed both bacterial cocci and yeast on cytology and crusts resolved with antimicrobial therapy.

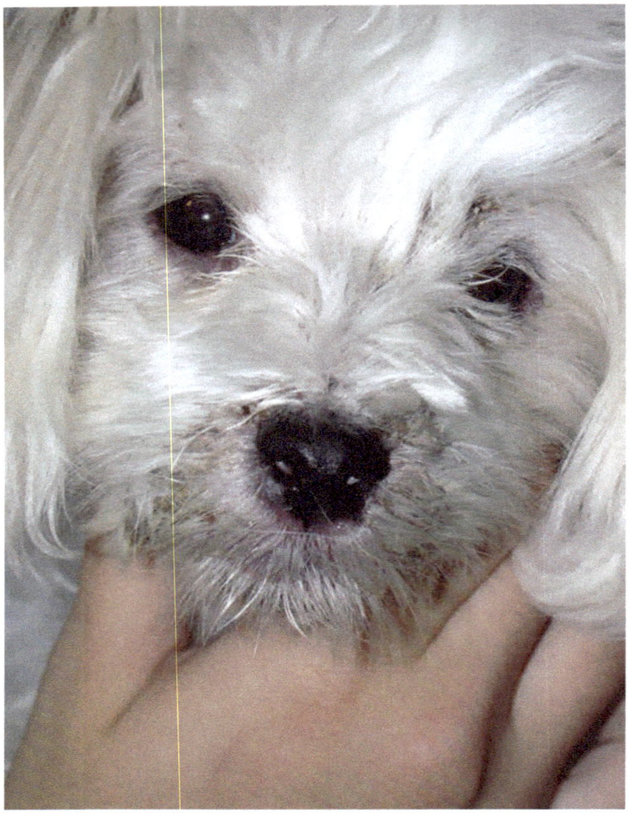

Figure 3.17 Crusting on the lips and eyelids of this puppy mimicked juvenile cellulitis but was due to *Demodex*.

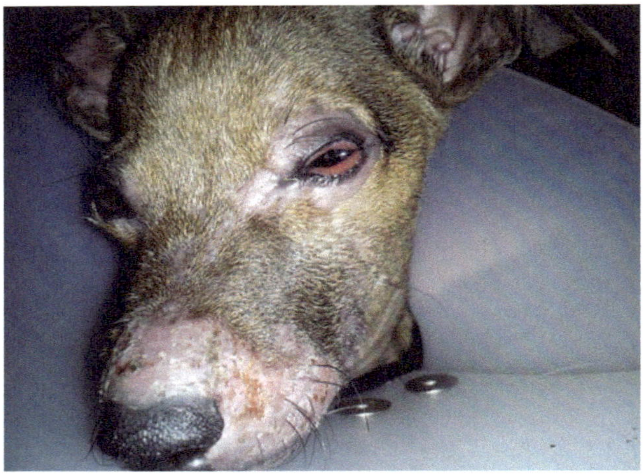

Figure 3.18 Alopecia and thickened skin in a puppy with chronically untreated juvenile cellulitis; lesions slowly resolved with immunosuppressive therapy.

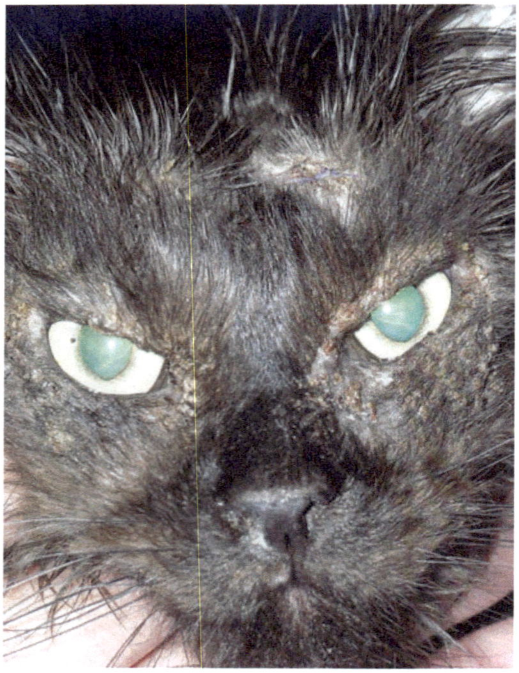

Figure 3.19 Eyelid crusting in this cat was due to pemphigus foliaceus.

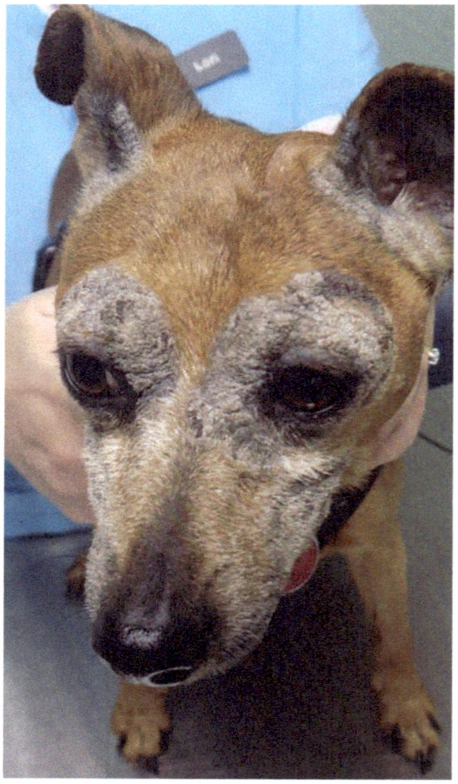

Figure 3.20 Symmetrical adherent crusting on the eyelids of a dog with zinc responsive dermatosis related to a deficient diet.

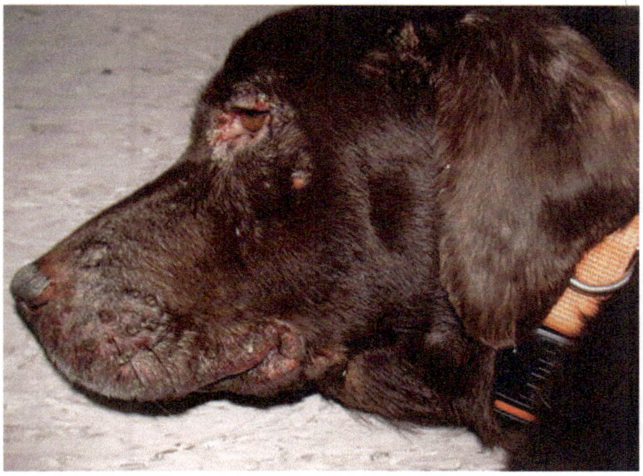

Figure 3.21 Lip crusting and erosion due to hepatocutaneous syndrome; paw pads and pressure points were all symmetrically affected.

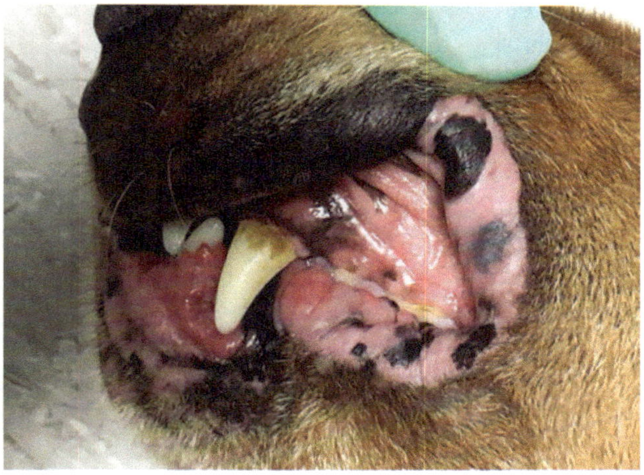

Figure 3.22 Patchy lip depigmentation due to cutaneous epitheliotropic lymphoma; unlike vitiligo the depigmentation was associated with intense erythema and erosion on other parts of the body.

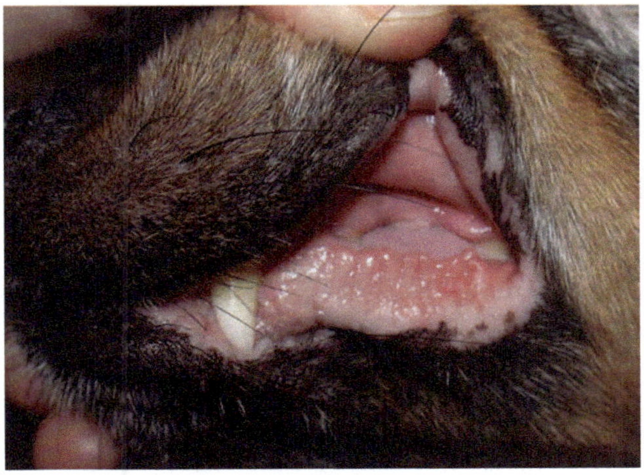

Figure 3.23 Patchy lip depigmentation due to vitiligo; there is no associated inflammation.

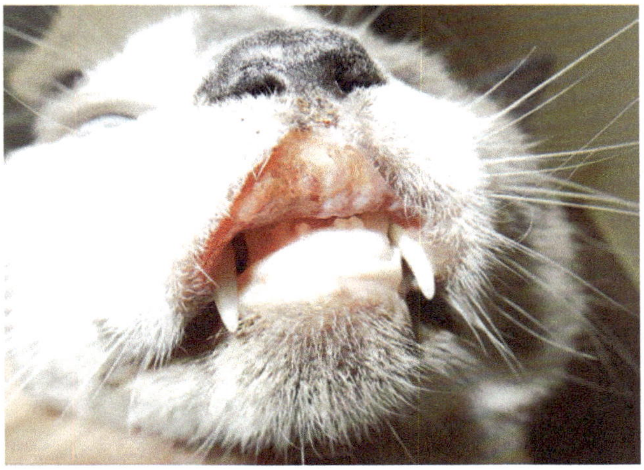

Figure 3.24 A severe rodent ulcer on the lip of a cat secondary to allergic dermatitis.

Muzzle (cont.)

b) Crusty
   - Infection (bacterial, dermatophyte, or *Demodex*, Figure 3.30A; feline herpesvirus dermatitis, Figure 3.30B)
   - Feline mosquito bite hypersensitivity (Figure 3.30C)
   - Immune-mediated disease (i.e. pemphigus foliaceus [Figure 3.31], juvenile cellulitis)
   - Metabolic disease (zinc responsive dermatosis, hepatocutaneous syndrome)

c) Ulcerated
   - Feline herpesvirus dermatitis
   - Immune-mediated disease (PF/PV/DLE/SLE/EM/vasculitis/drug eruption; Figure 3.32)
   - Neoplasia (cutaneous lymphoma, squamous cell carcinoma (SCC)

d) Acute erosive moist or crusted erythematous plaques on dorsal muzzle
   - Canine eosinophilic facial furunculosis (Figure 3.33)

e) Chin papules/pustules/furuncles
   - Acne (Figure 3.34), *Demodex* (Figure 3.35), dermatophyte, contact sensitivity

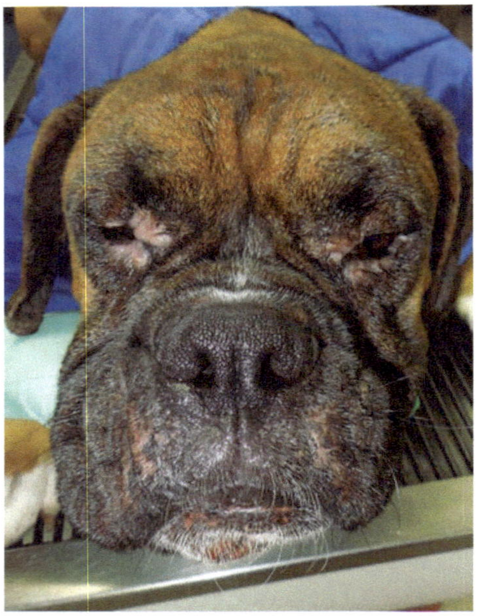

Figure 3.25 Acute erosions and crusts on the eyelids and lips of a dog with a drug eruption due to an antibiotic.

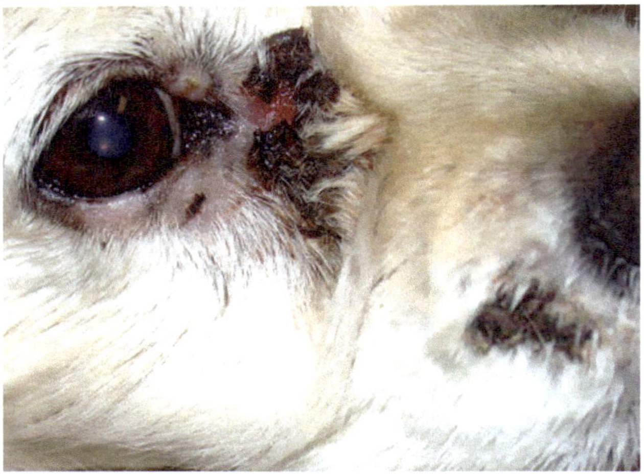

Figure 3.26A Eyelid and lip ulcers and crusts due to cutaneous lymphoma; note the depigmentation.

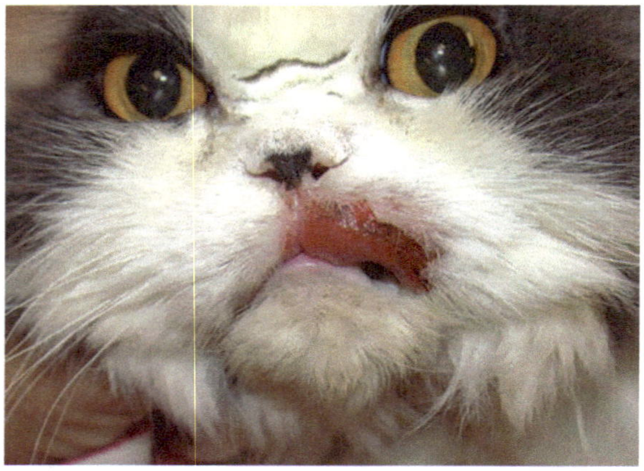

Figure 3.26B Asymmetrical chronic lip ulceration in an older cat due to squamous cell carcinoma.

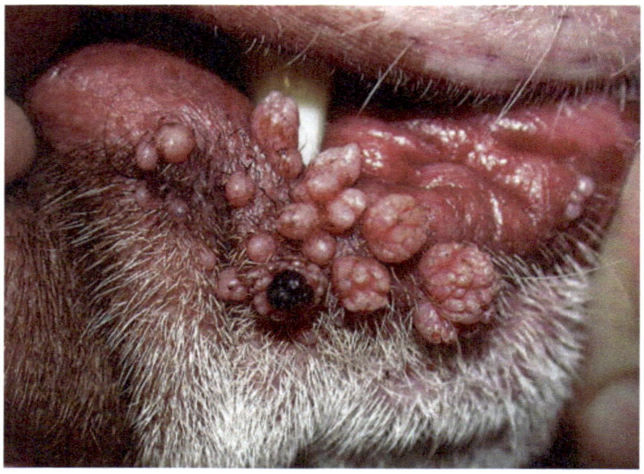

Figure 3.26C Multiple smooth to fronded exophytic pink lip masses due to canine oral viral papillomas.

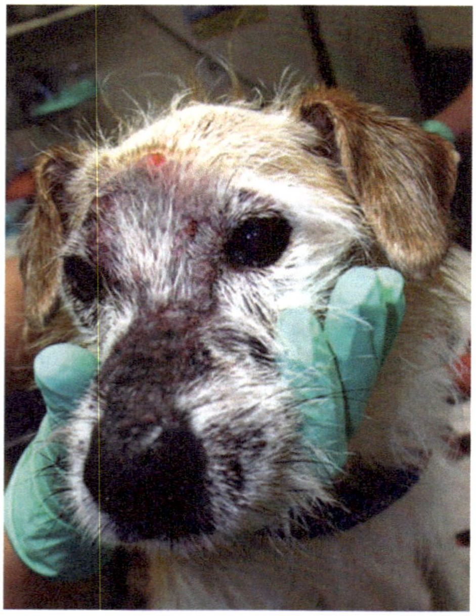

Figure 3.27A Patchy alopecia and hyperpigmentation with peripheral crusting on the muzzle due to dermatophytosis.

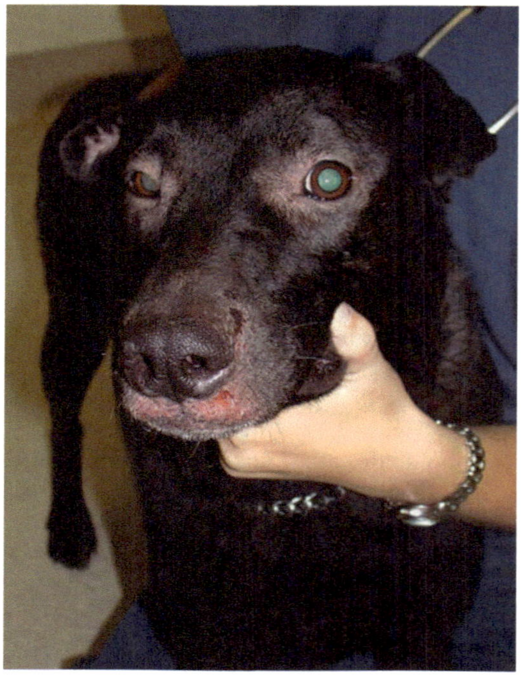

Figure 3.27B Distal muzzle barbering due to atopy.

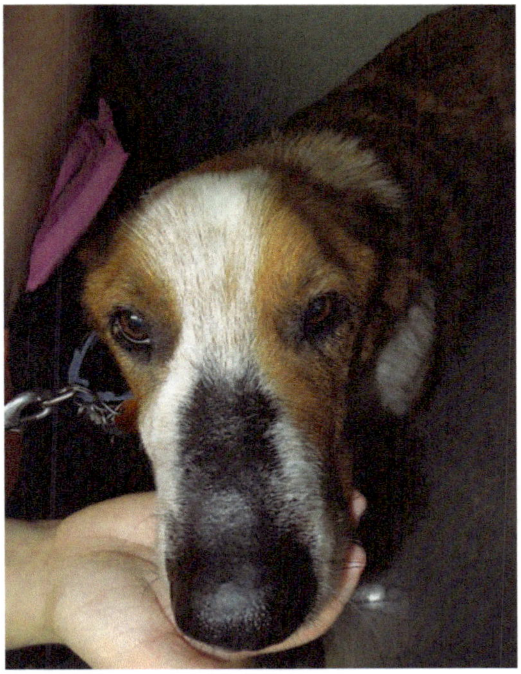

Figure 3.28 Non-inflammatory alopecia and hyperpigmentation on the dorsal muzzle can be a sign of hypothyroidism.

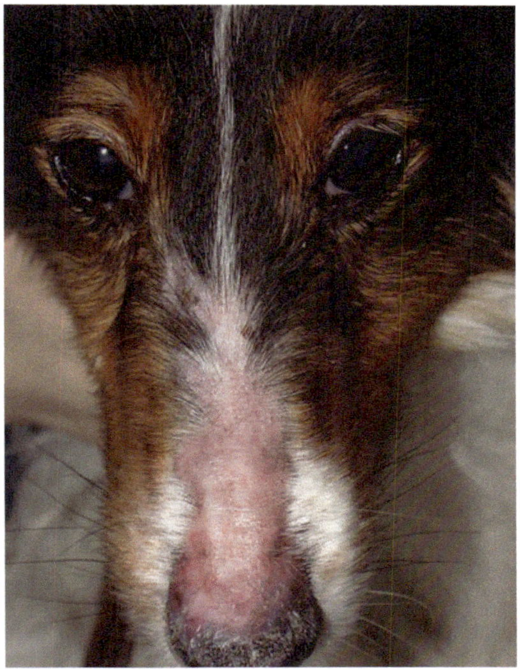

Figure 3.29 Scarring alopecia on the muzzle of a sheltie with dermatomyositis (DM).

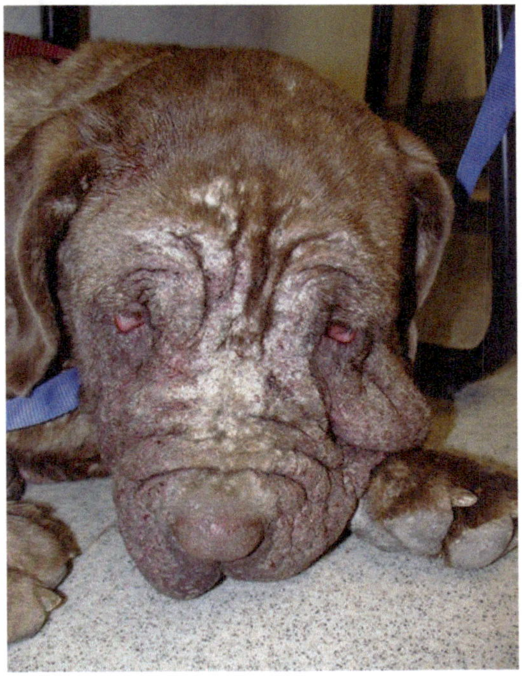

Figure 3.30A Severe muzzle alopecia and crusting due to demodicosis.

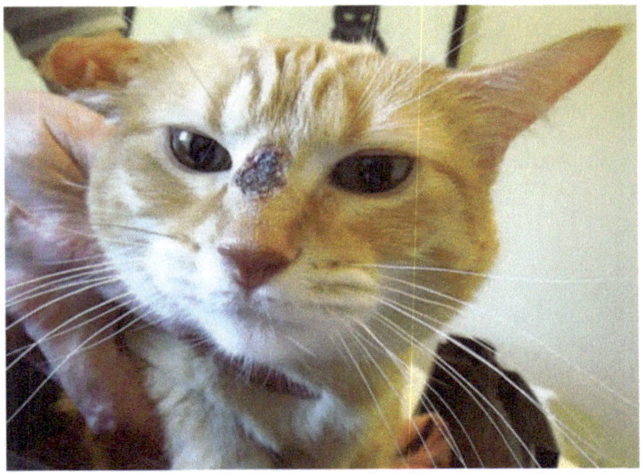

Figure 3.30B Adherent crusting on the dorsal muzzle of a cat due to herpesvirus dermatitis.

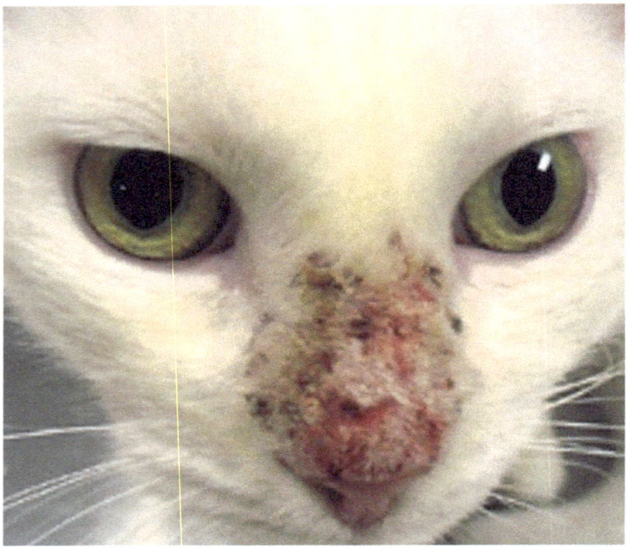

Figure 3.30C Crusts, papules, and erythema on the dorsal muzzle of a cat with mosquito bite hypersensitivity. Source: Photo courtesy Dr. Amy Shumaker, DACVD.

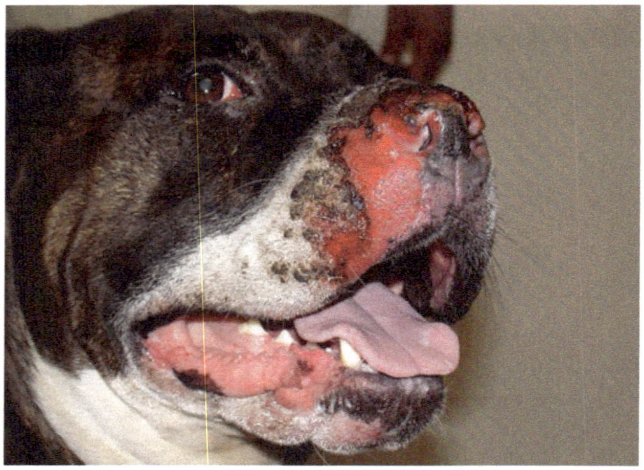

Figure 3.32 Acute muzzle ulceration due to a drug eruption.

3.2 Ears

3.2.1 Pinnal margin

a) Crusty +/− alopecic
   - Ear margin seborrhea, pinnal marginal dermatosis (Figure 3.36)
   - Pinnal vasculitis (Figures 3.37A and 3.37B)
   - Scabies (Figures 3.38A and 3.38B)
   - Barbering due to hypersensitivity dermatitis (atopy or food allergy, Figure 6.30)
   - Zinc responsive dermatosis (Figure 3.39)

b) Erosive/ulcerated
   - Immune-mediated disease (especially vasculitis [Figure 3.40], pinnal thrombovascular necrosis, cold agglutinin disease)

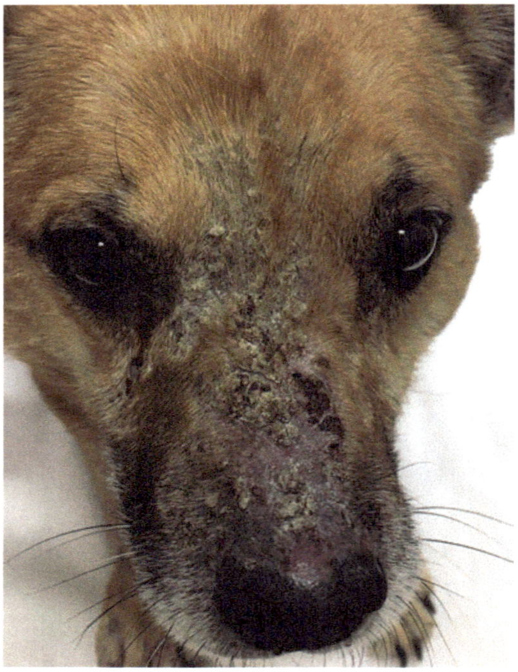

Figure 3.31 Muzzle crusting due to pemphigus foliaceus.

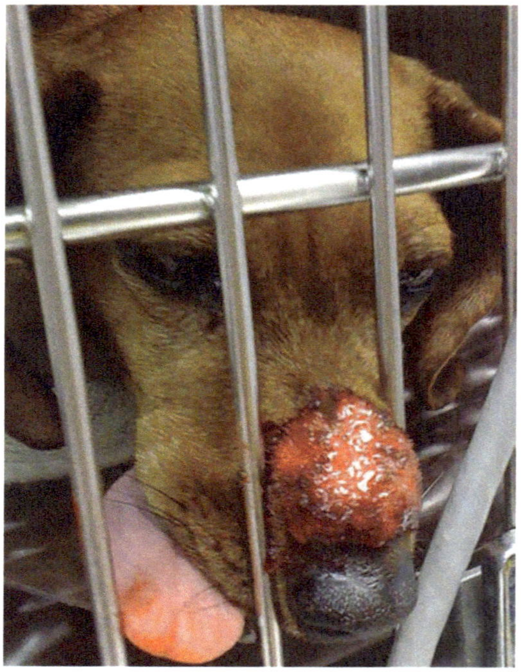

Figure 3.33 Acute plaque-like to nodular moist furunculosis on the dorsal muzzle is characteristic of canine eosinophilic facial furunculosis.

   - Neoplasia (sun-induced feline squamous cell carcinoma, Figure 3.41)
   - Frostbite

c) Mass
   - Neoplasia
   - Calcinosis circumscripta (post ear crop)

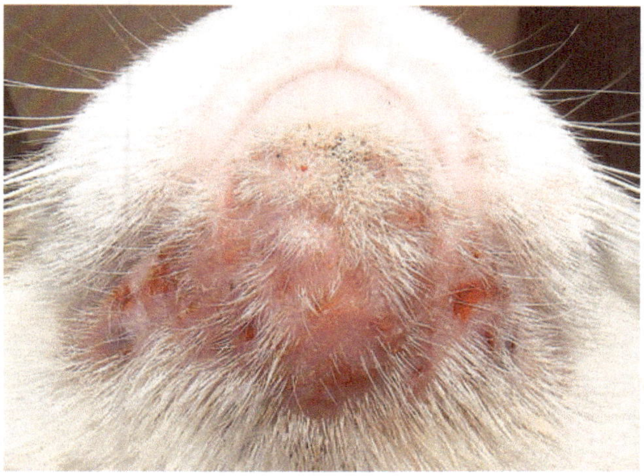

Figure 3.34 Severe feline acne characterized by draining furuncles.

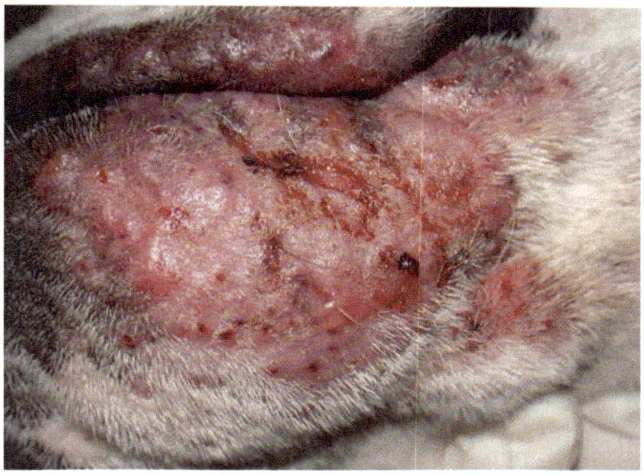

Figure 3.35 Chin furunculosis due to *Demodex*.

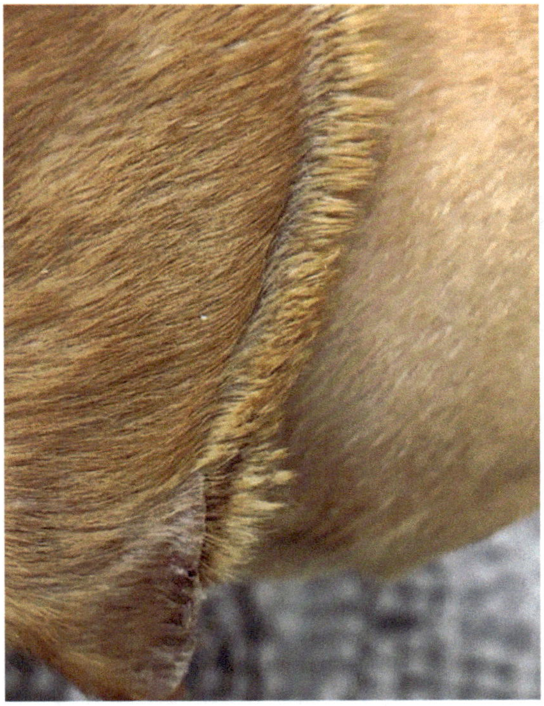

Figure 3.36 Ear margin seborrhea in a dachshund; follicular casts can be seen with careful examination.

3.2.2 Pinna

a) Crusty +/− alopecic
   - Immune-mediated disease (i.e. pemphigus foliaceus [Figures 3.42A and 3.42B], vasculitis [Figure 3.42C])
   - Infection (bacterial, *Demodex*, dermatophyte; Figure 3.43A)
   - Self-trauma/pruritus due to hypersensitivity dermatitis (atopy/food allergy/parasite, Figure 3.43B)
   - Metabolic disease (zinc responsive dermatosis, Figure 3.44)
   - Sebaceous adenitis (Figure 3.45)

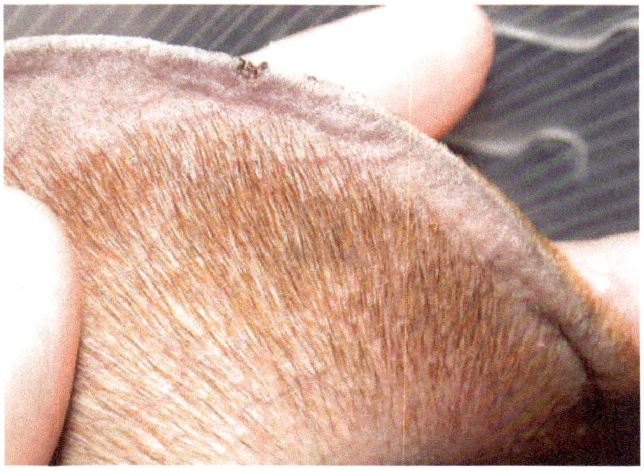

Figure 3.37A Early pinnal vasculitis characterized by alopecia and a tiny ulceration.

b) Erosive/ulcerated
   - Immune-mediated disease (i.e. vasculitis, pinnal thrombovascular necrosis, EM [Figure 3.46], cold agglutinin disease)
   - Frostbite

c) Alopecia with no inflammation/crusting
   - Pattern baldness (Figure 3.47)
   - Yorkie leather ear
   - Overuse of topical steroids (Figure 3.48)

d) Mass
   - Neoplasia
   - Histiocytosis (Figure 3.49A)
   - Leproid granuloma (Figure 3.49B)

3.2.3 Outer ear canal

a) Ulceration
   - Severe infection (esp. Pseudomonas)
   - Immune-mediated disease (i.e. PF, EM [Figure 3.50])

b) Adherent crusts
   - Sebaceous adenitis (Figure 3.51)

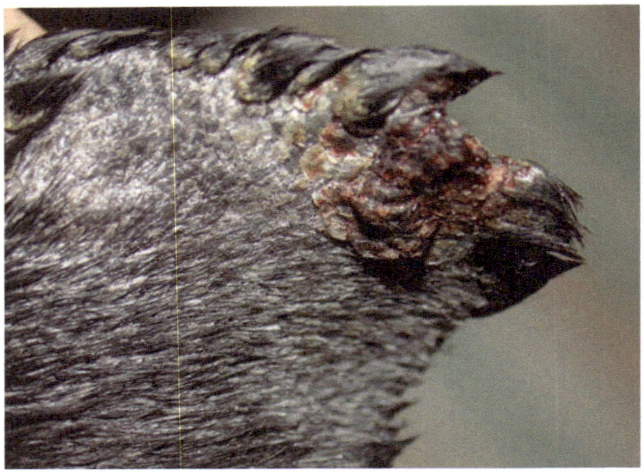

Figure 3.37B Pinnal vasculitis causing crusting and ulceration of the distal pinna.

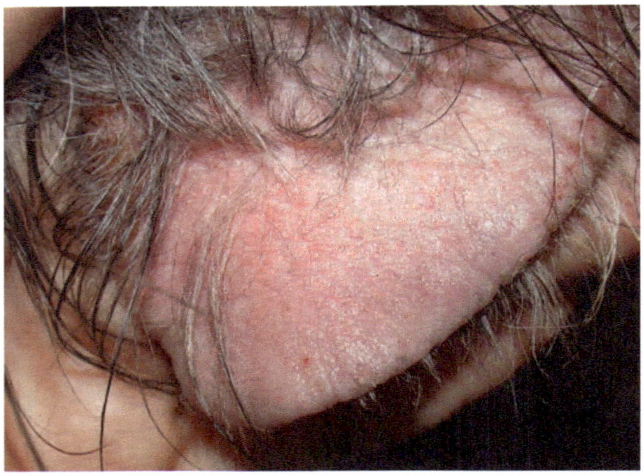

Figure 3.38A Canine sarcoptic mange causing pinnal marginal alopecia and severe pruritus.

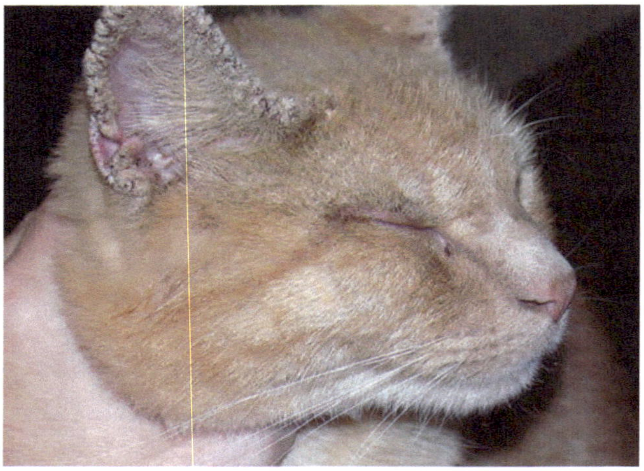

Figure 3.38B Feline *Notoedres* causing pinnal marginal crusting and pruritus.

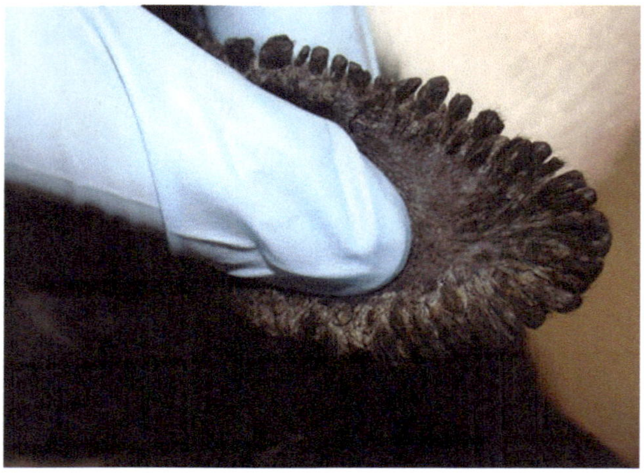

Figure 3.39 Zinc responsive dermatosis in a young Boston terrier, causing adherent fronded crusts on pinnal margins.

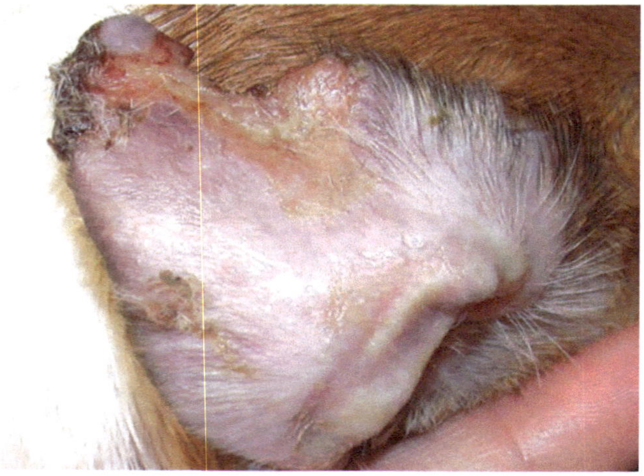

Figure 3.40 Ulceration of pinnal skin and cartilage caused by vasculitis triggered by rabies vaccination.

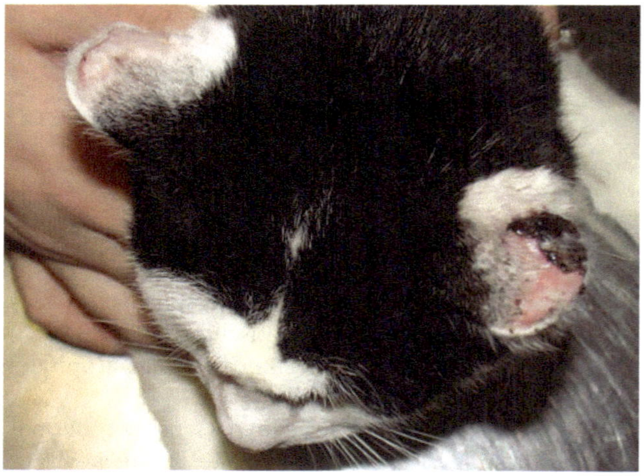

Figure 3.41 Pinnal ulceration and crusting in a cat due to solar-induced squamous cell carcinoma.

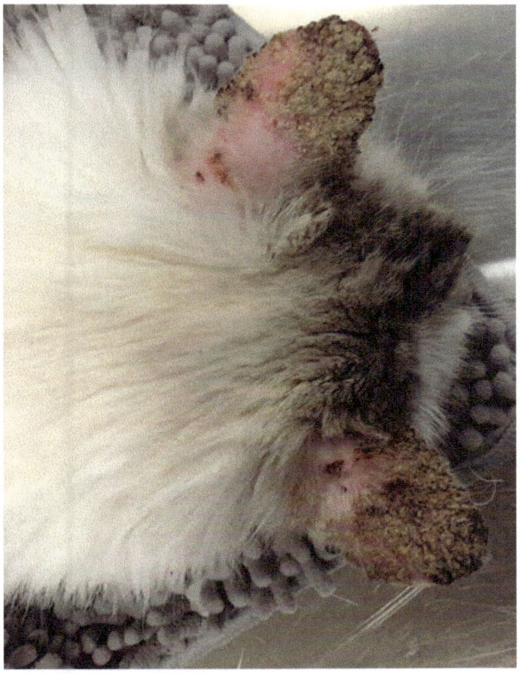

Figure 3.42A Pinnal crusting and alopecia due to pemphigus foliaceus.

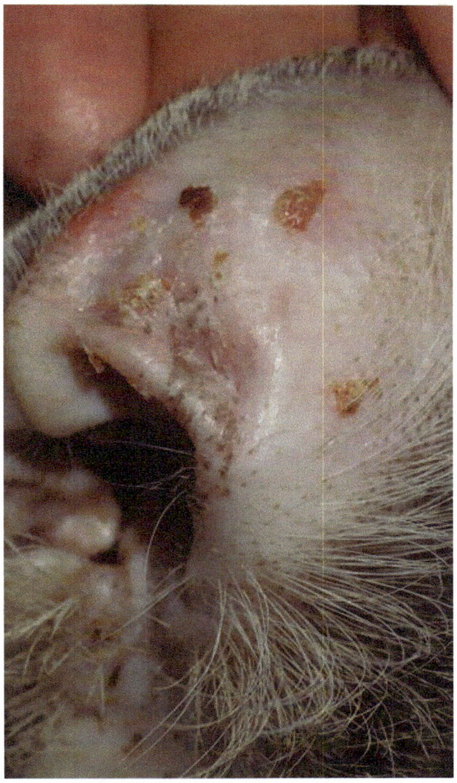

Figure 3.42B Crusts also involved the concave pinnal surface.

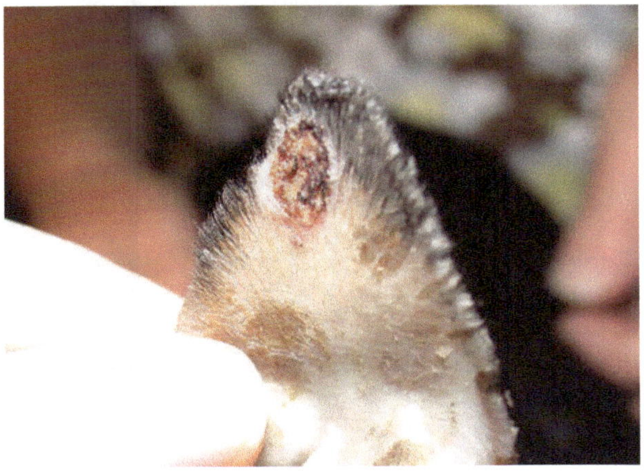

Figure 3.42C Ulceration on the distal concave pinna of a chihuahua due to rabies vaccine-induced vasculitis.

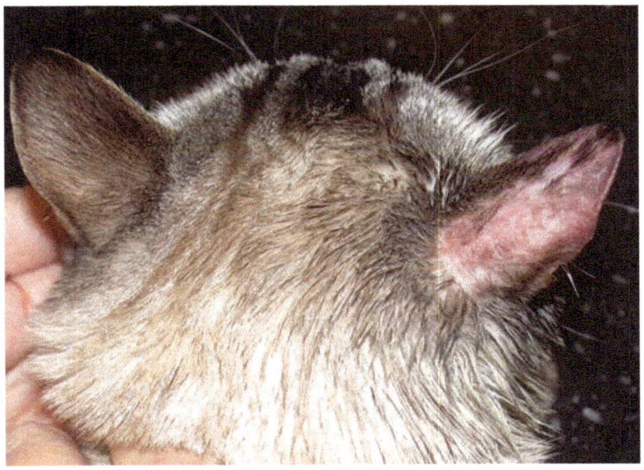

Figure 3.43A Asymmetrical pinnal alopecia and crusting due to dermatophytosis.

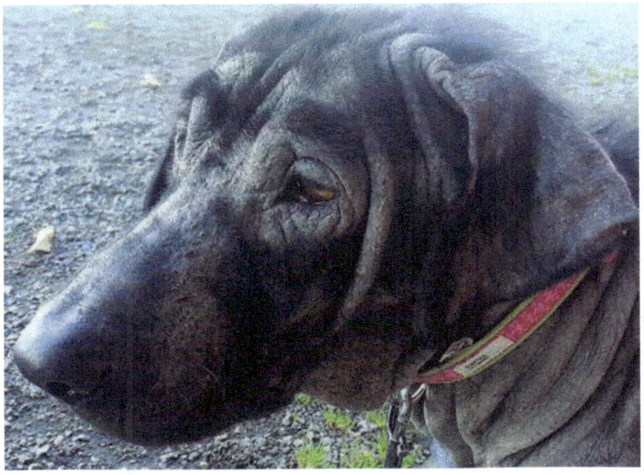

Figure 3.43B Pinnal barbering/crusting caused by self-trauma due to atopy and food allergy.

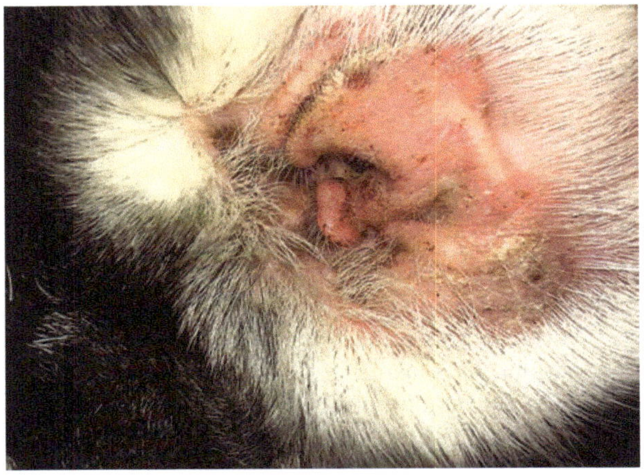

Figure 3.44 Crusting and scaling on the concave pinna of a Husky with zinc responsive dermatosis.

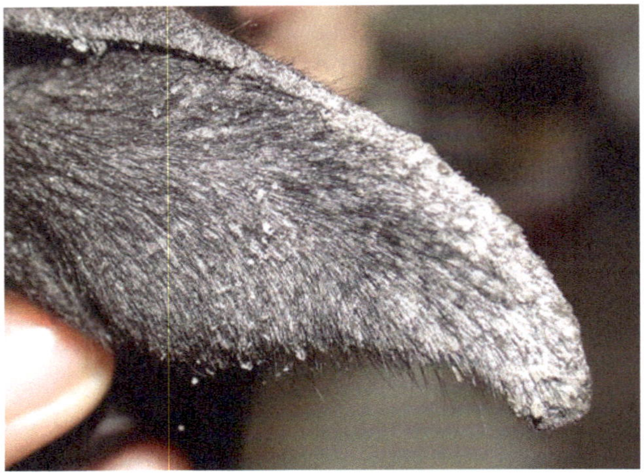

Figure 3.45 Pinnal scaling and follicular casting due to sebaceous adenitis.

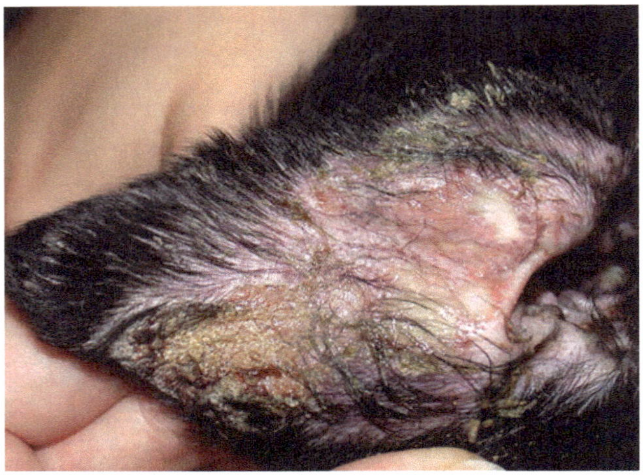

Figure 3.46 Pinnal ulceration due to erythema multiforme.

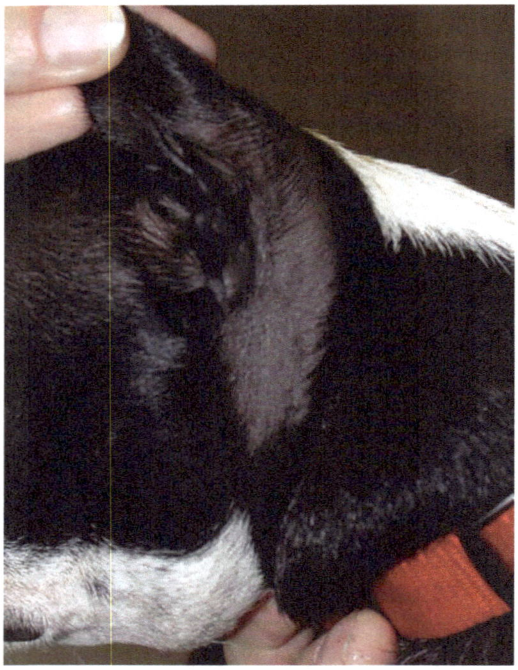

Figure 3.47 Non-inflammatory symmetrical caudal auricular alopecia in a Boston Terrier due to pattern baldness.

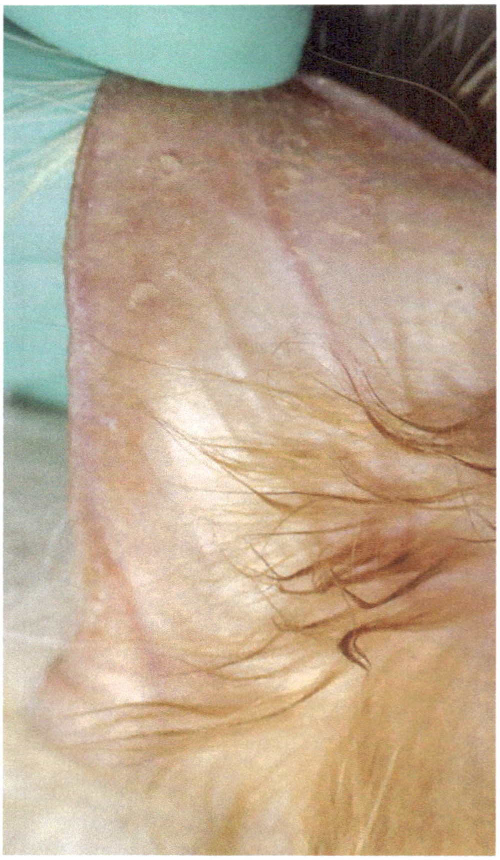

Figure 3.48 Marked pinnal alopecia and cutaneous atrophy due to overuse of topical steroids in a cat.

Outer ear canal (cont.)

c) Masses
   - Polyp (Figure 3.52)
   - Neoplasia (i.e. SCC [Figures 3.53A and 3.53B], ceruminous gland adenoma [Figure 3.54]/adenocarcinoma, plasmacytoma)
   - Apocrine cystadenomas (blue tinged cystic masses, Figure 19.18B)

3.3 Paws

3.3.1 Interdigital

a) Inflamed/moist/crusted
   - Hypersensitivity (atopy, food allergy, Figures 3.55A and 3.55B)

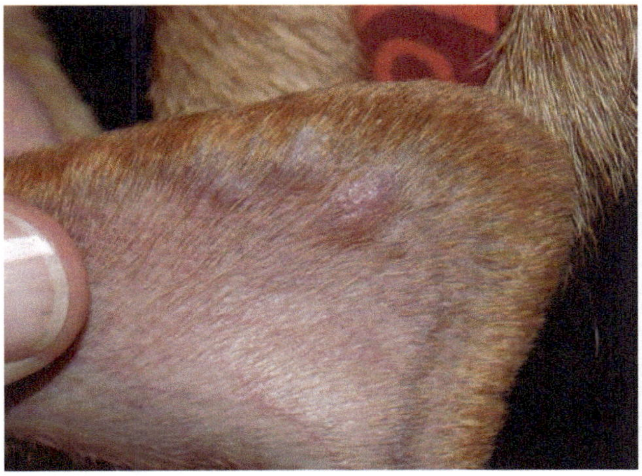

Figure 3.49A Hypotrichotic pink dermal pinnal masses due to reactive histiocytosis.

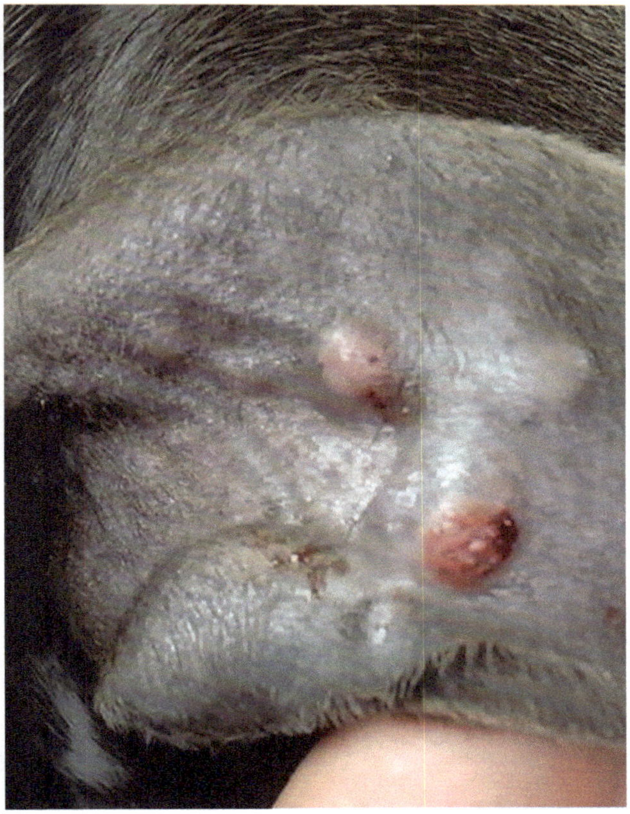

Figure 3.49B Similar masses in a different dog were due to leproid granulomas, a mycobacterial infection.

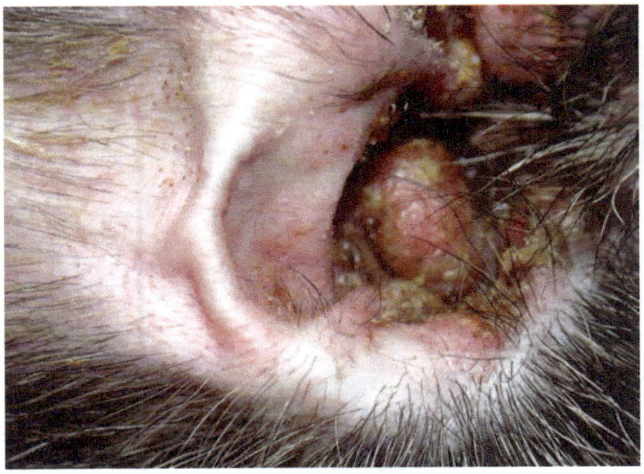

Figure 3.50 Ulceration and crusting in the ear canal of a dog with erythema multiforme.

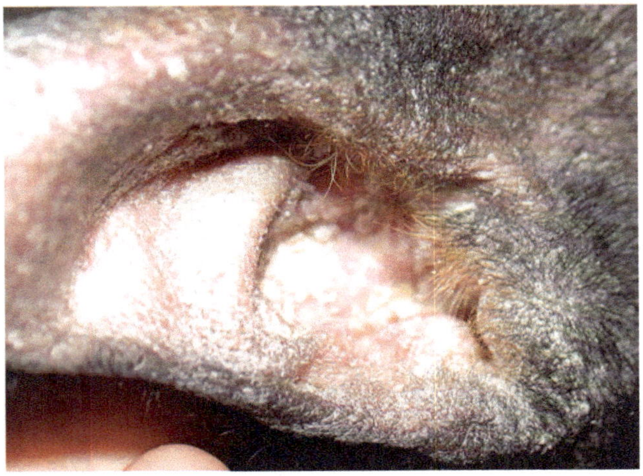

Figure 3.51 Adherent crusts and scales in the ear canal of a dog with sebaceous adenitis.

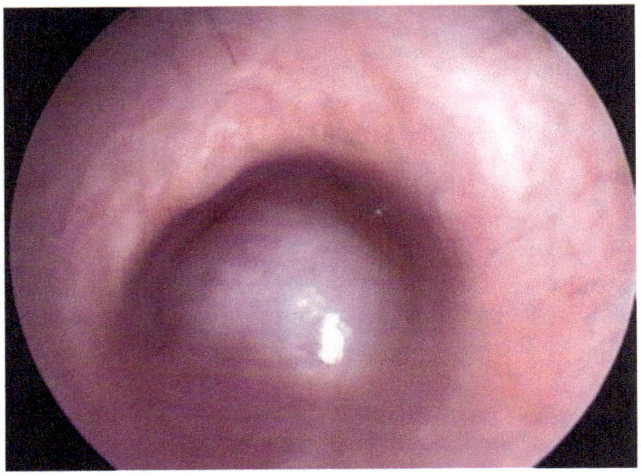

Figure 3.52 Otoscopic view of a cat with an inflammatory polyp.

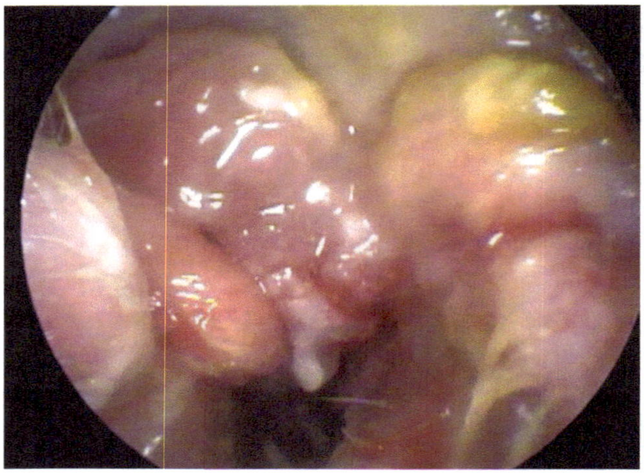

Figure 3.53A An inflamed ulcerated ear canal mass in a dog with recurrent otitis which was found on biopsy to be squamous cell carcinoma.

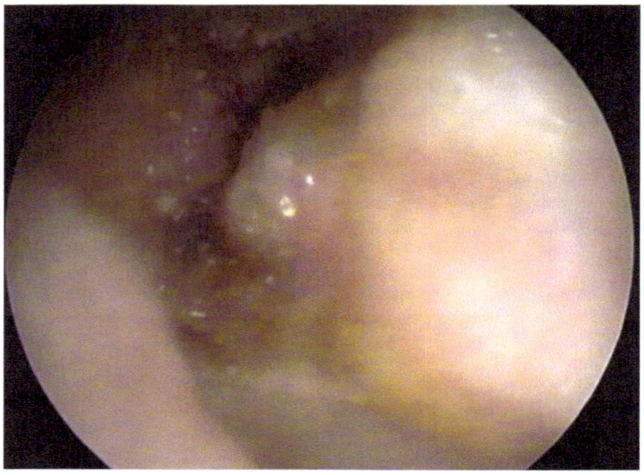

Figure 3.53B In this cat with chronic otitis, the canal is occluded by a diffuse squamous cell carcinoma.

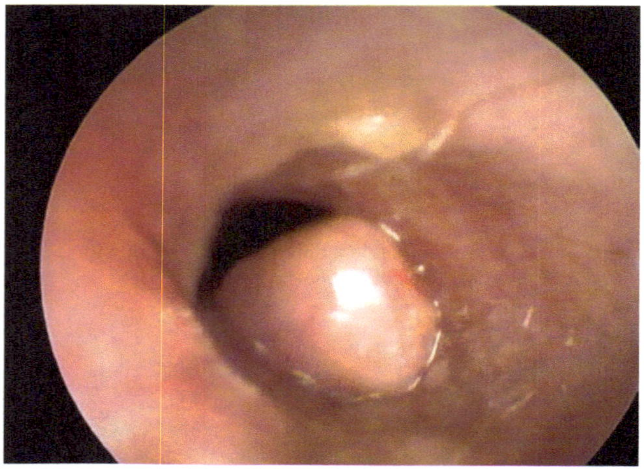

Figure 3.54 A smooth sessile canal mass in a dog which was found on excisional biopsy to be a ceruminous gland adenoma.

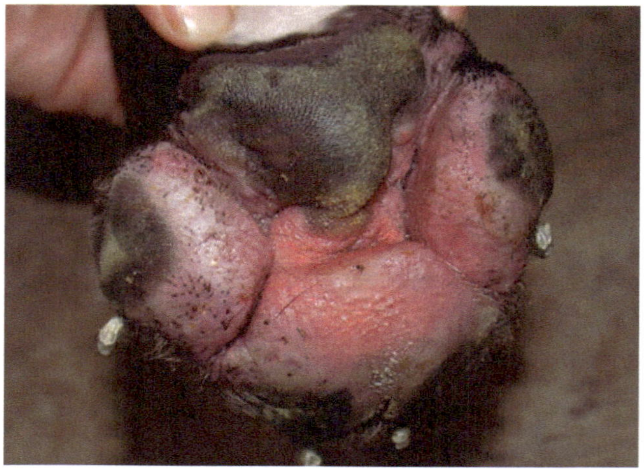

Figure 3.55A Severe interdigital erythema, swelling, and fibrosis due to atopic dermatitis.

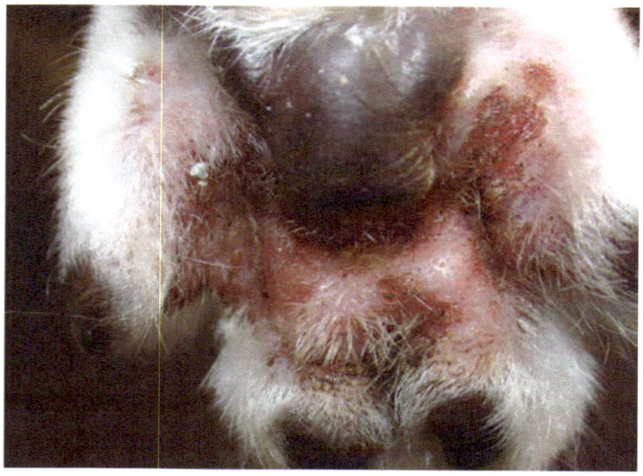

Figure 3.55B Interdigital erythema and crusted excoriations in a cat with atopic dermatitis.

Interdigital (cont.)

Infection (bacterial and/or *Malassezia* secondary to hypersensitivity; Figures 3.56 and 3.57)
Demodex (Figure 3.58)
Dermatophyte
Plant awn/grass foreign bodies (Figure 3.59)

b) Mass

Follicular cyst (dilated/inflamed interdigital hair follicle due to allergy/licking/secondary infection and/or conformational abnormality or obesity causing increased pressure on area, Figure 3.60)
Granuloma (due to grass awn or ruptured follicular cyst)
Viral papilloma (Figure 3.61)
Neoplasia

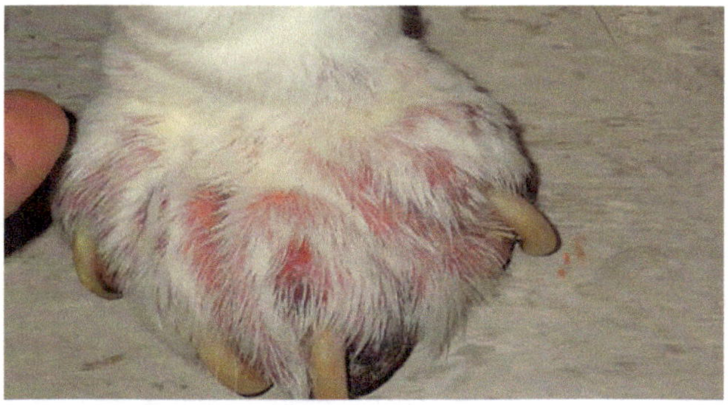

Figure 3.56 An atopic Bulldog with severe bacterial pododermatitis.

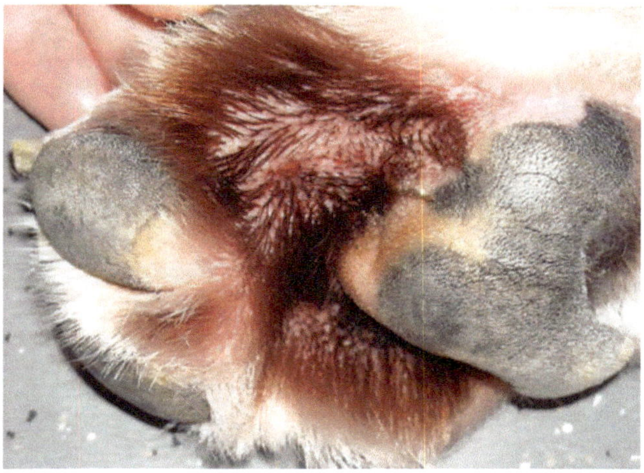

Figure 3.57 Interdigital inflammation and brown fur discoloration in an atopic dog with *Malassezia* pododermatitis.

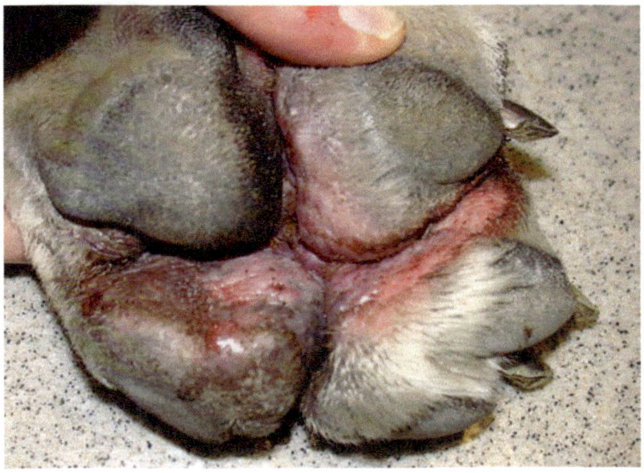

Figure 3.58 Severe interdigital swelling with draining tracts due to demodicosis.

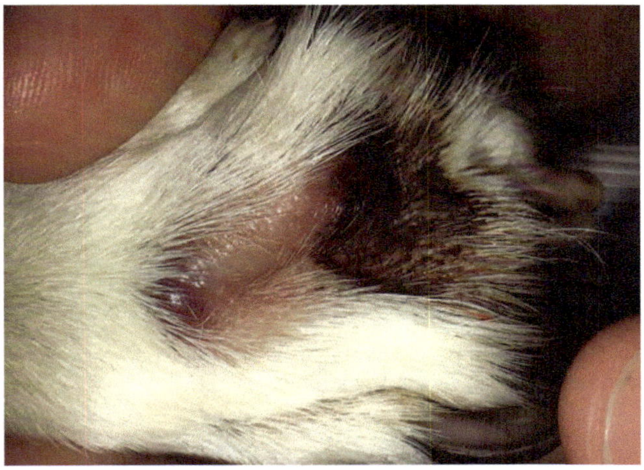

Figure 3.59 An interdigital draining tract due to a grass awn (foxtail).

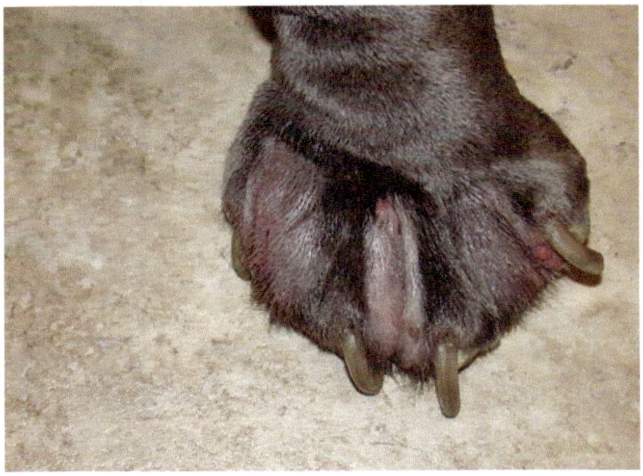

Figure 3.60 Draining dorsal interdigital cysts/granuloma due to atopic dermatitis.

3.3.2 Palmar metacarpal/plantar metatarsal

a) Inflamed/crusted +/– moist
   - Hypersensitivity (atopy, food allergy)
   - Canine metacarpal/metatarsal fistulas (Chapter 6, Figure 6.26; Chapter 11, Figure 11.21A–11.21C)

3.3.3 Paw pad

a) Crusty
   - Idiopathic nasodigital hyperkeratosis (Figure 6.14B)
   - Metabolic (zinc responsive [Figure 3.62], hepatocutaneous syndrome, Figure 3.63)
   - Immune-mediated (esp. pemphigus foliaceus, Figure 3.64)
   - Dermatophytosis (Figure 3.65)
   - Viral papilloma
   - Neoplasia (i.e. cutaneous lymphoma, Figure 3.66)
   - Parasitic (hookworm dermatitis, *Pelodera*)

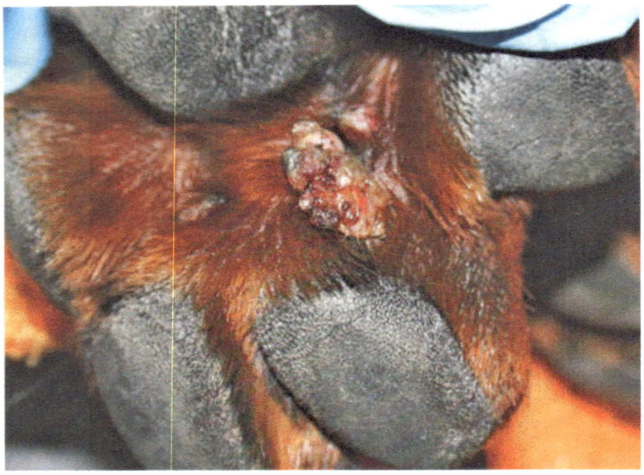

Figure 3.61 An acute fronded interdigital mass which was biopsied as a viral papilloma.

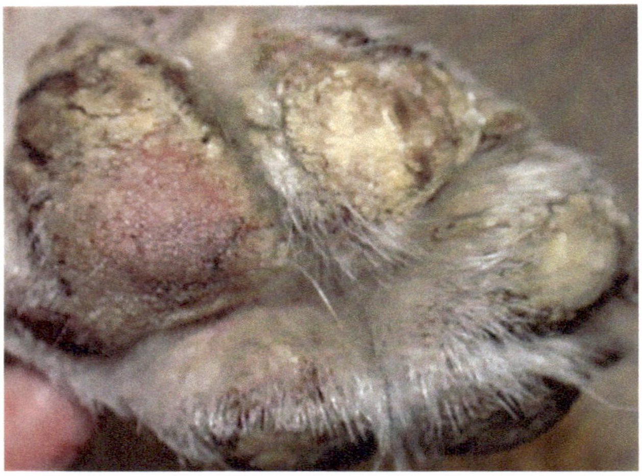

Figure 3.62 Paw pad crusting due to zinc responsive dermatosis in a Husky.

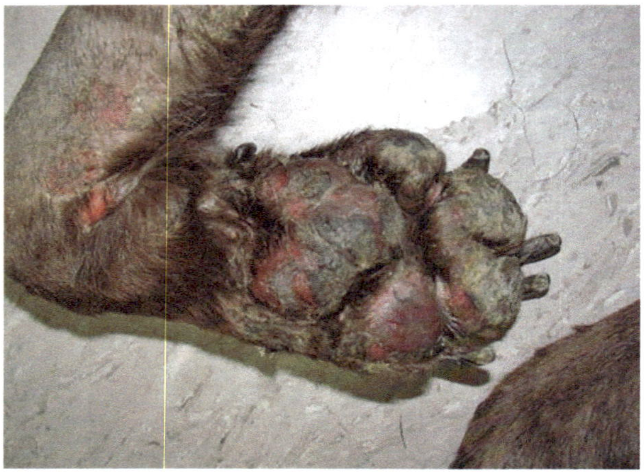

Figure 3.63 Crusting and ulceration affecting the paw pads of a dog with hepatocutaneous syndrome.

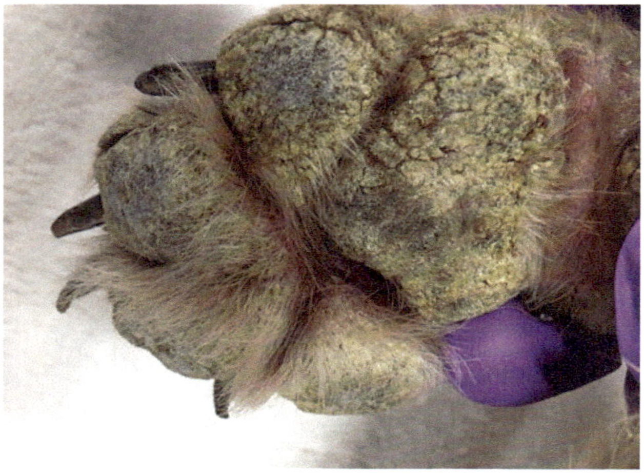

Figure 3.64 Paw pad crusting caused by pemphigus foliaceus.

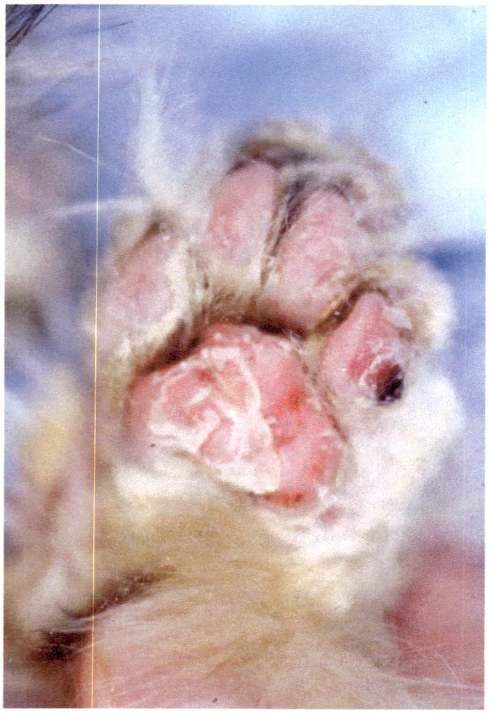

Figure 3.65 This cat's paw pad crusting and scaling was due to dermatophytosis.

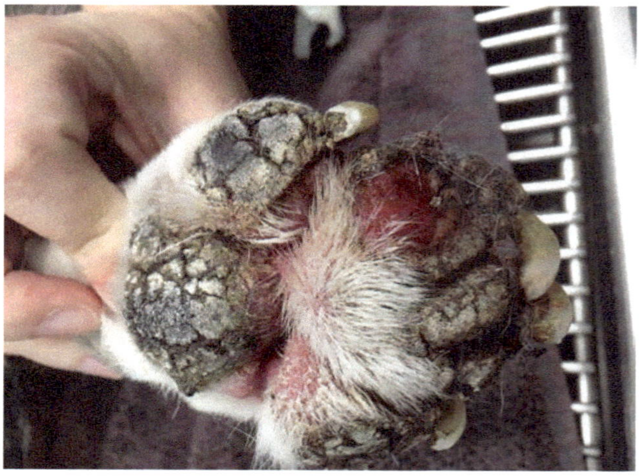

Figure 3.66 Severe paw pad crusting and ulceration in a dog with cutaneous epitheliotropic lymphoma.

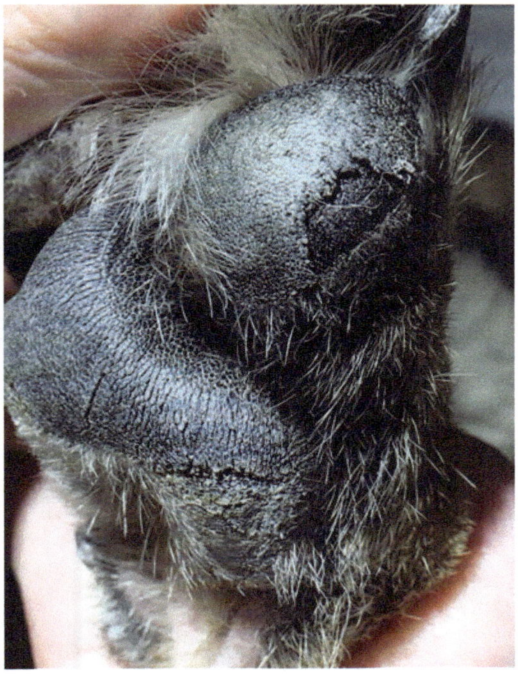

Figure 3.67 A young German Shepherd dog with chronic recurrent peripheral foot pad ulcerations which spontaneously heal, typical of split paw pad disease.

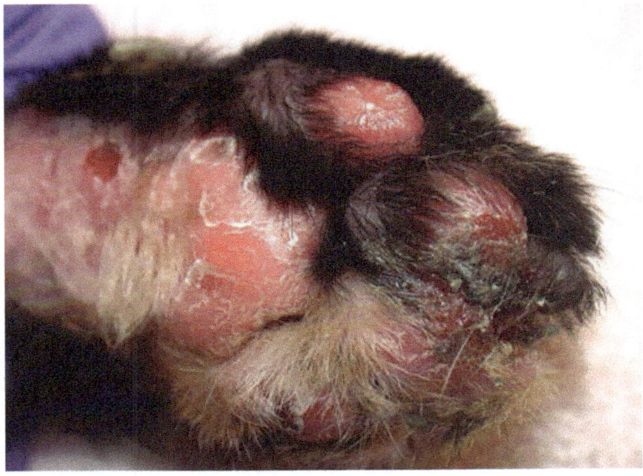

Figure 3.69 A cat with paw pad ulcers and crusts due to lymphoma.

Paw pad (cont.)

b) Ulcerated
   Trauma
   Split pawpad disease (Figure 3.67)
   Immune-mediated disease (i.e. vasculitis [Figure 3.68], plasma cell pododermatitis)
   Neoplasia (i.e. SCC, cutaneous lymphoma, Figure 3.69)
c) Depigmented
   Immune-mediated disease (i.e. vitiligo if non-ulcerated, vasculitis)
   Neoplasia (i.e. cutaneous lymphoma [Figure 3.70A], amelanotic melanoma)

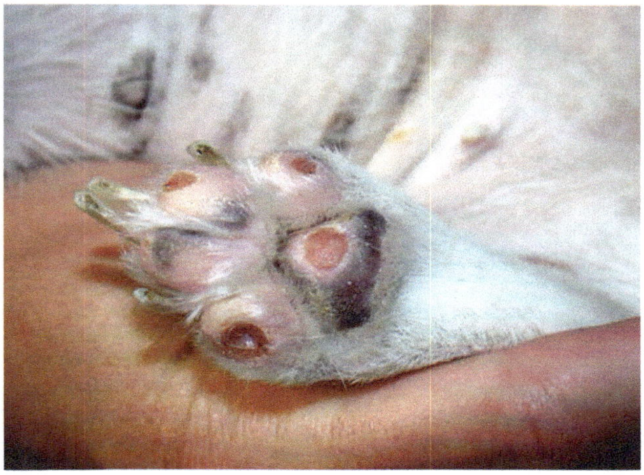

Figure 3.68 Central circular paw pad ulcerations in a terrier with rabies vaccine induced vasculitis.

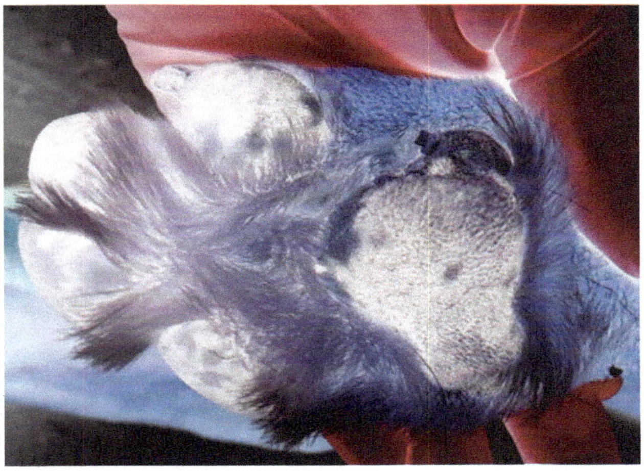

Figure 3.70A Paw pad depigmentation due to cutaneous lymphoma.

d) Mass or swelling
   Calcinosis circumscripta (Figure 3.70B)
   Fungal granuloma
   Neoplasia
   Plasma cell pododermatitis (Figures 3.70C and 3.70D)

3.3.4 Nailbed

a) Inflamed/moist/crusted
   Infection (bacterial and/or *Malassezia* secondary to hypersensitivity, Figures 3.71 and 3.72)
   Demodex
   Dermatophyte
   Immune-mediated (i.e. pemphigus [Figure 3.73], vasculitis, SLE)
b) Mass
   Neoplasia (i.e. SCC, melanoma, lymphoma, subungual keratoma)
   Viral papilloma

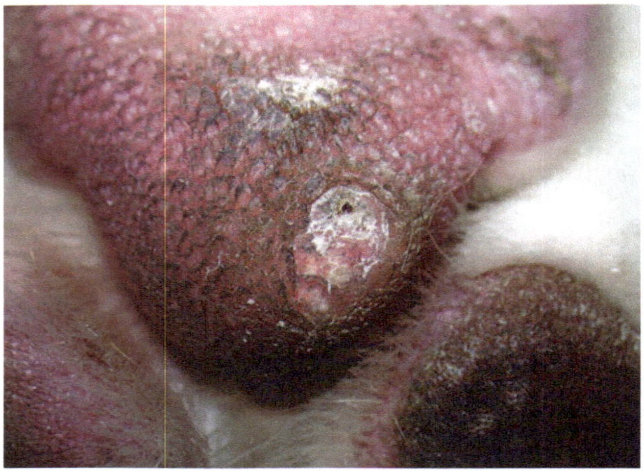

Figure 3.70B A firm, gritty pink to white mass on the paw pad caused by calcinosis circumscripta.

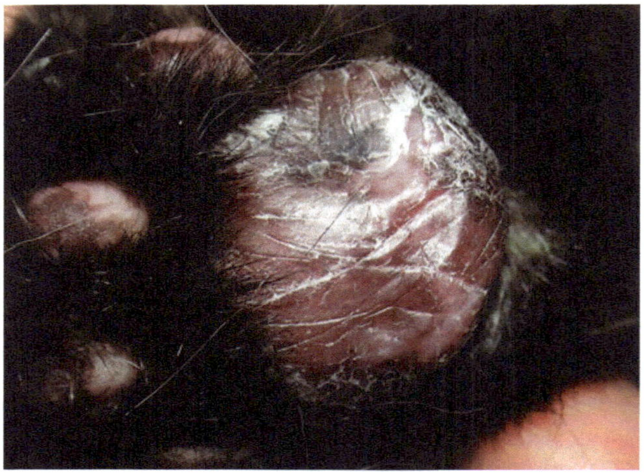

Figure 3.70C Diffuse spongy paw pad swelling and scaling in a cat with plasma cell pododermatitis.

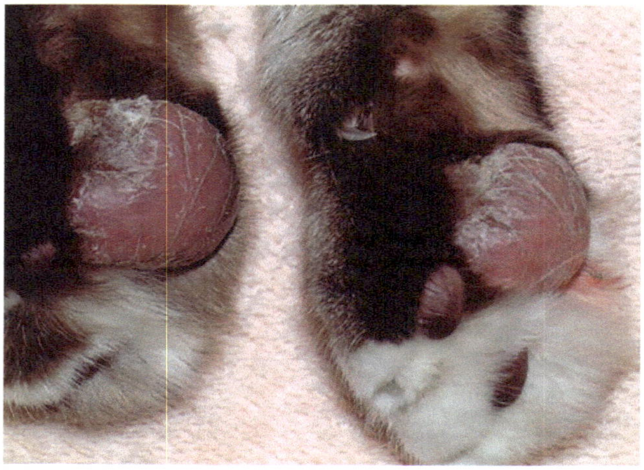

Figure 3.70D Plasma cell pododermatitis can affect one paw more severely or be bilaterally symmetric.

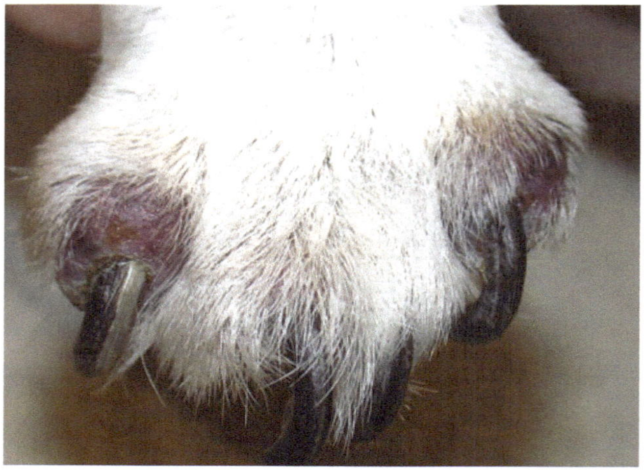

Figure 3.71A An atopic dog with bacterial paronychia.

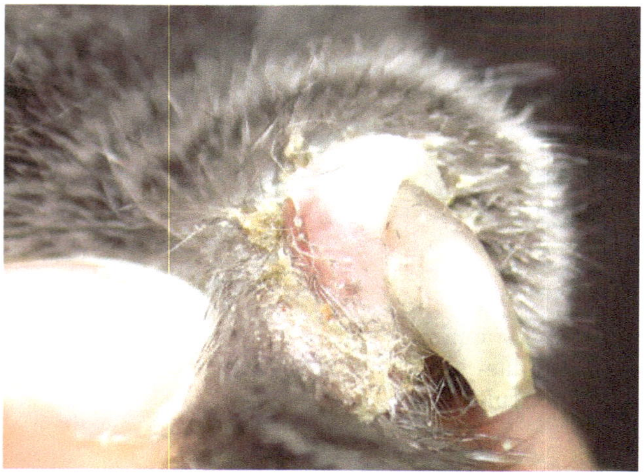

Figure 3.71B An atopic cat with bacterial paronychia.

3.4 Claws

a) Onychodystrophy/Onychogryphosis (abnormal, twisted, and or thickened)
   - One or two nails: dermatophytosis (Figure 3.74), trauma to nailbed, subungual keratoma, neoplasia (SCC/melanoma)
   - Multiple/most nails: Symmetric lupoid onychodystrophy (SLO) (Figure 3.75), vasculitis, severe dermatophytosis

b) Onychomadesis (nail loss)
   - One or two nails: dermatophytosis, trauma to nailbed, subungual keratoma, neoplasia
   - Multiple/most nails: SLO, vasculitis

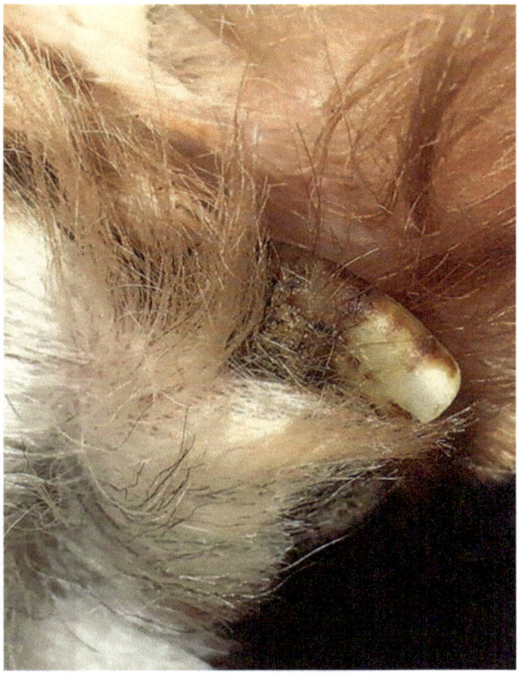

Figure 3.72 Brownish discoloration of the proximal toenail and nailbed due to *Malassezia* paronychia, secondary to atopy.

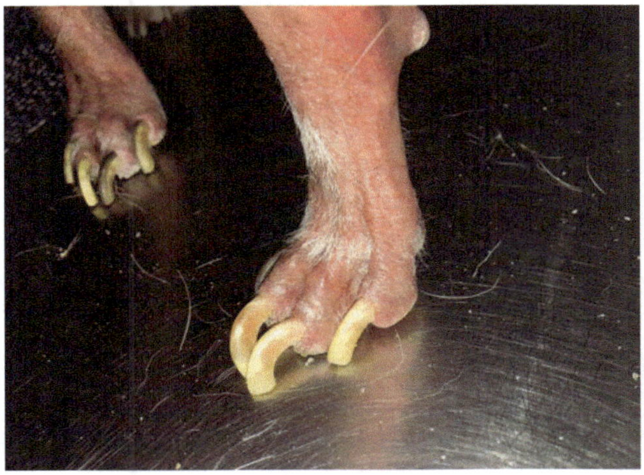

Figure 3.74 Thickened and yellowish toenails due to onychomycosis in a dog with generalized dermatophytosis.

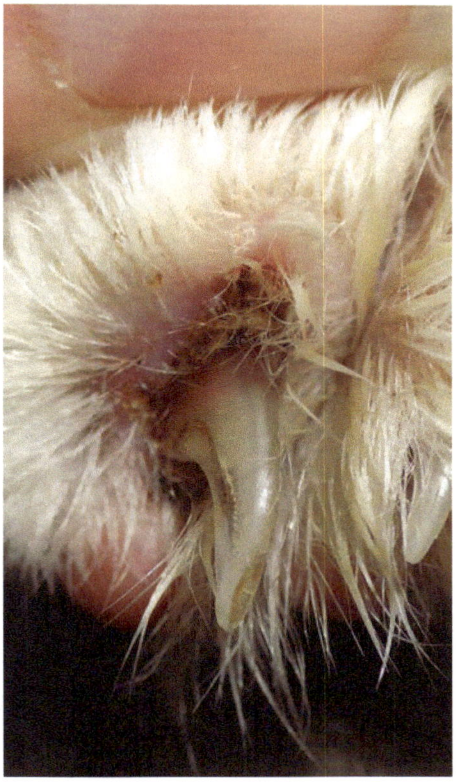

Figure 3.73 Purulent paronychia due to pemphigus foliaceus in a cat.

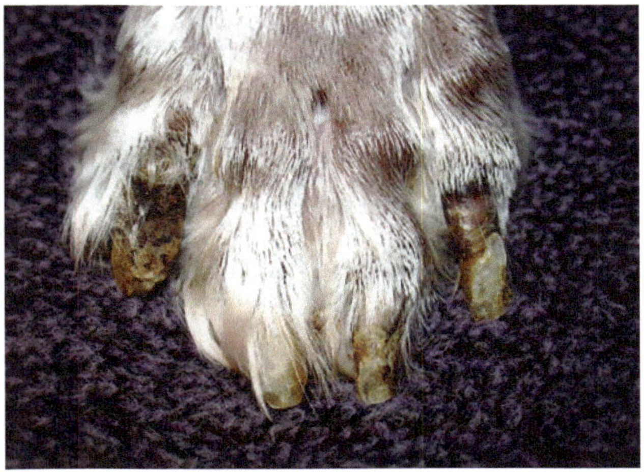

Figure 3.75 A dog with dystrophic, crumbly toenails due to lupoid onychodystrophy.

3.5 Perianal/perivulvar

a) Inflamed/moist/crusted +/– erosive
   - Infection (bacterial and/or *Malassezia* secondary to hypersensitivity, Figure 3.76)
   - Vulvar fold dermatitis due to conformation +/– urinary leakage
   - Immune-mediated disease (pemphigus/EM/mucous membrane pemphigoid/MCLE (mucocutaneous lupus erythematosus), Figure 3.77)

b) Draining tract
   - Anal sacculitis
   - Perianal fistula (Figure 3.78)
   - Deep bacterial or fungal infection

c) Mass
   - Neoplasia
   - Perianal adenoma

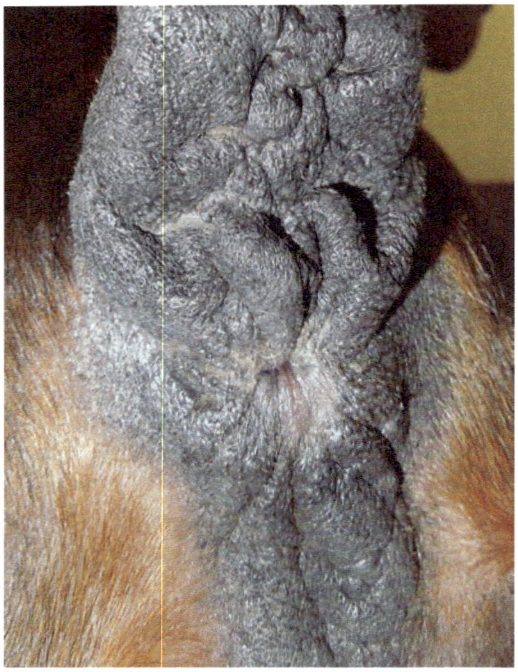

Figure 3.76 Perianal inflammation and lichenification due to chronic bacterial and yeast infection, secondary to atopy.

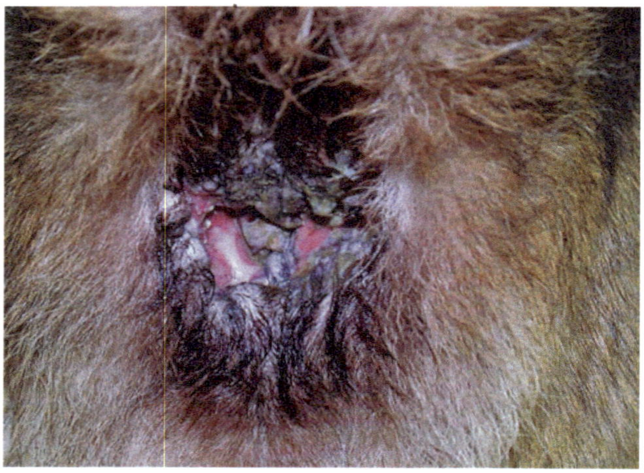

Figure 3.78 A German Shepherd with deep draining tracts due to perianal fistulas.

3.6 Tail

a) Alopecia
   - Endocrinopathy (hypothyroid [Figure 3.79], Cushing's, sex hormone, [Figure 3.80])
   - Vasculitis (tail tip, Figure 3.81)
   - Repetitive trauma ("happy tail," Figure 3.82)
   - Tail gland hyperplasia (focal alopecia on dorsal proximal tail, Figure 3.83)
   - Sebaceous adenitis (Figure 3.84)

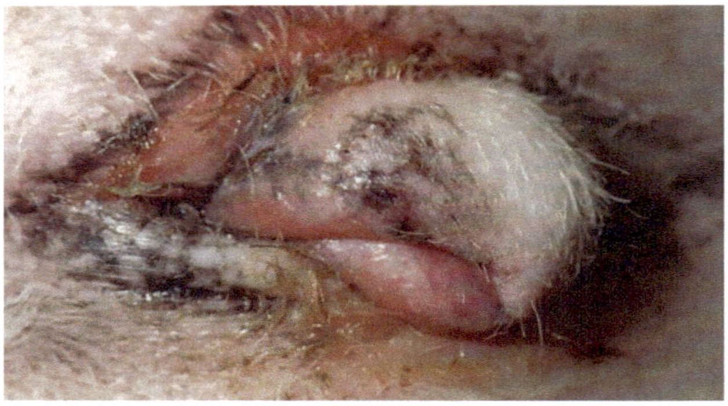

Figure 3.77 Vulvar and perivulvar ulceration and post-inflammatory hyperpigmentation in a dog with mucocutaneous lupus erythematosus (MCLE).

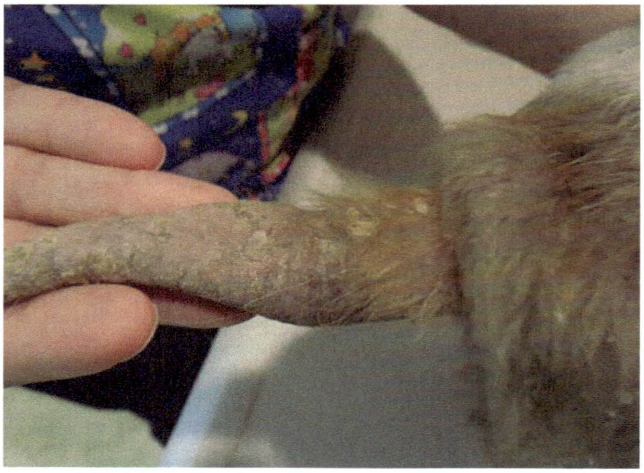

Figure 3.79 Tail alopecia due to hypothyroidism and secondary pyoderma.

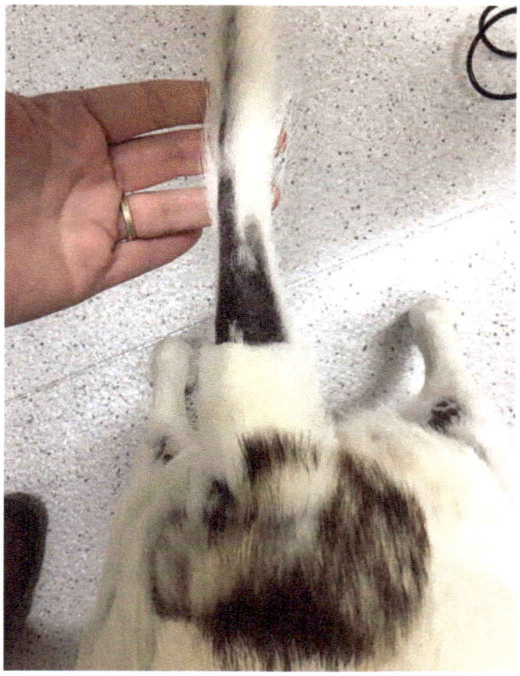

Figure 3.80 Tail alopecia due to sex hormone imbalance.

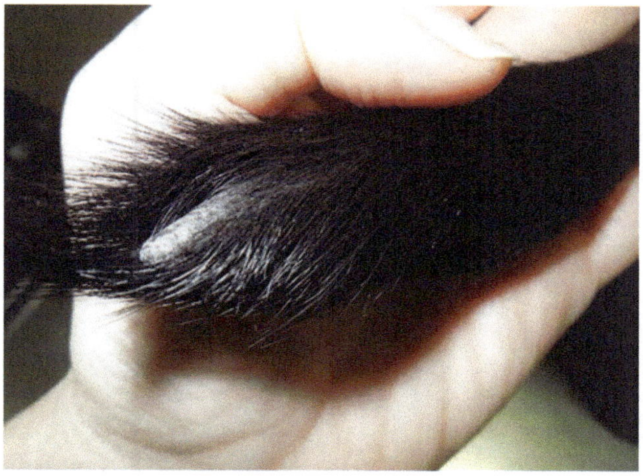

Figure 3.81 Tail tip scarring alopecia due to vasculitis.

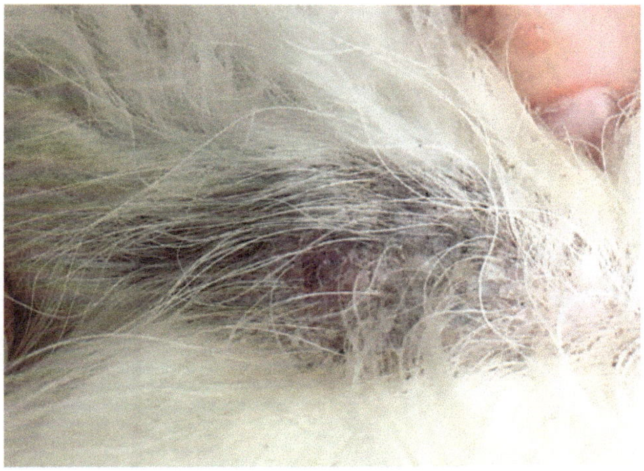

Figure 3.83 Hypotrichosis and comedone formation on the dorsal proximal tail due to tail gland hyperplasia.

Tail (cont.)

b) Scaling/crusting
   Infection (bacterial/fungal [Figure 3.85]/*Demodex*, [Figure 3.86])
   Sebaceous adenitis
   Pemphigus foliaceus (other areas will be affected)

3.7 Pressure points (elbows/hocks)

a) Callus (non-pruritic alopecic thickened lesion due to friction, common in large heavy dogs, Figure 3.87)
b) Pyoderma (pustules/draining tracts due to excessive friction pushing hairs into follicles, Figure 3.88)
c) Scabies (pruritic crusts/alopecia/excoriations, Figure 3.89)
d) Pressure sore (focal deep ulcer, often infected)
e) Calcinosis circumscripta (alopecic or haired dermal mass which contains white gritty acellular material on aspirate)

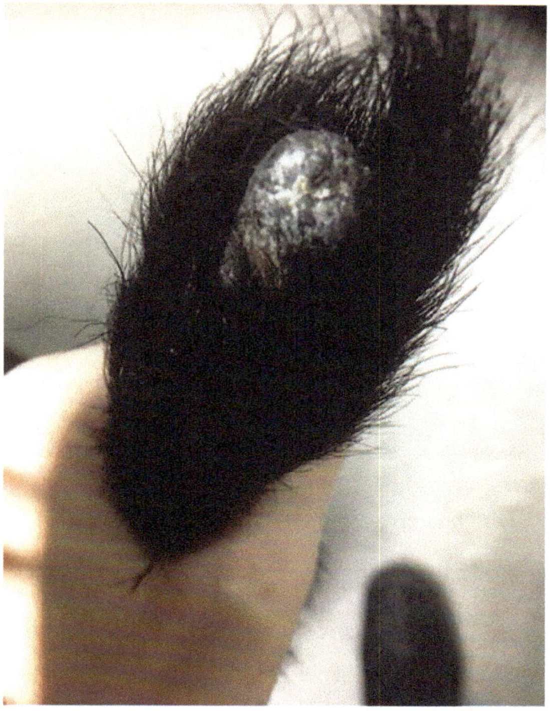

Figure 3.82 Tail tip swelling and scarring due to repetitive trauma ("happy tail").

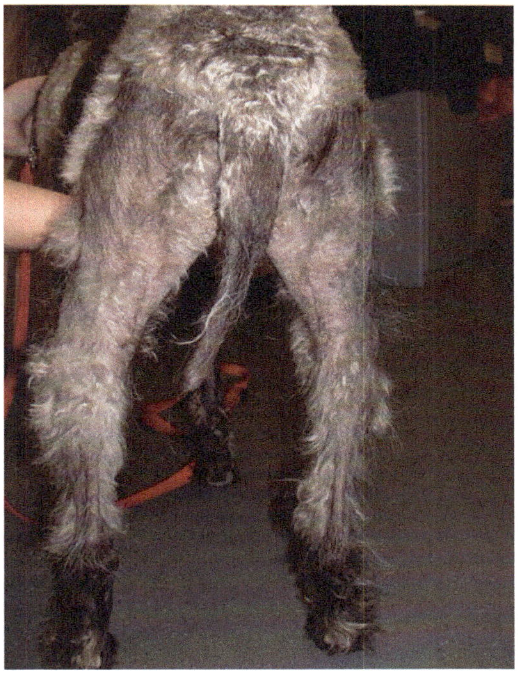

Figure 3.84 Tail hypotrichosis due to sebaceous adenitis.

f) Follicular cysts due to pressure (Figure 3.90A)
g) Vasculitis (crusted +/− ulcerated, Figure 3.90B)
h) Hepatocutaneous syndrome (crusted/inflamed; pawpads usually also affected; Figure 3.90C)

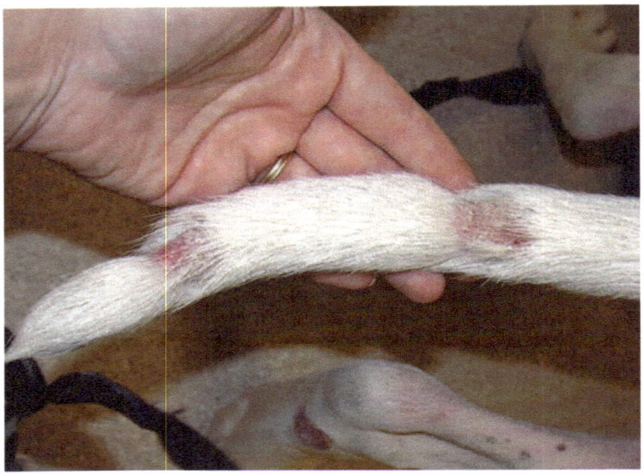

Figure 3.85 Multifocal areas of alopecia and scaling on the tail of a dog with dermatophytosis.

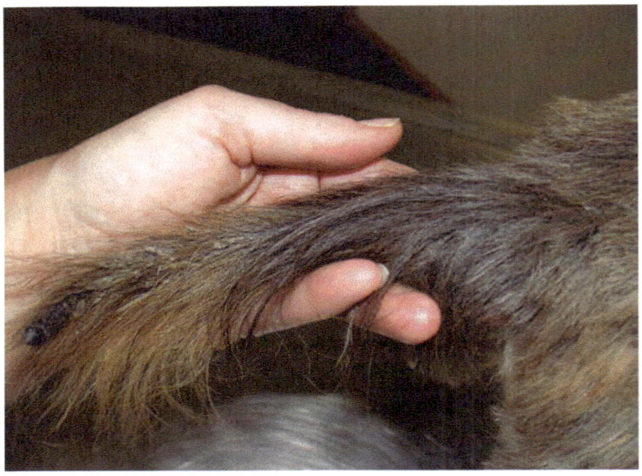

Figure 3.86 Crusting and hair loss on the tail due to generalized *Demodex*.

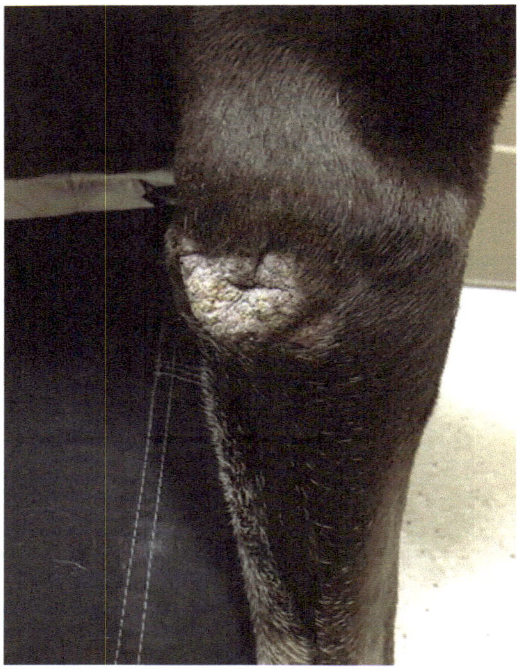

Figure 3.87 Elbow callus in a large-breed dog.

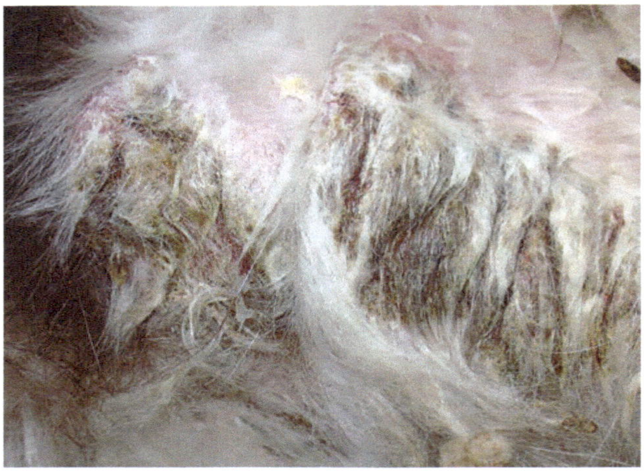

Figure 3.88 Severe elbow callus dermatitis and furunculosis in a dog with hepatocutaneous syndrome.

3.8 Trunk (dorsal and/or lateral)

a) Alopecia – symmetric, not inflamed or pruritic
   - Endocrinopathy (hypothyroid, hyperadrenocorticism, sex hormone dermatosis, Figures 3.91A and 3.91B)
   - Alopecia X (Figure 3.92)
   - Color dilution alopecia/black hair follicular dysplasia (Figure 3.93)
   - Canine recurrent flank alopecia (Chapter 2, Figure 2.32; Chapter 6, Figures 6.5, 6.23)

b) Alopecia – lumbar/tailhead
   - Flea bite hypersensitivity (Figures 3.94A and 3.94B)

c) Alopecia – asymmetric/patchy or focal
   - Infection (bacterial/fungal/*Demodex*; Figures 3.95–3.97)
   - Pruritus due to underlying hypersensitivity dermatitis (parasite/atopy/food, Figures 3.98A, 3.98B, and 3.99)
   - Solar dermatitis (white haired areas; Figure 3.100)
   - Immune-mediated (alopecia areata, [Figure 3.101], vaccine-induced localized vasculitis [Chapter 6, Figures 6.42, 6.43, and 6.58])

d) Papules/pustules/crusts
   - Infection (bacterial/fungal/*Demodex*; Figures 3.102–3.104)
   - Post-grooming furunculosis (occurs within 1–5 days post grooming, often due to *Pseudomonas*, very painful, multifocal draining ulcers, Figures 3.105A and 3.105B)

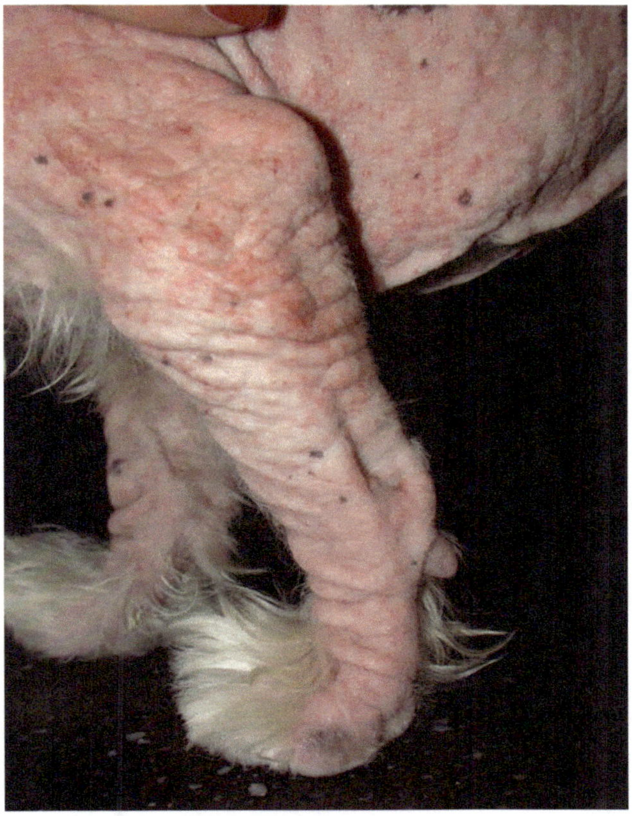

Figure 3.89 Scabies causes pruritus, alopecia, papules, and crusts which commonly affect elbows and hocks.

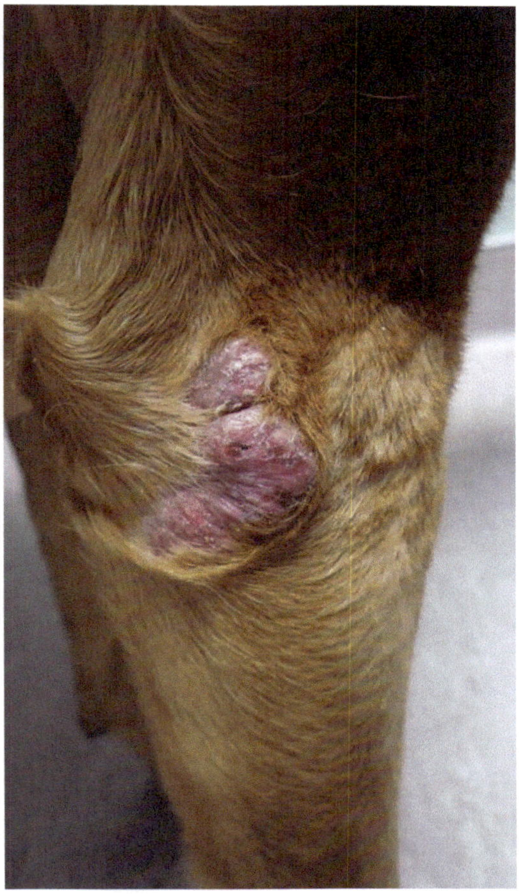

Figure 3.90A Raised pink alopecic nodules to plaques on the elbow of a large-breed dog which were determined to be follicular cysts which formed secondary to chronic friction and trauma to the hair follicles on this pressure point.

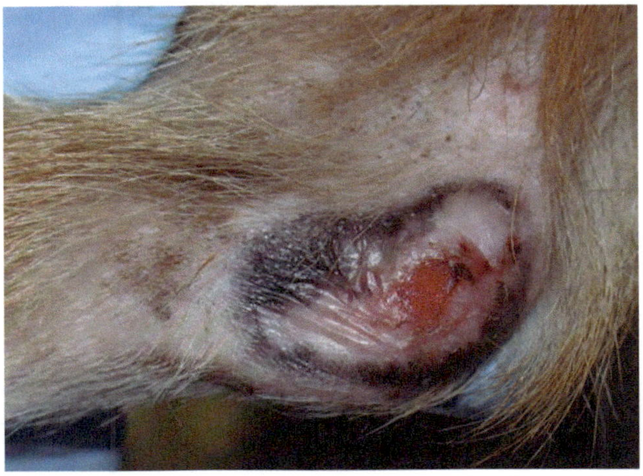

Figure 3.90B Erosions and crusts on the hock due to vasculitis.

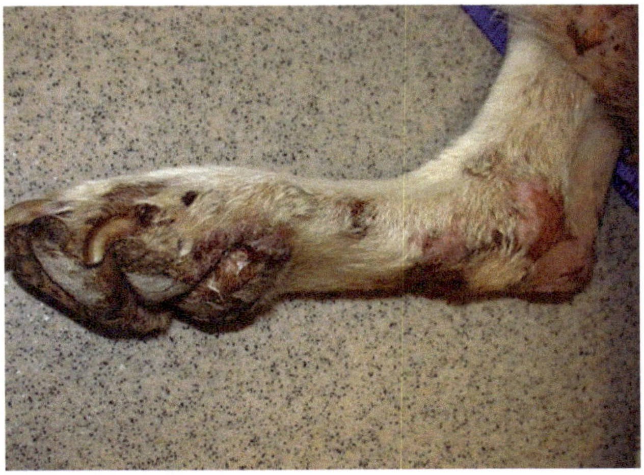

Figure 3.90C Hock crusts and ulcerations due to hepatocutaneous syndrome; note the marked paw pad hyperkeratosis.

Trunk – dorsal and/or lateral (cont.)

Pemphigus foliaceus (Figure 3.106)
Solar dermatosis (Figure 3.107)

e) Comedones

Schnauzer comedone syndrome (Figure 3.108)
Endocrinopathy (hypothyroid, hyperadrenocorticism, sex hormone dermatosis)

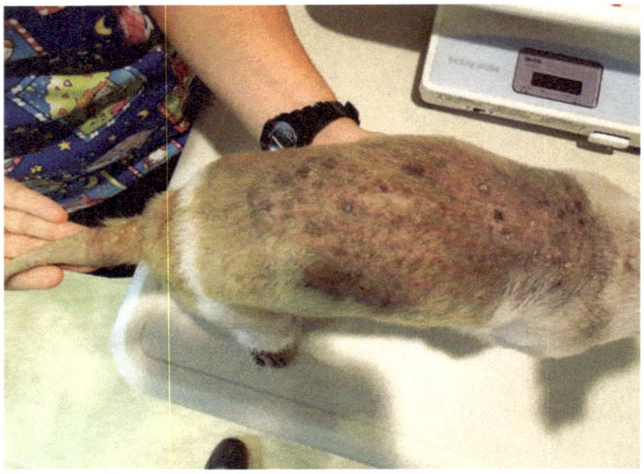

Figure 3.91A Truncal alopecia due hypothyroidism and a secondary bacterial pyoderma.

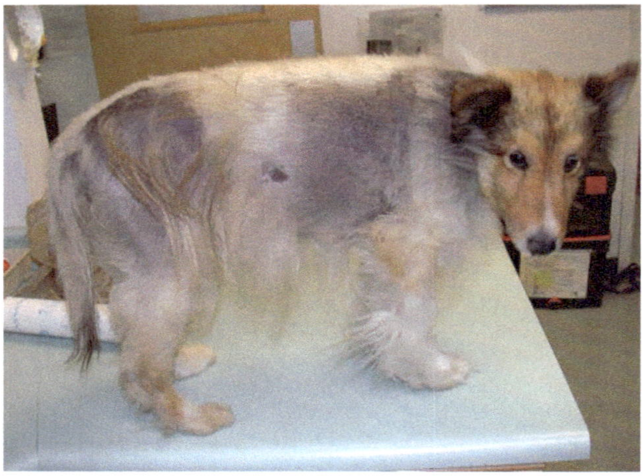

Figure 3.91B Truncal hypotrichosis due to Cushing's disease.

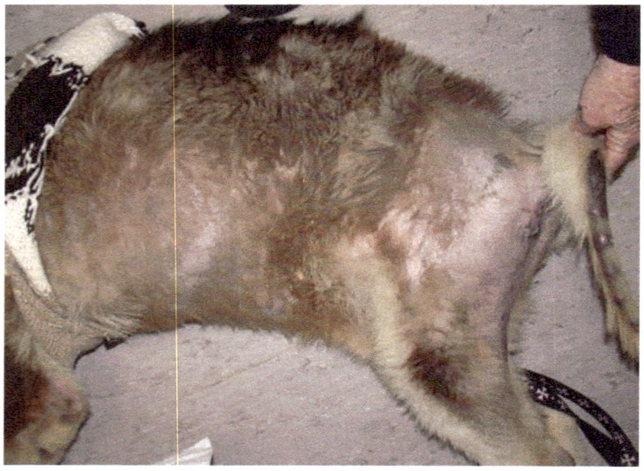

Figure 3.92 A Husky with alopecia involving the trunk, proximal limbs, and tail due to Alopecia X.

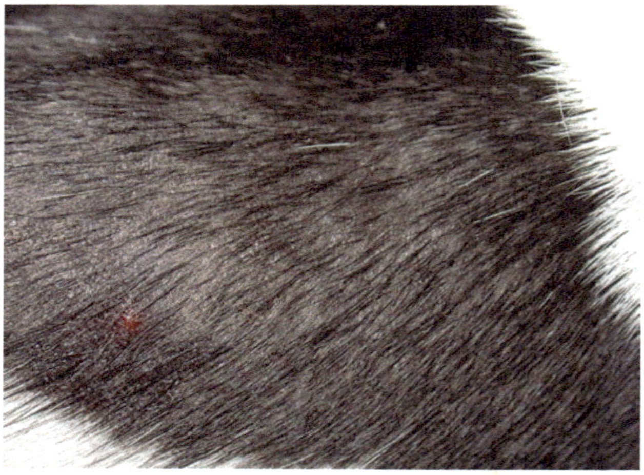

Figure 3.93 Truncal alopecia involving only the black hairs in a dog with black hair follicular dysplasia.

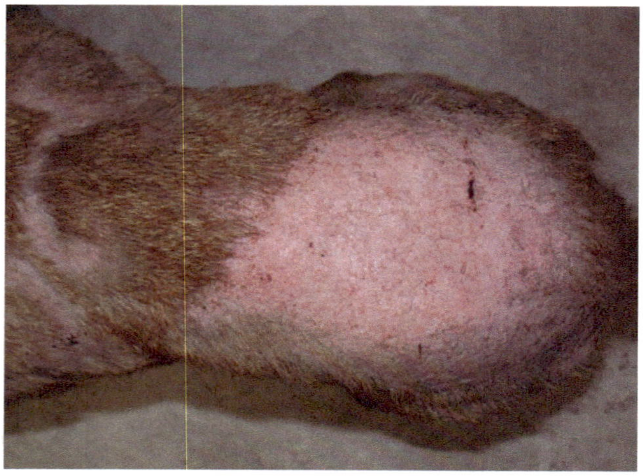

Figure 3.94A Lumbar alopecia and erythema in a dog caused by barbering due to flea bite hypersensitivity.

Trunk – dorsal and/or lateral (cont.)

Infection (bacterial/*Demodex*/dermatophyte, Chapter 2, Figures 2.43 and 2.44)
Solar dermatitis (white-skinned areas, Figure 3.109)

f) Follicular casting
   Sebaceous adenitis (Figure 3.110)
g) Greasy dorsal truncal haircoat
   Infection (bacterial, yeast, *Demodex injai*, [Figure 3.111])
h) Plaque
   Calcinosis cutis (Figure 3.112)
i) Easily torn skin
   Ehlers Danlos (Figure 3.113)
   Feline fragile skin syndrome (Figure 3.114)

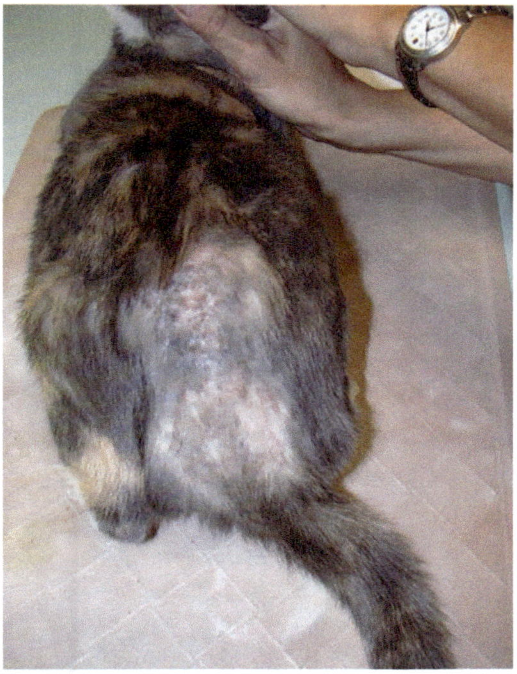

Figure 3.94B Lumbar alopecia and erythema in a cat caused by barbering due to flea bite hypersensitivity.

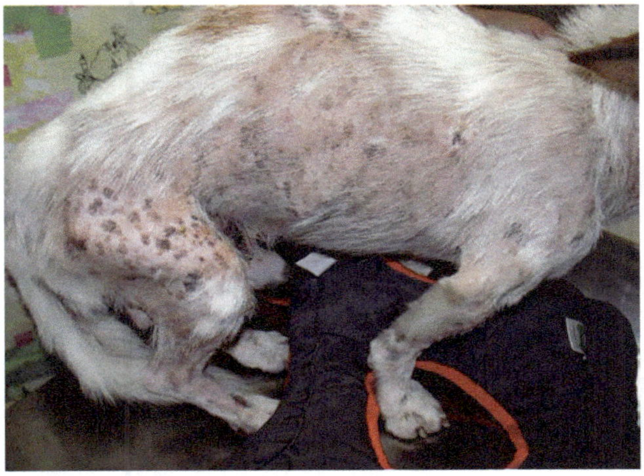

Figure 3.96 Patchy truncal alopecia due to generalized demodicosis.

Trunk – dorsal and/or lateral (cont.)

j) Draining tracts
   - Panniculitis – sterile/immune-mediated (Figures 3.115–3.118)
   - Panniculitis – infectious (mycobacterial, *Actinomyces* [Figure 3.119], *Nocardia*)
   - Foreign body (grass awn)

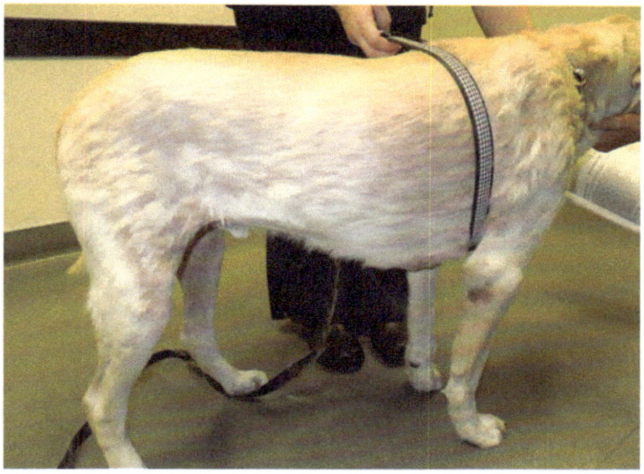

Figure 3.95 Patchy truncal hypotrichosis in a dog with bacterial folliculitis.

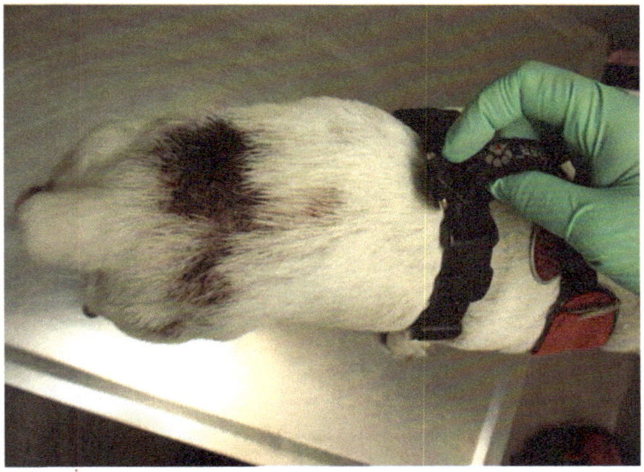

Figure 3.97 Scarring alopecia and hyperpigmentation on the trunk caused by dermatophytosis.

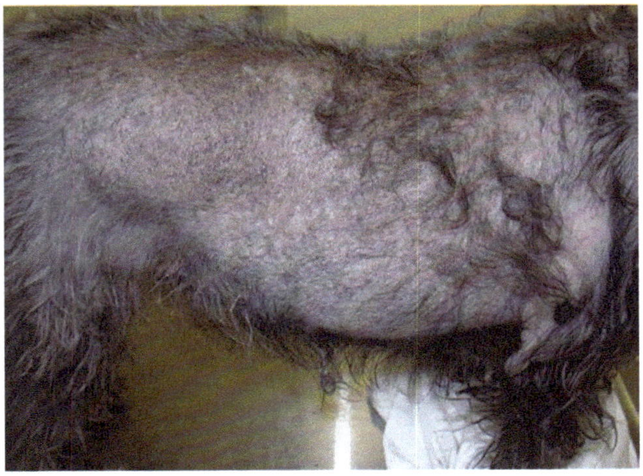

Figure 3.98A Truncal barbering due to atopic dermatitis in a dog.

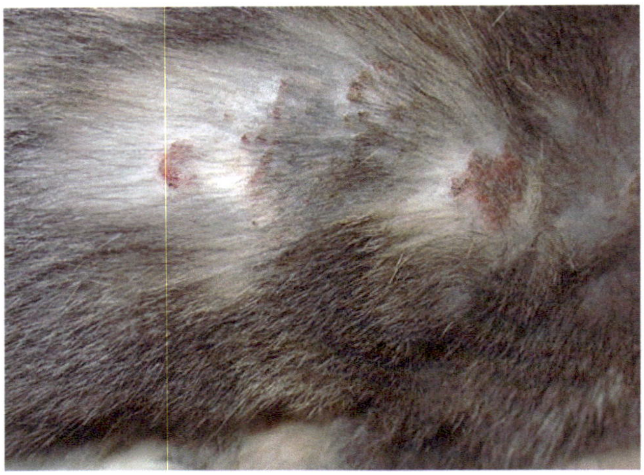

Figure 3.98B Truncal barbering due to atopic dermatitis in a cat.

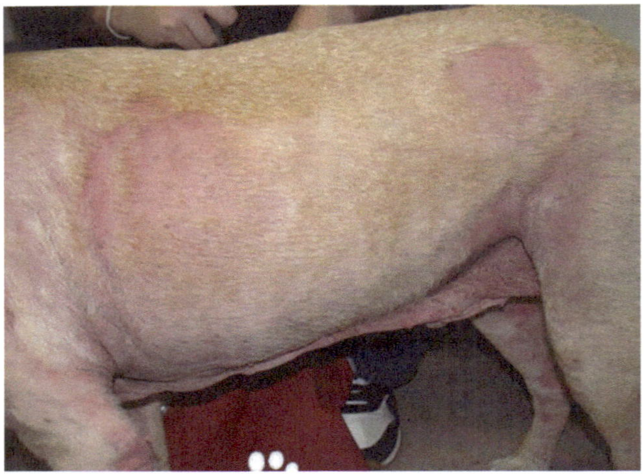

Figure 3.99 Patchy truncal barbering and erythema in a dog with food allergy.

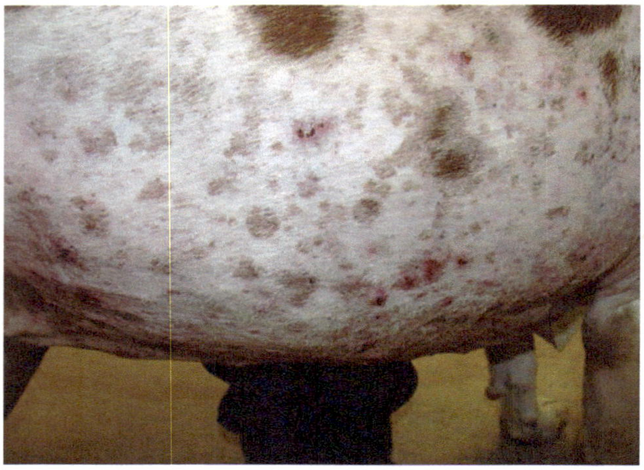

Figure 3.100 A Pit bull Terrier with truncal hypotrichosis and crusts due to solar dermatitis.

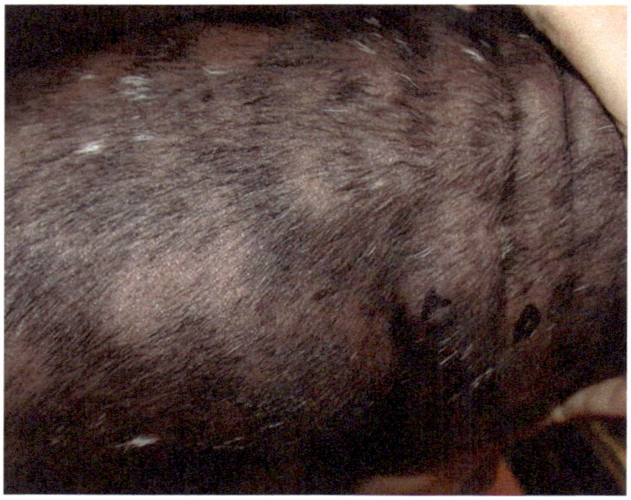

Figure 3.101 A dog with extensive non-pruritic truncal hypotrichosis which was determined on biopsy to be due to alopecia areata.

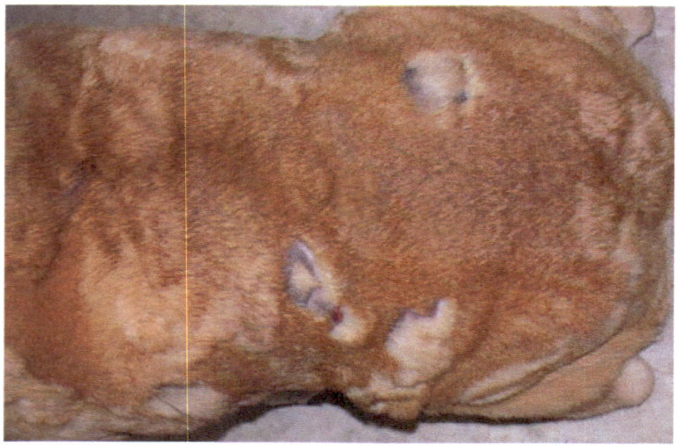

Figure 3.102A Patchy areas of truncal crusting and alopecia due to bacterial pyoderma in an atopic dog.

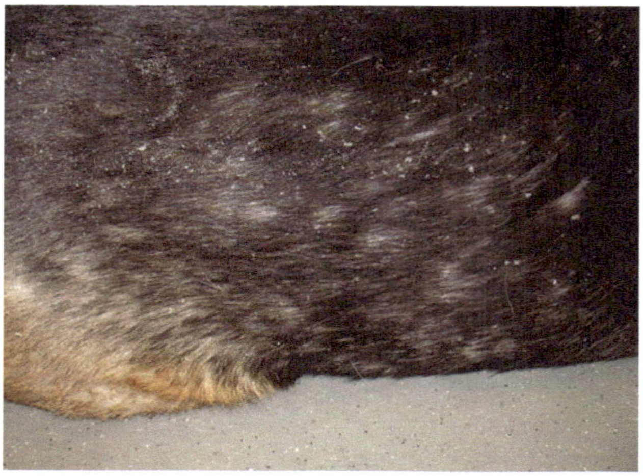

Figure 3.102B Patchy areas of truncal crusting and alopecia due to bacterial pyoderma in an atopic dog.

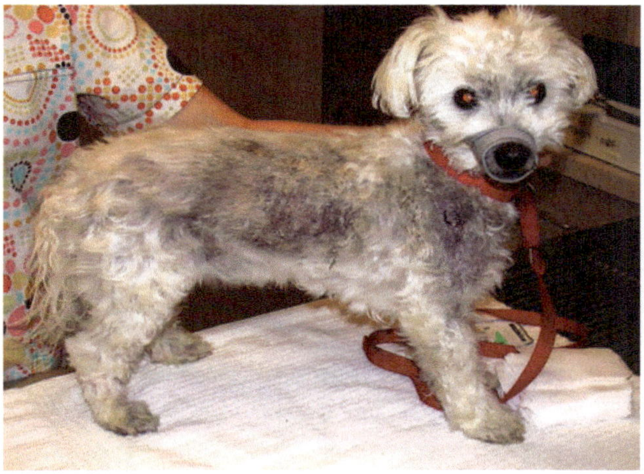

Figure 3.103 Truncal alopecia due to generalized demodicosis in a dog receiving chronic steroids for an autoimmune disorder.

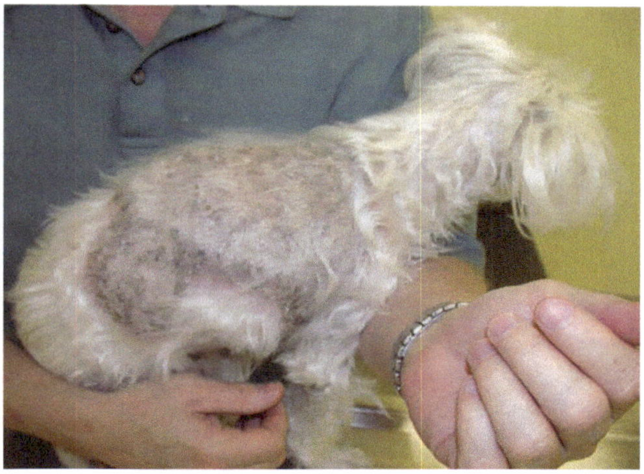

Figure 3.104 Extensive truncal crusting caused by dermatophytosis in a dog with Cushing's disease.

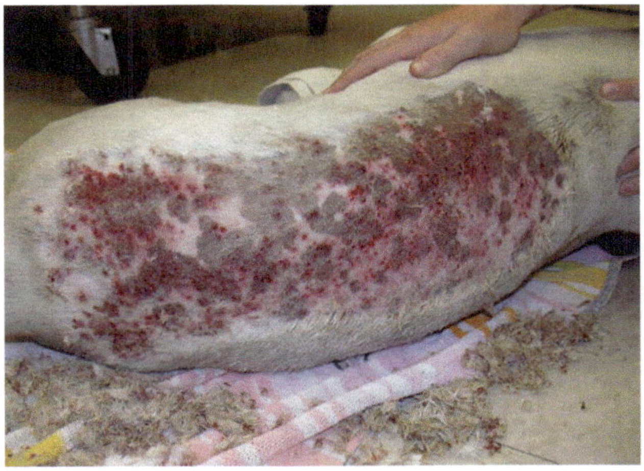

Figure 3.105A American Bulldog with post-grooming furunculosis; sedation was required for shaving due to marked pain.

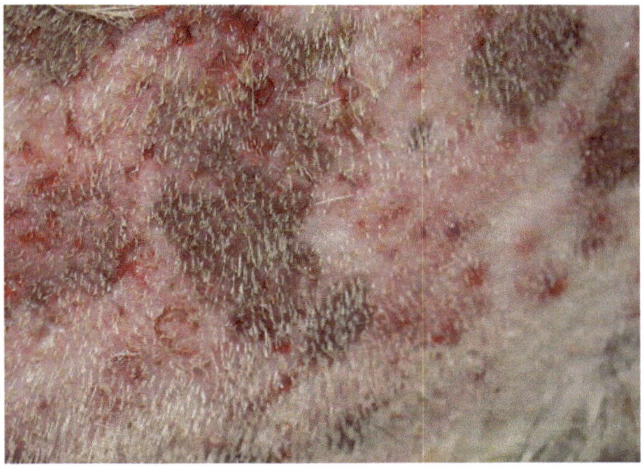

Figure 3.105B Close-up of the same dog demonstrating hemorrhagic ruptured follicles.

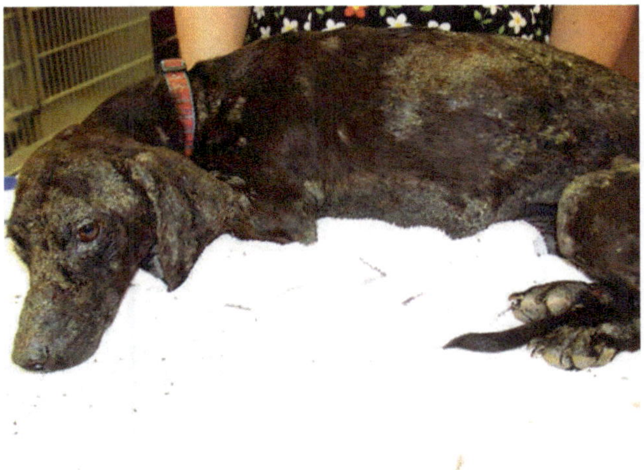

Figure 3.106 Severe generalized and truncal crusting due to pemphigus foliaceus.

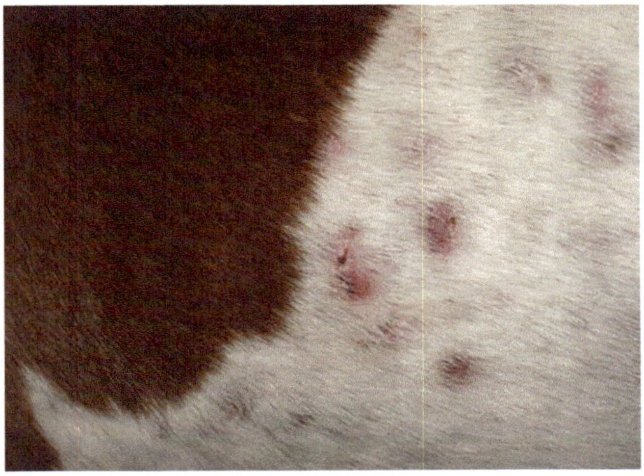

Figure 3.107 A dog with solar dermatosis; note the crusts and inflammatory bullae are restricted to non-pigmented areas.

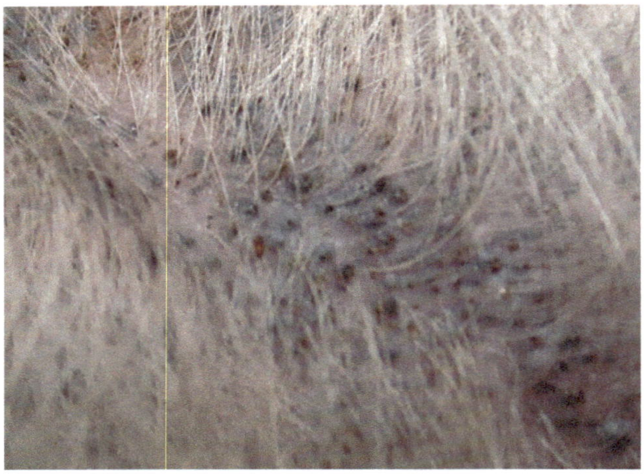

Figure 3.108 Comedones on the dorsal midline of a Miniature Schnauzer.

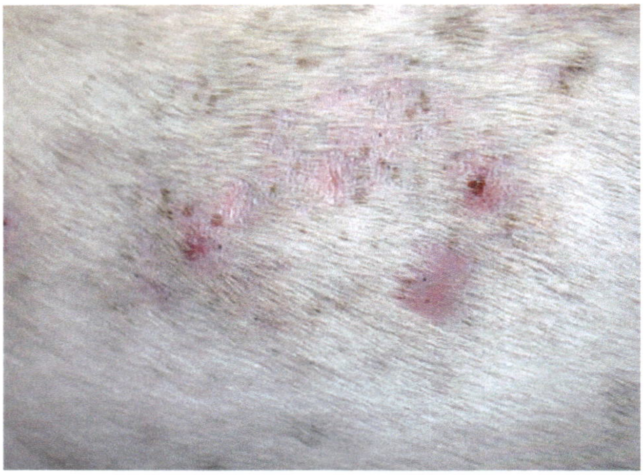

Figure 3.109 Comedones on the lateral trunk of a sunbathing American Bulldog indicative of solar dermatosis.

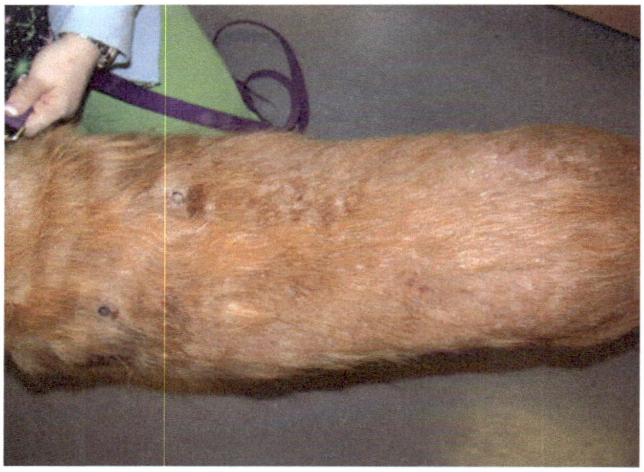

Figure 3.110 A dog with truncal hypotrichosis and follicular casting caused by sebaceous adenitis.

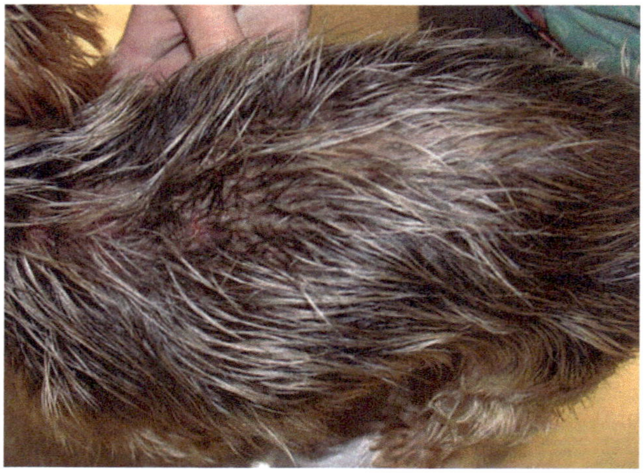

Figure 3.111 A Terrier with an extremely greasy truncal hair coat caused by *Demodex injai*.

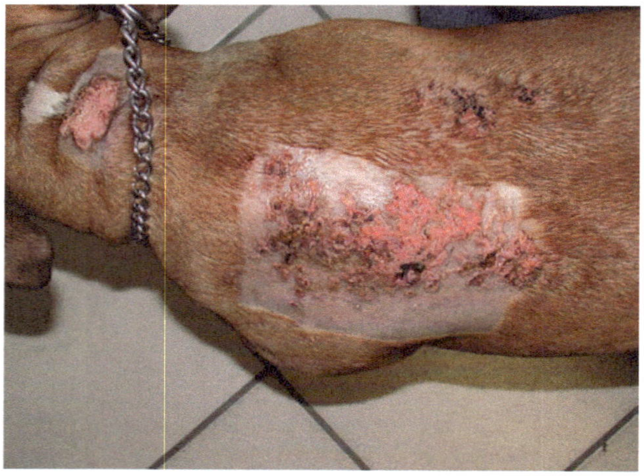

Figure 3.112 Raised inflamed, gritty, dorsal truncal plaques due to calcinosis cutis caused by prolonged steroid administration.

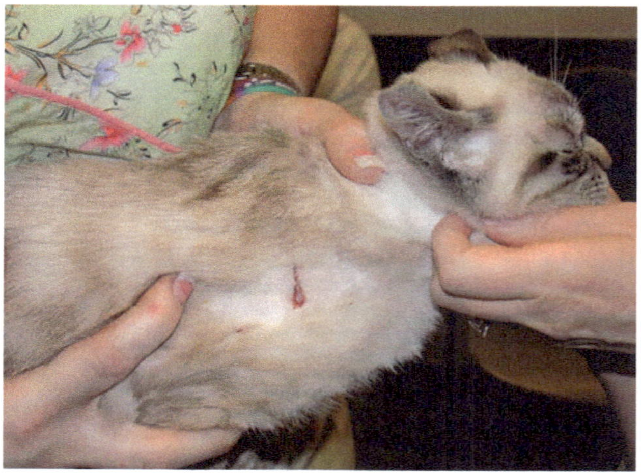

Figure 3.113 A young cat with no history of steroid exposure, but easily torn skin due to Ehlers Danlos.

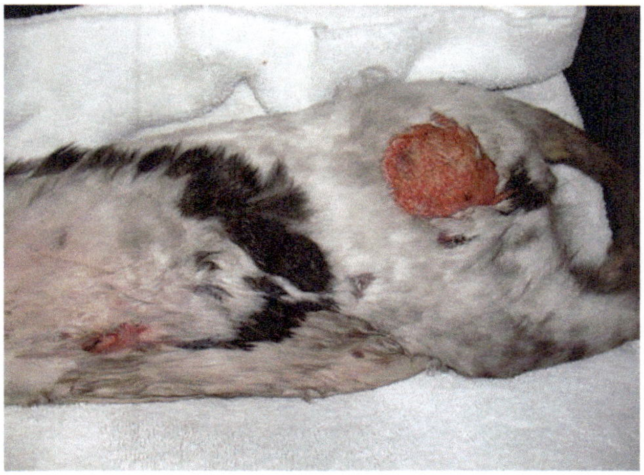

Figure 3.114 Feline fragile skin syndrome due to Cushing's disease causing large areas of skin tearing.

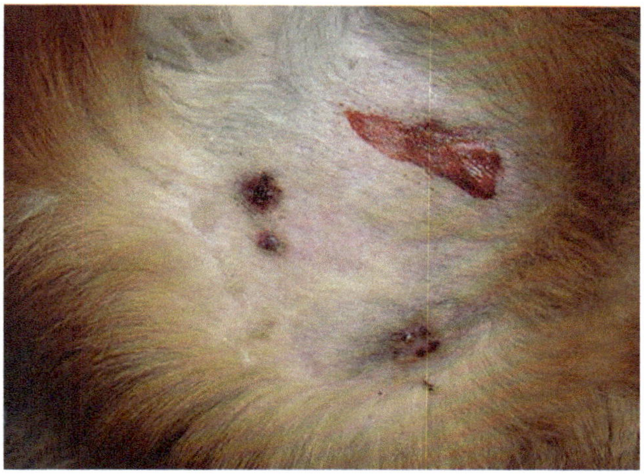

Figure 3.115 A Sheltie with truncal draining tracts due to sterile panniculitis.

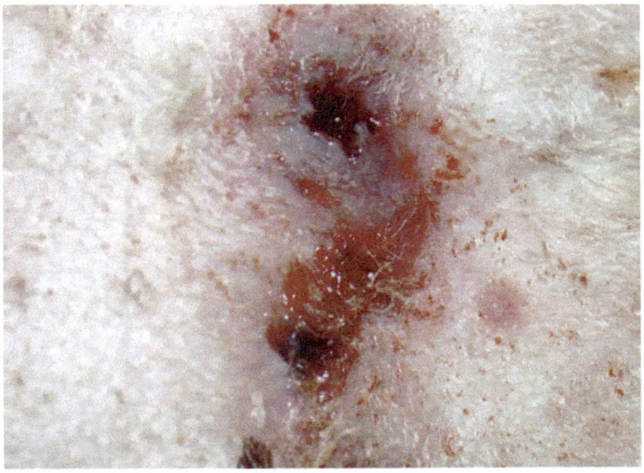

Figure 3.116 Truncal draining tracts due to sterile panniculitis.

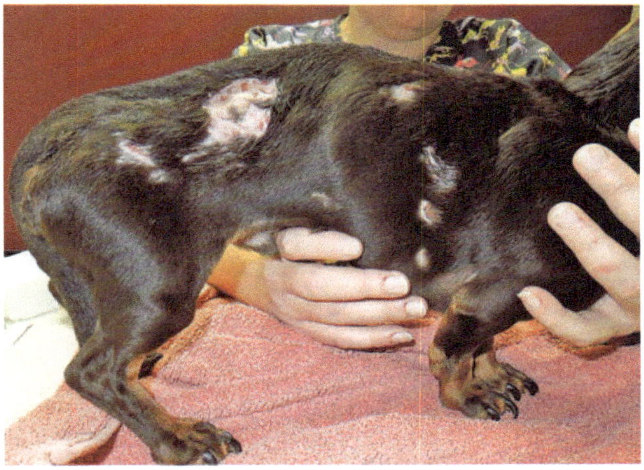

Figure 3.117 A Miniature Dachshund with truncal draining tracts and scarring due to sterile panniculitis.

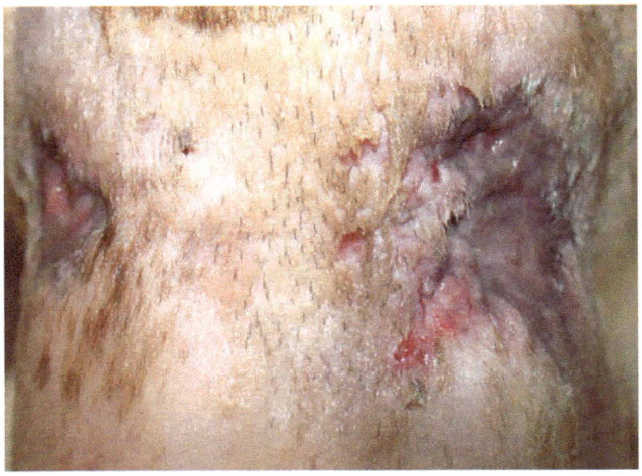

Figure 3.118 Truncal draining tracts due to sterile panniculitis complicated by methicillin resistant Staph infection.

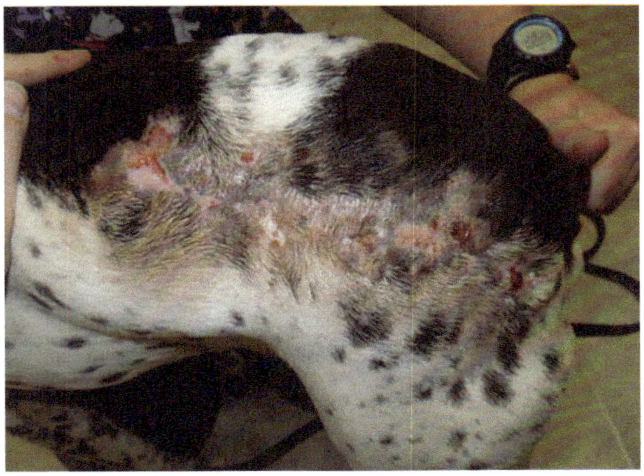

Figure 3.119 Truncal draining tracts and scarring in this hunting dog were due to actinomycosis likely carried in by a migrating foxtail.

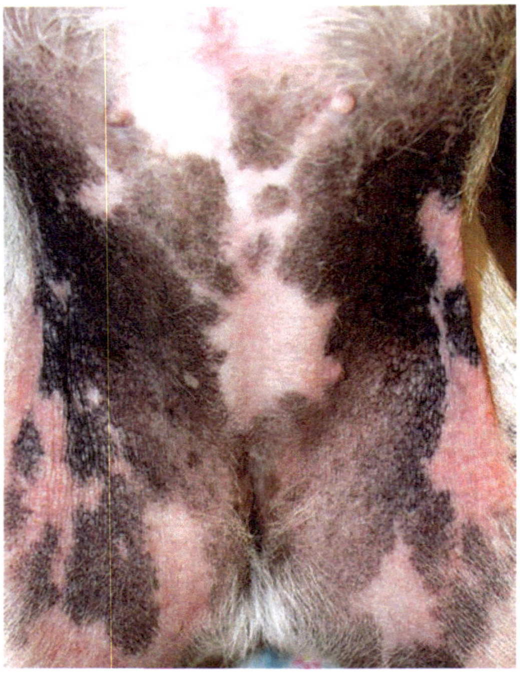

Figure 3.120A Inguinal erythema due to atopic dermatitis.

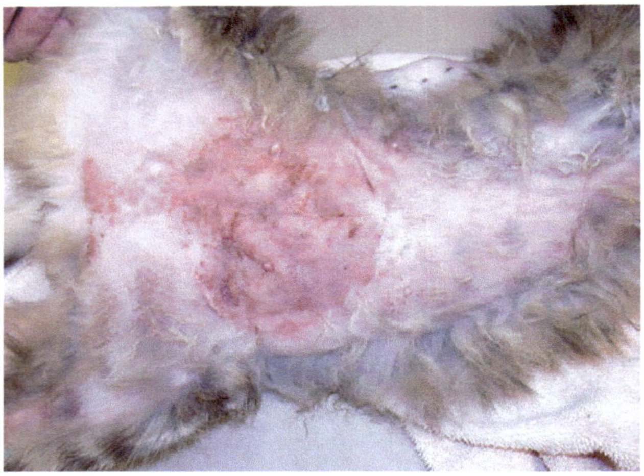

Figure 3.120B Inguinal erythema and moist dermatitis caused by overgrooming in an atopic cat.

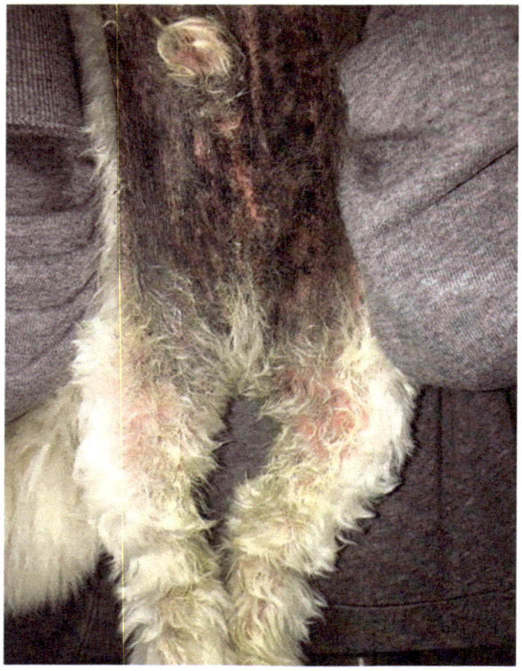

Figure 3.121 Intense inguinal erythema and post-inflammatory hyperpigmentation caused by bacterial overgrowth in an atopic dog.

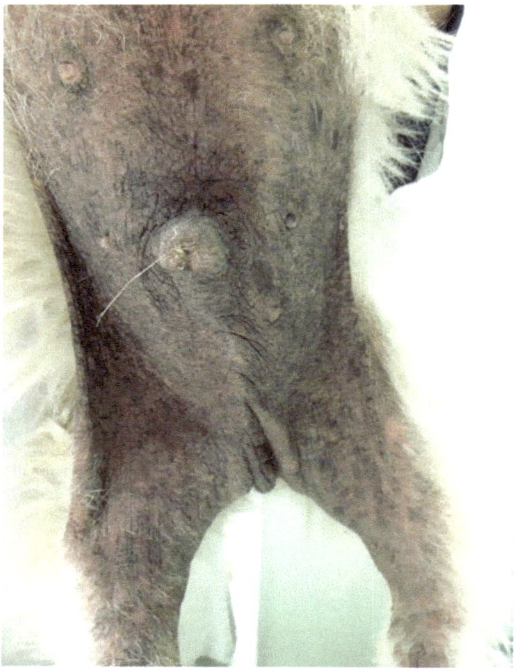

Figure 3.122A Inguinal erythema and lichenification due to *Malassezia* dermatitis triggered by food allergy.

3.9 Inguinal/axillary

a) Erythema
   Hypersensitivity dermatitis (atopy [Figures 3.120A and 3.120B], food allergy, contact)
   Infection (bacterial/fungal/*Demodex*, Figures 3.121, 3.122A, and 3.122B)
   Solar dermatosis

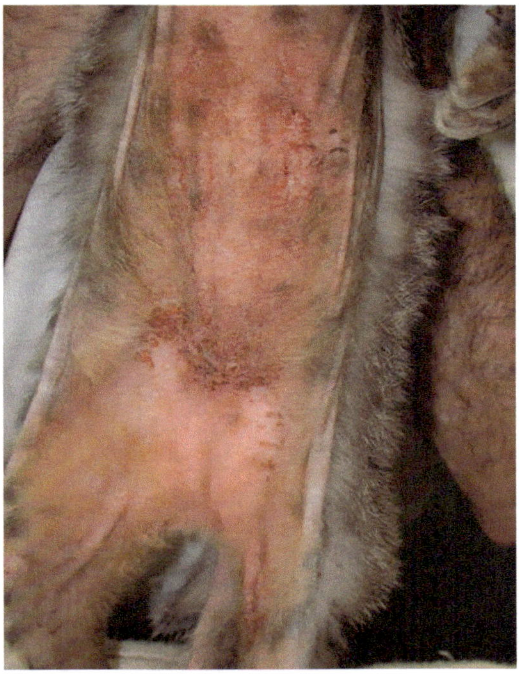

Figure 3.122B An atopic cat with inguinal *Malassezia* dermatitis.

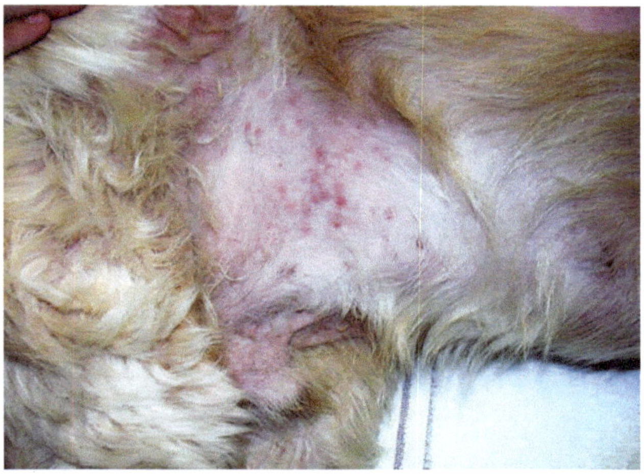

Figure 3.123 Inguinal papulocrusting dermatitis caused by a bacterial folliculitis in an atopic dog.

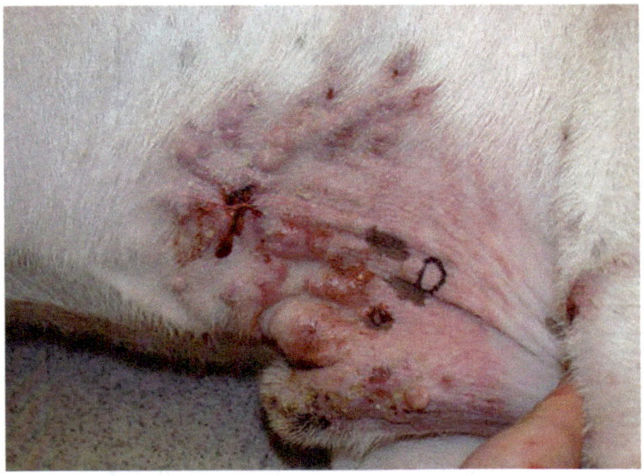

Figure 3.124 Inguinal crusts and bullae due to chronic solar dermatosis.

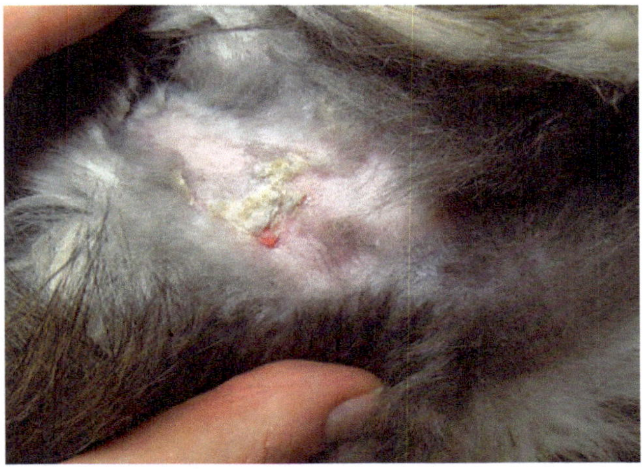

Figure 3.125 Periareolar crusting in a cat with pemphigus foliaceus.

Inguinal/axillary (cont.)

b) Papules/pustules/crusts
   - Infection (bacterial/fungal/*Demodex*; Figure 3.123)
   - Solar dermatosis (Figure 3.124)
   - Immune-mediated disease (i.e. periareolar crusting in feline pemphigus foliaceus, Figure 3.125)

c) Lichenification
   - Bacterial and/or *Malassezia* overgrowth (Figure 3.126A and 3.126B)

d) Comedones
   - Endocrinopathy (hypothyroidism, hyperadrenocorticism, sex hormone dermatosis; Figures 3.127A and 3.127B)
   - Infection (bacterial/*Demodex*/dermatophyte, Chapter 2, Figures 2.43 and 2.44)
   - Solar dermatosis

e) Plaques
   - Calcinosis cutis (Figure 3.128)
   - Eosinophilic plaque (Figure 3.129)

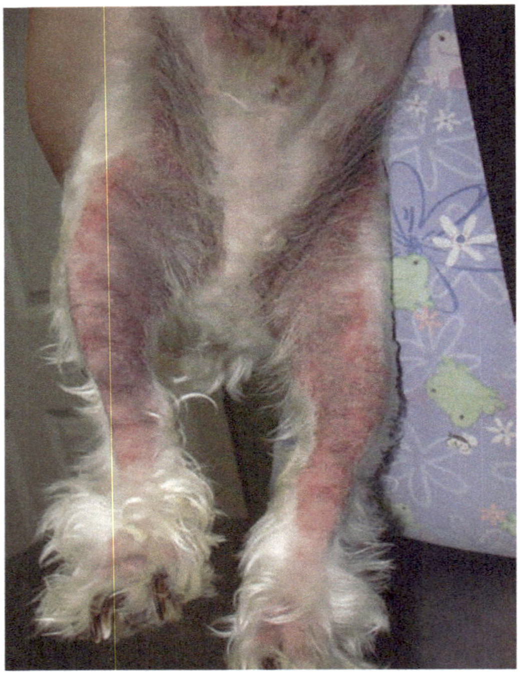

Figure 3.126A Inguinal lichenification due to bacterial overgrowth in an atopic dog.

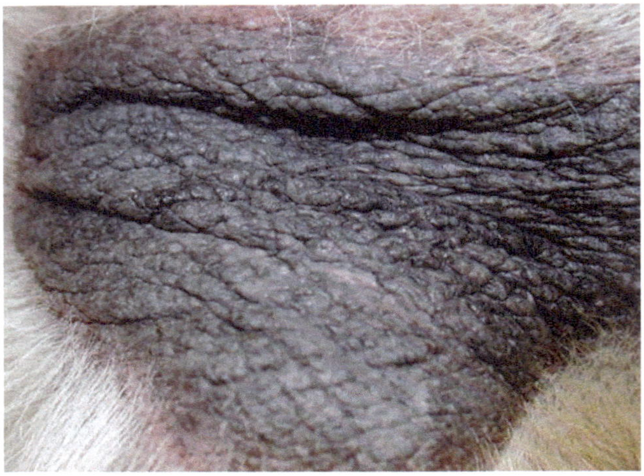

Figure 3.126B Inguinal lichenification and hyperpigmentation due to *Malassezia* dermatitis triggered by atopy.

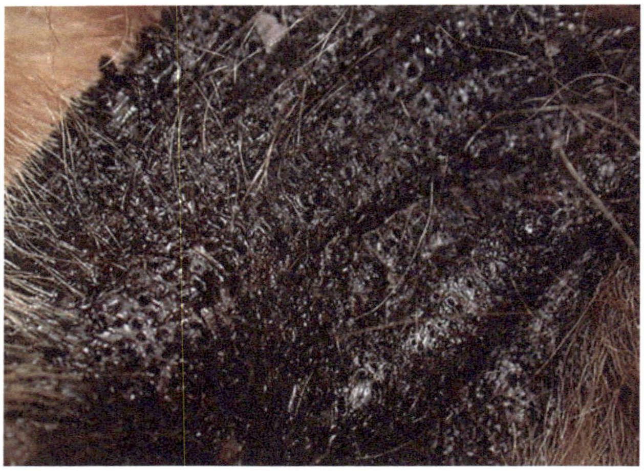

Figure 3.127A Marked inguinal comedone formation as well as hyperpigmentation due to hypothyroidism.

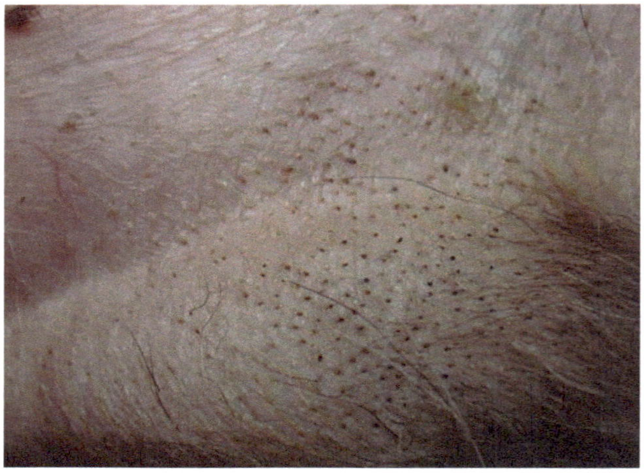

Figure 3.127B Inguinal comedones induced by chronic exogenous steroid treatment.

Inguinal/axillary (cont.)

f) Ulceration
   Immune-mediated disease (i.e. erythema multiforme [Figure 3.130A], VCLE [Figure 3.130B])
g) Linear preputial dermatosis (Figure 3.131) due to testicular tumor or exposure to human transdermal hormone replacement creams
h) Draining tracts
   Mycobacteriosis (Figures 3.132 and 8.16A and B)
   Lymphangiosarcoma (Figure 3.133)
i) Localized to multifocal areas of cutaneous atrophy/easily torn skin/milia
j) Overuse of topical steroid creams or sprays (Figures 3.134A and 3.134B)

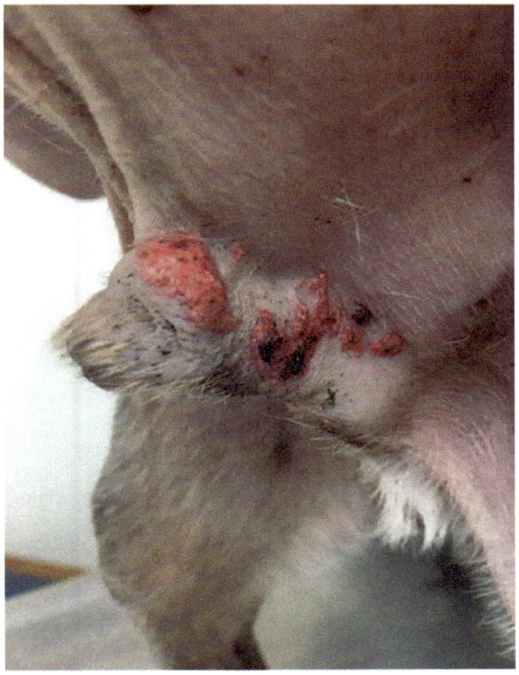

Figure 3.128 Raised, inflamed, gritty inguinal plaques caused by calcinosis cutis in a Cushingoid dog.

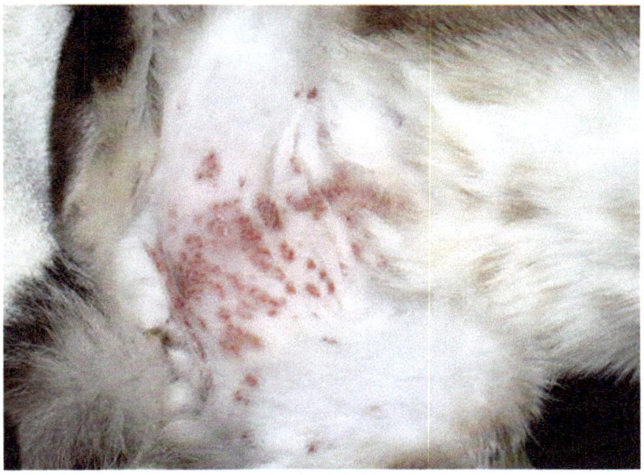

Figure 3.129 Numerous oval to linear eosinophilic plaques in an atopic cat.

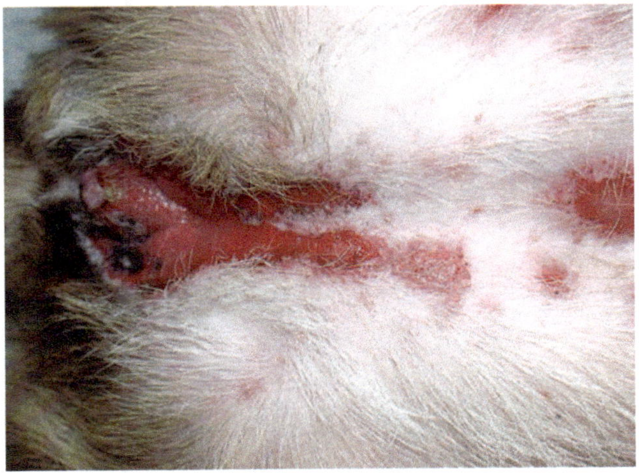

Figure 3.130A Inguinal and perivulvar ulcerations in a dog with erythema multiforme.

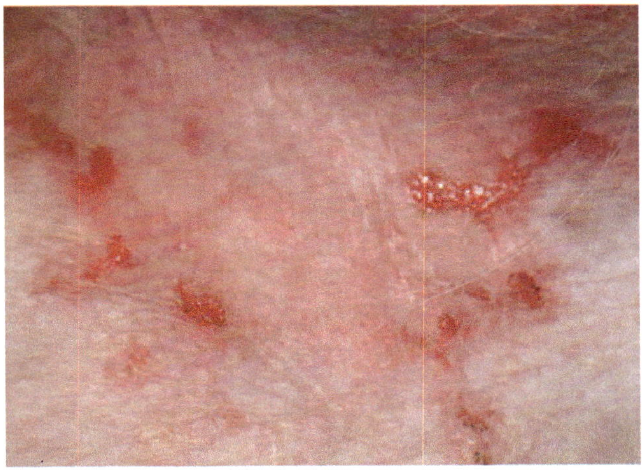

Figure 3.130B Serpiginous inguinal ulcerations in a sheltie with vesicular cutaneous lupus erythematosus.

3.10 Oral cavity

a) Erythema
   - Gingivitis/periodontal disease
   - Epitheliotropic lymphoma (Figure 3.135)

b) Plaque or mass
   - Oral eosinophilic granuloma (Figure 3.136)
   - Fungal granuloma
   - Foreign body granuloma

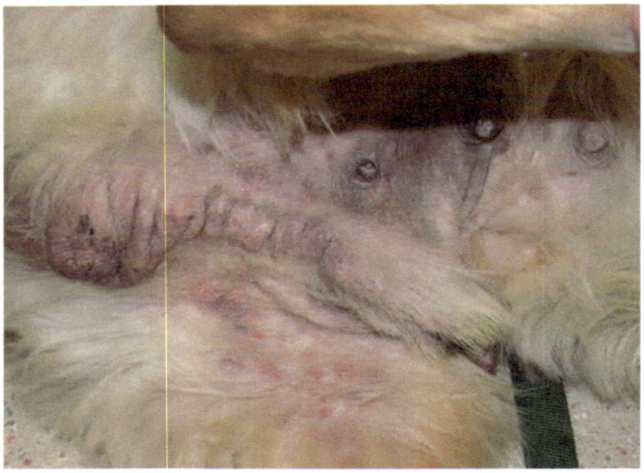

Figure 3.131 This intact male dog with an enlarged testicle due to a Sertoli cell tumor has enlarged nipples and pathognomic linear preputial dermatosis.

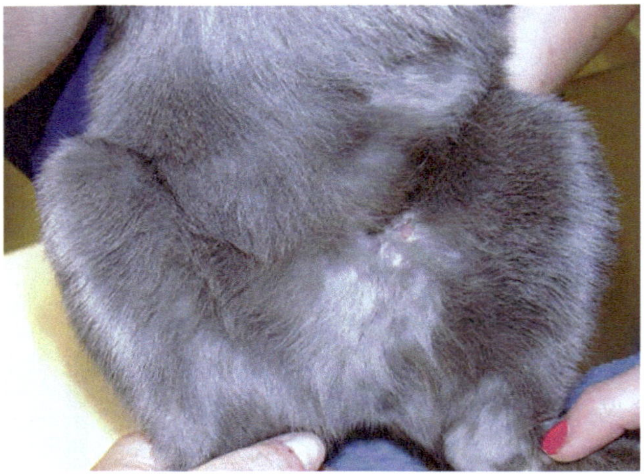

Figure 3.132 A cat with a crusted draining inguinal nodule due to mycobacteriosis.

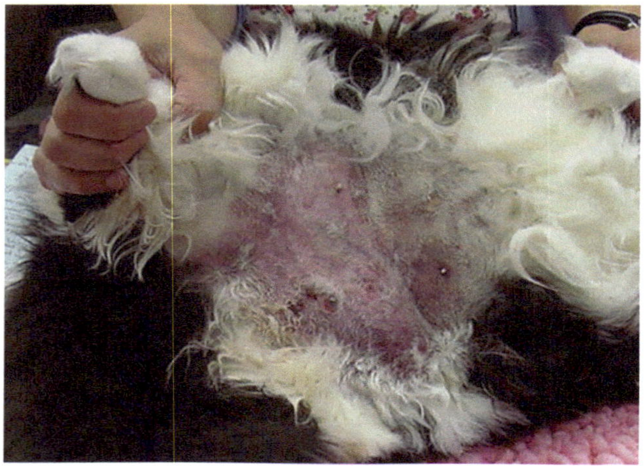

Figure 3.133 Diffuse purplish discoloration of fat with serosanguinous oozing due to an inguinal lymphangiosarcoma.

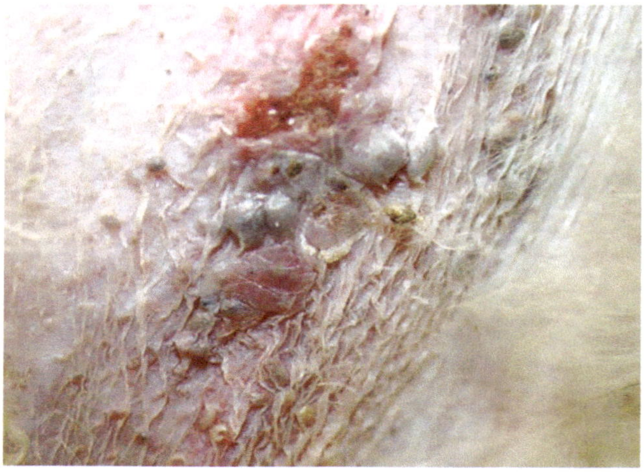

Figure 3.134A Inguinal cutaneous atrophy with milia and easily torn skin caused by overuse of a steroid spray.

Oral cavity (cont.)

Calcinosis circumscripta (tongue, Figures 19.44B and C)
Granulomatous glossitis due to burdock ingestion (Figure 18.6E)
Neoplasia

c) Ulceration
   Burn
   Ingestion of caustic substance
   Canine chronic ulcerative paradental stomatitis (CUPS)
   Oral cavity (cont.)
   Feline stomatitis
   Feline herpes (Figure 9.3) or calicivirus
   Immune-mediated disease (drug reaction, erythema multiforme [Figure 3.137], vasculitis

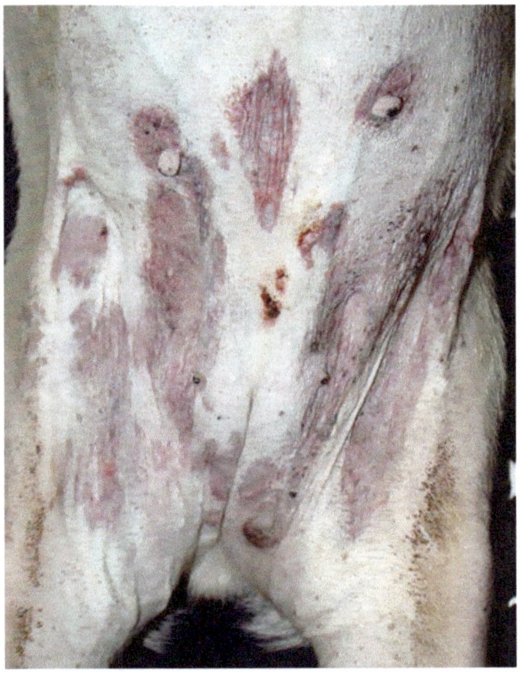

Figure 3.134B In this dog, a potent steroid spray was used 2–3 times a week for six months, causing marked hair loss, cutaneous atrophy, and separation of a prior spay incision on the ventral midline; the darker pink areas are underlying muscle.

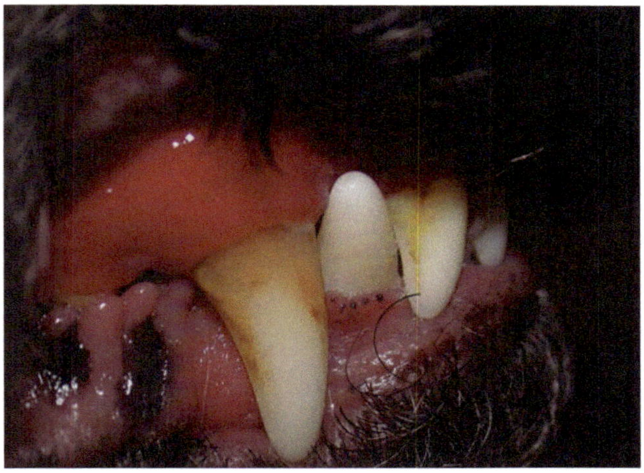

Figure 3.135 Marked gingival mucosal hyperemia in a dog with cutaneous epitheliotropic lymphoma.

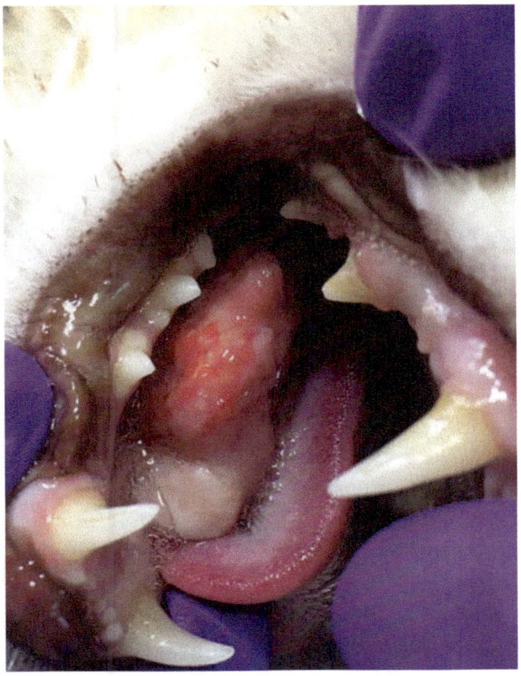

Figure 3.136 A raised sublingual eosinophilic granuloma triggered by food allergy in a cat.

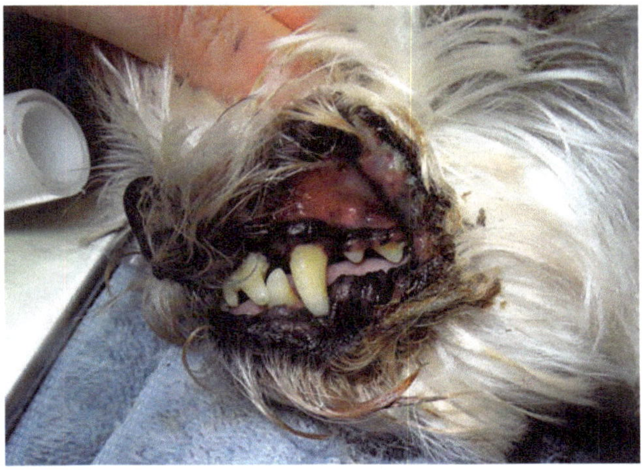

Figure 3.137 Oral and lip mucosal ulcerations in a dog with erythema multiforme triggered by an antibiotic.

Oral cavity (cont.)

[Figure 3.138], toxic epidermal necrolysis, pemphigus vulgaris [Figure 3.139], epidermolysis bullosa acquisita (Figures 11.8A–C), SLE)

Congenital immunobullous disease (epidermolysis bullosa)

Neoplasia (Figures 3.140A and 3.140B)

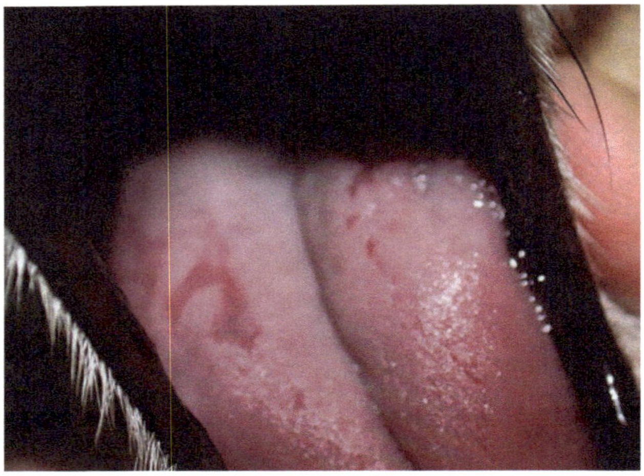

Figure 3.138 Linear lingual erosions in a dog with vasculitis.

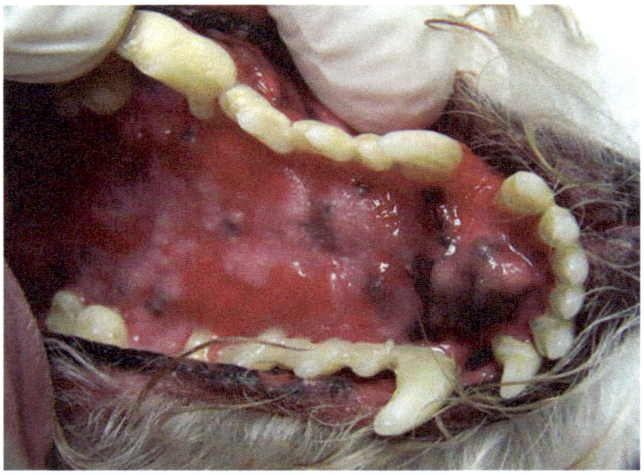

Figure 3.139 Extensive ulceration of the hard palate in a dog with pemphigus vulgaris.

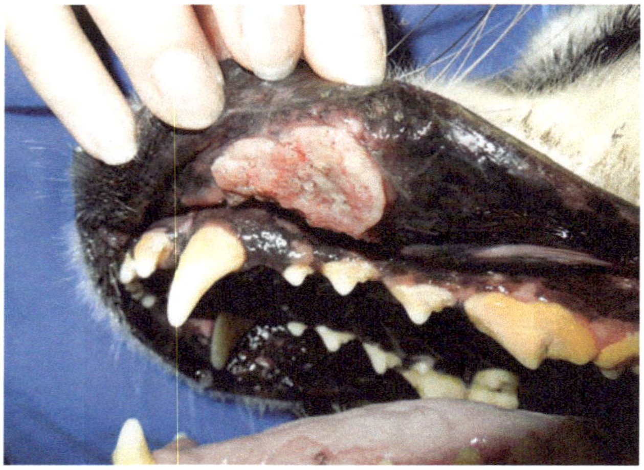

Figure 3.140A An ulcerated lip mucosal mass which was revealed on biopsy to be a squamous cell carcinoma.

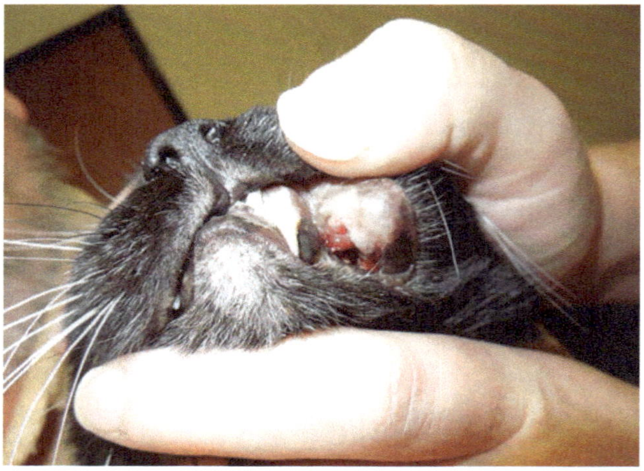

Figure 3.140B An ulcerated oral squamous cell carcinoma in a cat.

Further reading

Beco, L., Guagere, E., Lorente Mendez, C. et al. (2013). Suggested guidelines for using systemic antimicrobials in bacterial skin infections (1): diagnosis based on clinical presentation, cytology and culture. *Vet. Rec.* 172 (3): 72–78.

Coyner, K. (2007). Diagnosis and treatment of solar dermatitis in dogs. *Vet. Med.* 102 (8): 511–515.

Coyner, K. (2011). Skills laboratory: how to perform skin scraping and skin surface cytology. *Vet. Med.* 106 (11): 554–563.

Miller, W.H., Griffen, C.E., and Campbell, K.L. (2013). *Muller and Kirk's Small Animal Dermatology*, 7e. Elsevier Mosby: St Louis, MO.

Meckenburg, L., Linke, M., and Tobin, D. (2009). *Hair Loss Disorders in Domestic Animals*. Wiley-Blackwell: Ames, IA.

Olivry, T. (2006). A review of autoimmune skin diseases in domestic animals: I – superficial pemphigus. *Vet. Dermatol.* 17 (5): 291–305.

4

Causes and workup for pruritus in dogs and cats

Kimberly S. Coyner, DVM, DACVD

Dermatology Clinic for Animals, Lacey, WA, USA

A) Pruritus is a common reason for pet owners to present their animals for veterinary care. The list of possible causes for pruritus is long and can be daunting but, in the majority of cases, causes for pruritus in dogs and cats can be broken down into three main categories:
- Parasites (fleas, mites).
- Infections (bacterial, fungal).
- Allergies (to fleas, food, or environmental allergens, less commonly contact allergy).
  - Many animals have a combination of these three factors.

Less common causes for pruritus include:
- Immune-mediated disorders such as pemphigus foliaceus.
- Keratinization disorders such as sebaceous adenitis.
- Cutaneous epitheliotropic lymphoma.
- Paraneoplastic disorders.
  - All of these also have crusting, scaling, or follicular casting which does not resolve with treatment for infection.
- Cats may overgroom due to behavioral causes or pain.

B) To identify the cause of the pruritus and prescribe appropriate treatment, in each case it is important to perform the basic dermatologic diagnostics:
- Flea combing.
- Skin scrapings for mites.
- Skin cytology to evaluate if bacteria or yeast are present, as well as to evaluate inflammatory cell types present.
  - If bacteria are present on cytology despite empiric antibiotic treatment, then aerobic bacterial skin culture is indicated.
  - If pruritic crusting lesions suggestive of infection are present and inflammatory cells are found on cytology but no organisms, then consider dermatophyte culture and/or skin biopsies for dermatopathology.

C) Treat infection with appropriate anti-infective oral and topical therapies (see Chapter 8), and even if no mites are found on skin scrapings, trial treat with an antiparasitic medication such as an isoxazoline effective for fleas and mites such as *Sarcoptes* in dogs or *Demodex* in cats; these mites can be difficult to find on scrapings and can mimic allergies.
- A short course (two to three weeks) of oral anti-inflammatory steroids or oclacitinib (dogs) can be given if needed for relief of pruritus while infection and parasites are treated, but avoid long acting steroid injections and continue antibiotics beyond when steroids or oclacitinib have finished.

D) If pruritus persists despite infection and parasite control, and if any prior crusts associated with infection have resolved, then begin the allergy workup and symptomatic antipruritic medications to keep the pet comfortable while the underlying allergy is addressed.
- If symptoms are non-seasonal begin hypoallergenic diet trial.
- If symptoms are seasonal/intermittent then consider allergy testing/desensitization therapy vs. medical management for atopy, see Chapter 10.

E) If pruritus with crusts/scales persist despite infection treatment/cytologically verified clearance of infection and parasite control, then biopsy for dermatopathology (stop steroids two to four weeks prior).

F) See the following algorithms (Algorithms 4.1 and 4.2) for further details on causes and workup of pruritus in dogs and cats.

Clinical Atlas of Canine and Feline Dermatology, First Edition. Edited by Kimberly S. Coyner.

Companion website: www.wiley.com/go/coyner/dermatology

Algorithm 4.1 Pruritic dog – Causes/Workup.

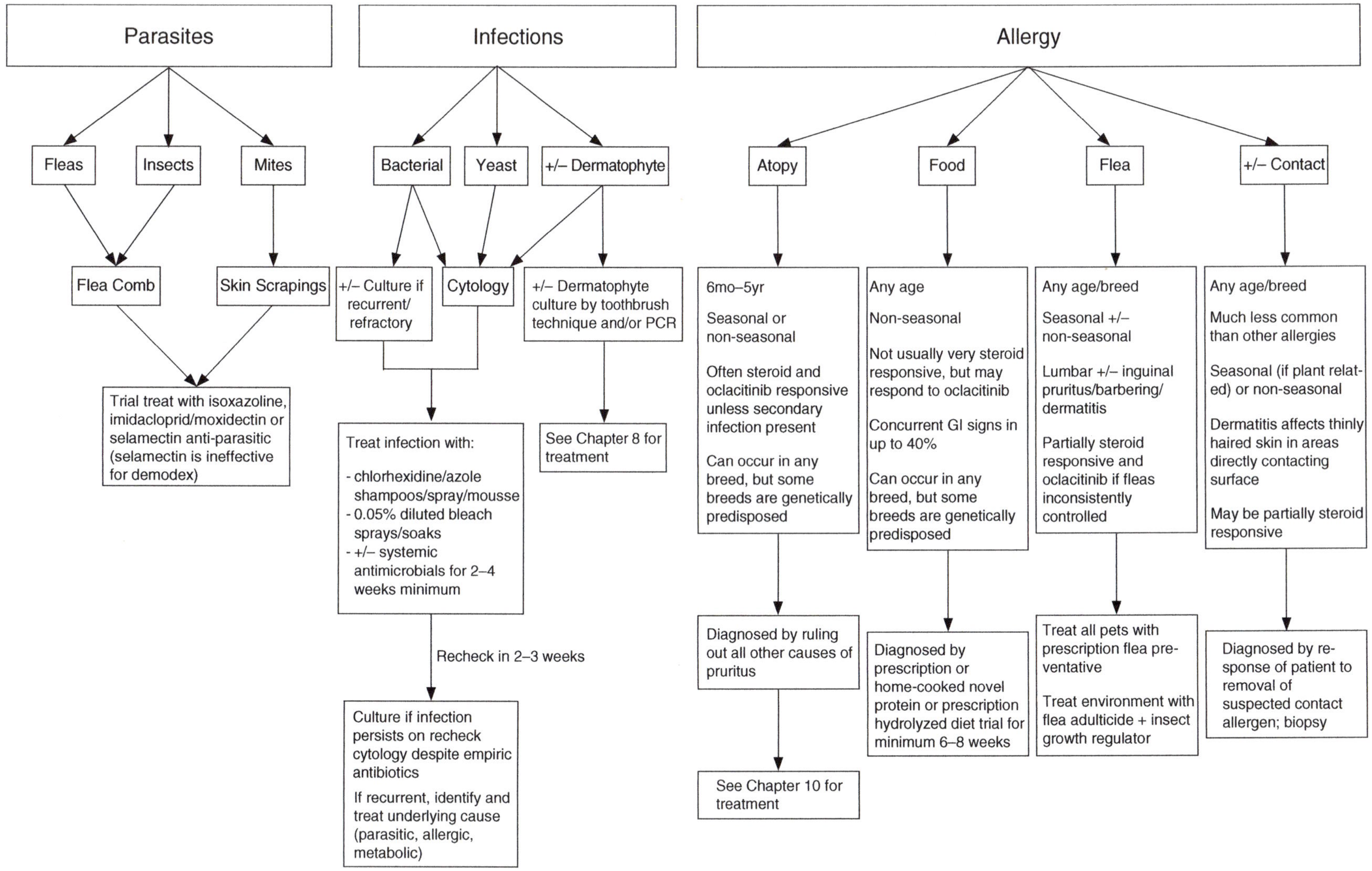

*Less common causes for pruritus: Pemphigus foliaceus, cutaneous epitheliotropic lymphoma, sebaceous adenitis

Algorithm 4.2 Pruritic cats – Causes/Workup.

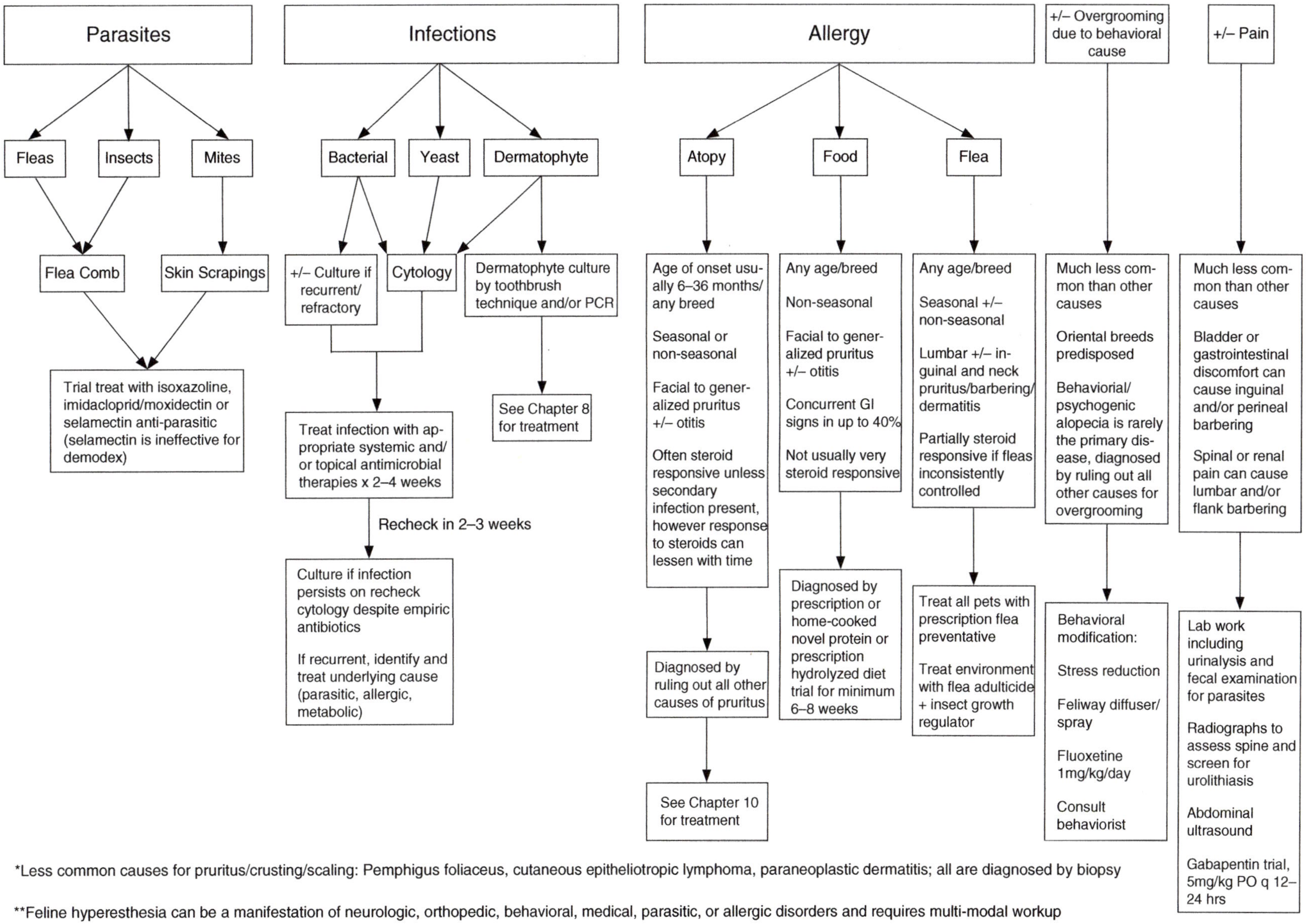

*Less common causes for pruritus/crusting/scaling: Pemphigus foliaceus, cutaneous epitheliotropic lymphoma, paraneoplastic dermatitis; all are diagnosed by biopsy

**Feline hyperesthesia can be a manifestation of neurologic, orthopedic, behavioral, medical, parasitic, or allergic disorders and requires multi-modal workup

5

Causes and workup for alopecia in dogs and cats

Kimberly S. Coyner, DVM, DACVD

Dermatology Clinic for Animals, Lacey, WA, USA

A) Alopecia is another common reason for pet owners to present their animals for examination, and can be localized, regional, or generalized, and may or may not be associated with pruritus, crusting, or scaling.
- Location or distribution of alopecia can be a helpful clue in determining etiology; see Chapter 3.
- Self-induced alopecia due to pruritus or associated with crusting/scaling suggests hypersensitivity and/or infection, less commonly immune-mediated diseases or keratinization disorders; see Chapter 4.

B) Non-pruritic symmetric alopecia involving the trunk and tail in dogs can be due to follicular, keratinization, or endocrine disorders, and age of onset, breed, and hair color of the dog should be considered prior to diagnostics such as labwork or skin biopsies.
- See Algorithm 5.1 describing causes and workup for canine non-inflammatory alopecia.
- See Chapter 12 for further discussion of endocrine alopecia and Chapter 13 for further discussion of non-inflammatory/non-infectious alopecia in dogs and cats.

C) Multifocal punctate, patchy, or circular alopecia in dogs is often due to infectious causes of folliculitis (bacterial, *Demodex*, dermatophyte) and is usually associated with scaling/crusting +/− comedones; pruritus may or may not be present.
- These infections are often secondary to an underlying allergy, endocrine, or keratinization disorder.
- To identify the cause of the alopecia and prescribe appropriate treatment, in each case it is important to perform the basic dermatologic diagnostics:
  - Flea combing.
  - Skin scrapings for mites.
  - Skin cytology to evaluate if bacteria or yeast are present, as well as to evaluate inflammatory cell types present.
    - If bacteria are present on cytology despite empiric antibiotic treatment, then aerobic bacterial skin culture is indicated; see Chapter 8.
- If alopecia with crusting lesions suggestive of infection are present and inflammatory cells are found on cytology but no organisms, then consider dermatophyte culture (see Chapter 8) and/or skin biopsies for dermatopathology.
- Less commonly, immune-mediated skin or follicular diseases and canine solar dermatitis can also cause focal to multifocal alopecia which may or may not be crusty or pruritic, and are diagnosed by ruling out infection and biopsy/dermatopathology; see Chapters 11 and 18.
- See Algorithm 5.2 describing causes and workup for canine focal to multifocal alopecia.

D) Causes and workup for alopecia in cats are similar to dogs, with a few exceptions.
- Endocrine alopecia is very rare in cats.
- Alopecia caused by overgrooming due to behavioral causes or pain can occur but is uncommon compared to parasitic, allergic, and infectious causes of alopecia.
- Paraneoplastic alopecia due to liver or pancreatic neoplasia is a rare disorder unique in older cats, causing extensive alopecia and easily epilated fur on the ventral trunk/medial limbs; underlying skin has a shiny appearance.
  - Facial and pedal hairloss and crusting may also be present.
  - Secondary bacterial and yeast infections are common.
  - Weight loss and systemic illness are also present.
- See Algorithm 5.3 describing causes and workup for feline alopecia and Chapter 13 for further discussion of non-inflammatory/non-infectious alopecia.

Clinical Atlas of Canine and Feline Dermatology, First Edition. Edited by Kimberly S. Coyner.

Companion website: www.wiley.com/go/coyner/dermatology

Algorithm 5.1 Canine non-inflammatory truncal alopecia – Causes/Workup.

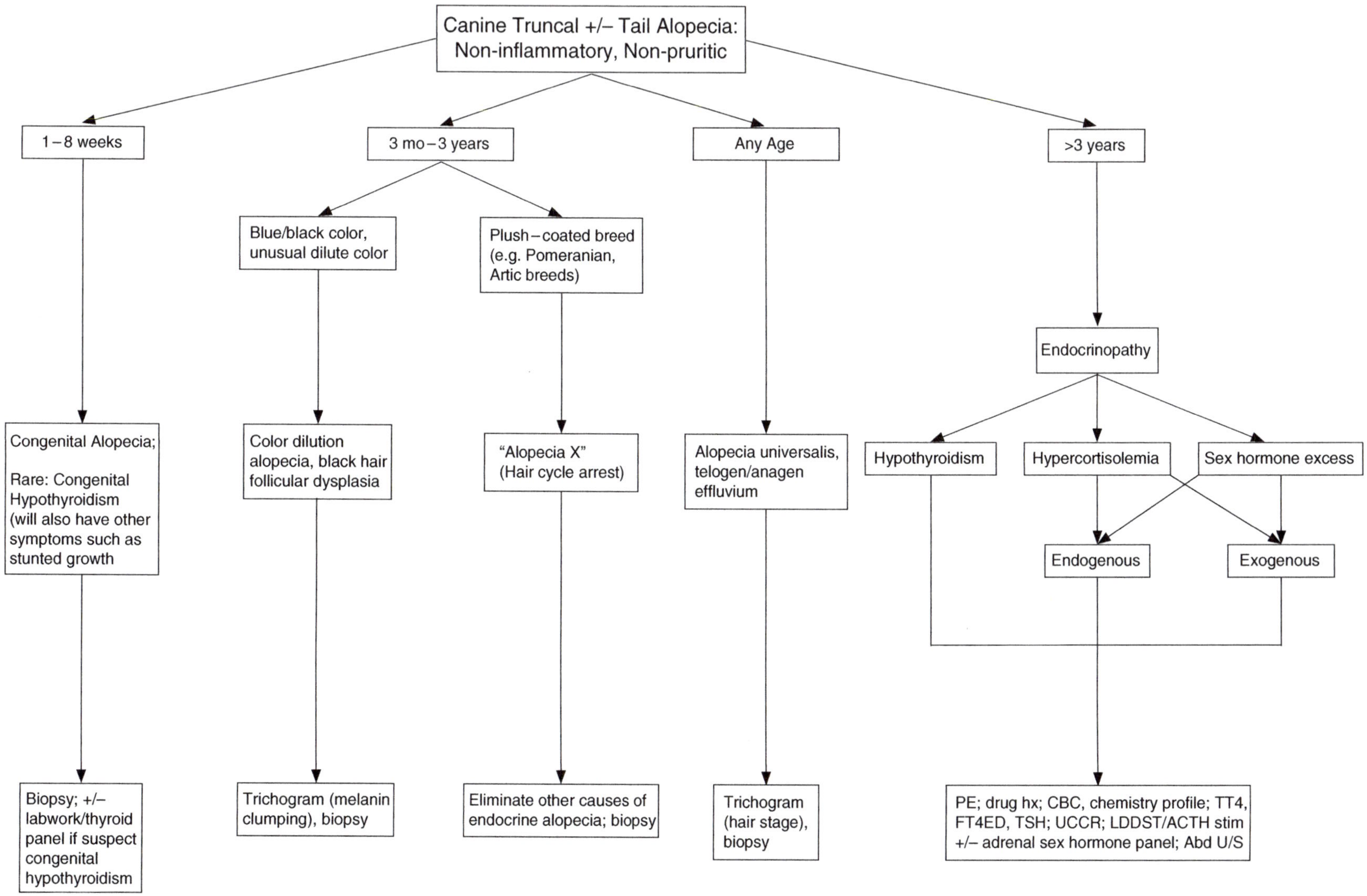

PE: Physical examination; CBC: complete blood count; TT4: total thyroid level; FT4ED: free T4 by equilibrium dialysis; TSH: thyroid stimulating hormone; UCCR: urine cortisol/creatinine ratio; LDDST: low dose dexamethasone suppression test; ACTH stim: adrenocorticotropic hormone stimulation test; Abd U/S: abdominal ultrasound

Algorithm 5.2 Canine multifocal alopecia – Causes/Workup.

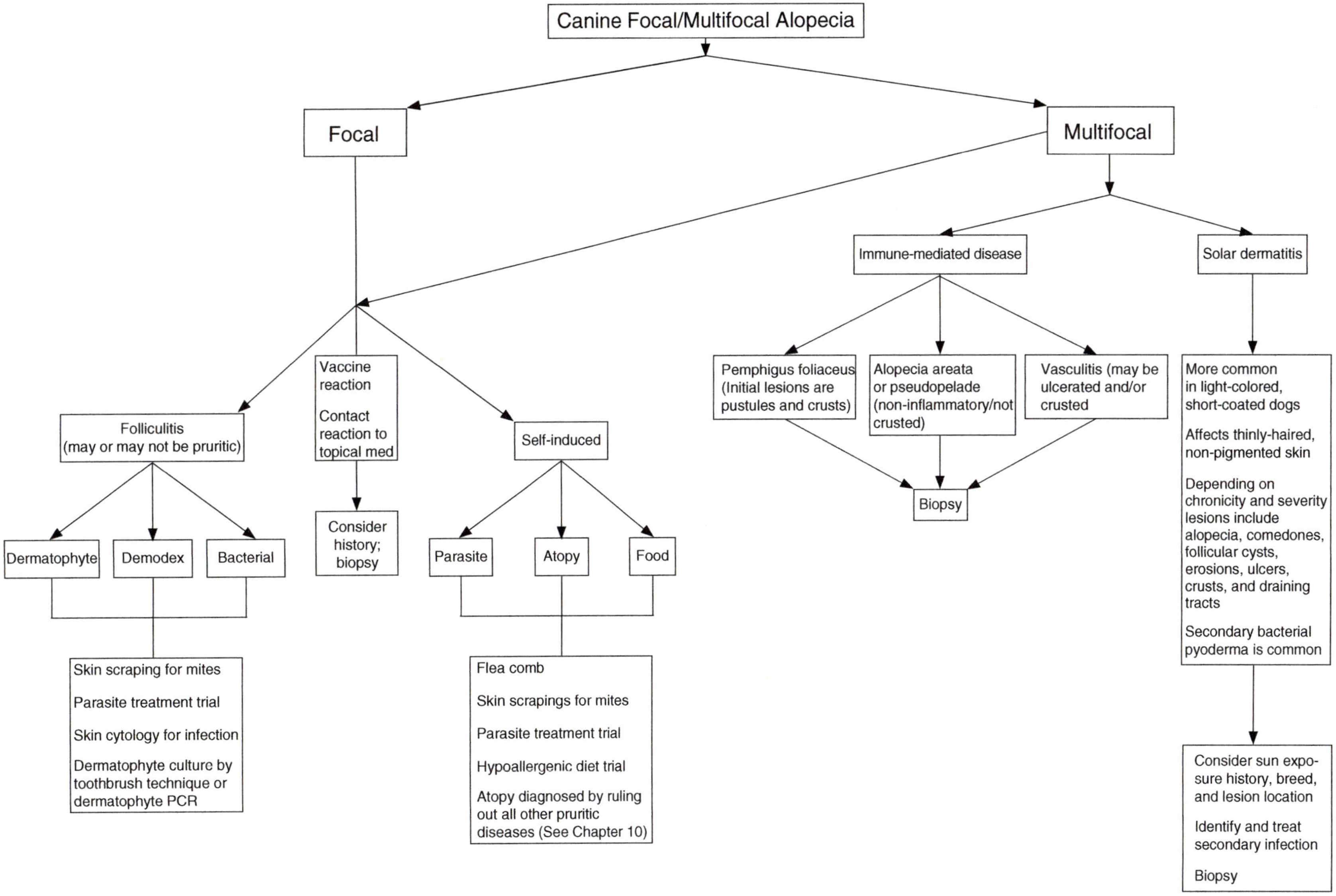

Algorithm 5.3 Feline alopecia – Causes/Workup.

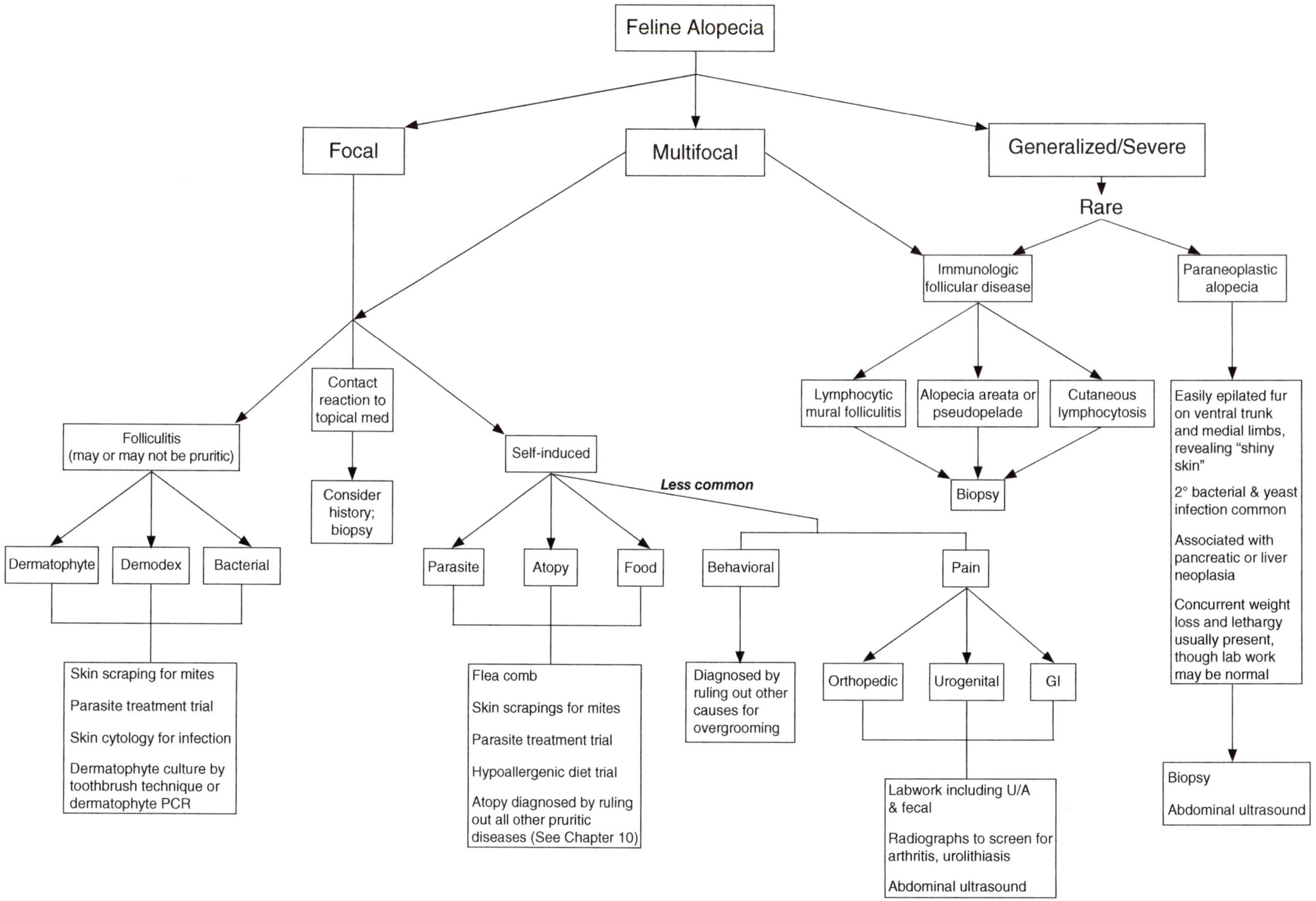

6

Breed-related dermatoses

Kimberly S. Coyner, DVM, DACVD

Dermatology Clinic for Animals, Lacey, WA, USA

Table 6.1 Canine breed-related dermatoses.

Dog breed	Common condition	Figures
Afghan	Fluffy haircoat change post neutering (this occurs to some extent in most double coated dogs but is more noticeable in Afghans and setters)	
Airedale	Canine recurrent flank alopecia	
Akita	Sebaceous adenitis, pemphigus foliaceus, uveodermatologic syndrome	Figures 6.1A and 6.1B
American Bulldog	Ichthyosis, solar dermatitis, atopy/food allergy	Figure 6.2
Belgian Tervuren/ Malinois	Vitiligo	Figure 6.3
Bernese Mountain Dog	Systemic and malignant histiocytosis	
Boston Terrier	Zinc responsive dermatosis, atopy/food allergy	Figure 6.4
Boxer	Canine recurrent flank alopecia, dermoid cysts on head, mast cell tumors, distal pinnal ulcers often secondary to pruritus/repetitive ear flopping due to atopy/food allergy	Figures 6.5 and 6.6
Bull Terrier	Lethal acrodermatitis, solar dermatitis	
Cavalier King Charles Spaniel	Oral eosinophilic granulomas, primary secretory otitis media, syringomyelia induced head/neck pruritus, congenital keratoconjunctivitis sicca and ichthyosiform dermatosis	Figures 6.7A–6.7C
Cairn Terrier	Ichthyosis	
Chihuahua	Rabies vaccine-induced pinnal vasculitis, sterile panniculitis, pattern baldness, color dilution alopecia, atopy/food allergy	Figures 6.8–6.11A and 6.11B
Chinese Crested	Comedones/follicular cysts	Figure 6.12
Chow	Pemphigus foliaceus, Alopecia X, uveodermatologic syndrome	Figure 6.13
Cocker Spaniel	Proliferative otitis and recurrent pyoderma due to atopy/food allergy, vitamin A responsive dermatosis, idiopathic nasodigital hyperkeratosis	Figures 6.14A and 6.14B
Collie/Sheltie	Dermatomyositis, discoid lupus erythematosus, systemic lupus erythematosus, vesicular lupus erythematosus, reactive histiocytosis, superficial spreading pyoderma	Figures 6.15 and 6.16
Curly Coated Retriever	Follicular dysplasia	

(*Continued*)

Clinical Atlas of Canine and Feline Dermatology, First Edition. Edited by Kimberly S. Coyner.

Companion website: www.wiley.com/go/coyner/dermatology

Table 6.1 Canine breed-related dermatoses (Continued)

Dog breed	Common condition	Figures
Dachshund	Alopecia areata, pinnal marginal dermatosis and vasculitis, sterile panniculitis, pattern baldness	Figures 6.17–6.19
Dalmatian	Atopy, solar dermatitis	
Doberman Pinscher	Acral lick dermatitis, follicular dysplasia, color dilution alopecia, hypothyroidism, vitiligo	Figures 6.20 and 6.21
English Bulldog	Acrochordonous plaques, canine recurrent flank alopecia, pododermatitis/interdigital cysts, intertrigo, atopy/food allergy	Figures 6.22–6.25
Flat Coated Retriever	Systemic and malignant histiocytosis	
German Shorthair Pointer	Acral mutilation, exfoliative cutaneous lupus erythematosus	Figures 16.8A–D
German Shepherd	Metatarsal/metacarpal fistulas, perianal fistulas, nodular dermatofibrosis, lupoid onychodystrophy, discoid lupus erythematosus, systemic lupus erythematosus, mucocutaneous lupus erythematosus, vitiligo, mucocutaneous pyoderma, deep pyoderma, pinnal marginal scaling due to atopy/food allergy	Figures 6.26–6.30
Golden Retriever	Ichthyosis, reactive histiocytosis, atopy/food allergy	Figure 6.31
Greyhound	Bald thigh syndrome, corns	Figure 6.32
Fox Terrier	*Demodex injai*, atopy/food allergy	
Havanese	Sebaceous adenitis	Figures 6.33A and 6.33B
Husky	Zinc responsive dermatosis, uveodermatologic syndrome, eosinophilic granulomas	Figure 6.34
Irish Setter	Fluffy haircoat change post neutering	Figure 6.35
Irish Water Spaniel	Follicular dysplasia	
Jack Russell Terrier	Ichthyosis, rabies vaccine-induced pinnal vasculitis, *Trichophyton* dermatophytosis	Figures 6.36A, 6.36B, and 6.37
Keeshond	Intracornifying epitheliomas (ICE tumors), Alopecia X	Figure 6.38
Labrador Retriever	Nasal parakeratosis, atopy/food allergy, color dilution alopecia (silver labs)	Figures 6.39 and 6.40
Malamute	Alopecia X, zinc responsive dermatosis	Figure 6.41
Maltese	Rabies vaccine-induced injection site alopecia	Figure 6.42
Miniature Pinscher	Pattern baldness	
Miniature Poodle	Alopecia X, rabies vaccine-induced injection site alopecia	Figure 6.43
Miniature Schnauzer	Schnauzer comedo syndrome, aurotrichia, canine recurrent flank alopecia, superficial suppurative necrolytic dermatitis, viral pigmented plaques	Figures 6.44–6.46
Norfolk Terrier	Ichthyosis	
Norwegian Elkhound	Intracornifying epitheliomas (ICE tumors)	
Pitbull Terrier	Solar dermatitis, atopy/food allergy	Figures 6.47A, 6.47B, and 6.48
Pomeranian	Alopecia X	Figure 6.49
Pug	Pigmented viral plaques, mast cell tumor, atopy/food allergy	Figures 6.50 and 6.51

Table 6.1 Canine breed-related dermatoses (Continued)

Dog breed	Common condition	Figures
Portuguese Water Dog	Follicular dysplasia	
Rhodesian Ridgeback	Dermoid sinus	Figure 16.6A
Rottweiler	Vitiligo, lupoid onychodystrophy	Figure 6.52
Samoyed	Sebaceous adenitis, Alopecia X, uveodermatologic syndrome	
Schipperke	Alopecia X-like disorder	
Shar-Pei	Mucinosis, atopy/food allergy	Figures 6.53A and 6.53B
Shih Tzu	*Demodex injai*, *Malassezia* dermatitis, atopy/food allergy	Figure 6.54
St. Bernard	Nasal arteritis	Figure 6.55
Standard Poodle	Sebaceous adenitis	Figures 6.56A and 6.56B
Standard Schnauzer	Nasal arteritis, canine recurrent flank alopecia	
Vizsla	Sebaceous adenitis	
West Highland White Terrier	*Malassezia* dermatitis secondary to atopy/food allergy, previously termed epidermal dysplasia; ichthyosis	Figure 6.57
Yorkshire Terrier	Rabies vaccine-induced injection site alopecia, atopy/food allergy, dermatophytosis, color dilution/black hair follicular dysplasia, "leather ear"	Figures 6.58 and 6.59

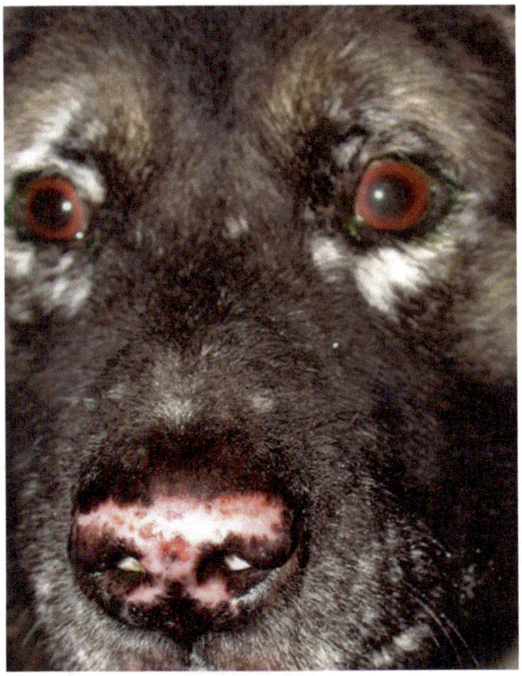

Figure 6.1A An Akita with uveodermatologic syndrome causing depigmentation of the nasal planum and eyelid fur as well as uveitis.

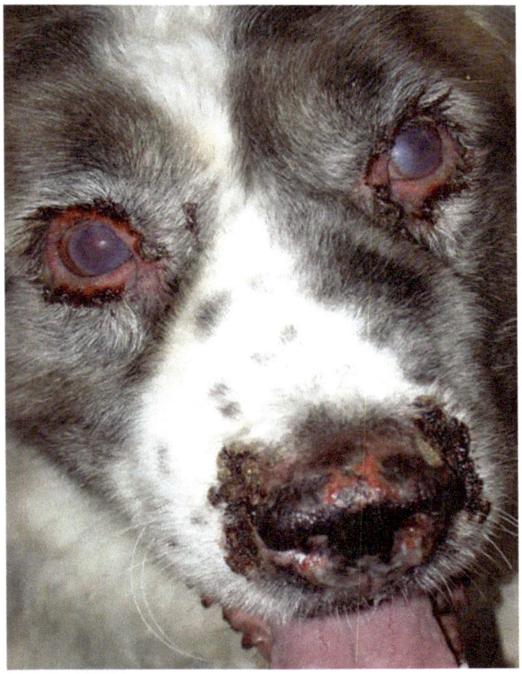

Figure 6.1B An Akita with uveodermatologic syndrome, causing uveitis as well as depigmentation and crusting of the nasal planum and eyelids.

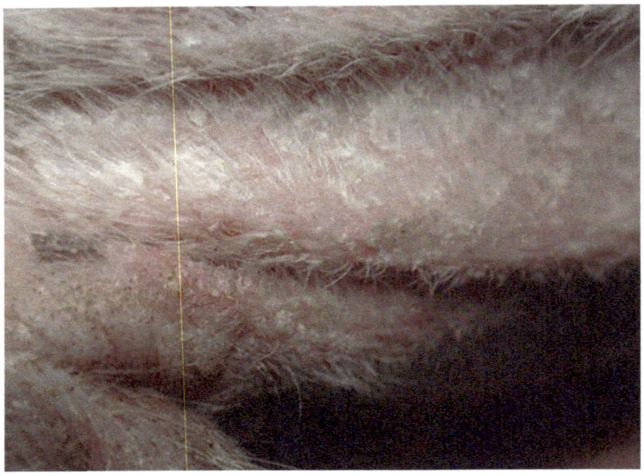

Figure 6.2 An American Bulldog puppy with ichthyosis, causing the typical "fish scale" lesions.

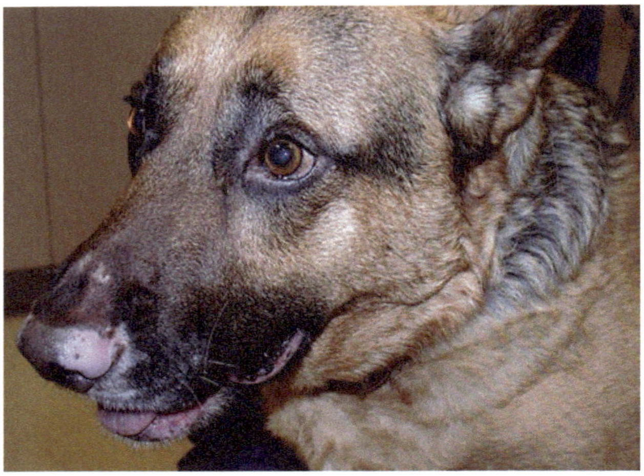

Figure 6.3 A Belgian Malinois with patchy depigmentation of the nasal planum, lips, and muzzle due to vitiligo.

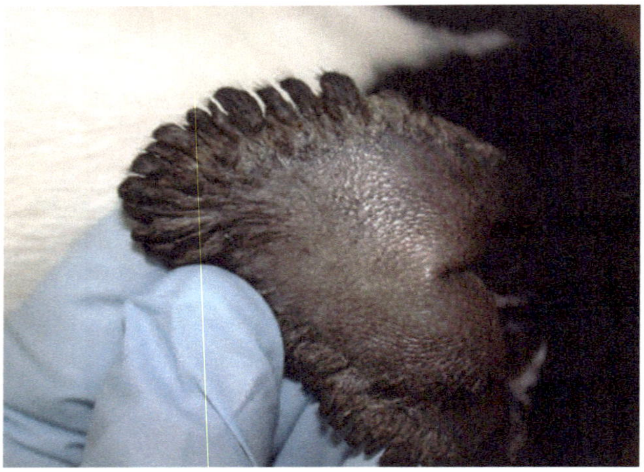

Figure 6.4 A Boston Terrier puppy with adherent pinnal hyperkeratosis due to zinc responsive dermatosis.

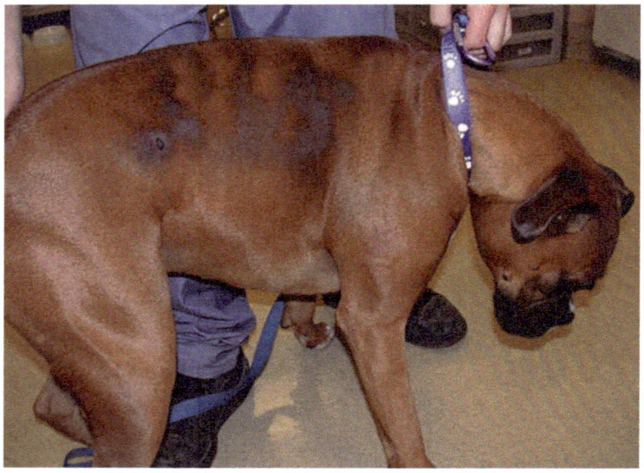

Figure 6.5 A Boxer with patchy truncal hypotrichosis and hyperpigmentation due to canine recurrent flank alopecia.

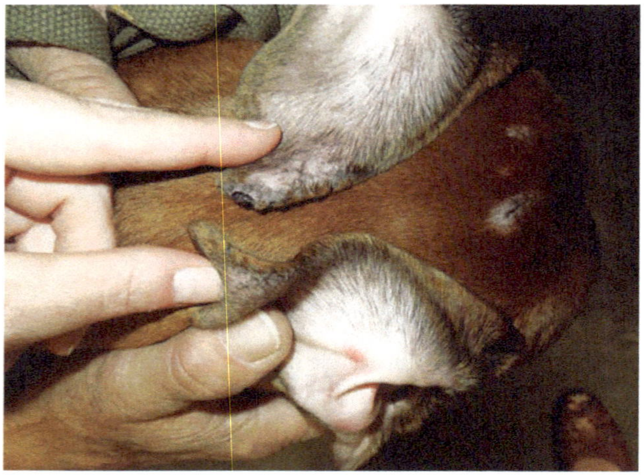

Figure 6.6 A Boxer with distal pinnal crusts and ulcerations triggered by repetitive ear flapping due to atopy and food allergy.

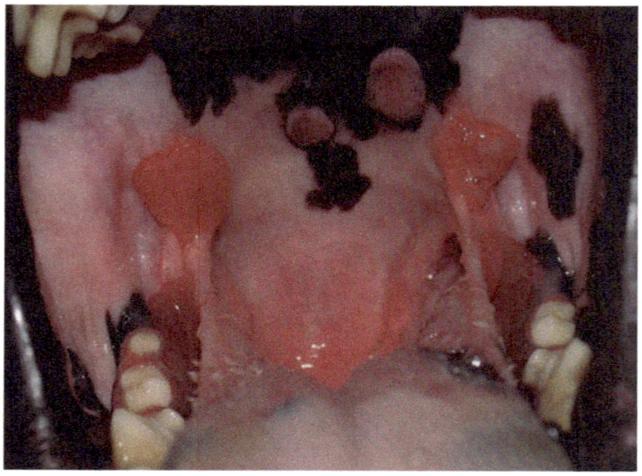

Figure 6.7A Oral eosinophilic granulomas in a Cavalier King Charles Spaniel.

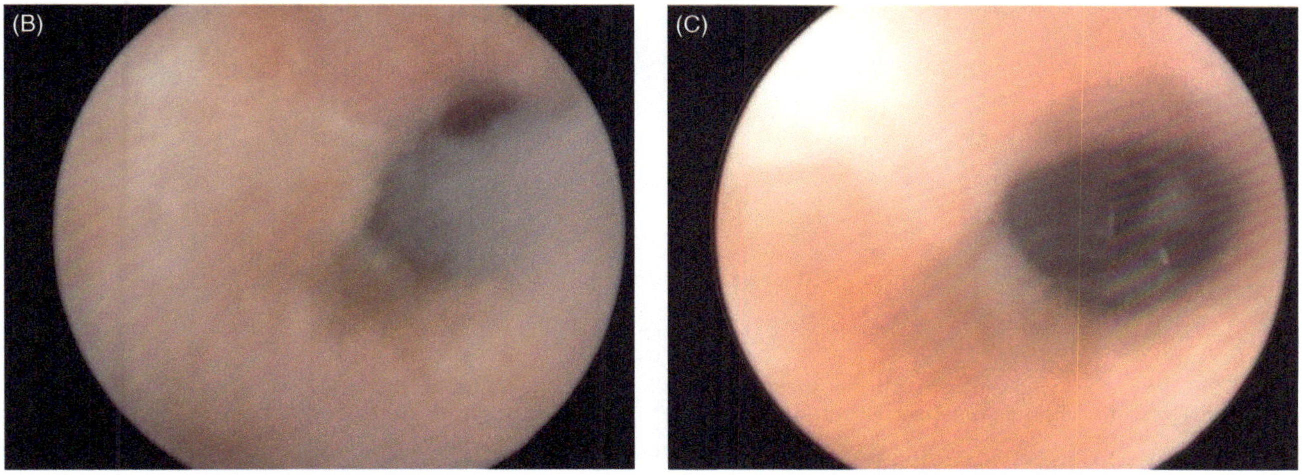

Figures 6.7B and C Primary secretory otitis media, during and post middle ear flush to remove mucous.

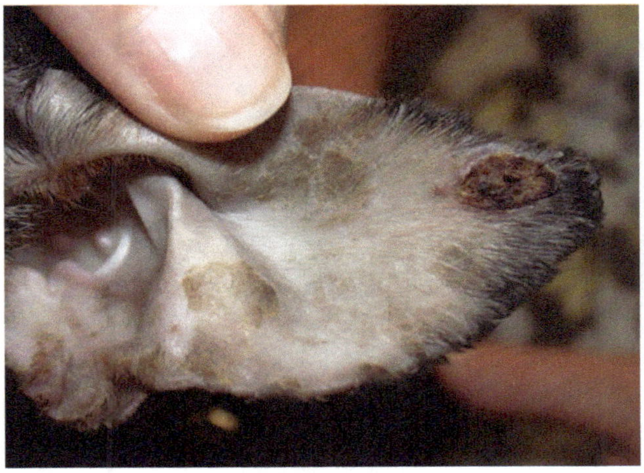

Figure 6.8 Distal pinnal crusted ulceration in a Chihuahua due to rabies vaccine-induced vasculitis.

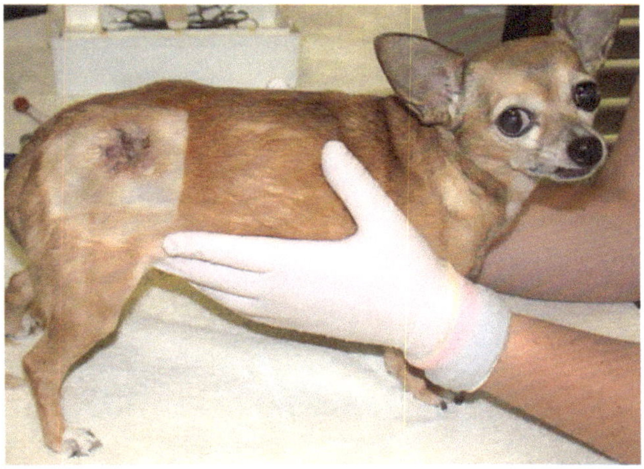

Figure 6.9 A Chihuahua with sterile panniculitis causing deep truncal ulcerations and draining tracts; the immune-mediated disease was complicated by secondary deep bacterial infection.

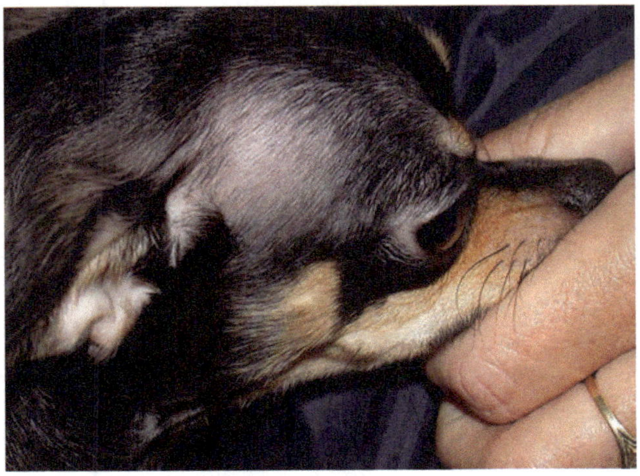

Figure 6.10 Non-inflammatory temporal hypotrichosis in a Chihuahua due to pattern baldness.

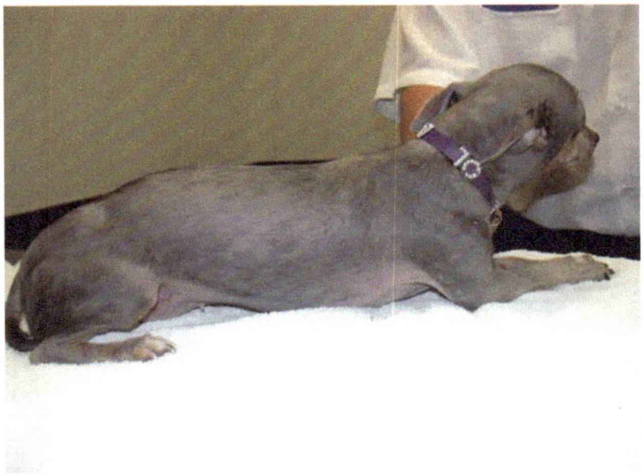

Figure 6.11A Generalized non-inflammatory hypotrichosis in a blue Chihuahua due to color dilution alopecia.

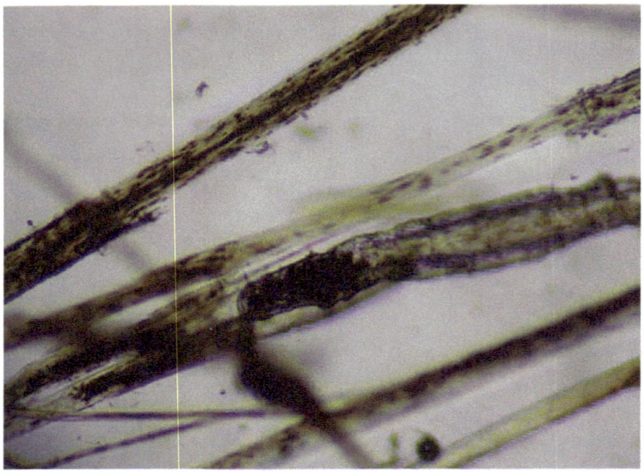

Figure 6.11B Trichogram of remaining hairs demonstrate pigment clumping in hair shafts consistent with color dilution (4×).

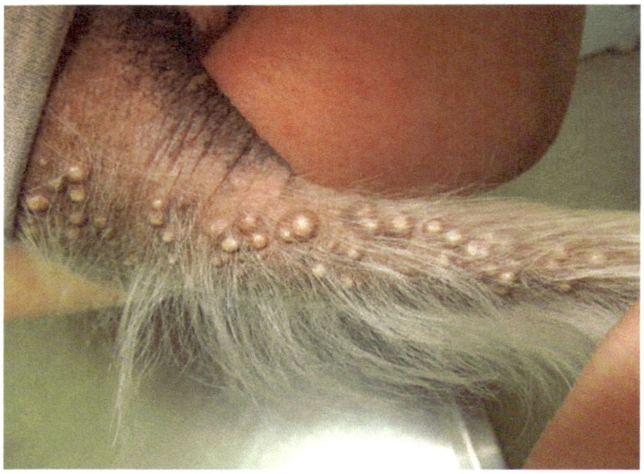

Figure 6.12 Numerous small follicular cysts in a Chinese Crested dog; lesions are present symmetrically on all limbs.

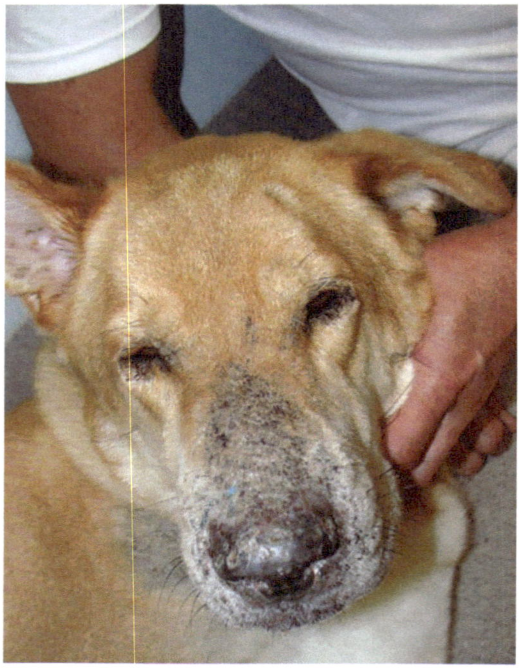

Figure 6.13 Pemphigus foliaceus causing crusting on the muzzle and nasal planum of a Chow.

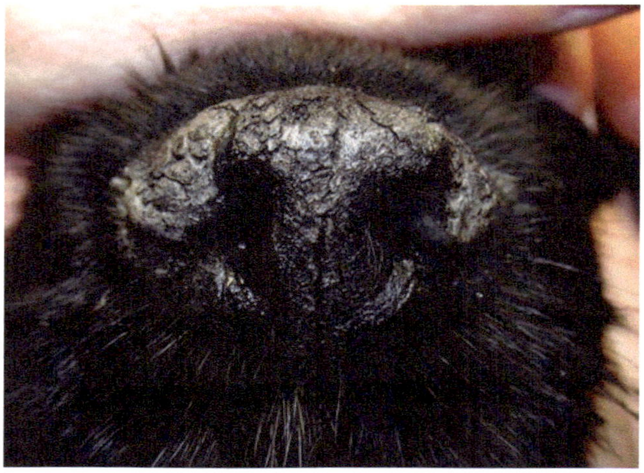

Figure 6.14A Idiopathic nasal planum hyperkeratosis in a Cocker Spaniel.

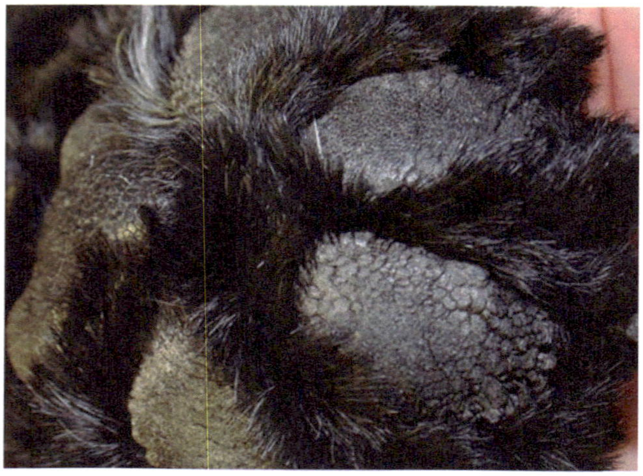

Figure 6.14B Hyperkeratotic paw pads were present in the same dog.

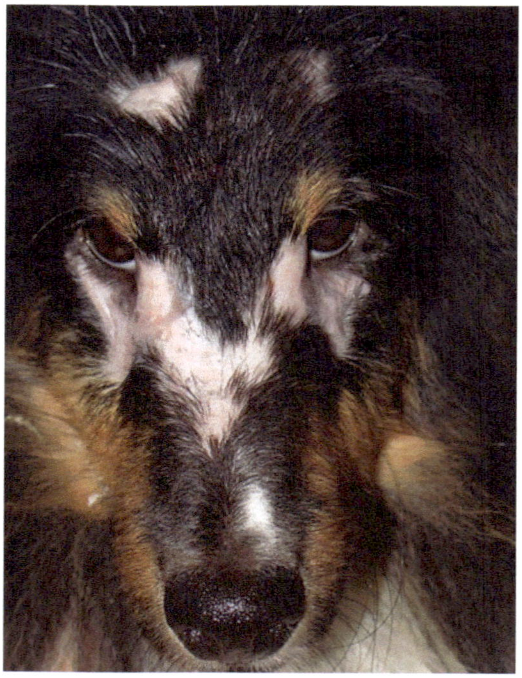

Figure 6.15 A young Sheltie with dermatomyositis causing patchy facial alopecia and scarring.

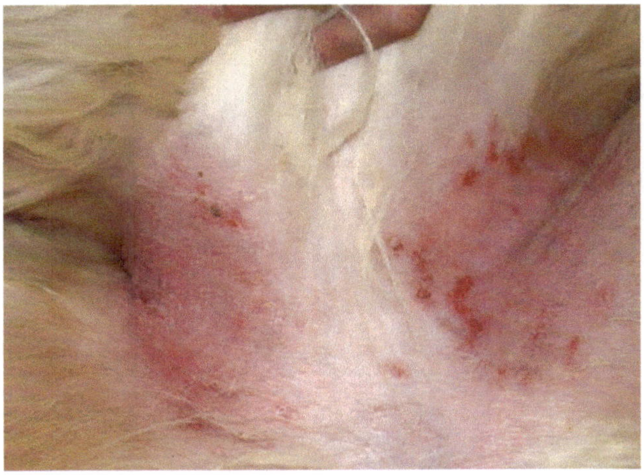

Figure 6.16 Oval to serpiginous inguinal erosions and crusts in a Sheltie due to vesicular cutaneous lupus erythematosus.

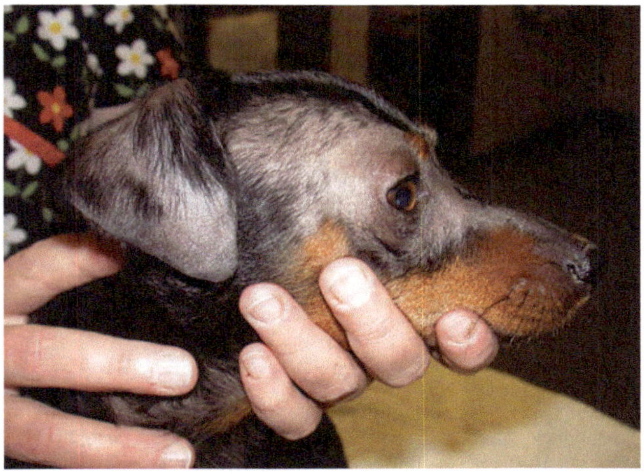

Figure 6.17 A Miniature Dachshund with non-inflammatory alopecia and hyperpigmentation due to alopecia areata.

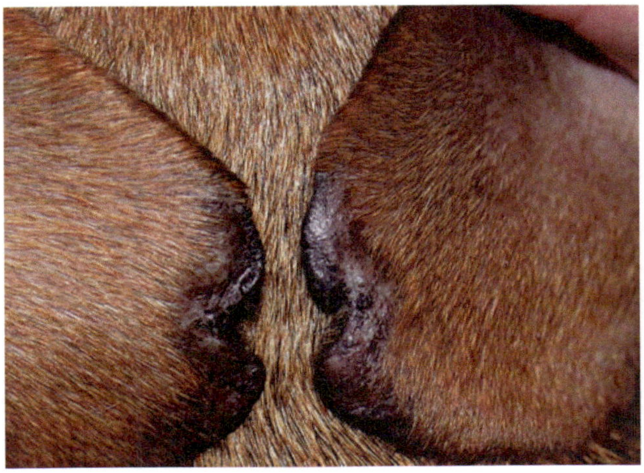

Figure 6.18 Distal pinnal alopecia, scarring, and cartilage deformation in a Miniature Dachshund with pinnal vasculitis; lesions were previously ulcerative but healing has occurred post immunosuppressive therapy.

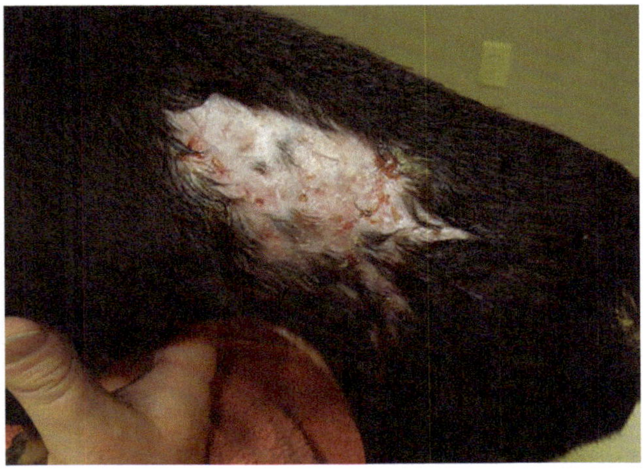

Figure 6.19 Patchy truncal scarring alopecia and draining tracts due to sterile panniculitis in a Miniature Dachshund.

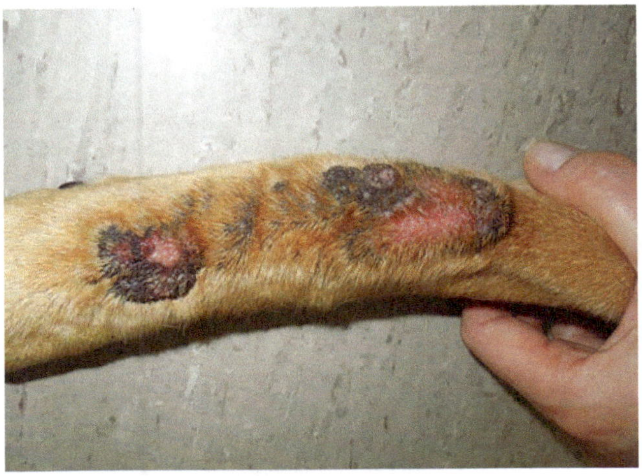

Figure 6.20 Acral granuloma in a Doberman Pinscher.

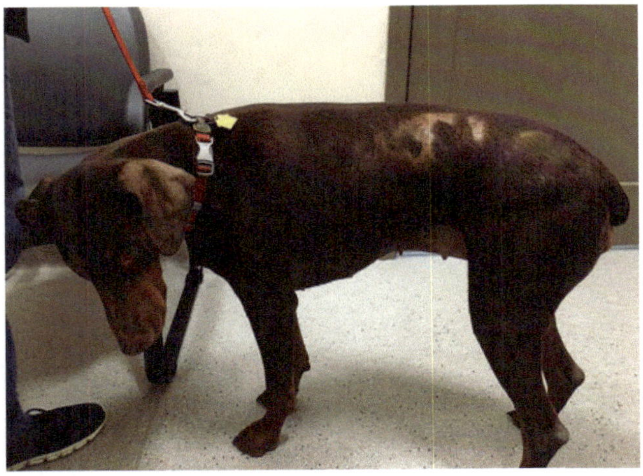

Figure 6.21 Patchy non-inflammatory flank alopecia in a young Doberman Pinscher due to follicular dysplasia.

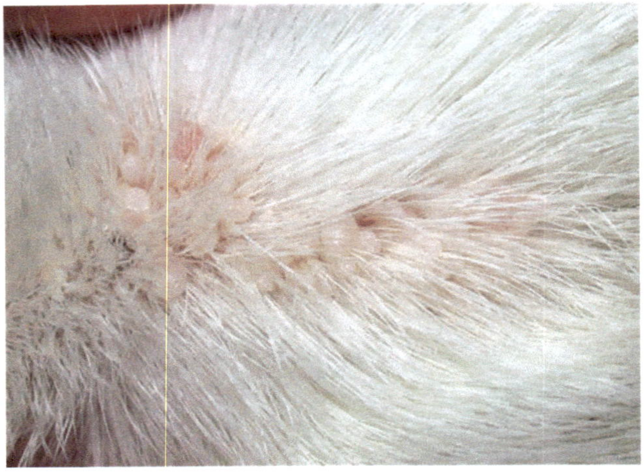

Figure 6.22 Raised rubbery dermal masses (acrochordons) on the dorsal neck of a food allergic English Bulldog; lesions virtually resolved after a hypoallergenic diet was instituted.

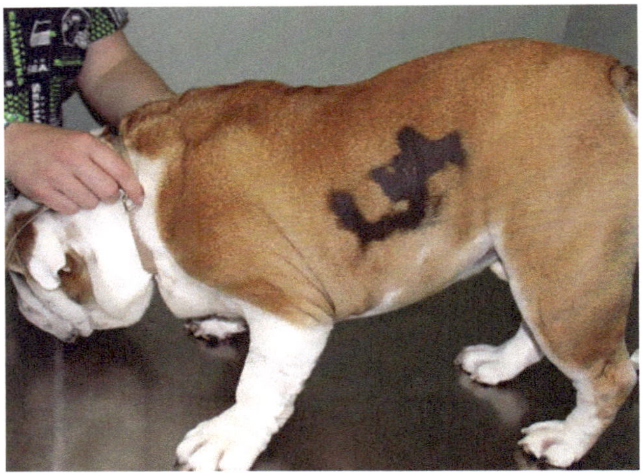

Figure 6.23 The same Bulldog also had patchy flank alopecia and hyperpigmentation due to canine recurrent flank alopecia.

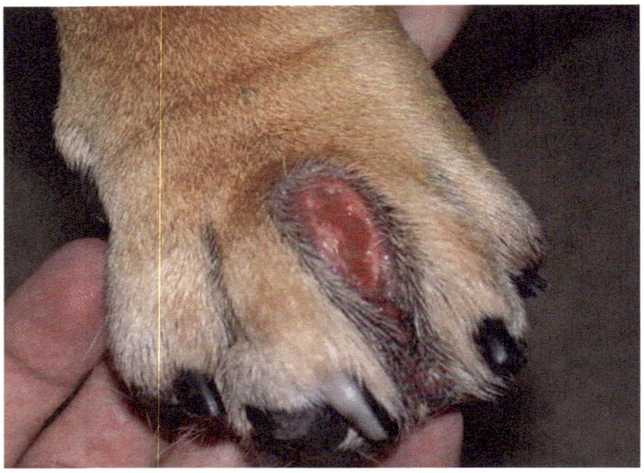

Figure 6.24 An atopic English Bulldog with a ruptured and infected interdigital cyst/granuloma.

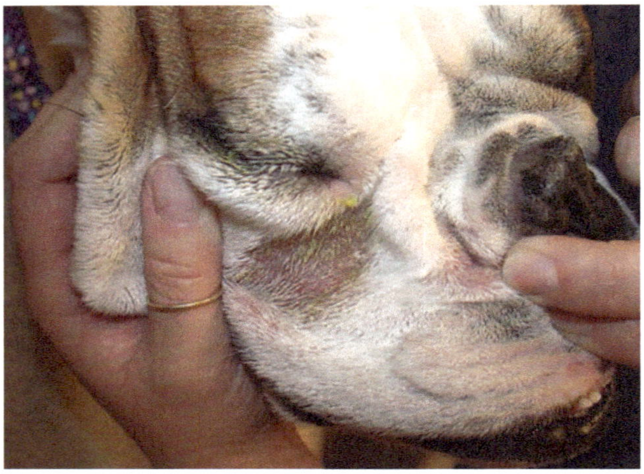

Figure 6.25 A Bulldog with facial fold intertrigo.

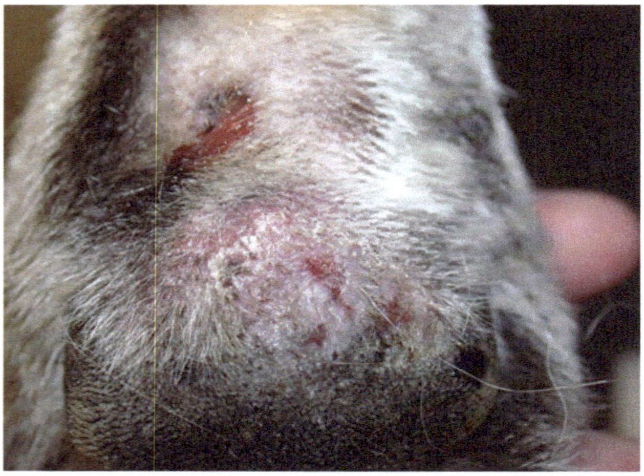

Figure 6.26 Firm swelling with draining tracts and serosanguinous discharge in a German Shepherd with metatarsal/metacarpal fistulas.

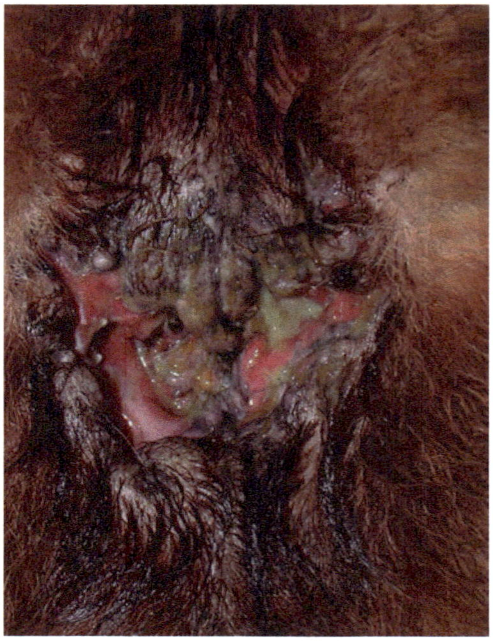

Figure 6.27 Perianal fistulas in a German Shepherd causing crateriform ulcerations and purulent drainage.

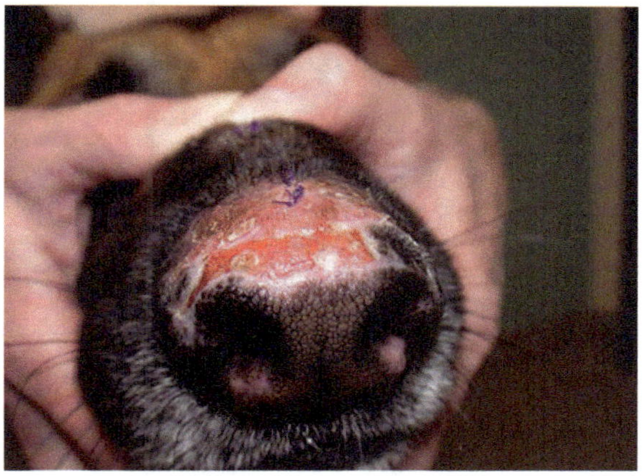

Figure 6.28 Discoid lupus erythematosus in a German Shepherd causing pigmentation and erosion on the dorsal nasal planum extending to haired skin; early lesions with just depigmentation and loss of nasal reticular pattern are present on the ventral nares.

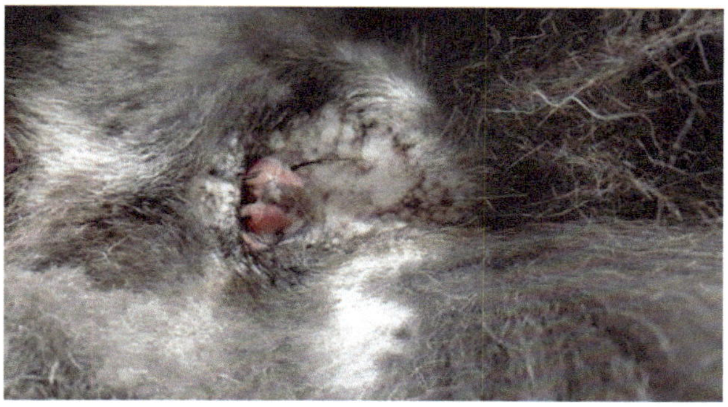

Figure 6.29 A German Shepherd dog with mucocutaneous lupus erythematosus; note the vulvar erosions/ulcerations and perivulvar latticework hyperpigmentation common to this disorder; similar lesions were present on the anal and perianal area.

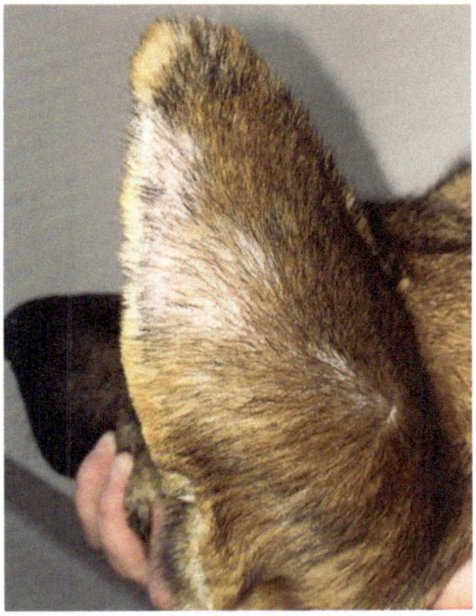

Figure 6.30 Patchy pinnal marginal and outer pinnal hypotrichosis and scaling in an atopic German Shepherd; lesions and pinnal-pedal response when pinnal margins were scraped mimic sarcoptic mange, and trial treatment for scabies was performed with no improvement but complete resolution occurred with treatment for atopy.

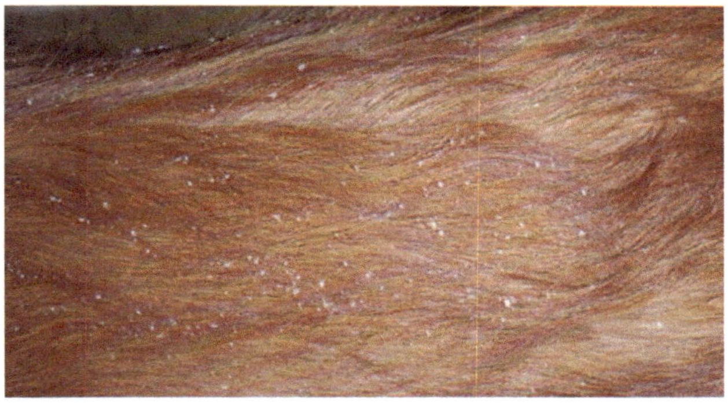

Figure 6.31 Diffuse non-pruritic truncal scaling in a Golden Retriever with ichthyosis.

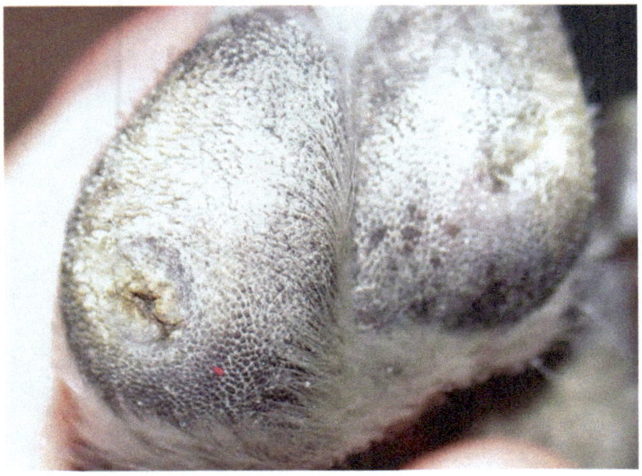

Figure 6.32 A Greyhound footpad corn; note the round area of toepad smoothness with associated fissuring; the dog presented for lameness.

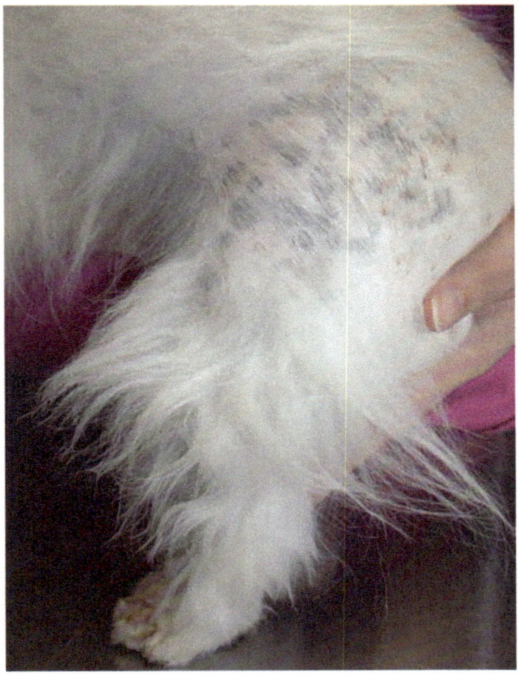

Figure 6.33A A Havanese with sebaceous adenitis which caused hypotrichosis and scaling involving the trunk, thighs, and head.

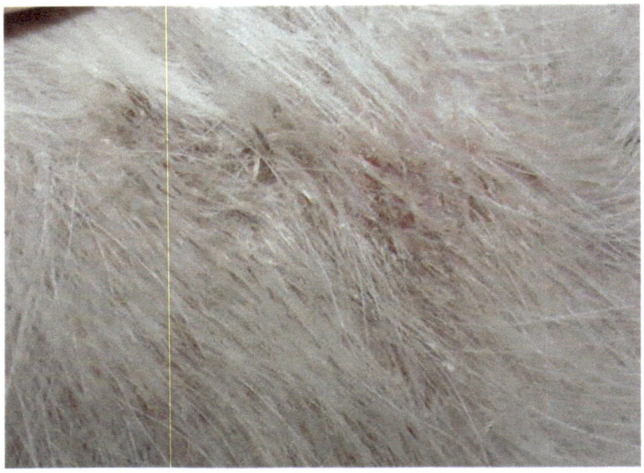

Figure 6.33B On close examination, adherent scaling and follicular casting is present. Skin scrapings for mites and cytology were negative, diagnosis was made on biopsy/dermatopathology.

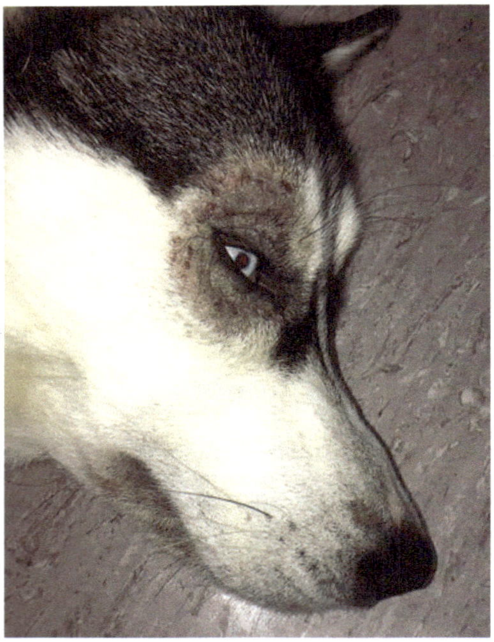

Figure 6.34 Periocular alopecia, erythema, and adherent crusting in a husky with zinc responsive dermatosis.

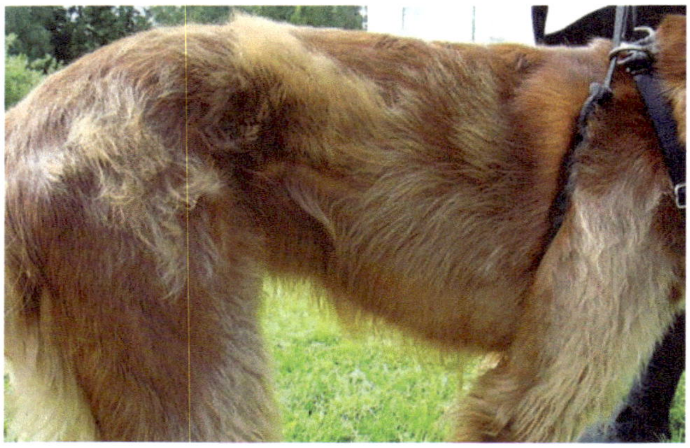

Figure 6.35 An Irish Setter with a fuzzy truncal coat which developed after neutering; this occurs to some extent in most double coated dogs but is more noticeable in Setters and Afghans. *Source:* Photo courtesy of Dr. Babette Taugbol.

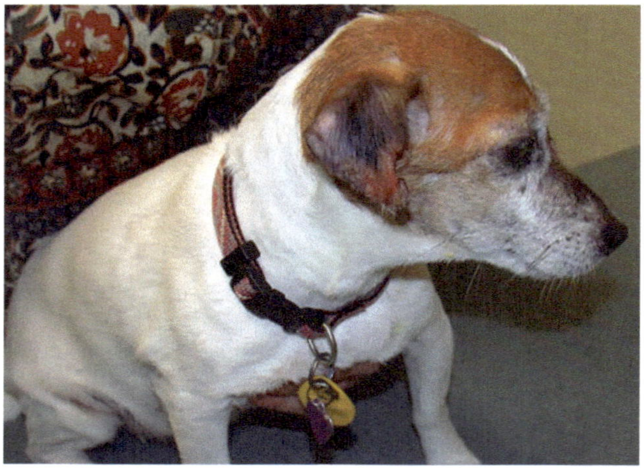

Figure 6.36A Pinnal ulceration in a Jack Russell Terrier caused by vasculitis post rabies vaccination.

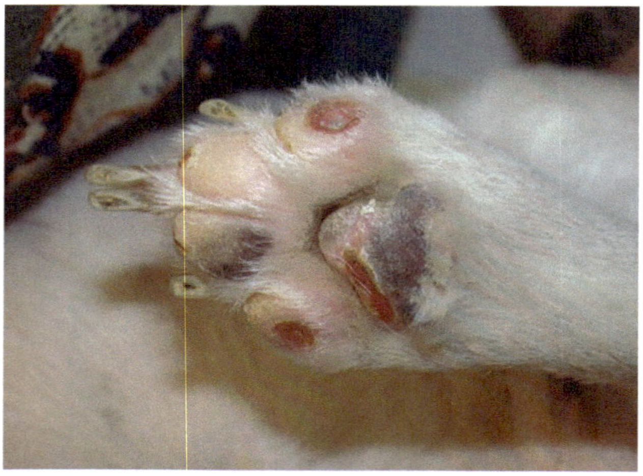

Figure 6.36B This dog also had central paw pad ulcerations.

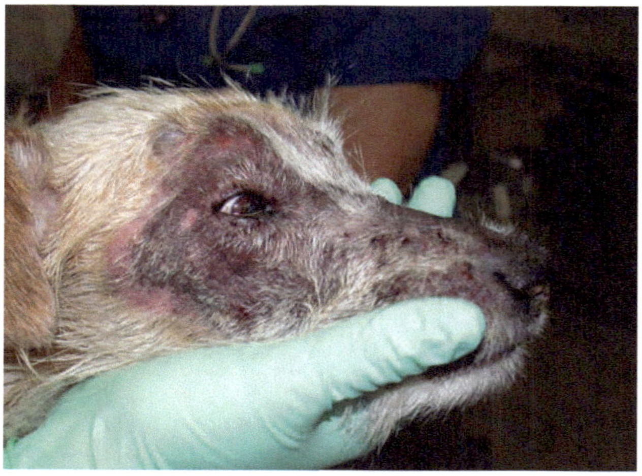

Figure 6.37 A Jack Russell Terrier with alopecia, crusting, and hyperpigmentation on the face and muzzle caused by *Trichophyton mentagrophytes*; the dog had a prior history of seasonal atopy, was intensely pruritic and had been unsuccessfully treated for allergies with immunomodulating medications for one year prior to presentation.

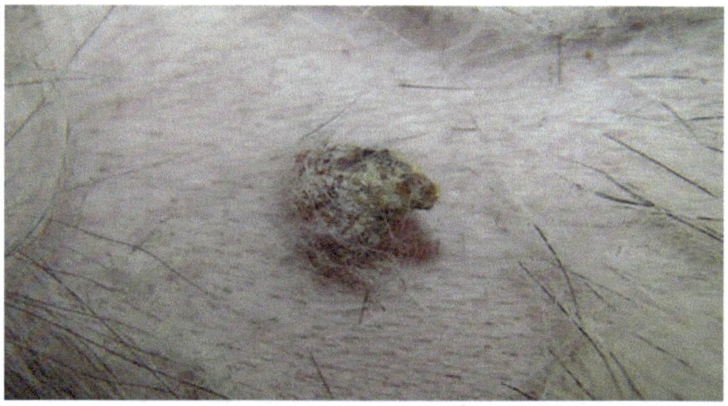

Figure 6.38 A Norwegian Elkhound with numerous raised, often hyperkeratotic sometimes cystic, dermal masses on the trunk which biopsy confirmed as intracornifying epitheliomas (ICE tumors).

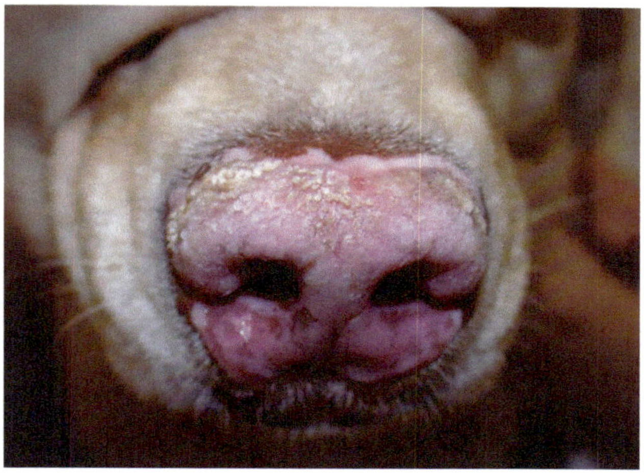

Figure 6.39 Nasal planum hypopigmentation and dorsal planum adherent hyperkeratosis in a young Labrador with nasal parakeratosis.

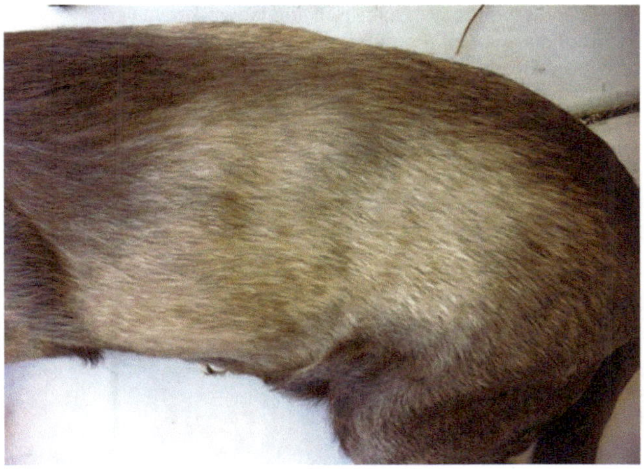

Figure 6.40 A Silver Labrador with color dilution alopecia characterized by non-pruritic truncal hypotrichosis, coarse wiry primary hairs, and increased lighter fuzzy secondary hairs.

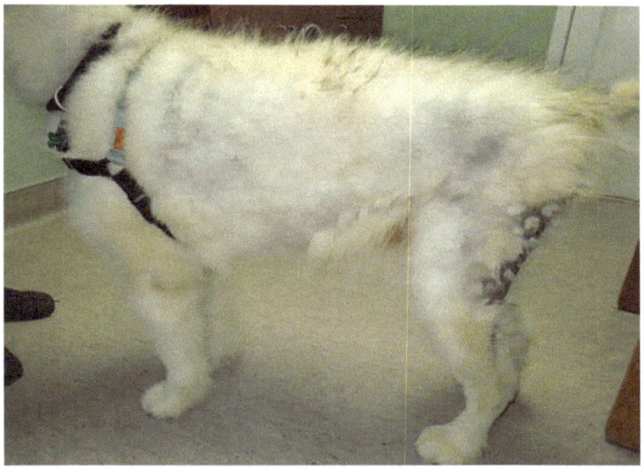

Figure 6.41 A Malamute with Alopecia X characterized by non-pruritic truncal, neck, and tail hypotrichosis with loss of primary hairs/retention of fuzzy secondary hairs, non-inflammatory alopecia, and hyperpigmentation on the caudal thighs. Full labwork, thyroid panel, and urine cortisol creatinine ratio were normal.

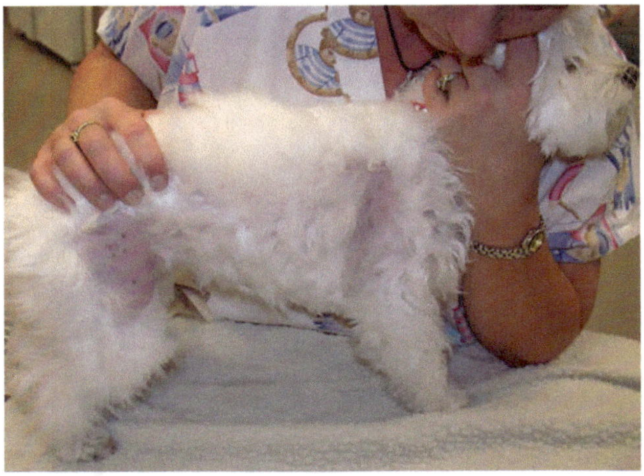

Figure 6.42 A Maltese with scarring alopecia on the right thigh and shoulder associated with prior rabies vaccinations in both locations.

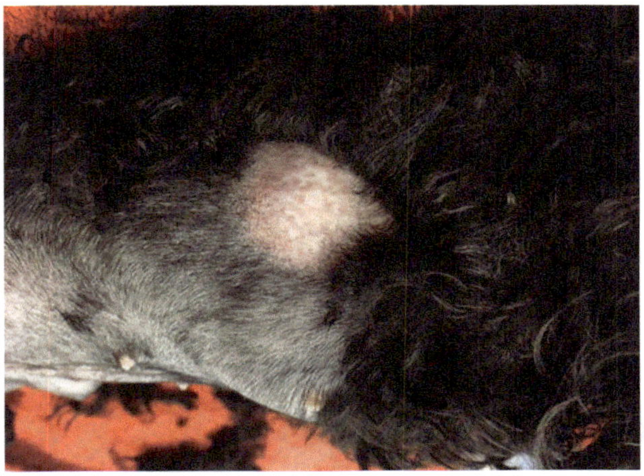

Figure 6.43 A Miniature Poodle with focal alopecia and indurated skin on the lateral thorax which occurred six weeks post rabies vaccination; biopsy revealed marked nodular lymphocytic to granulomatous inflammation associated with crystalline vaccine adjuvant and overlying follicular damage.

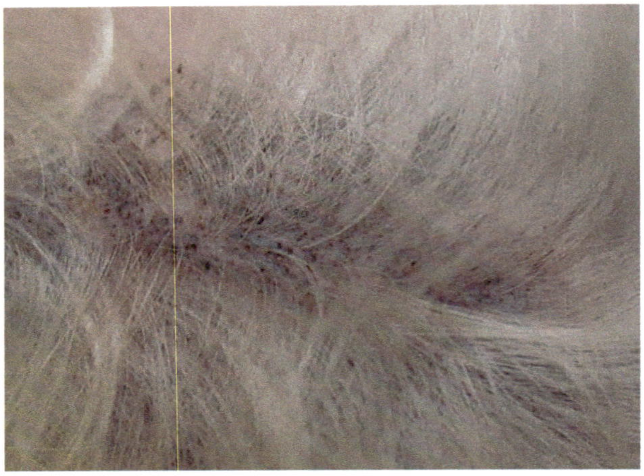

Figure 6.44 Numerous comedones and mild hypotrichosis on the dorsal midline of a Miniature Schnauzer with Schnauzer comedo syndrome.

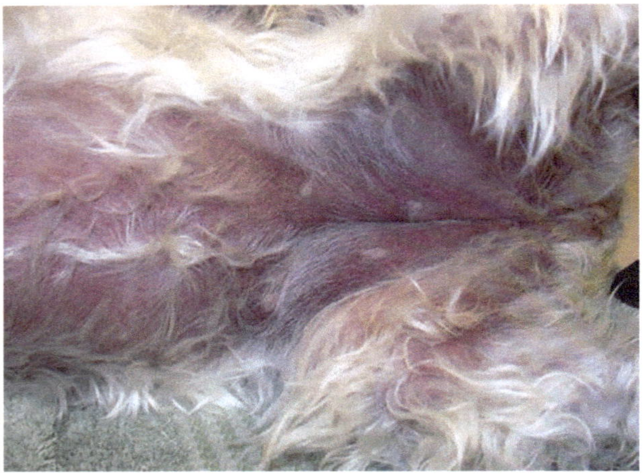

Figure 6.45 A Miniature Schnauzer with superficial suppurative necrolytic dermatitis (a.k.a. sterile pustular erythroderma of Miniature Schnauzers) causing severe generalized violaceous erythema which progressed to erosions and crusting on the pinnae; disease occurred after a limonene shampoo. The dog was febrile and severely systemically ill and labwork revealed neutrophilia, hypoalbuminemia, and elevated liver enzymes; she recovered after prolonged hospitalization for supportive care including steroids and plasma transfusion.

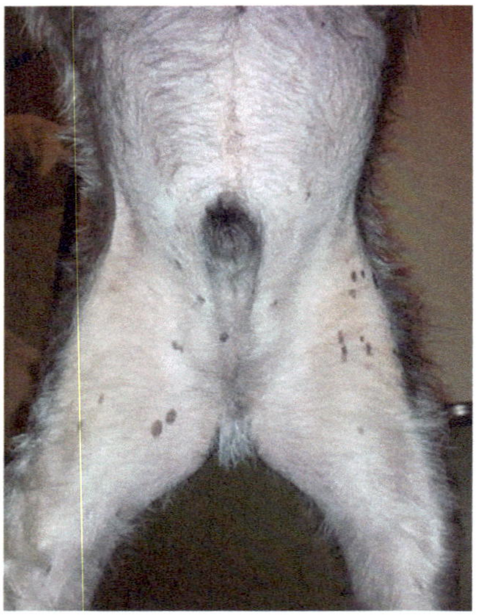

Figure 6.46 Numerous pigmented macules and small plaques caused by papilloma virus infection in a Miniature Schnauzer; lesions progressed after treatment with oclacitinib for the dog's atopic dermatitis.

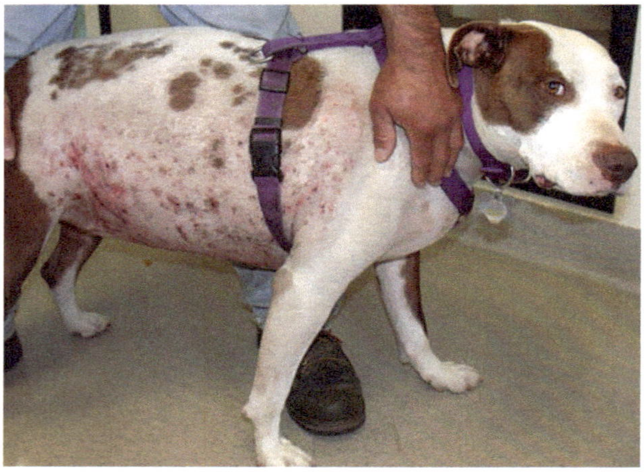

Figure 6.47A A Pitbull Terrier with solar dermatitis causing minimally pruritic ventrolateral truncal hypotrichosis, scarring, erythema, papules, and crusts which had been previously unsuccessfully treated as atopic dermatitis.

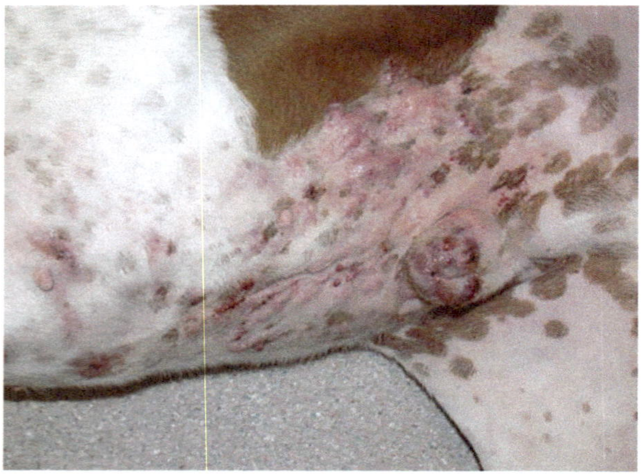

Figure 6.47B A more severely affected Pitbull Terrier with solar dermatitis causing raised, painful, sometimes draining, and crusted bullae on the inguinal area.

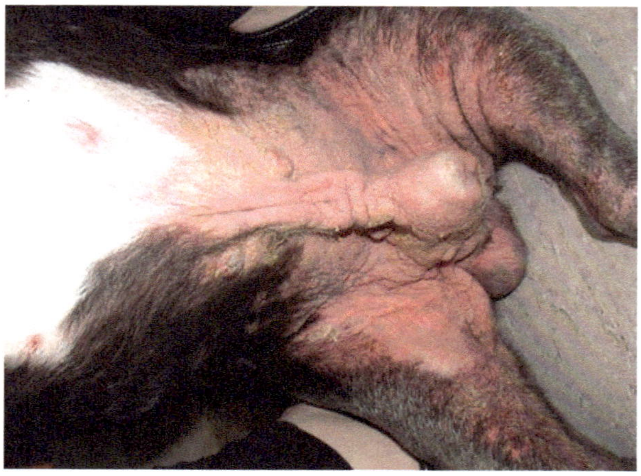

Figure 6.48 An atopic Pitbull Terrier with secondary severe pyoderma caused by MRSP.

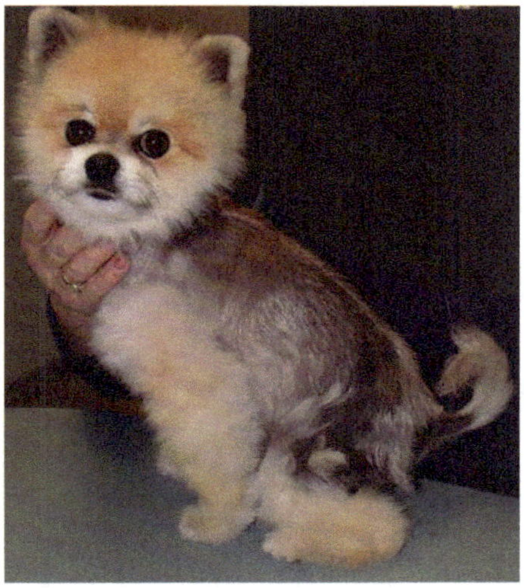

Figure 6.49 A Pomeranian with Alopecia X causing truncal, neck, and tail hypotrichosis and hyperpigmentation. Full labwork, thyroid panel, and urine cortisol creatinine ratio were normal.

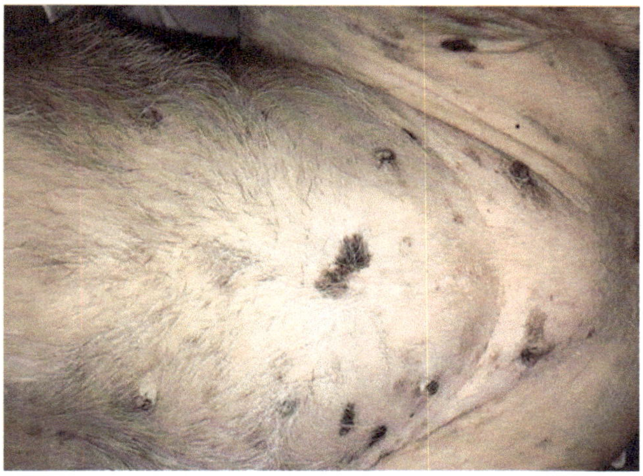

Figure 6.50 Numerous inguinal pigmented macules and plaques in a Pug caused by papilloma virus infection; lesions progressed after chemotherapy for mast cell tumor.

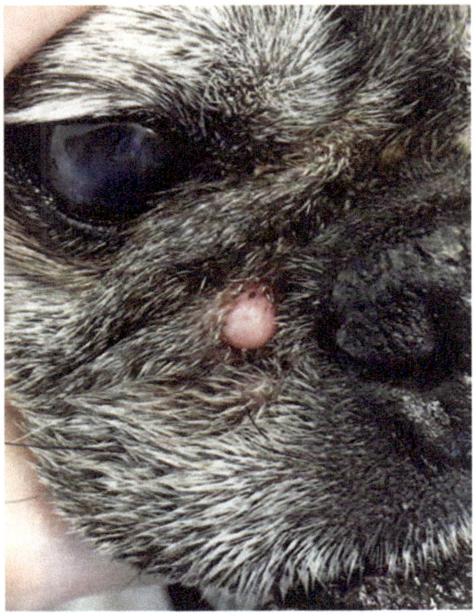

Figure 6.51 A pink raised mass on the face of a Pug; cytology determined it was a mast cell tumor.

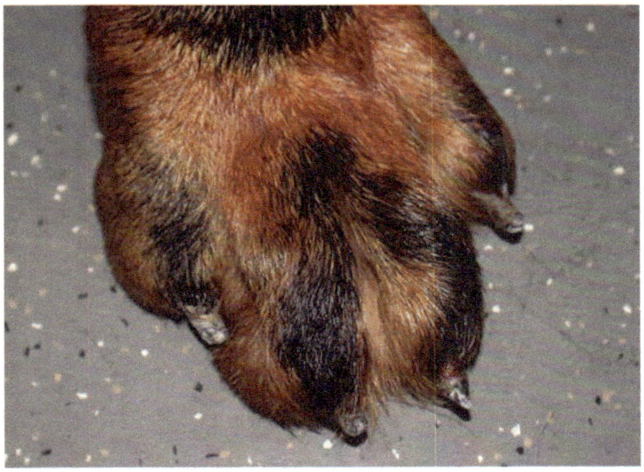

Figure 6.52 Stubby dystrophic toenails in a Rottweiler with symmetric lupoid onychodystrophy.

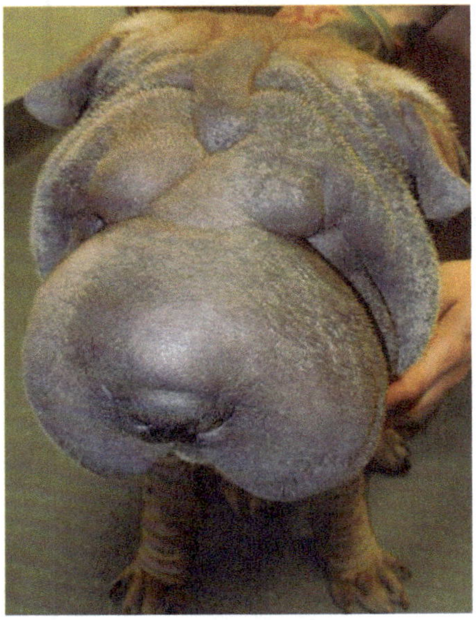

Figure 6.53A A young Shar-Pei with severe diffuse swelling of muzzle and eyelids caused by mucinosis.

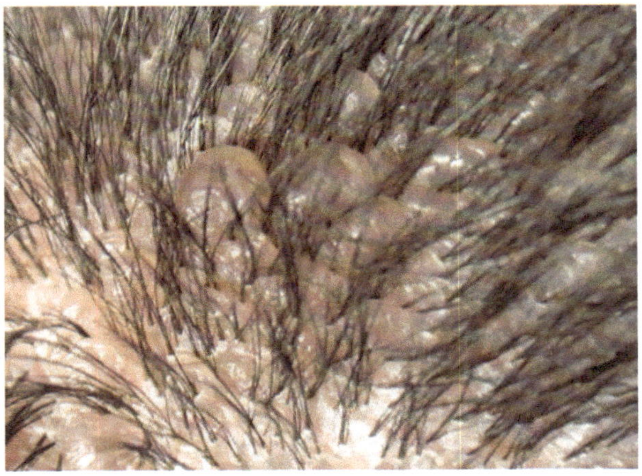

Figure 6.53B The same dog had innumerable small mucinotic vesicles on the trunk and legs which would ooze viscous clear fluid when ruptured.

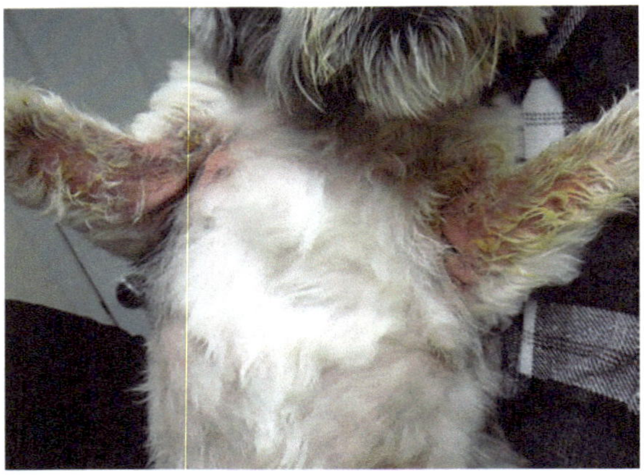

Figure 6.54 A Shih Tzu with *Malassezia* dermatitis due to underlying atopy; note the erythema, hypotrichosis, and sticky yellowish crusts on the medial limbs and axillae. Yeast were found on recheck skin cytology after the dog was treated for prior cytologically diagnosed bacterial overgrowth.

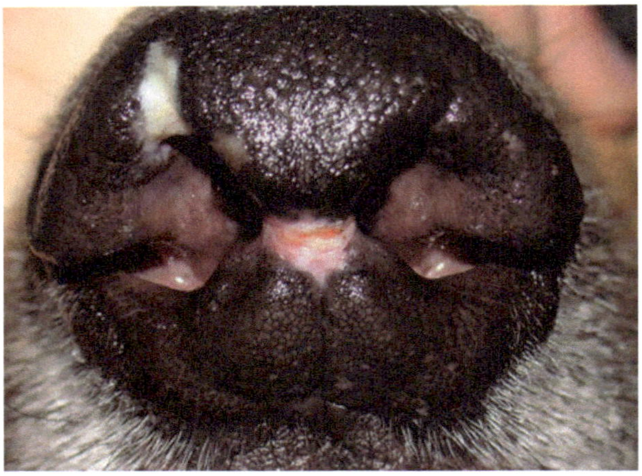

Figure 6.55 Nasal arteritis in a St. Bernard dog; the central nasal ulceration had been present and slowly progressive for 18 months prior to arterial rupture which prompted owners to seek medical care.

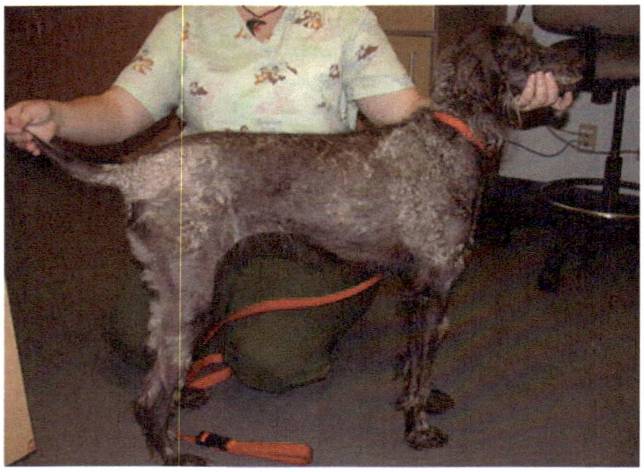

Figure 6.56A A Standard Poodle with sebaceous adenitis causing generalized hypotrichosis on the trunk, limbs, tail, and head including the pinnae; remaining hair is wispy and straight rather than curly.

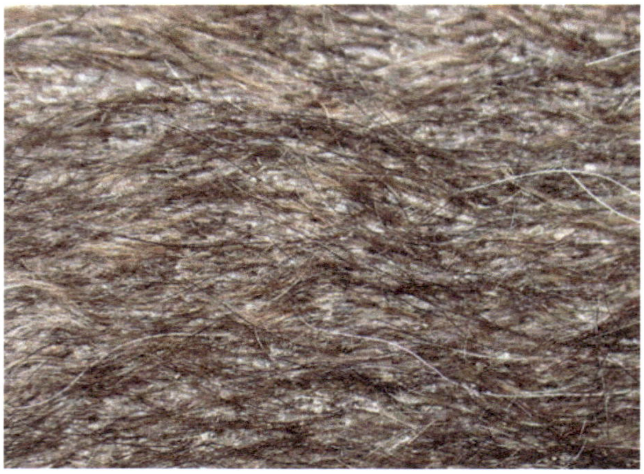

Figure 6.56B Closer examination of affected skin reveals adherent scaling and follicular casting. Skin scrapings for mites and cytology were negative; diagnosis was made on biopsy/dermatopathology.

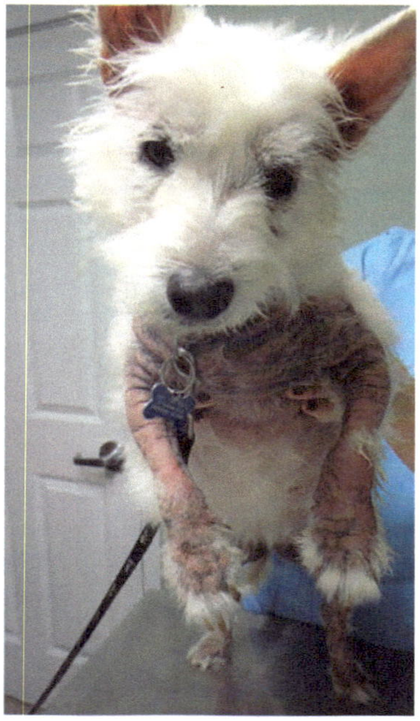

Figure 6.57 Severe ventral truncal and limb alopecia, lichenification, and hyperpigmentation in an atopic West Highland White Terrier caused by *Malassezia* dermatitis as well as MRSP infection.

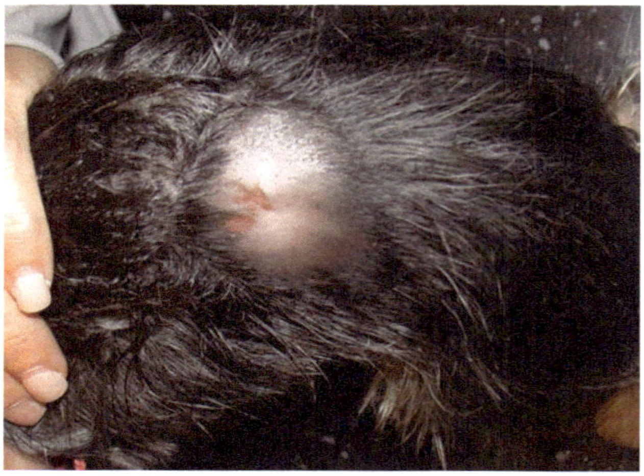

Figure 6.58 Focal scarring alopecia on the shoulder of a Yorkshire Terrier post rabies vaccination.

Table 6.2 Feline breed-related dermatoses.

Cat breed	Common condition	Figures
Abyssinian	Psychogenic alopecia, atopy, food allergy	Figure 6.60
Bengal	Atopy, food allergy, ulcerative nasal dermatitis	Figures 6.61A and 6.61B
Burmese	Congenital hypotrichosis, cutaneous asthenia (Ehlers–Danlos-like syndrome)	
Persian	Dermatophytosis, facial fold dermatitis, idiopathic facial dermatitis (dirty face syndrome)	Figures 6.62 and 6.63
Rex	*Malassezia* dermatitis, follicular dysplasia	Figure 6.64
Siamese	Vitiligo, food hypersensitivity, psychogenic alopecia	Figure 6.65
Sphynx	*Malassezia* dermatitis, allergic dermatitis, urticaria pigmentosa	Figures 6.66–6.68

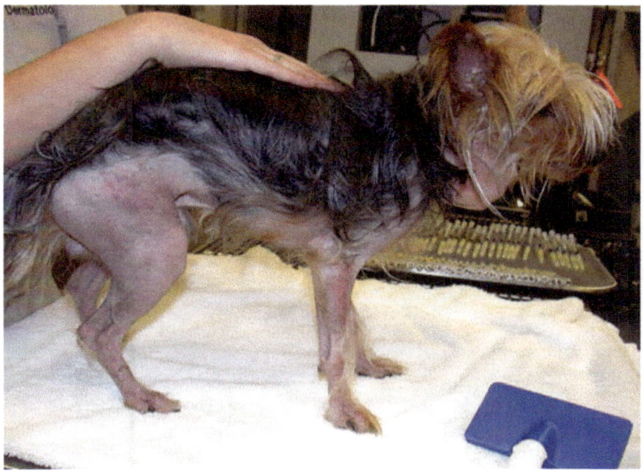

Figure 6.59 An atopic Yorkie with marked barbering and erythema present on the limbs and ventral trunk.

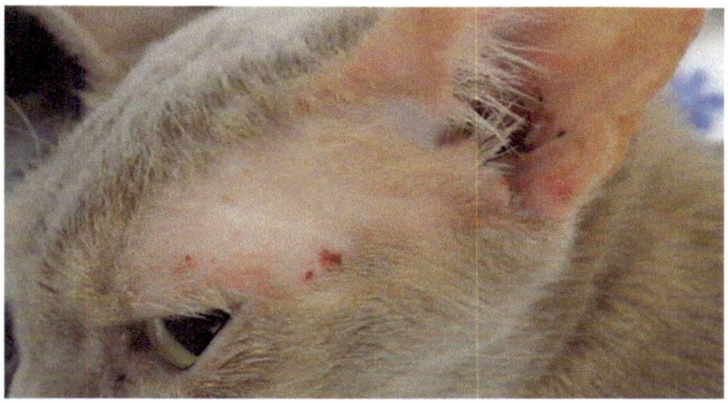

Figure 6.60 An atopic and food allergic Abyssinian cat with temporal excoriations; a hypoallergenic diet partially improved her pruritus then allergy immunotherapy based on intradermal testing caused complete remission of her pruritus.

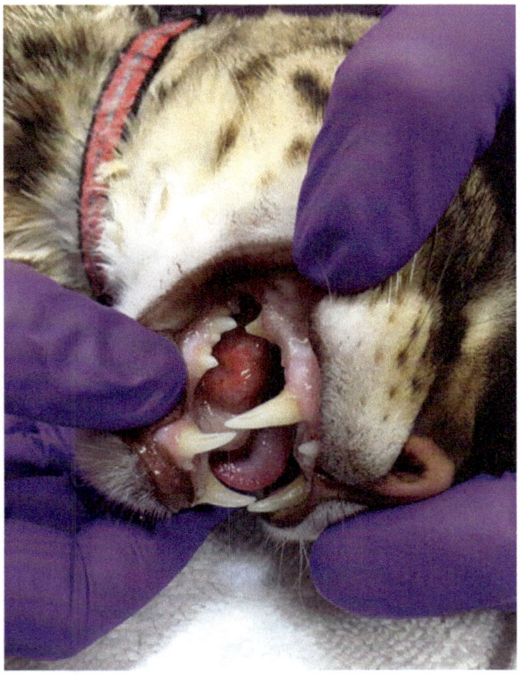

Figure 6.61A A food allergic Bengal cat with an oral eosinophilic granuloma.

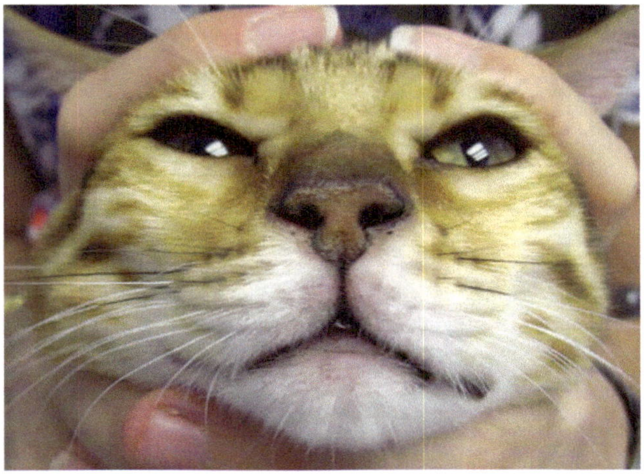

Figure 6.61B A Bengal cat with ulcerative nasal dermatitis. *Source:* Image courtesy of VIN and Cherry Douglas DVM.

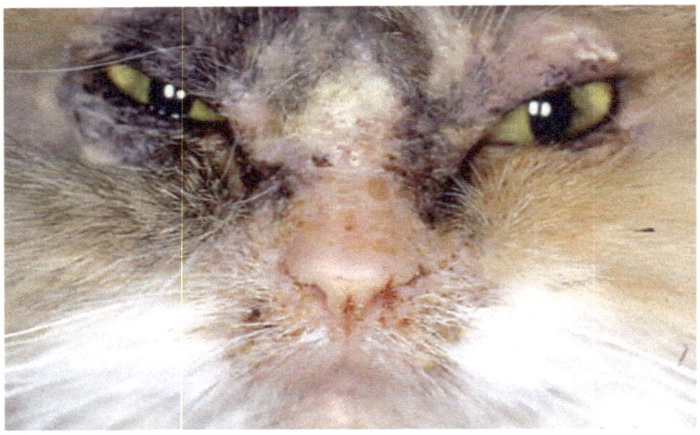

Figure 6.62 A Persian cat with patchy facial alopecia and crusting due to dermatophytosis.

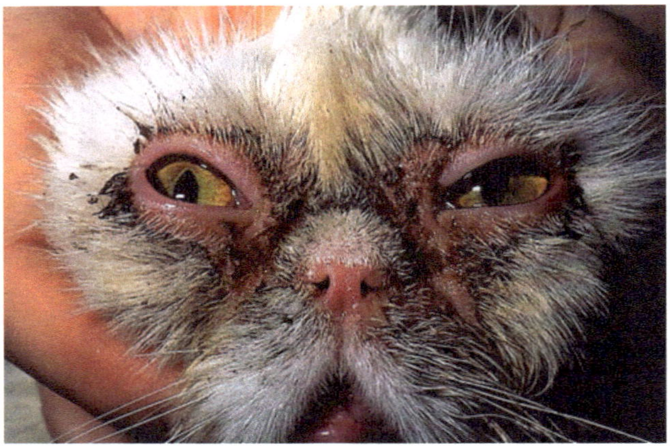

Figure 6.63 Severe moist facial dermatitis in a Persian cat with idiopathic facial dermatitis.

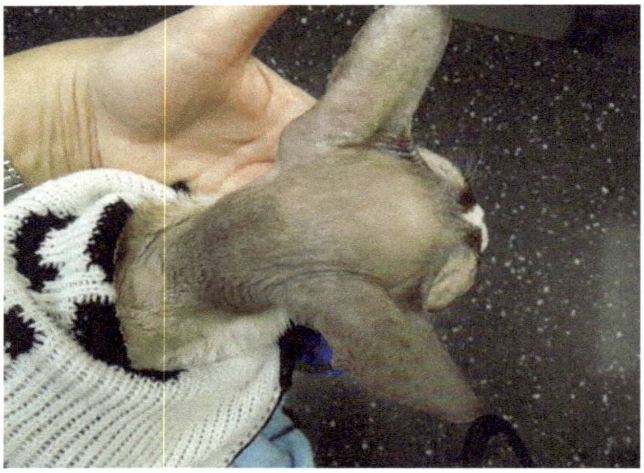

Figure 6.64 A Rex cat with non-inflammatory alopecia on the head/ears which also involved the dorsal tail.

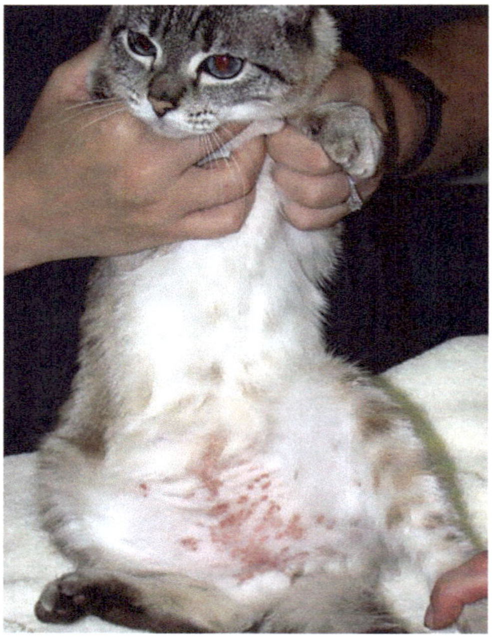

Figure 6.65 A Siamese cat with atopic dermatitis complicated by psychogenic/behavioral overgrooming.

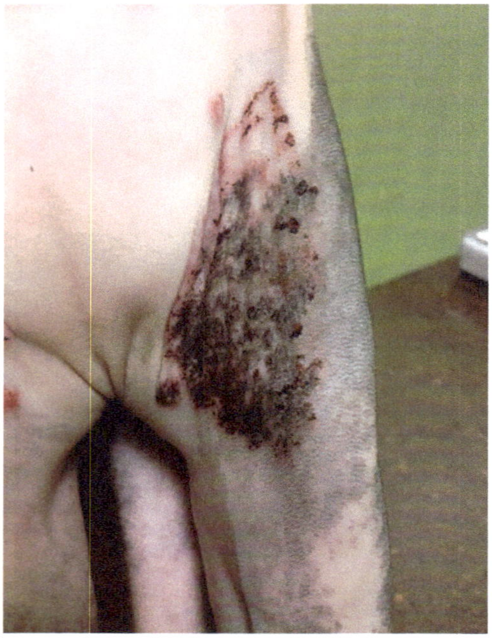

Figure 6.66 A Sphynx cat with *Malassezia* dermatitis secondary to atopy. *Source:* Photo courtesy of Dr. Ann Trimmer, DACVD.

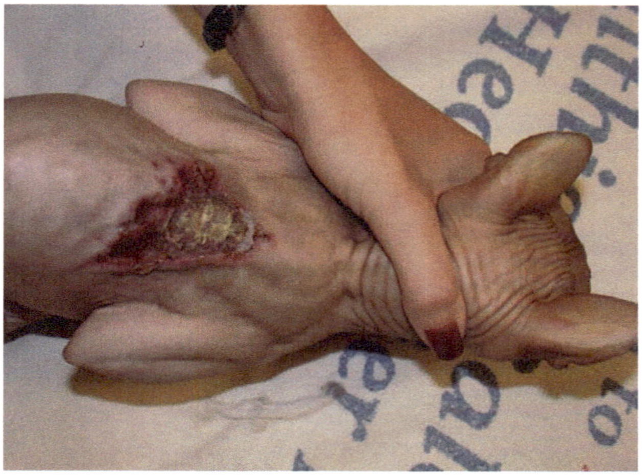

Figure 6.67 A Sphynx cat with severe pruritus and self-trauma to the dorsal shoulders caused by a hypersensitivity dermatitis.

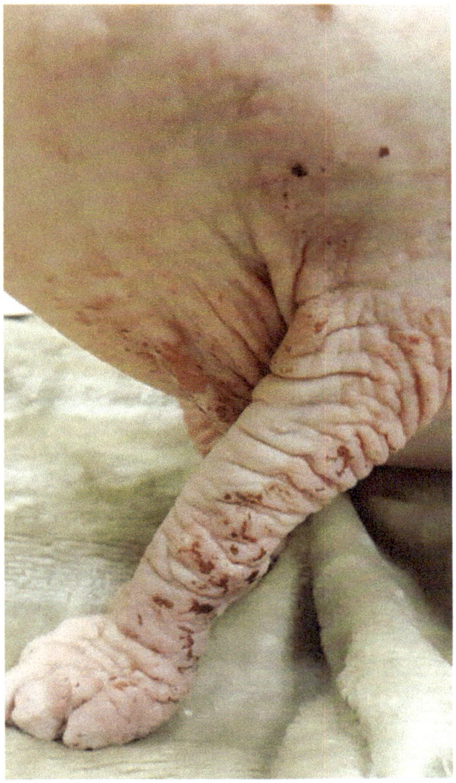

Figure 6.68 Urticaria pigmentosa in a Sphynx kitten. *Source:* Photo courtesy of Dr. Amy Shumaker, DACVD.

Further reading

Bryden, S.L., White, S.D., Dunston, S.M. et al. (2005). Clinical, histopathological and immunological characteristics of exfoliative cutaneous lupus erythematosus in 25 German short-haired pointers. *Vet. Dermatol.* 16 (4): 239–252.

Clark, R.D. and Stainer, J.R. (1994). *Medical and Genetic Aspects of Purebred Dogs*. Fairway, KS: Forum Publications Inc.

Clark, R.D. (1992). *Medical and Genetic and Behavioral Aspects of Purebred Cats*. Fairway, KS: Forum Publications Inc.

Hernblad Tevell, E., Bergvall, K., and Egenvall, A. (2008). Sebaceous adenitis in Swedish dogs, a retrospective study of 104 cases. *Acta Vet. Scand.* 50 (1): 11.

Jackson, H.A. (2004 Feb). Eleven cases of vesicular cutaneous lupus erythematosus in Shetland sheepdogs and rough collies: clinical management and prognosis. *Vet. Dermatol.* 15 (1): 37–41.

Leeb, T., Muller, E.J., Roosie, P., and Welle, M. (2017). Genetic testing in veterinary dermatology. *Vet. Dermatol.* 28 (1): 4–e1.

Mauldin, E. (2013 Jan). Canine ichthyosis and related disorders of cornification in small animals. *Vet. Clin. North Am. Small Anim. Pract.* 43 (1): 89–97.

Miller, W.H., Griffen, C.E., and Campbell, K.L. (2013). *Muller and Kirk's Small Animal Dermatology*, 7e. St Louis, MO: Elsevier Mosby.

Moriello, K.A., Coyner, K., Paterson, S., and Mignon, B. (2017 Jun). Diagnosis and treatment of dermatophytosis in dogs and cats: Clinical Consensus Guidelines of the World Association for Veterinary Dermatology. *Vet. Dermatol.* 28 (3): 266–e68.

Narama, I., Kobayashi, Y., Yamagami, T. et al. (2005). Pigmented cutaneous papillomatosis (pigmented epidermal nevus) in three pug dogs; histopathology, electron microscopy and analysis of viral DNA by the polymerase chain reaction. *J. Comp. Pathol.* 132: 132–138.

Olivry, T., Rossi, M.A., Banovic, F., and Linder, K.E. (2015). Mucocutaneous lupus erythematosus in dogs (21 cases). *Vet. Dermatol.* 26 (4): 256–e55.

Torres, S.M., Brien, T.O., and Scott, D.W. (2002). Dermal arteritis of the nasal philtrum in a Giant Schnauzer and three Saint Bernard dogs. *Vet. Dermatol.* 13 (5): 275–281.

White, S.D., Bourdeau, P., Rosychuk, R.A. et al. (2001). Zinc-responsive dermatosis in dogs: 41 cases and literature review. *Vet. Dermatol.* 12 (2): 101–109.

7

Parasitic skin diseases

Heide Newton, DVM, DACVD

Dermatology for Animals, Tucson, AZ, USA

All treatments listed for parasites other than fleas and ticks are extra-label unless otherwise specified. Only one of the listed antiparasitic treatments should be employed at a time with the option to change to another treatment if adverse effects or inefficacy is noted.

Clinical Atlas of Canine and Feline Dermatology, First Edition. Edited by Kimberly S. Coyner.

Companion website: www.wiley.com/go/coyner/dermatology

Table 7.1 Canine and feline ectoparasites.

Disease	Clinical signs	Diagnosis	Treatment
Canine demodicosis (Figures 7.1A–7.18B, 2.42, 2.43, 3.30A, 3.58, 3.111) *Demodex canis* *Demodex injai* *Demodex cornei* (short bodied *Demodex* mite) has been shown to be a variant of *D. canis*. Juvenile (<4 yr) and adult (>4 yr) onset. Predisposed breeds: American Staffordshire Terrier, English Bulldog, Staffordshire Bull Terrier, Shar-Pei, West Highland White Terrier; for *D. injai*, Fox Terrier and Shih Tzus are predisposed.	Localized: Patch(es) of hypotrichosis +/− comedones, erythema and/or scaling and variable pruritus often on face, forelimbs, and/or bilateral ceruminous otitis externa. Generalized: Numerous patches of hypotrichosis, erythema, follicular hyperkeratosis, comedones, and follicular casts; +/− peripheral lymphadenopathy; secondary bacterial folliculitis and furunculosis in some cases. *D. injai*: Greasy seborrhea of dorsum and face and variable pruritus. Pododermatitis: Interdigital and digital erythema, alopecia, furunculosis, edema, and often secondary bacterial infection.	Mite identification via skin scraping most commonly; tape preparation, hair plucks, cytology of exudate from furuncles; rarely, biopsy may be needed for very scarred areas such as paws. Cytology to rule out secondary bacterial infections. Adult onset cases: Screen labwork and thyroid panel for underlying immunosuppressive disease.	Localized: In most cases spontaneous resolution will occur within a few months and no treatment is required; Goodwinol (rotenone) ointment and benzoyl peroxide gel may be used. Otic *Demodex*: Use a topical otic product containing ivermectin or milbemycin as labeled for treatment of ear mites, or instill 0.1 ml 0.1% ivermectin into affected ear once daily until 2 weeks beyond negative ear swab. Isoxazoline insecticides also likely effective. In cases of generalized, *D. canis*, *D. injai*, and demodectic pododermatitis, treat for 4 weeks beyond negative skin scraping (no live or dead mites or eggs): 1. First-line treatment: Isoxazoline insecticides: Fluralaner 25 mg/kg PO q12w. Afoxolaner 2.5 mg/kg PO q4w. Sarolaner 2 mg/kg PO q4w. 2. Second-line treatment options: Avermectins[a] (caution with herding breeds): 1% Ivermectin 0.4–0.6 mg/kg PO q24h. 1% Doramectin 0.6 mg/kg PO/SQ q7d. 0.1% Moxidectin 0.2–0.4 mg/kg PO q 24h. 2.5% Moxidectin topically q7d (Advantage Multi®). 3. Other treatment options: Milbemycin 1–2 mg/kg PO q24h. Amitraz dips (0.03–0.05% or 250 ppm) q1–2w (licensed treatment, but rarely used due to superior efficacy and safety of isoxazoline insecticides). [a] Systemic avermectins cannot be used in combination with ketoconazole or spinosad insecticides (Comfortis®, Trifexis®) due to risk of severe toxicity. Bathe with benzoyl peroxide-containing shampoo for follicular flushing of mites; follow with conditioner to avoid overdrying. Control secondary bacterial infections with chlorhexidine shampoos 1–2 times weekly alternating with benzoyl peroxide shampoo and/or chlorhexidine wipes/mousse/spray +/− systemic antibiotics for severe generalized or deep pyoderma. Avoid immunosuppressive medications.

Feline demodicosis *Demodex cati* (Figures 7.19A–7.19C)	Localized: Patch(es) of hypotrichosis, erythema, scale and variable pruritus often at face, head, cervical region, and/or bilateral ceruminous otitis externa. Generalized: Alopecia, scale, erythema, crust, and hyperpigmentation, with variable pruritus at face, head, neck, trunk, and limbs; often associated with underlying systemic disease or immunosuppression.	Mite identification via skin scraping, tape preparation, fecal floatation. Screen labwork for underlying immunosuppressive metabolic or retroviral disease.	Treat for 4 weeks beyond negative skin scraping (no live or dead mites or eggs): 1. First-line treatment options: Isoxazoline insecticides: Fluralaner 40 mg/kg topically q12w. 2–4% lime sulfur dips q7d. 2. Second-line treatment options: 2.5% Moxidectin topically q7d (Advantage Multi). 1% ivermectin 0.3 mg/kg PO q24h. 1% doramectin 0.4–0.6 mg/kg PO or SQ once weekly. Milbemycin 1–2 mg/kg PO q24h. Address underlying immunosuppression.
Feline demodicosis *Demodex gatoi* (Figures 7.20A–B)	Pruritus, alopecia, erythema, and scale often at lateral thorax, ventral and lateral abdomen, and medial limbs; contagious to other cats.	Mite identification via skin scraping, tape preparation, fecal floatation.	Same as *D. cati.* Treat all in contact cats simultaneously.
Canine scabies *Sarcoptes scabiei* (Figures 7.21–7.24B, 3.38A, 3.89)	Progressive and intense pruritus involving ventral trunk, elbows, hocks, paws, face, and pinnae with papules, crusts, erythema, and alopecia; with chronicity, bacterial pyoderma, lichenification, and hyperpigmentation occur.	Definitive diagnosis can be difficult and may rest on clinical signs and response to treatment. Skin scraping (mites difficult to find). Positive pinnal-pedal reflex. Cytology to rule out secondary bacterial or *Malassezia* infections.	Selamectin (licensed treatment Revolution®) dosed topically extralabel at q2w × 3tx. Moxidectin (licensed treatment Advantage Multi®) topically q30d × 2tx. Fluralaner 25 mg/kg PO q12w. Afoxolaner 2.5 mg/kg PO q4w. Sarolaner 2 mg/kg PO q4w. 1% ivermectin 0.2–0.4 mg/kg PO or SQ q7d × 3tx. Milbemycin 1–2 mg/kg PO q7–14d × 3 tx. 2–3% lime sulfur dips q 1–2w × 4–6w. 1% doramectin 0.2 mg/kg SQ or PO q7d × 4–6w. Fipronil spray 2 pumps per lb. q14d × 3tx. Treat all in contact dogs simultaneously. Control secondary bacterial or *Malassezia* infections with miconazole/chlorhexidine shampoos or sprays/mousse/wipes every 1–2 days on affected areas. Tapering 2–3 week course of prednisone (starting at 0.5 mg/kg/d) or oclacitinib 0.4–0.6 mg/kg PO BID × 7–14 days then once daily × 7–14 days (use in dogs >1 yr of age only).

(Continued)

Table 7.1 Canine and feline ectoparasites (Continued)

Disease	Clinical signs	Diagnosis	Treatment
Feline scabies *Notoedres cati* (Figures 7.25–7.27, 3.38B)	Progressive pruritus, crusts, thickened skin and hypotrichosis at pinnae, head, neck and can spread to rest of body.	Definitive diagnosis can be difficult and may rest on clinical signs and response to treatment. Skin scrapings (mites may be difficult to find).	Selamectin topically q2w × 3tx (Revolution®) Moxidectin topically q2–4 weeks × 3tx (Advantage Multi). 1% ivermectin 0.2–0.3 mg/kg SQ q14d × 4–6w. 1% doramectin 0.2–0.3 mg/kg SQ q 1–2w for 4–6w. 2–4% lime sulfur dips q7d × 6w. Fluralaner likely effective. Treat all in contact cats simultaneously.
Ear mites *Otodectes cynotis* (Figures 7.28–7.30)	Otic pruritus with dark dry "coffee grounds" otic debris. Ectopic mites can cause pruritus on face, neck, and trunk which can mimic allergy. Contagious to other mammals. Secondary yeast or bacterial otitis externa common.	Mite identification in otic debris. Cytology for secondary yeast or bacterial otitis externa.	Selamectin (licensed treatment Revolution) dosed topically at q2–4w × 3tx. Moxidectin topically q30d (licensed treatment Advantage Multi). Fluralaner 25 mg/kg PO or 40 mg/kg topically q12w. Ivermectin 0.2–0.3 mg/kg SQ q14d × 2tx or PO q7d × 3tx. Topical otic preparations with ivermectin, milbemycin, or mineral oil can be used, but systemic therapy still recommended for ectopic mites. Treat all in contact dogs and cats simultaneously.
Cat fur mite *Lynxacarus radovskyi* (Figure 7.31)	Variable depending on chronicity and extent of infestation ranging from minimal pruritus and "salt and pepper" appearance with dull, dirty coat to intense pruritus with generalized maculopapular to exfoliative dermatitis and alopecia. Can be contagious to others from direct contact or fomites.	Mite or egg identification on hair shafts (trichogram), superficial scrapings or acetate tape preparations. Caudal body sites may yield more mites.	Moxidectin/imidacloprid (Advantage Multi) topically q14d × 2tx. Fluralaner 25–50 mg/kg PO once. Fipronil topically q2w or lime sulfur dips q7d.
Cheyletiellosis *Cheyletiella sp.* (Figures 7.32–7.34) Predisposed breeds: Cocker Spaniel	Variable to no pruritus, dorsal dry scale, variable hair loss, erythema, and/or papules. Contagious to other mammals (not species specific).	Mite identification in hair/scale samples.	Selamectin topically q2w × 3tx. 2–3% lime sulfur dips q7d × 3–4tx. Fipronil spray 6 ml/kg q14d × 4–6w. 1% ivermectin 0.2–0.3 mg/kg SQ q14d × 2tx or PO q7d × 3tx. Milbemycin 2 mg/kg PO q7d × 3tx. Fluralaner 25 mg/kg PO q12w. Treat all in contact dogs and cats simultaneously.

Pediculosis (Lice) Dog: *Trichodectes canis* (Figure 7.35) *Linognathus setosus* (Figure 7.36) Cat: *Felicola subrostratus* (Figure 7.37)	Scale and pruritus with secondary excoriations, papules, and crusts. Contagious among same mammal species (host specific).	Louse identification in hair/scale samples collected by flea combing or tape preparation.	Fipronil spray 6 ml/kg q14d × 2tx. Selamectin topically q2w × 2tx. Imidacloprid topically q14d × 2tx. Moxidectin (Advantage Multi) topically q2w × 2tx. 1% ivermectin 0.2–0.3 mg/kg SQ q14d × 2tx or PO q7d × 3tx. 1% doramectin 0.2–0.4 mg/kg PO/SQ weekly × 4w. Groom and clip away mats. Treat all in contact dogs/cats simultaneously and thoroughly clean environment and fomites.
Trombiculosis "Chiggers" *Eutrombicula alfreddugesi* *Neotrombicula autumnalis* (Figure 7.38)	Seasonal (late summer and fall) pruritus, papules, crusts at legs, paws, head, ears, ventrum; orange-red mites may be tightly attached to skin; history of environmental exposure in woods or fields.	Clinical signs, mite identification.	Fipronil spray q14d (dogs and cats). Permethrin spray or spot on (dogs only). Avoid exposure to outdoor environments or reinfestation can occur.
Hookworm Dermatitis *Ancylostoma braziliense* *Ancylostoma caninum* *Uncinaria stenocephala*	Papules, erythema, hyperkeratosis, alopecia, interdigital and pawpad swelling, with variable amounts of pruritus or pain, affecting body parts in contact with ground especially paws, distal limbs, and ventrum. History of poor sanitation in grass or dirt kennels or exposure to unsanitary dog parks.	Clinical signs, hookworm eggs on fecal flotation, and history of poor sanitation.	Antihelminthic treatment such as pyrantel, fenbendazole, ivermectin, or milbemycin for all in contact dogs. Clean kennels and premises with emphasis on feces removal. Routine monthly heartworm prevention products are protective.
***Cuterebra* sp.** (Figures 7.39A–7.39C)	Localized swelling with fistula, often at cervical region and observed during August, September, and October.	Clinical signs and identification of larva removed from fistula.	Incise or spread fistula and gently extract larva with forceps using care to avoid crushing larva and extract completely, then treat as any open wound.
Myiasis (infection with fly larvae, a.k.a. maggots) (Figure 7.40)	Larvae visible on or in the skin with punched out round holes often near neglected wounds or nose, eyes, mouth, anus, or genitalia. Often is a disease of neglect.	Identification of larvae in wounds.	Clip hair and clean lesions, surgically debride affected tissue, and manage wound care. First-line treatment (achieve fastest kill of larvae): Nitenpyram or spinosad/milbemycin at label doses. Second-choice treatment (due to slower kill of larvae): spinosad or afoxolaner at label doses. Treat underlying predisposing factors such as poor hygiene or living conditions. Avoid fly exposure (house indoors) and eliminate fly attracting and breeding sites (such as manure piles).

(*Continued*)

Table 7.1 Canine and feline ectoparasites (Continued)

Disease	Clinical signs	Diagnosis	Treatment
Fly bite dermatitis (Figures 7.41A and 7.41B)	Erythema and hemorrhagic crusts at tips or folds of pinnae. Variable pruritus. Black fly bites can appear as peracute round target red to purple lesions on the ventral trunk; lesions are not raised, non-painful, and non-pruritic and resolve within a few days.	Clinical signs and history of outdoor exposure to flies.	Topical antibiotic and corticosteroid-containing ointments. Fly repellents or permethrin containing flea products to prevent fly bites. Avoid fly exposure (house indoors) and eliminate fly attracting and breeding sites (such as manure piles).
***Pelodera* dermatitis** (a.k.a. rhabditic dermatitis, cutaneous infestation with larvae of *Pelodera strongyloides*)	Ventral (paws, limbs, perineum, ventral thorax, and abdomen) erythema and alopecia with variable pruritus, papules and crusts, and secondary bacterial or yeast infections.	Clinical signs, identification of nematode larvae on trichogram, skin scrapings and/or biopsy, and history of exposure to filthy, damp decaying organic material. Cytology to evaluate secondary bacterial or yeast infections.	Moxidectin 2.5%/imidacloprid 10% topically q2w × 2tx. Avoid exposure to decaying organic material that may harbor nematode larvae. Treat secondary bacterial or yeast infections with appropriate topical or systemic therapies.
Dracunculiasis *Dracunculus insignis* Rare and reported in dogs and cats.	Single to multiple painful or pruritic nodules on limbs, head, or abdomen that ulcerate and do not heal, sometimes adult worms are seen in fistulae.	Clinical signs and identification of adult nematodes or larvae on cytology or histopathology.	Surgical excision of nodules. Avoid contact with contaminated water and avoid ingestion of intermediate host.
Spider bite Brown recluse (*Loxosceles*) spiders occur predominately in the South Central region of the United States, although there are reported sightings as far north as Illinois and as far as the east and west coast areas (Figure 7.42). They live in dark, warm, dry places such as woodpiles, crevices, barns, in attics, trees, and in small corners or in shoes, clothing, or bedding.	Bites are painless or minimally painful; initially a small area of localized inflammation occurs which subsequently spreads then localized necrosis and ulceration develop due to cytotoxicity from venom components (sphingomyelinase D) and localized production of cellular inflammatory mediators.	Clinical signs, history of a spider bite, if known. Definitive diagnosis is usually impossible, and misdiagnosis is frequent.	Immediate wound care (if witnessed) should include cleansing, cold compresses, confinement and elevation of the bitten extremity if possible, oral analgesics and antihistamines; pentoxifylline may be helpful to increase circulation and reduce vascular inflammation. Dapsone (an inhibitor of neutrophil function) has been used in some people with anecdotal benefit, though is controversial in humans. The use of hyperbaric oxygen has been shown useful in small clinical studies but is also controversial. Early excision of bite lesions and oral or intralesional injection of corticosteroids could worsen necrosis and are contraindicated. Wound care of necrotic or ulcerated lesions includes debridement of necrotic tissues, culture-directed antibiotic therapy for secondary infections, and delayed excision of eschars, with skin grafting if indicated. With proper wound management, necrotic wounds will heal over in 1–8 weeks; scarring may occur.

Fleas *Ctenocephalides felis felis* (Figures 7.43 and 7.44) *Echidnophaga gallinacea* (sticktight fleas)	Identification of fleas and/or flea feces ("flea dirt") and/or *Dipylidium caninum* (tapeworm) on physical examination. For individuals with hypersensitivity to flea saliva allergens: variable pruritus, often at caudal trunk. Anemia due to blood loss, especially in small patients with heavy infestations. Sticktight fleas are usually found embedded in the skin on pinnae, eyelid, and between the toes.	Flea and/or flea feces ("flea dirt") identification. *Dipylidium caninum* (tapeworm) identification in patient feces or fecal flotation. Clinical signs and exposure warrant therapeutic trial of flea control.	Routine use of topical or oral flea control product(s) per label instructions (see Table 7.2) for all pets in household, selected based on client ability and willingness to administer, flea burden, and other ectoparasite exposure. Environmental treatments: Indoors: thorough vacuuming of all floors and furniture, washing of pet beds, pesticide treatments of home with sodium borate or combination of pyrethrins/pyrethroids and insect growth regulator, professional extermination recommended for best results. Outdoors: Remove organic debris, restrict pet access to infested areas.
Ticks (Figures 7.45 and 7.46) *Rhipicephalus sanguineus* *Dermacentor variabilis* *Ixodes scapularis* *Amblyomma americanum* *Otobius megnini* (spinose ear tick)	Identification of ticks on physical examination. Less commonly, progressive ascending flaccid paralysis ("tick paralysis"). Spinose ear tick found on otoscopic examination, can trigger secondary otitis externa.	Tick identification.	Manual removal of attached ticks. Routine use of topical or oral tick control product(s) per label instructions (see Table 7.3) for all pets in household, selected based on client ability and willingness to administer, tick burden, and other ectoparasite exposure.

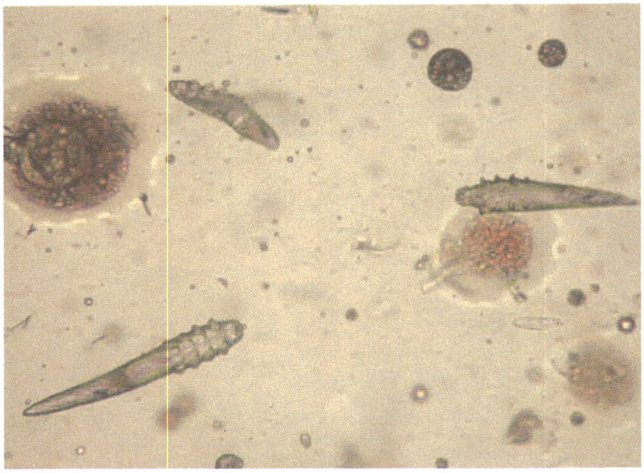

Figure 7.1A *Demodex canis* mites and nymphs (10×).

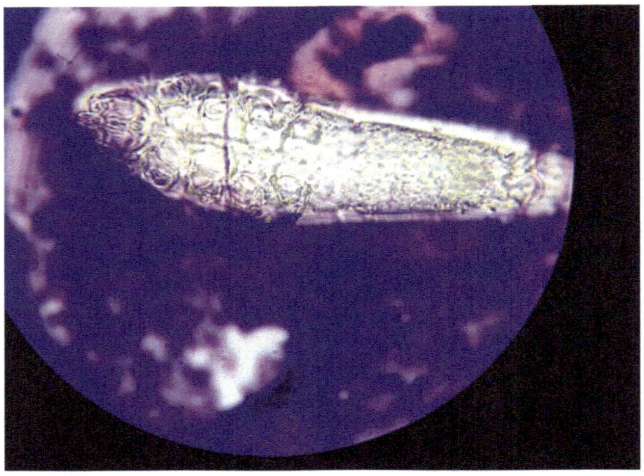

Figure 7.1B A canine *Demodex* mite found on cytology of an inflamed paw, (100×).

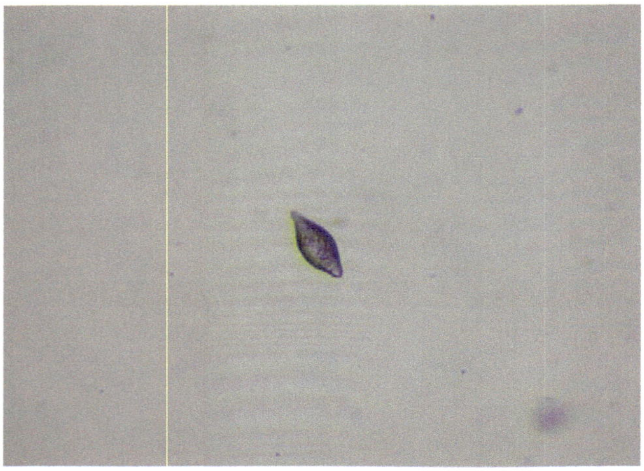

Figure 7.2 *Demodex canis* egg (10× with digital zoom).

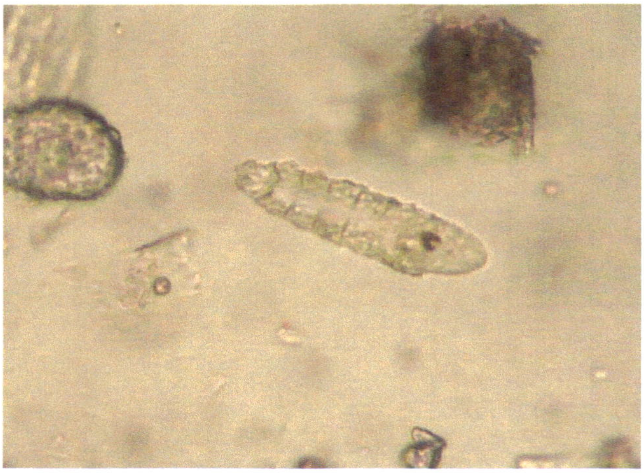

Figure 7.3A Short bodied form of *Demodex canis* (40×).

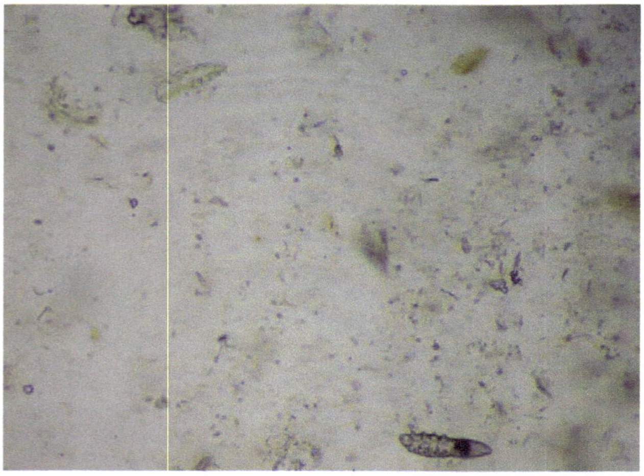

Figure 7.3B Size comparison between the short bodied (top of photo) and typical (bottom of photo) *Demodex canis* mites; the short bodied form is also more translucent (4×).

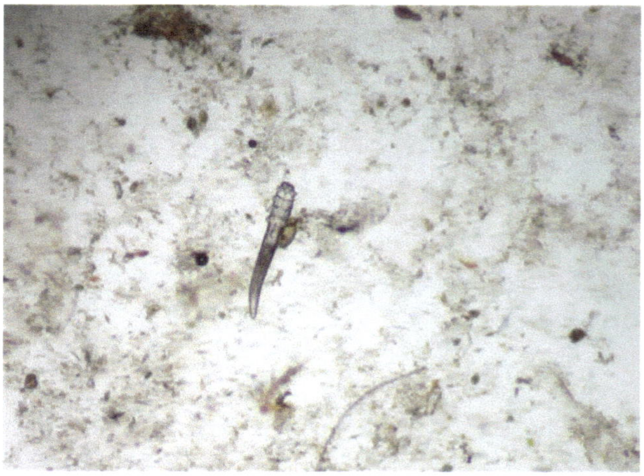

Figure 7.4A *Demodex injai*, the long bodied *Demodex* (4×).

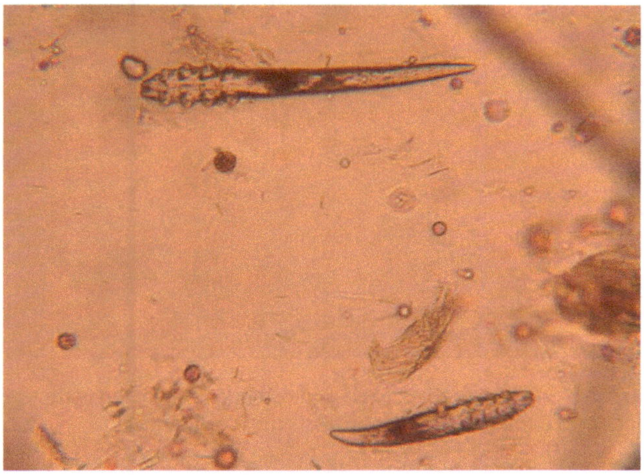

Figure 7.4B This dog had a mixed *Demodex* mite infection; *Demodex injai* is at the top of the photo and *Demodex canis* at the bottom (10×).

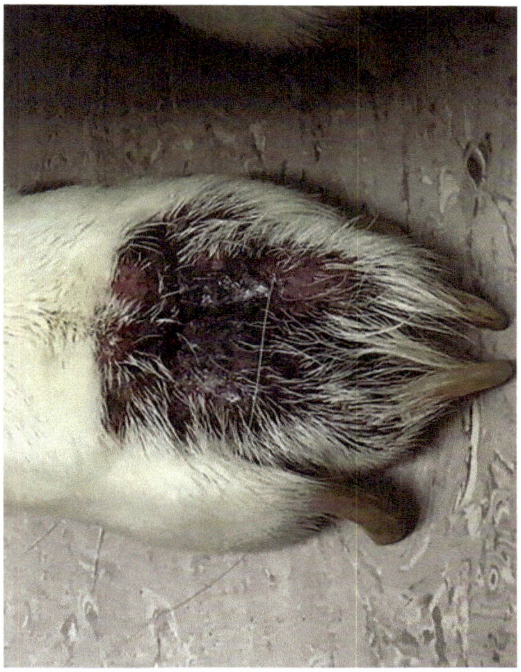

Figure 7.5 An elderly dog with demodicosis localized to one paw.

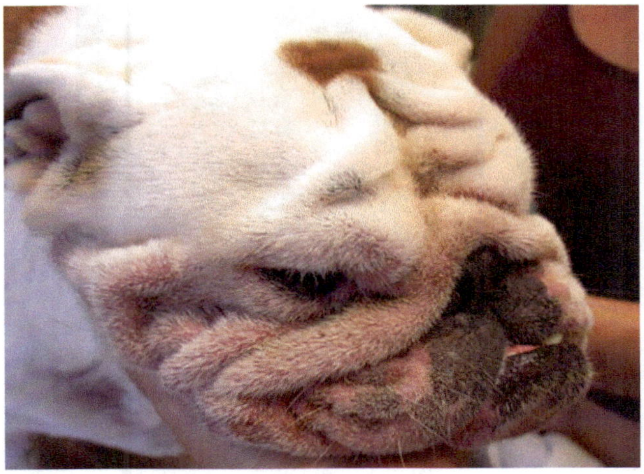

Figure 7.6 A young Bulldog with generalized demodicosis; a secondary *Malassezia* infection was present as well.

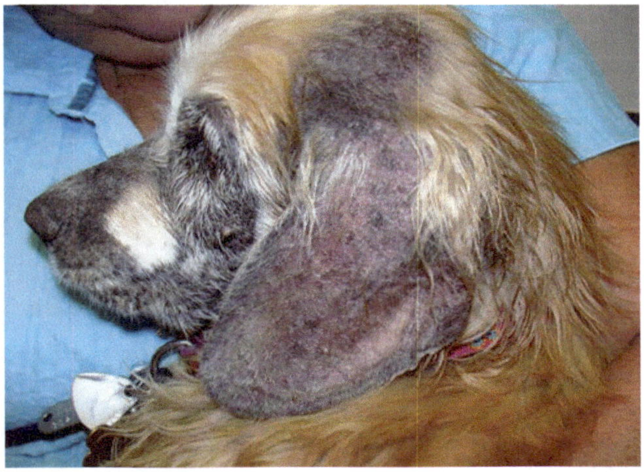

Figure 7.7 An elderly Cocker Spaniel with generalized demodicosis which also affected the ear pinna.

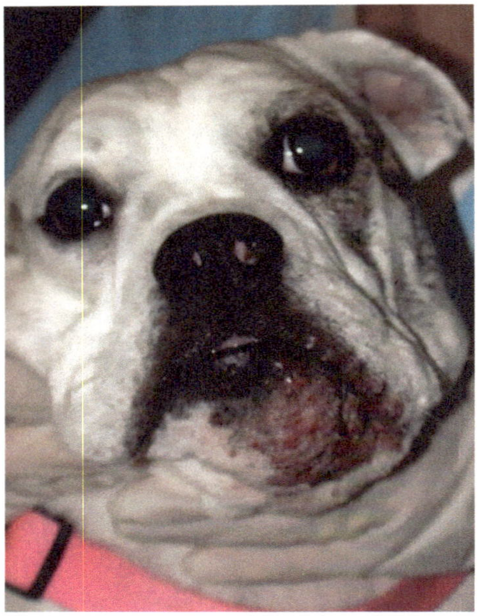

Figure 7.8 A young Bulldog with localized *Demodex* on the lip and chin.

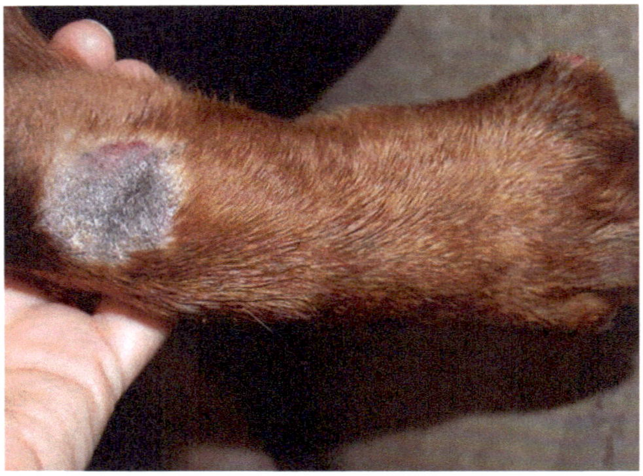

Figure 7.9A Localized alopecia and comedones in a dog with localized *Demodex*; dermatophytosis can look identical.

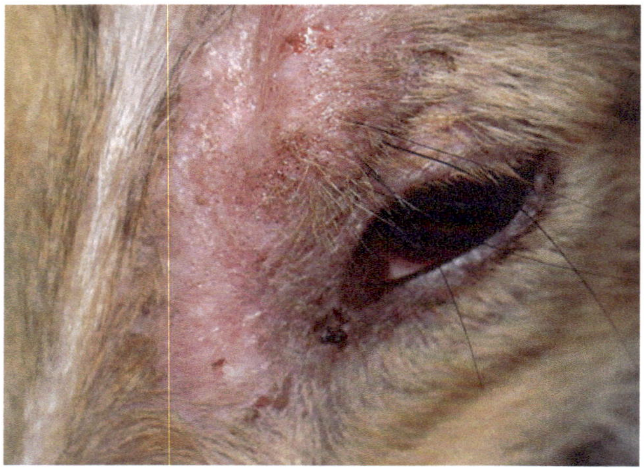

Figure 7.9B A young Sheltie with localized demodicosis on the eyelid.

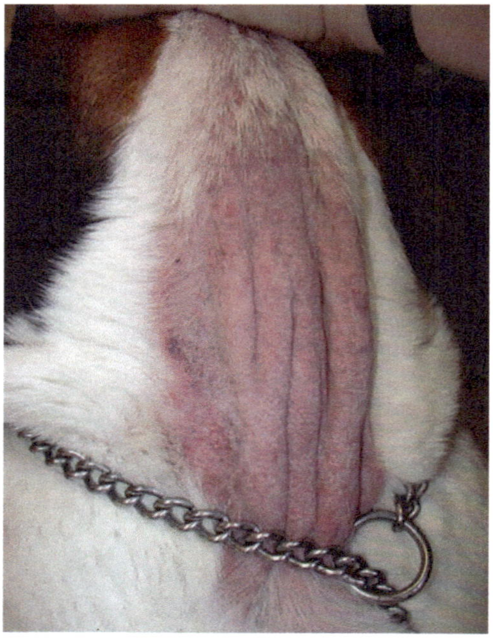

Figure 7.10 *Demodex* and *Malassezia* infections caused this Basset Hound's ventral neck dermatitis.

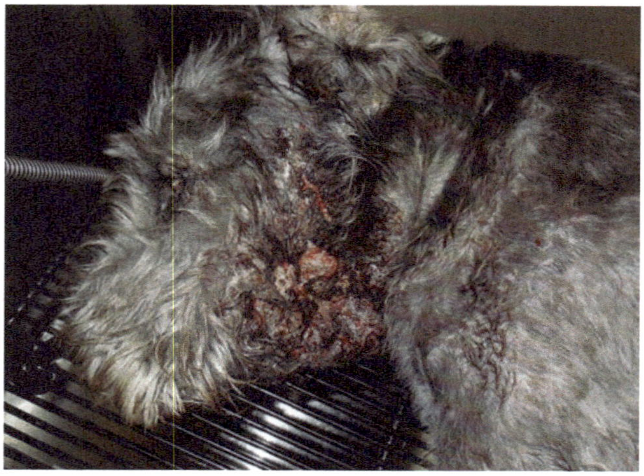

Figure 7.11A Severe crusting and ulceration on the ventral neck of a Wolfhound puppy with generalized demodicosis; the dog was intensely painful and pruritic due to secondary methicillin resistant staph deep pyoderma.

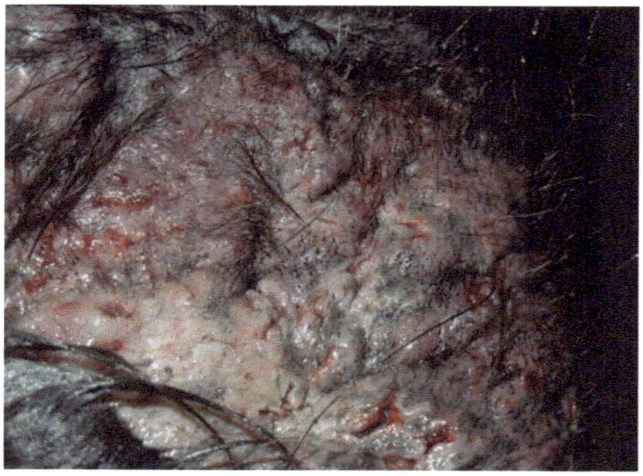

Figure 7.11B The same dog after sedation for hydrotherapy to remove accumulated exudate.

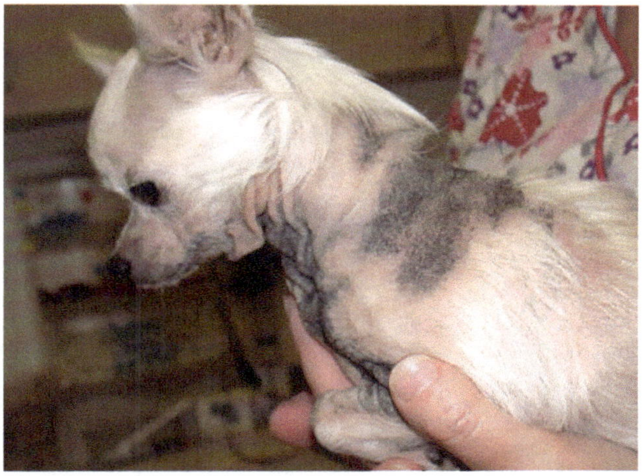

Figure 7.12 Demodicosis in this Chihuahua caused patchy alopecia and hyperpigmentation.

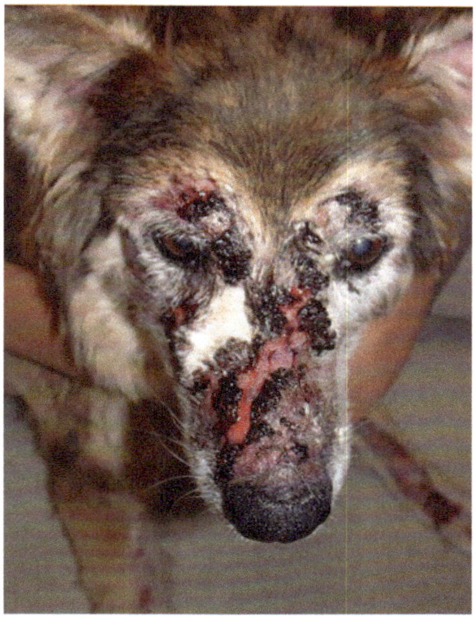

Figure 7.13 An elderly dog with severe demodicosis and secondary deep pyoderma on the face.

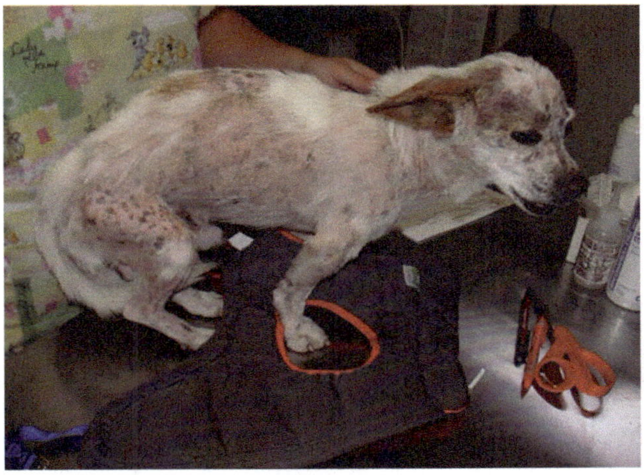

Figure 7.14 An elderly Terrier mix with generalized demodicosis triggered by internal neoplasia.

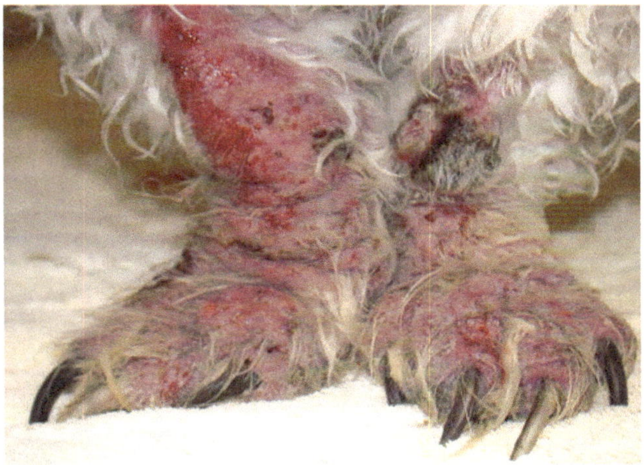

Figure 7.15 Painful pododermatitis caused by demodicosis and secondary deep pyoderma.

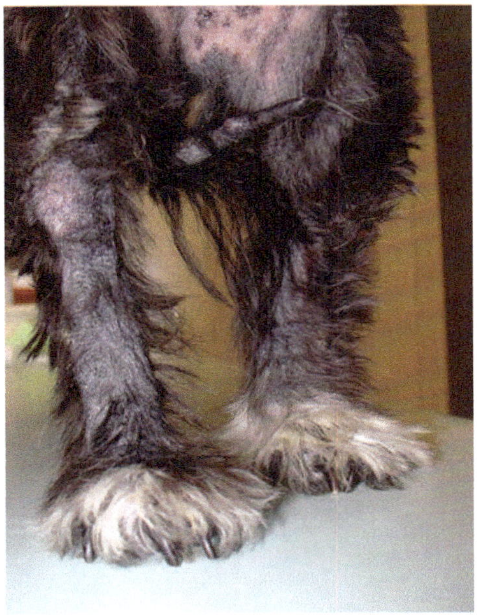

Figure 7.16 Demodicosis in a hypothyroid dog causing alopecia, hyperpigmentation, and comedones on the limbs and trunk.

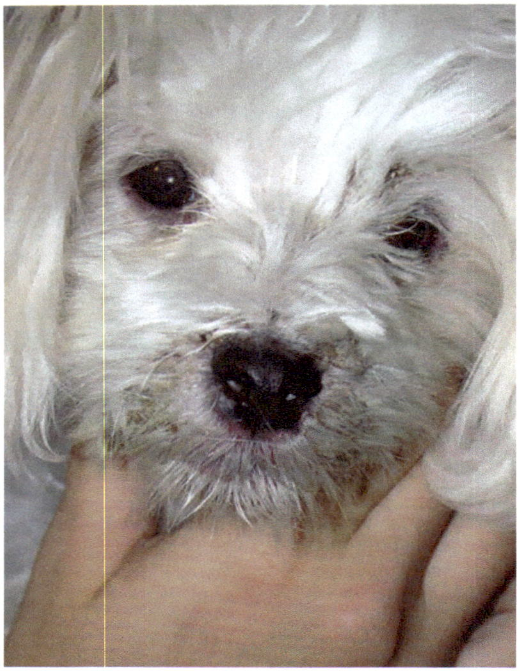

Figure 7.17A A young Maltese puppy with demodicosis that mimics juvenile cellulitis.

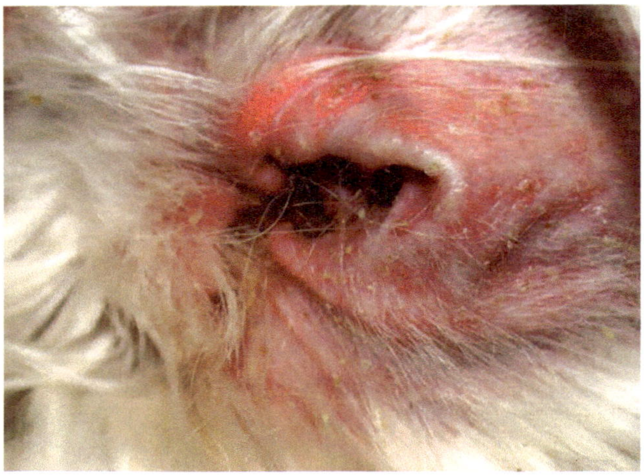

Figure 7.17B The same puppy had *Malassezia* otitis triggered by demodectic otitis.

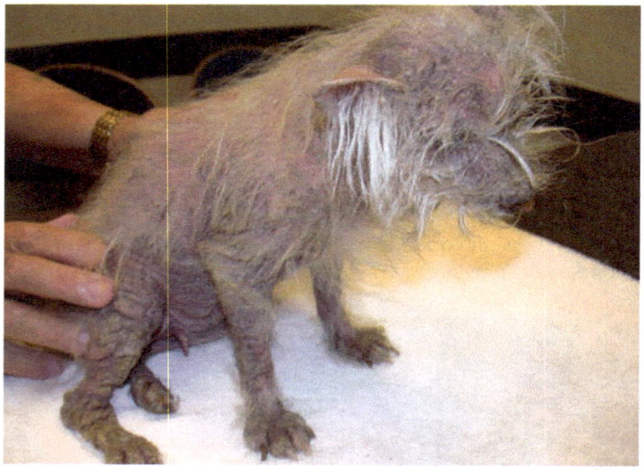

Figure 7.18A Severe generalized demodicosis and *Malassezia* dermatitis in Chihuahua mix.

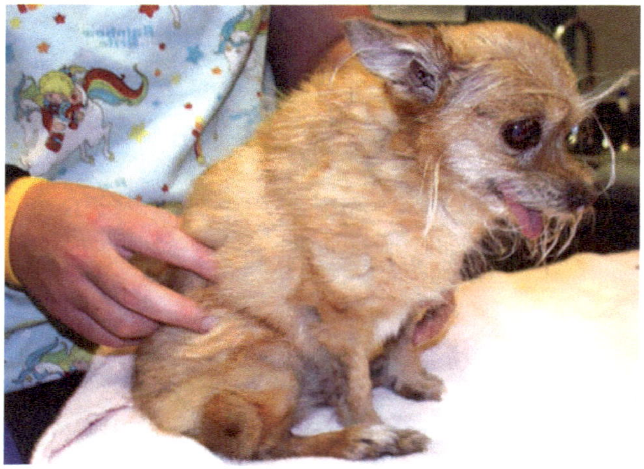

Figure 7.18B The same dog after treatment with ivermectin for four months.

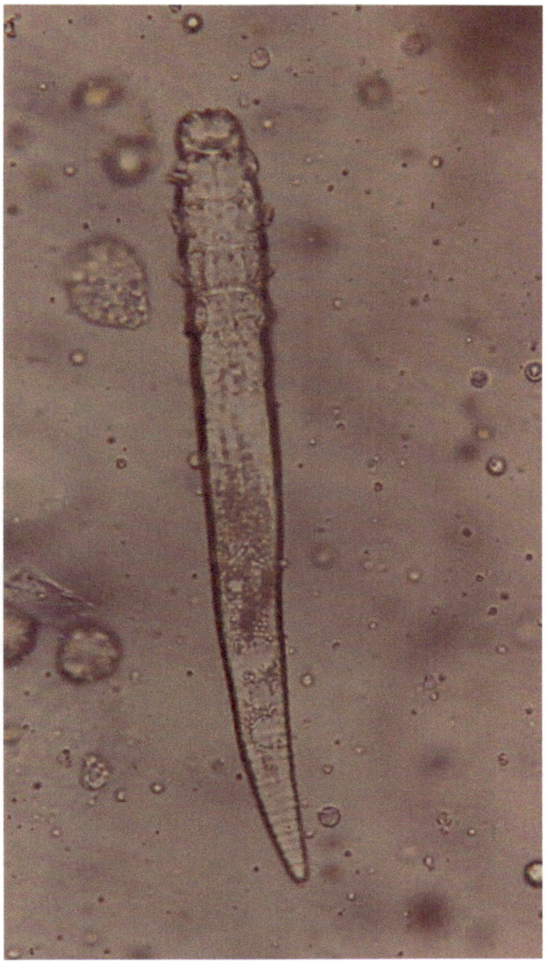

Figure 7.19A *Demodex cati* (10× with digital zoom).

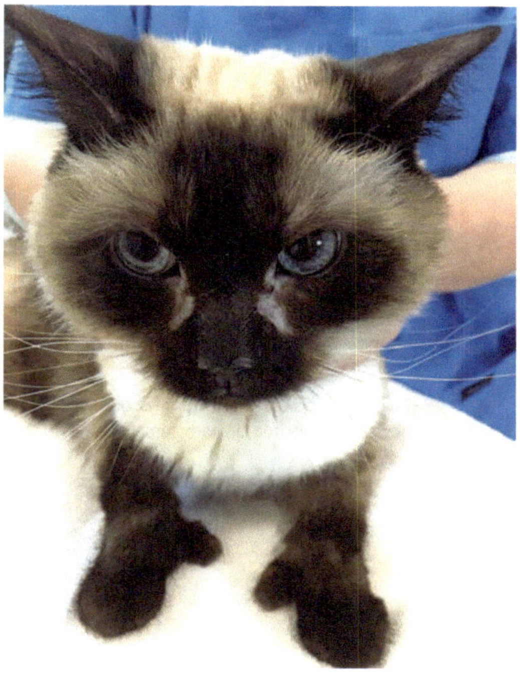

Figure 7.19B Linear facial alopecia due to *Demodex cati* which was triggered by a steroid inhaler for asthma.

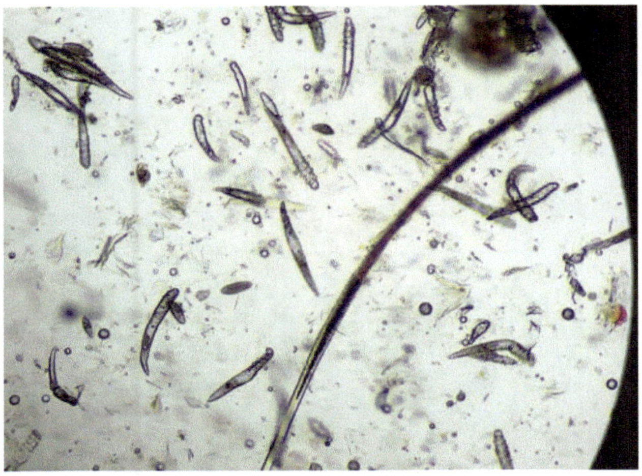

Figure 7.19C On skin scraping from this cat numerous *Demodex cati* mites, nymphs, and eggs were found (4×).

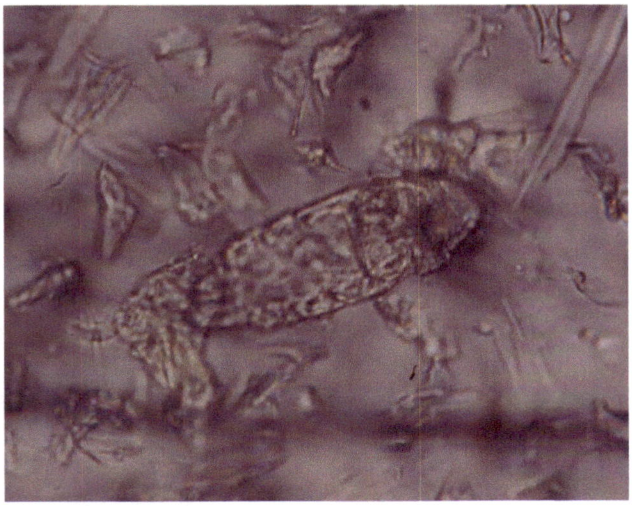

Figure 7.20A *Demodex gatoi* (40×).

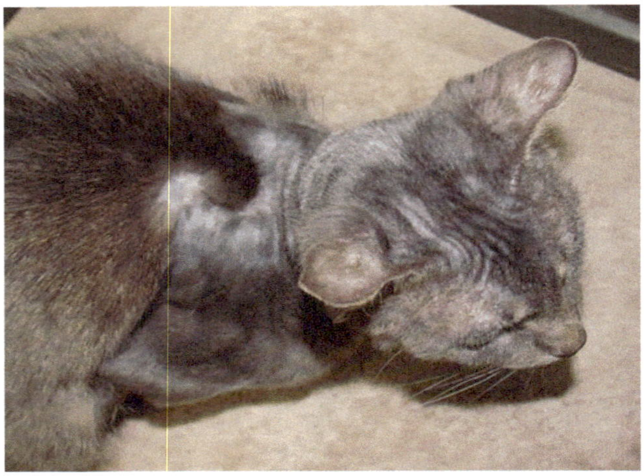

Figure 7.20B A cat with demodicosis caused by *D. gatoi*: note the extensive hypotrichosis on the outer pinnae, dorsal neck, and shoulders.

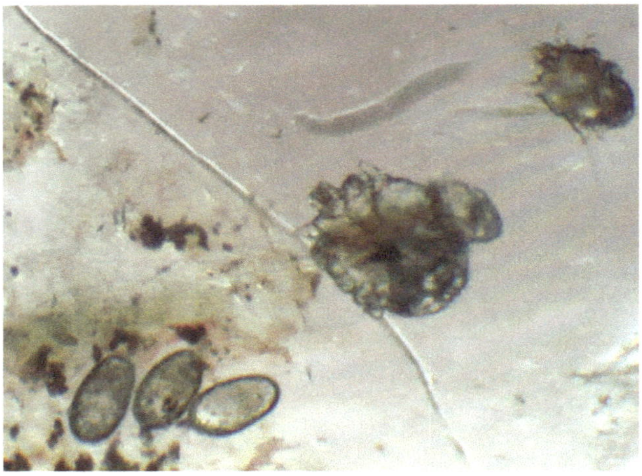

Figure 7.21 *Sarcoptes scabiei* adult mite (in the center), nymph (upper right corner), and eggs (lower left corner) (10×).

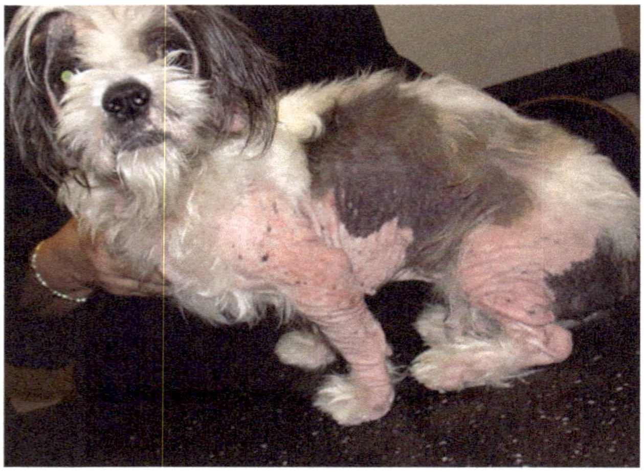

Figure 7.22A A Shih Tzu with sarcoptic mange; the involvement of the hocks and elbows is pathognomonic.

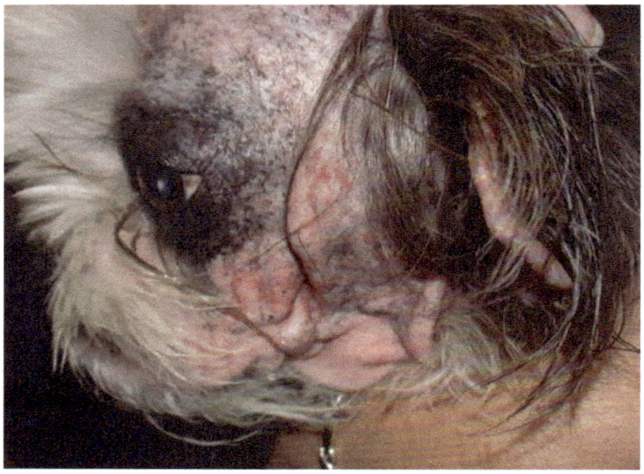

Figure 7.22B The same dog also had pinnal marginal alopecia typical for scabies and atypical facial alopecia.

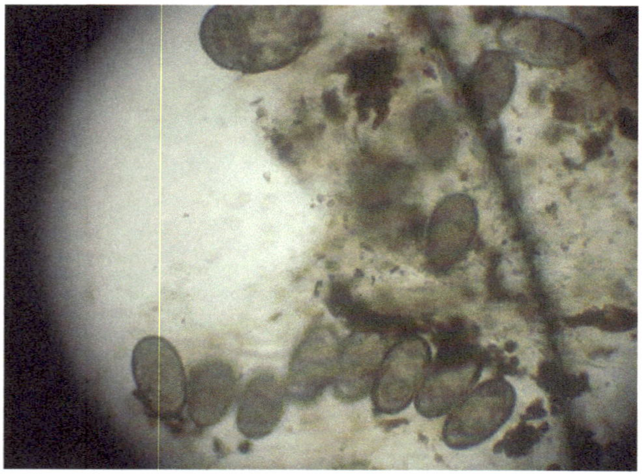

Figure 7.23 Numerous scabies eggs in an immunosuppressed dog (10×).

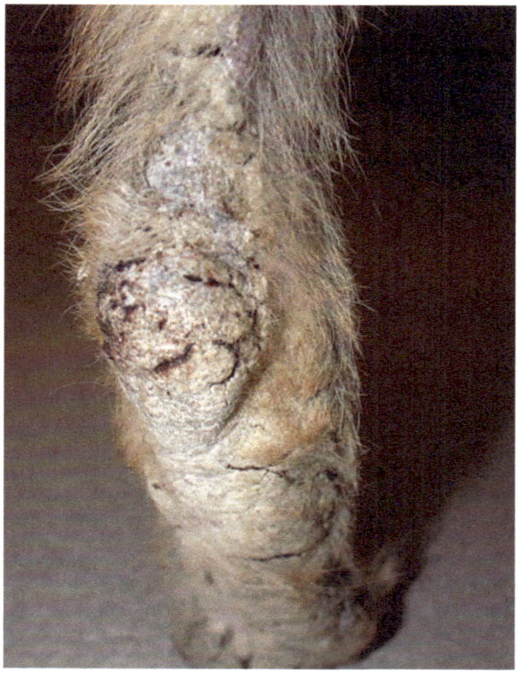

Figure 7.24A Alopecia and severe crusting on the hock of a dog with severe chronic untreated scabies.

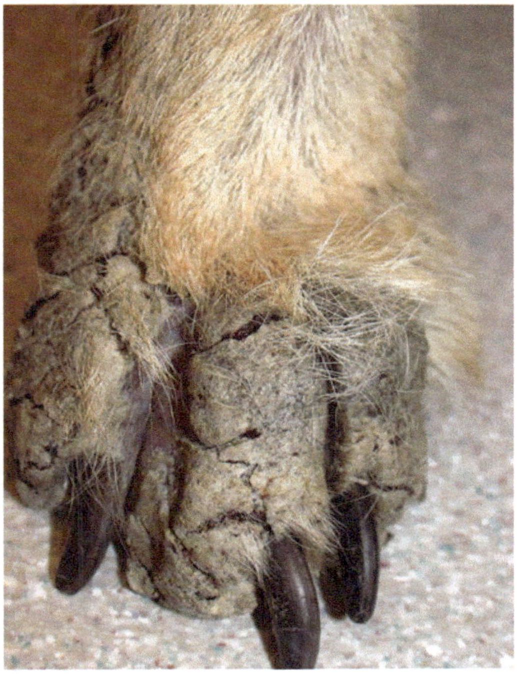

Figure 7.24B Crusting also involved the toes of the same dog.

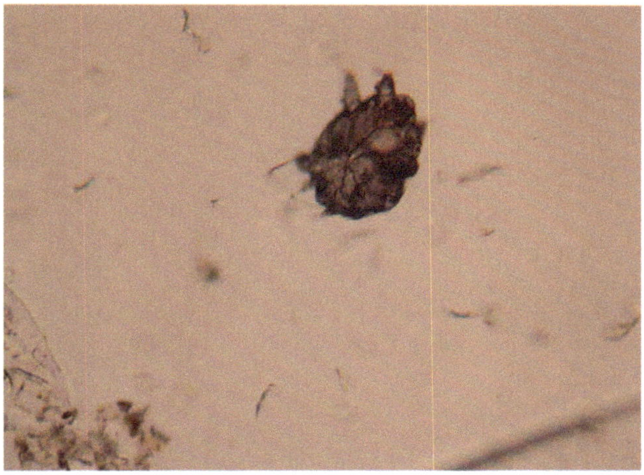

Figure 7.25 A *Notoedres cati* mite (10×).

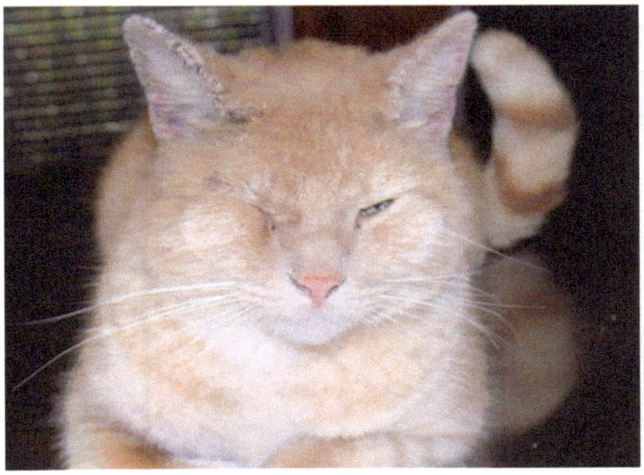

Figure 7.26 Pinnal marginal crusting in a cat with notoedric mange.

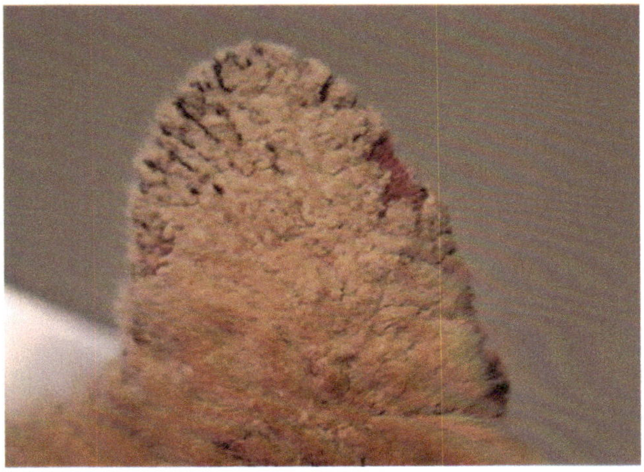

Figure 7.27 Crusting encompassed the caudal aspect of the pinna.

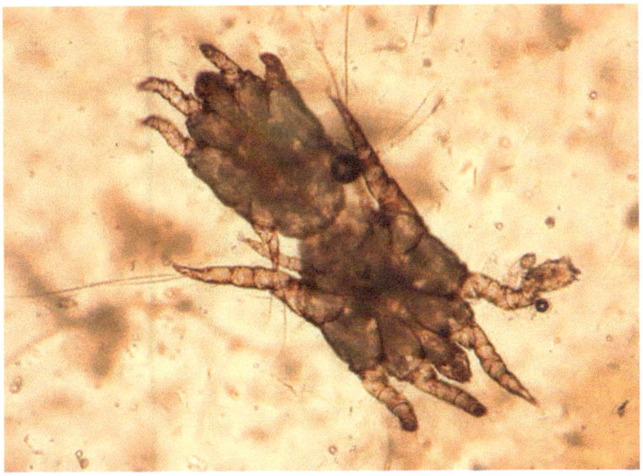

Figure 7.28A *Otodectes cynotis* nymph and adult (10×).

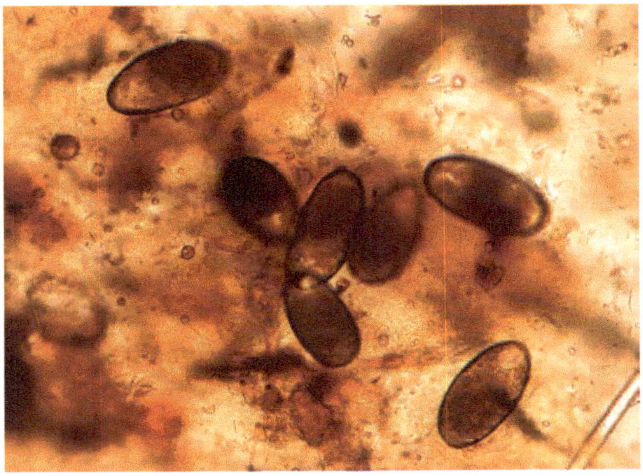

Figure 7.28B *Otodectes cynotis* eggs (10×).

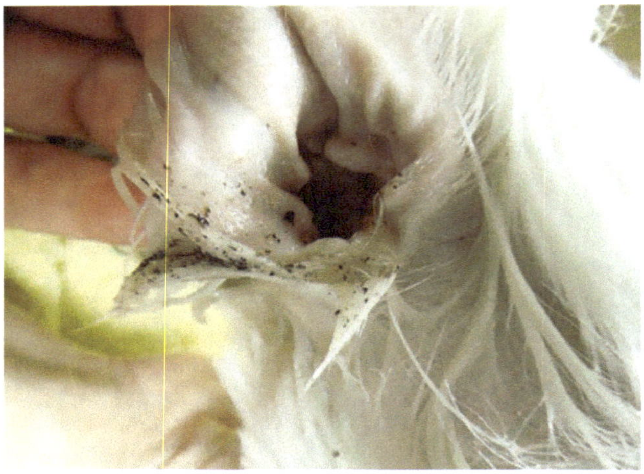

Figure 7.29 Black granular otic discharge typical for *Otodectes* otitis.

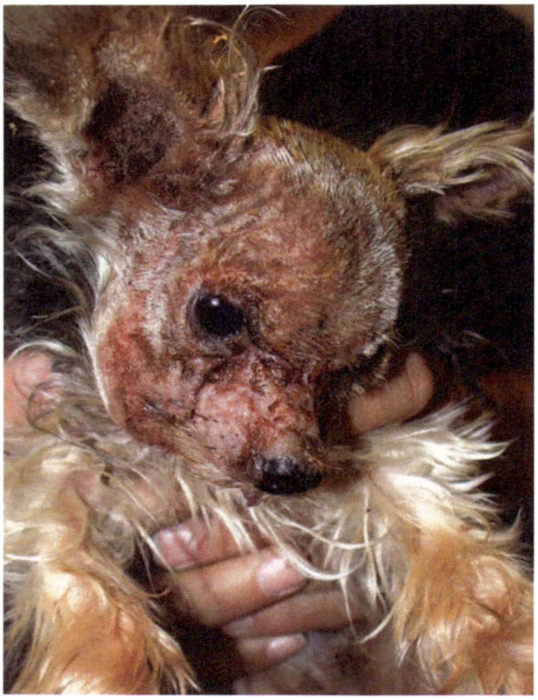

Figure 7.30 A Yorkshire Terrier with severe *Otodectes* infestation of ears and head.

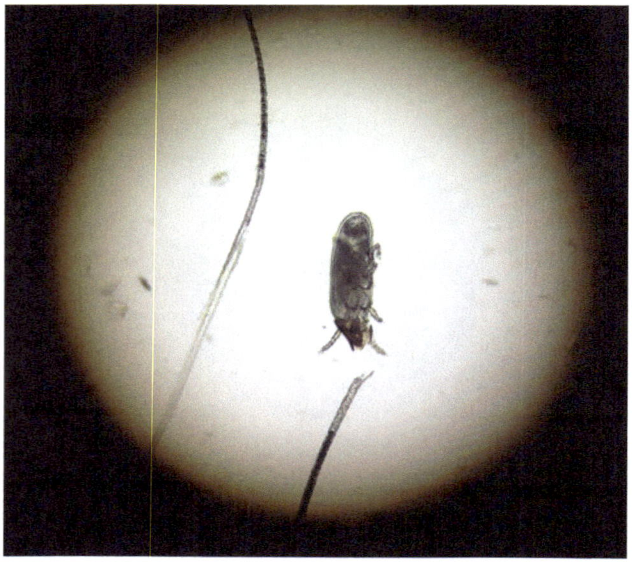

Figure 7.31 The cat fur mite, *Lynxacarus radovskyi* (4×). *Source:* Image courtesy of VIN and Cindy Krach, DVM.

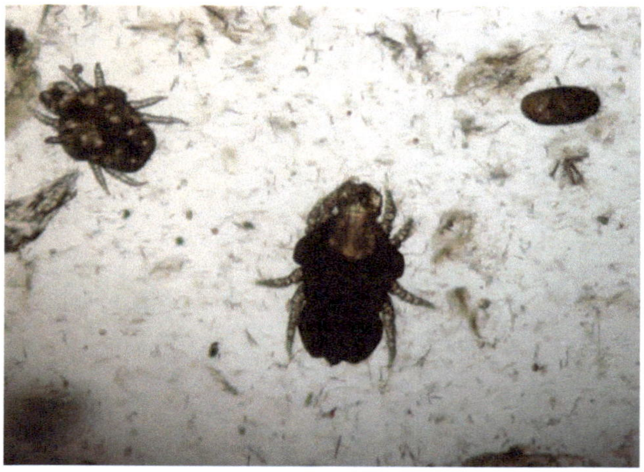

Figure 7.32 *Cheyletiella* mites (adult in the center, nymph in top left) and an egg (10×).

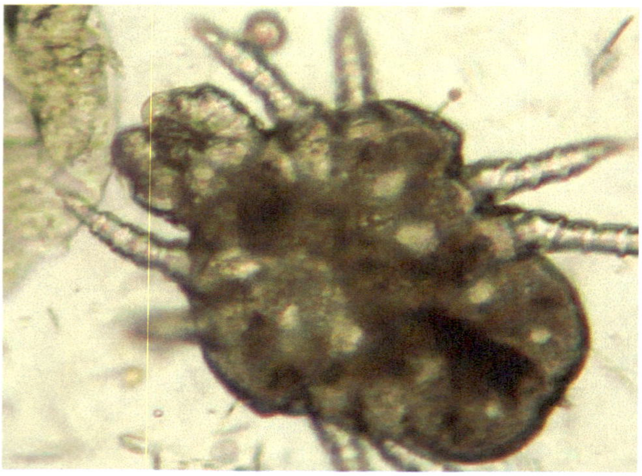

Figure 7.33 A closeup of a *Cheyletiella* mite, notice the clasping mouth parts (10× with digital zoom).

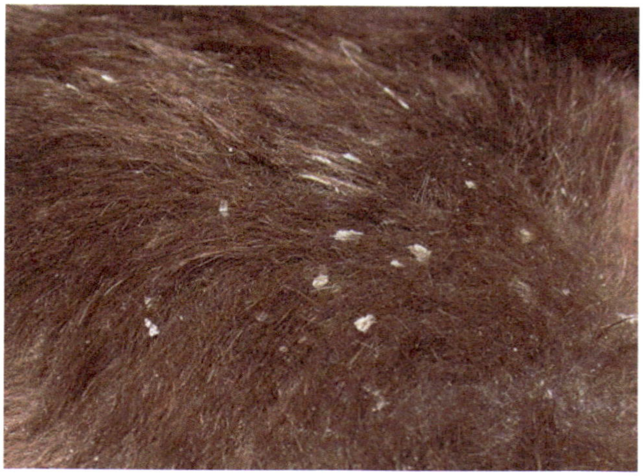

Figure 7.34 A Cocker Spaniel with dry dorsal truncal scaling due to *Cheyletiella* infestation.

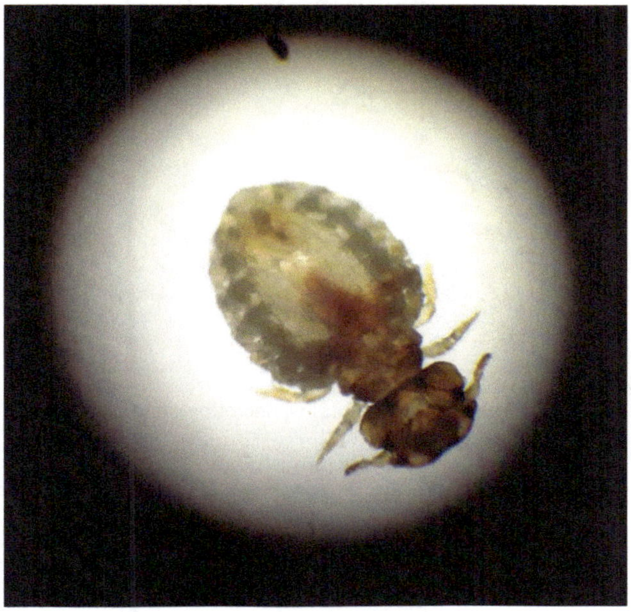

Figure 7.35 *Trichodectes canis*, the chewing dog louse (4×). *Source:* Image courtesy of VIN and Jaime Logan, DVM.

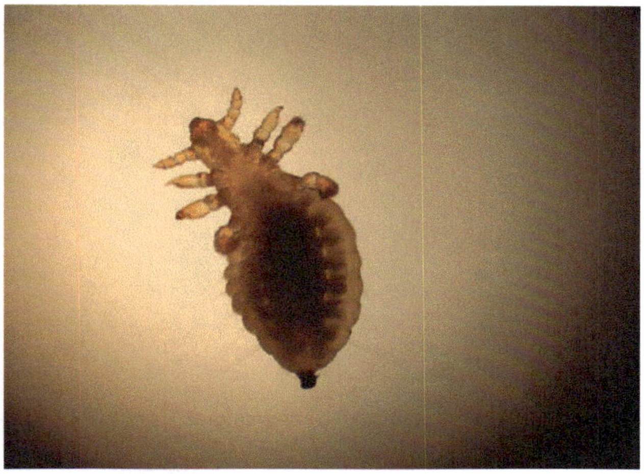

Figure 7.36 *Linognathus setosus*, the sucking dog louse (4×).

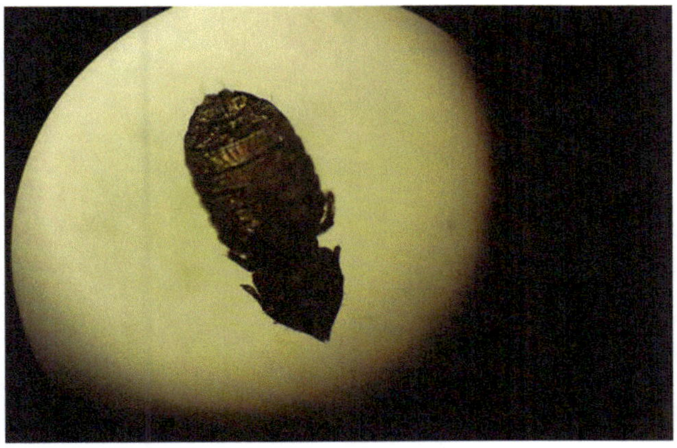

Figure 7.37 *Felicola subrostratus*, the feline louse (4×). *Source:* Image courtesy of VIN and Megan Petroff, DVM.

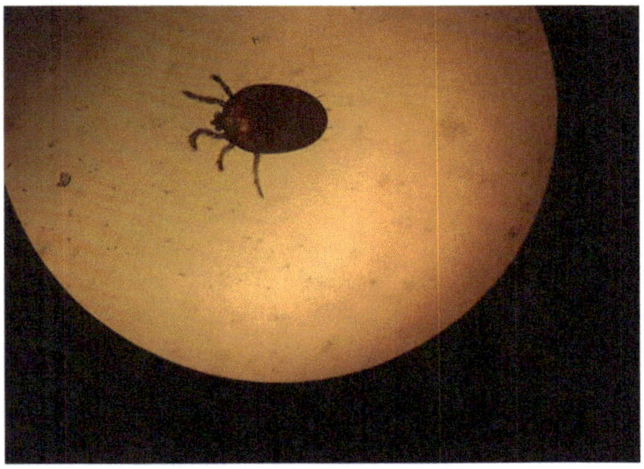

Figure 7.38 A chigger, likely *Eutrombicula alfreddugesi* (4×). *Source:* Image courtesy of VIN and Sam Elder, DVM.

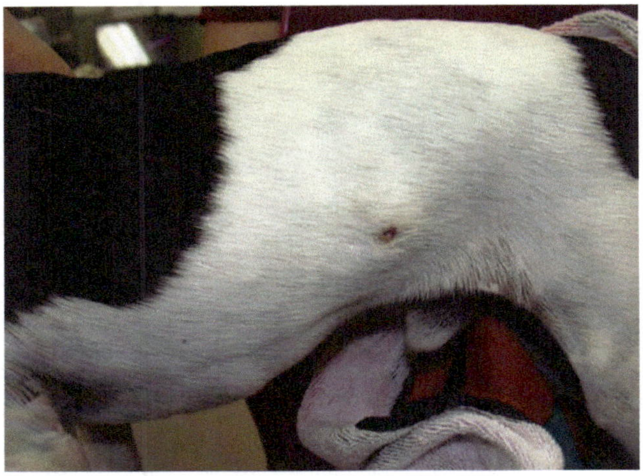

Figure 7.39A A small fistulated wound on the flank of a dog caused by *Cuterebra*.

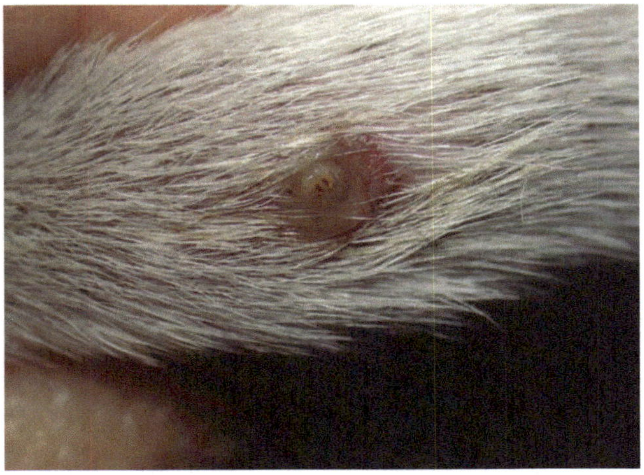

Figure 7.39B Closeup of the same dog, note the cuterebra peeking out from the fistula opening.

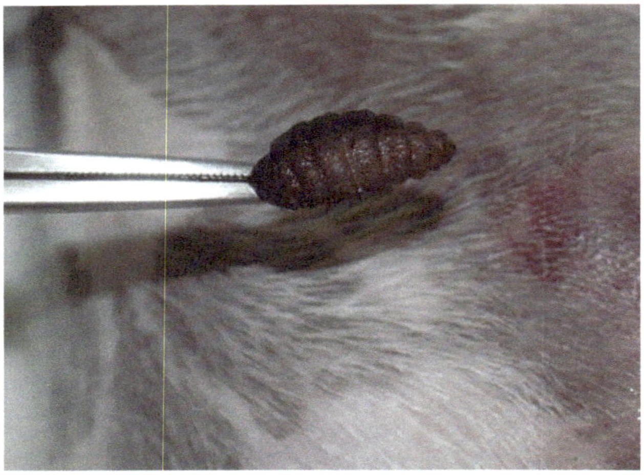

Figure 7.39C The cuterebra larva after removal.

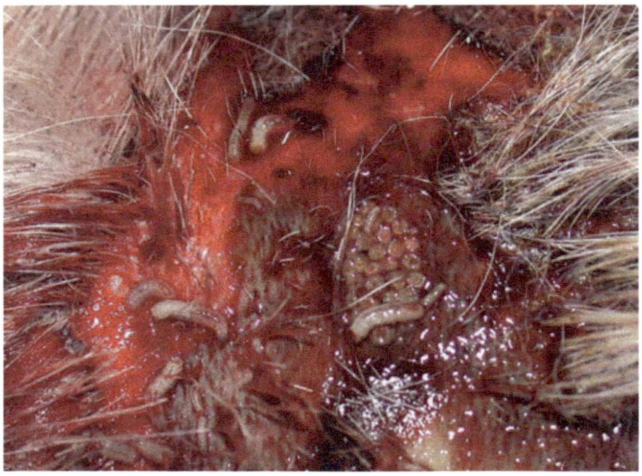

Figure 7.40 Numerous maggots in a necrotic wound on a dog.

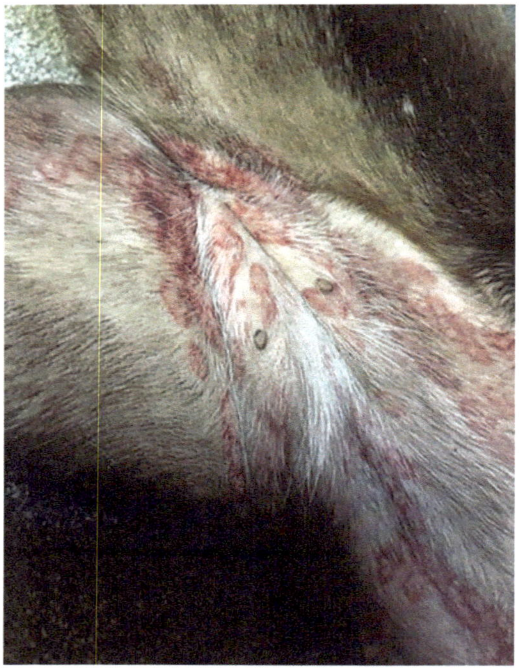

Figure 7.41A Acute red target lesions on the groin of a dog due to black fly bites. *Source:* Image courtesy of Dr. Brad Green, ACVIM.

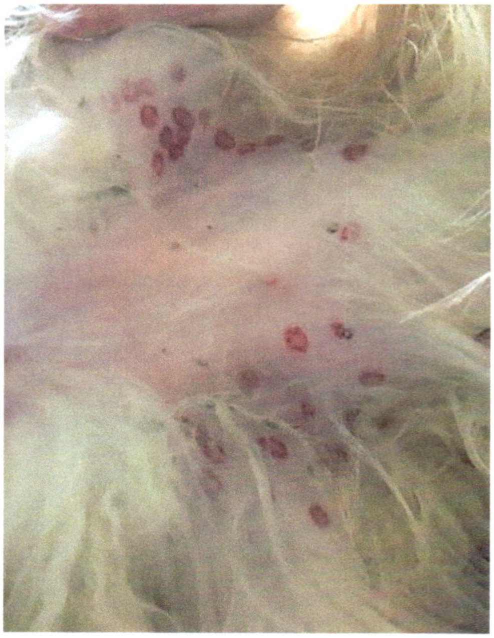

Figure 7.41B The housemate of the dog in Figure 7.41A. *Source:* Image courtesy of Dr. Brad Green, ACVIM.

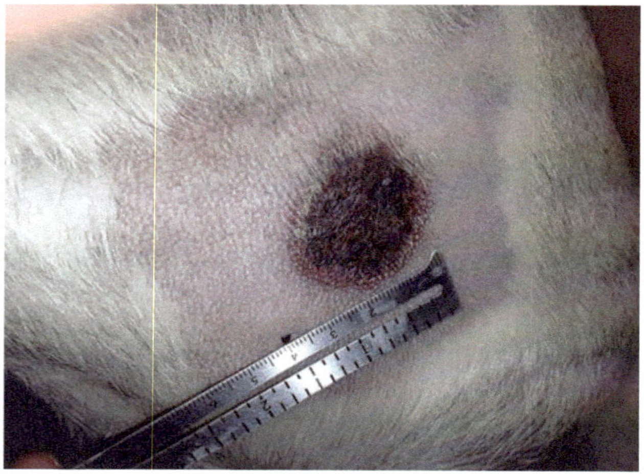

Figure 7.42 A circular necrotic eschar suspected to be a spider bite on the flank of a dog. *Source:* Image courtesy of VIN and Lewis Verner, DVM.

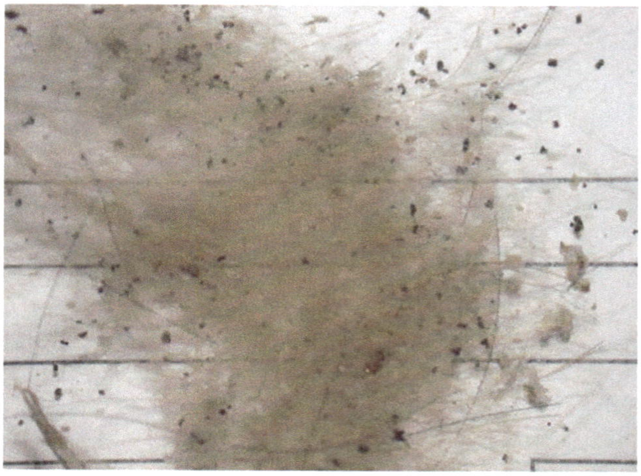

Figure 7.43A Numerous fragments of flea feces found on flea combing of a dog with fleabite hypersensitivity.

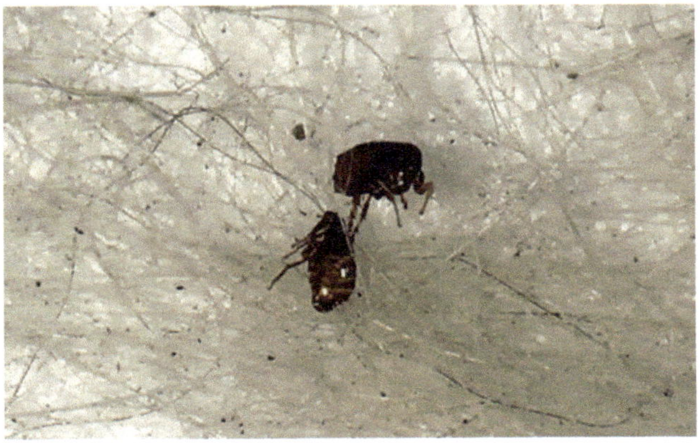

Figure 7.43B *Ctenocephalides felis* fleas.

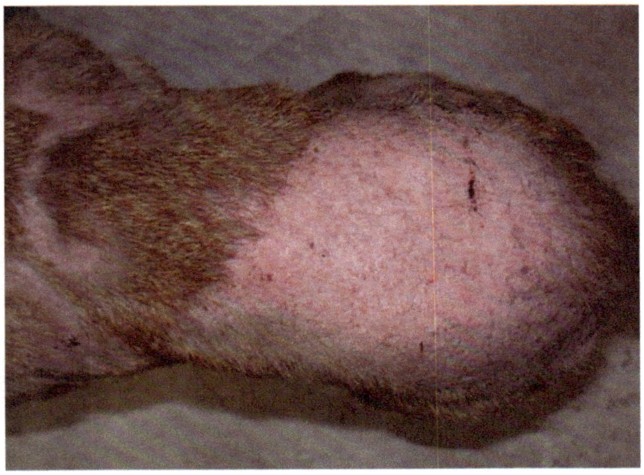

Figure 7.44 Barbering erythema and excoriations on the dorsal lumbar area of a dog with fleabite hypersensitivity.

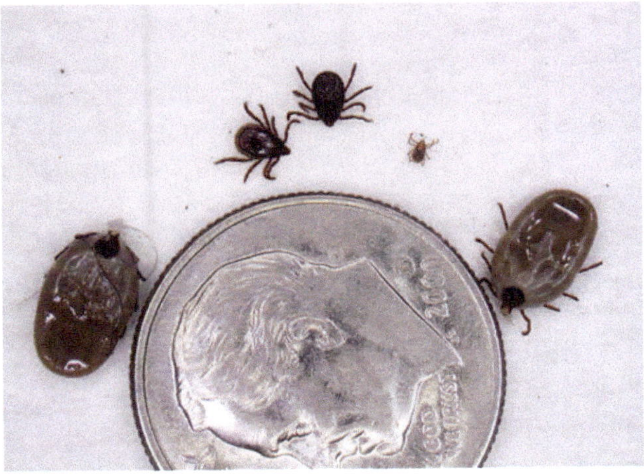

Figure 7.45 *Rhipicephalus sanguineus* adult females, males, and a nymph. *Source:* Image courtesy of VIN and Dr. David Jones.

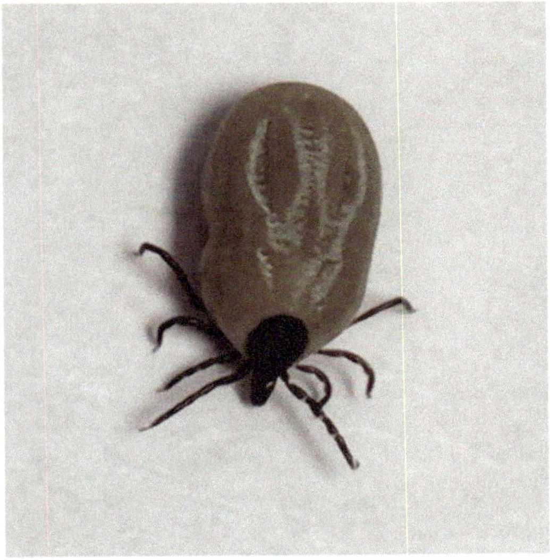

Figure 7.46 *Ixodes scapularis* adult female. *Source:* Image courtesy of VIN and Alanna Holmes, DVM.

Table 7.2 Flea control product options.

	Route		Labeled efficacy		
Flea control products	Topical	Oral	*Ctenocephalides felis felis*	*C. felis felis* eggs	*C. felis felis* larvae
Afoxolaner		X	X		
Dinotefuran/permethrin/pyriproxyfen	X		X	X	X
Fipronil/s-methoprene	X		X	X	X
Fipronil/pyriproxyfen/s-methoprene	X		X	X	X
Flumethrin/imidacloprid	X		X		
Fluralaner		X	X		
Imidacloprid/pyriproxyfen	X		X	X	
Imidacloprid/permethrin/pyriproxyfen	X		X	X	X
Nitenpyram		X	X		
Sarolaner		X	X		
Selamectin	X		X	X	
Spinetoram	X		X		
Spinosad		X	X		

Table 7.3 Tick control product options.

	Labeled efficacy			
Tick control products	*Amblyomma americanum* (Lone Star tick)	*Dermacentor variabilis* (American dog tick)	***Ixodes scapularis*** (Black-legged tick)	*Rhipicephalus sanguineus* (brown dog tick)
Afoxolaner	X	X	X	X
Amitraz collar		Species not specified		
Deltamethrin collar		X	X	X
Dinotefuran/permethrin/pyriproxyfen	X	X	X	X
Fipronil/s-methoprene	X	X	X	X
Fipronil/pyriproxyfen/s-methoprene	X	X	X	X
Flumethrin/imidacloprid collar	X	X	X	X
Fluralaner	X	X	X	X
Imidacloprid/permethrin/pyriproxyfen	X	X	X	X
Sarolaner	X	X		X
Selamectin		X		

Further reading

Becskei, C., Cuppens, O., and Mahabir, S.P. (2018). Efficacy and safety of sarolaner in the treatment of canine ear mite infestation caused by *Otodectes cynotis*: a non-inferiority study. *Vet. Dermatol.* 29 (2): 100–e39.

Becskei, C., De Bock, F., Illambas, J. et al. (2016). Efficacy and safety of a novel oral isoxazoline, sarolaner (Simparica™), for the treatment of sarcoptic mange in dogs. *Vet. Parasitol.* 222: 56–61.

Beugnet, F., Halos, L., and Larsen, D. (2016). Efficacy of oral afoxolaner for the treatment of canine generalised demodicosis. *Parasite* 23: 14.

Bowman, D. (ed.) (2014). *Georgi's Parasitology for Veterinarians, 10*e. St Louis, MO: Elsevier.

Căpitan, R.G.M. and Noli, C. (2017). Trichoscopic diagnosis of cutaneous *Pelodera strongyloides* infestation in a dog. *Vet. Dermatol.* 28 (4): 413–e100.

Frédéric Beugnet, F., Halos, L., Larsen, D. et al. (2016). Efficacy of oral afoxolaner for the treatment of canine generalized demodicosis. *Parasit. Vectors* 9: 392.

Fourie, J.J., Liebenberg, J.E., Horak, I.G. et al. (2015). Efficacy of orally administered fluralaner (Bravecto™) or topically applied imidacloprid/moxidectin (advocate®) against generalized demodicosis in dogs. *Parasit. Vectors* 28 (8): 187.

Han, H.S., Chen, C., Schievano, C., and Noli, C. (2018 May 6). The comparative efficacy of afoxolaner, spinosad, milbemycin, spinosad plus milbemycin, and nitenpyram for the treatment of canine cutaneous myiasis. *Vet. Dermatol.* [Epub ahead of print].

Han, H.S., Noli, C., and Cena, T. (2016). Efficacy and duration of action of oral fluralaner and spot-on moxidectin/imidacloprid in cats infested with *Lynxacarus radovskyi*. *Vet. Dermatol.* 27 (6): 474–e127.

Hutt, J.H., Prior, I.C., and Shipstone, M.A. (2015). Treatment of canine generalized demodicosis using weekly injections of doramectin: 232 cases in the USA (2002–2012). *Vet. Dermatol.* 26 (5): 345–349, e73.

Johnstone, I.P. (2002). Doramectin as treatment for canine and feline demodicosis. *Aust. Vet. Pract.* 32: 98–103.

Lerpen Duangkaew, L. and Hoffman, H. (2018). Efficacy of oral fluralaner for the treatment of *Demodex* gatoi in two shelter cats. *Vet. Dermatol.* 29 (3): 262.

Lucio-Forster, A., Eberhard, M.L., Cama, V.A. et al. (2014). First report of *Dracunculus insignis* in two naturally infected cats from the northeastern USA. *J. Feline Med. Surg.* 16 (2): 194–197.

Miller, W.H., Griffen, C.E., and Campbell, K.L. (2013). *Muller and Kirk's Small Animal Dermatology*, 7e. St Louis, MO: Elsevier Mosby.

Ordeix, L., Bardagí, M., Scarampella, F. et al. (2009). *Demodex injai* infestation and dorsal greasy skin and hair in eight wirehaired fox terrier dogs. *Vet. Dermatol.* 20 (4): 267–272.

Paterson, T.E., Halliwell, R., Fields, P.J. et al. (2014). Canine generalized demodicosis treated with varying doses of a 2.5% moxidectin+10% imidacloprid spot-on and oral ivermectin: parasiticidal effects and long-term treatment outcomes. *Vet. Parasitol.* 205: 687–696.

Sastre, N., Ravera, I., Villanueva, S. et al. (2012). Phylogenetic relationships in three species of canine *Demodex* mite based on partial sequences of mitochondrial 16S rDNA. *Vet. Dermatol.* 23 (6): 509–e101.

Short, J. and Gram, D. (2016). Successful treatment of *Demodex gatoi* with 10% Imidacloprid/1% Moxidectin. *J. Am. Anim. Hosp. Assoc.* 52 (1): 68–72.

Silbermayr, K., Joachim, A., Litschauer, B. et al. (2013). The first case of *Demodex gatoi* in Austria, detected with fecal flotation. *Parasitol. Res.* 112 (8): 2805–2810.

Six, R.H., Becskei, C., Mazaleski, M.M. et al. (2016). Efficacy of sarolaner, a novel oral isoxazoline, against two common mite infestations in dogs: *Demodex* spp. and *Otodectes cynotis*. *Vet. Parasitol.* 222: 62–66.

Taenzler, J., Liebenberg, J., Roepke, R.K.A. et al. (2016). Efficacy of fluralaner administered either orally or topically for the treatment of naturally acquired *Sarcoptes scabiei* var. *canis* infestation in dogs. *Parasit. Vectors* 23: 14.

Taenzler, J., de Vos, C., Roepke, R.K.A. et al. (2017). Efficacy of fluralaner against *Otodectes cynotis* infestations in dogs and cats. *Parasit. Vectors* 10: 30.

8

Bacterial, fungal, oomycete, and algal infections

Kimberly S. Coyner, DVM, DACVD

Dermatology Clinic for Animals, Lacey, WA, USA

Table 8.1 Superficial bacterial skin infections.

Superficial or surface pyoderma	Clinical signs	Diagnosis	Treatment
Impetigo Often seen in young puppies.	Non-pruritic pustules not associated with follicles, on sparsely haired areas of the skin such as inguinal area; rupture of pustules results in epidermal collarettes and scaling.	Clinical signs. Cytology. Skin scrapings to rule out *Demodex*.	Topical antibacterial therapy i.e. chlorhexidine. Rarely, refractory lesions may require oral antibiotics for 10–14 days.
Pyotraumatic dermatitis (Figures 8.1A and 8.1B) Often occurs in thickly coated dogs with underlying flea allergy or atopy.	Areas of acute, painful, moist, inflammatory dermatitis created by self-trauma. Peripheral papules/pustules or thickened lesions indicate pyotraumatic folliculitis.	Clinical signs. Cytology +/− aerobic bacterial culture if bacteria are present despite prior or current antibiotics. Skin scrapings to rule out *Demodex*.	May need sedation to clip/clean, follow with a 1–2 week course of oral anti-inflammatory steroid and topical astringents/antibacterial products +/− topical steroids or pramoxine, avoid alcohol containing products. If peripheral papules/pustules noted, or if lesion is thickened, then a 2–4 week course of systemic antibiotics would be indicated. In recurrent cases identify and treat underlying allergic cause.
Intertrigo (Figures 8.2A–8.2G)	Dermatitis occurs in areas of skin folding such as face folds, lipfold, tail fold, and vulvar area. Lesions are areas of moist inflammatory dermatitis with surface bacterial overgrowth.	Clinical signs. Cytology +/− aerobic bacterial culture if bacteria are present despite prior or current antibiotics. Skin scrapings/hair plucks to rule out *Demodex*.	Cleanse area q 1–3 days with antibacterial wipe, flush, or shampoo; apply topical antibiotic cream or solution daily for 5–7 days. Refractory cases may require surgical excision of excessive folds.
Mucocutaneous pyoderma (Figures 8.3A–8.3E)	Erythema, inflammation, crusting +/− depigmentation of lip margins, eyelids, nares, or anus.	Clinical signs. Cytology +/− aerobic bacterial culture if bacteria are present despite prior or current antibiotics. Skin scrapings/hair plucks to rule out *Demodex*.	Topical antibacterial therapy i.e. mupirocin BID × 14 days. +/− for severe cases systemic antibiotics × 3–4 weeks. In recurrent cases identify and treat underlying cause (see Table 8.4).

(*Continued*)

Clinical Atlas of Canine and Feline Dermatology, First Edition. Edited by Kimberly S. Coyner.

Companion website: www.wiley.com/go/coyner/dermatology

Table 8.1 Superficial bacterial skin infections (Continued)

Superficial or surface pyoderma	Clinical signs	Diagnosis	Treatment
Bacterial overgrowth syndrome (Figures 8.4A–8.4M)	Lesions of erythema, scaling, lichenification, hyperpigmentation, odor, pruritus, and eventual alopecia. Often present on the ventral trunk, axillary, and inguinal areas. No papules, pustules, or epidermal collarettes are present. Mimics *Malassezia* dermatitis.	Clinical signs. Cytology +/− aerobic bacterial culture if bacteria are present despite prior or current antibiotics. Skin scrapings to rule out *Demodex*.	Antibacterial shampoos, conditioners, and/or sprays in combination with a 3-week minimum course of systemic antibiotics. In recurrent cases identify and treat underlying cause (see Table 8.4 and Algorithm 8.1).
Bacterial folliculitis (Figures 8.5A–8.5P)	Primary lesions are papules (small [1–2 mm] raised, sometimes crusted pink or red bumps) and pustules. As the lesions mature and progress, expanding areas of alopecia and surrounding scaling (epidermal collarettes), hyperpigmentation, and lichenification can develop.	Clinical signs. Cytology +/− aerobic bacterial culture if bacteria are present despite prior or current antibiotics. Skin scrapings to rule out *Demodex*. +/− Dermatophyte culture.	Antibacterial shampoos, conditioners, and/or sprays in combination with a 3-week minimum course of systemic antibiotics (1 week beyond complete healing). In recurrent cases identify and treat underlying cause (see Table 8.4 and Algorithm 8.1). Rare idiopathic cases of recurrent bacterial folliculitis may respond to immunomodulating bacterins (Staphage Lysate®, Delmont Labs; ImmunoRegulin®, Neogen Corp).

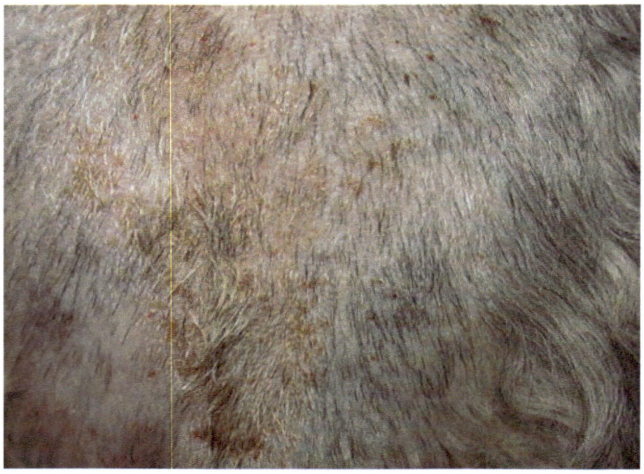

Figure 8.1A An area of acute moist dermatitis, which occurred due to contact reaction to shampoo.

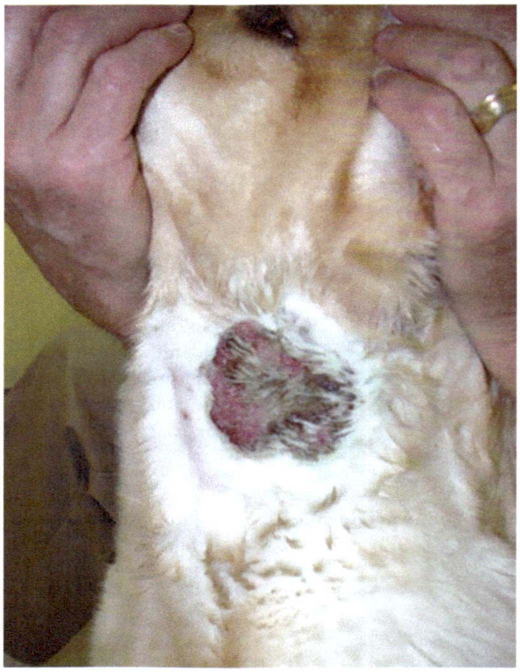

Figure 8.1B Pyotraumatic folliculitis secondary to atopy in a Labrador.

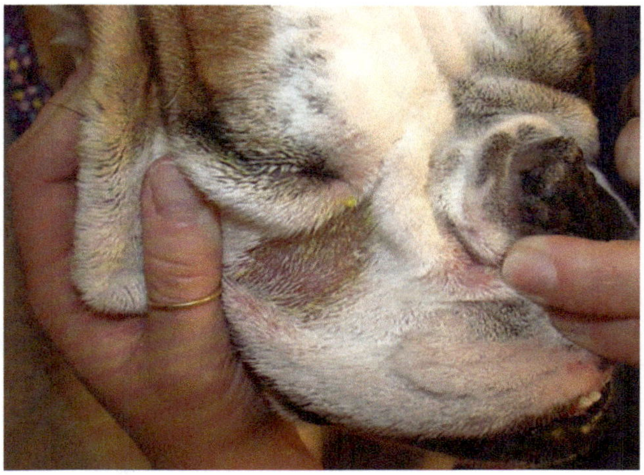

Figure 8.2A Face fold intertrigo in a Bulldog.

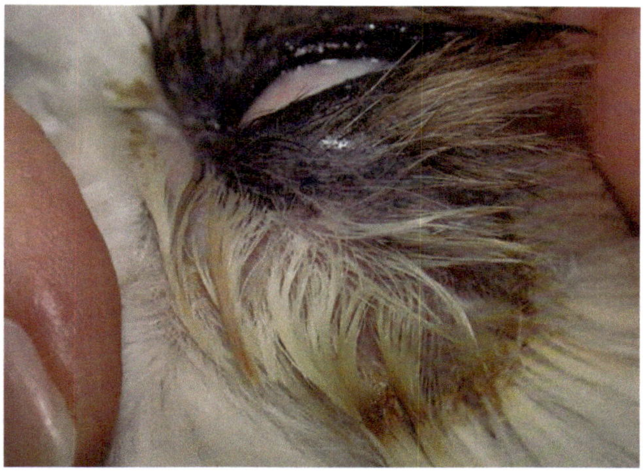

Figure 8.2B Bacterial and *Malassezia* face fold intertrigo in an atopic Shih Tzu.

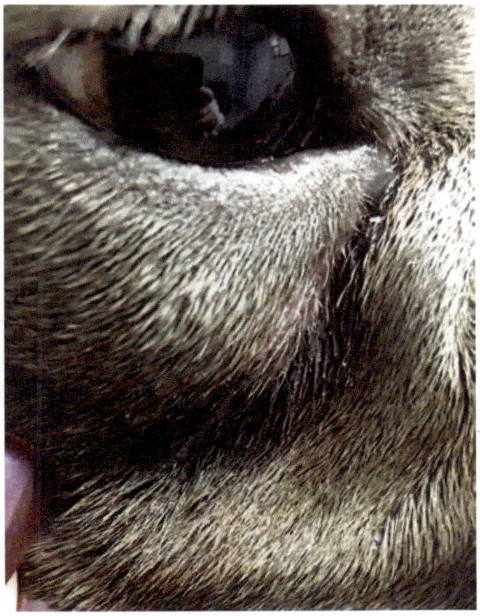

Figure 8.2C Moist facial fold dermatitis in an allergic French Bulldog.

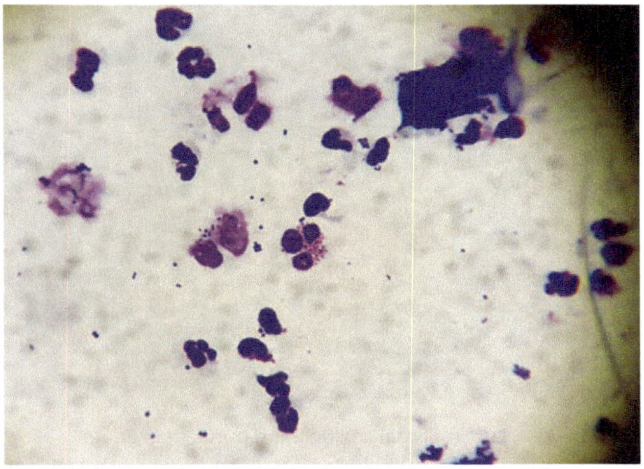

Figure 8.2D Face fold cytology of the dog in Figure 8.2C revealed neutrophils, eosinophils, and cocci bacteria (100×).

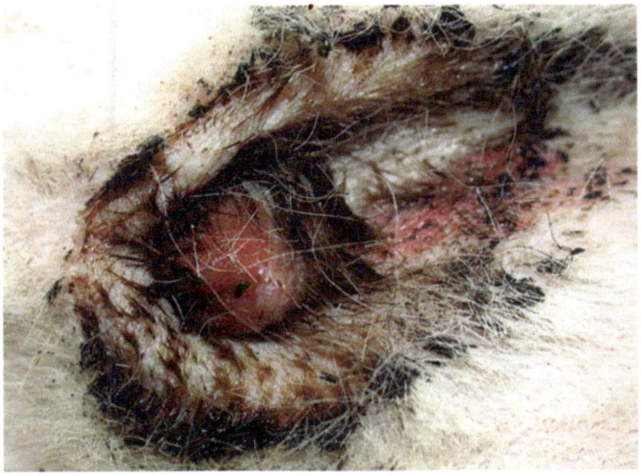

Figure 8.2E Vulvar fold dermatitis caused by *Pseudomonas* infection.

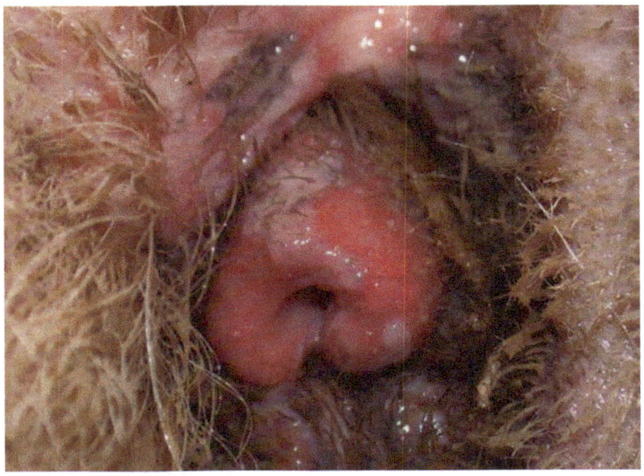

Figure 8.2F Severe vulvar fold intertrigo with ulceration; *Pseudomonas* was also cultured from this dog.

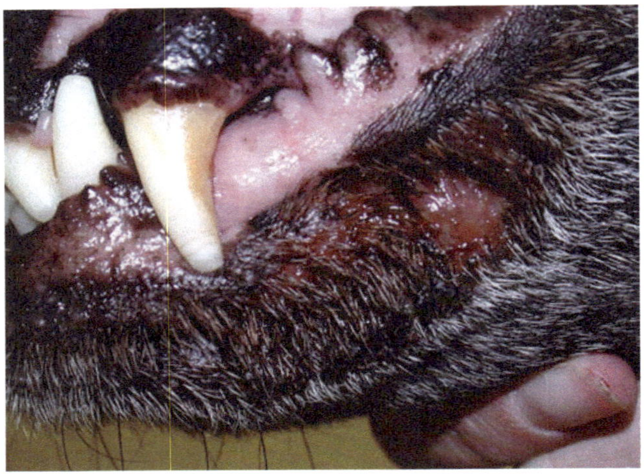

Figure 8.2G Lip fold pyoderma in an allergic dog.

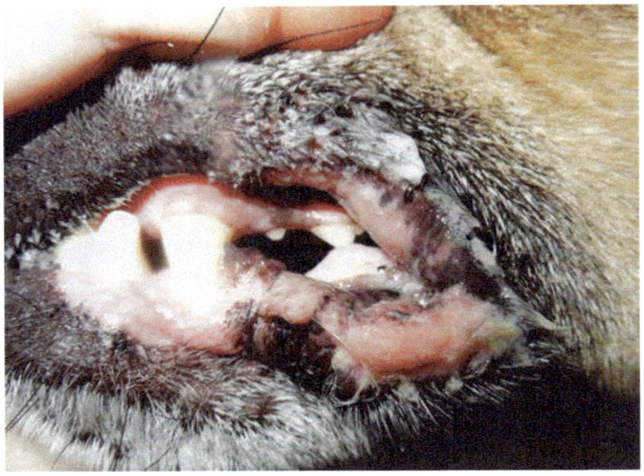

Figure 8.3A Lip mucocutaneous erosion and exudation in a food allergic Boxer.

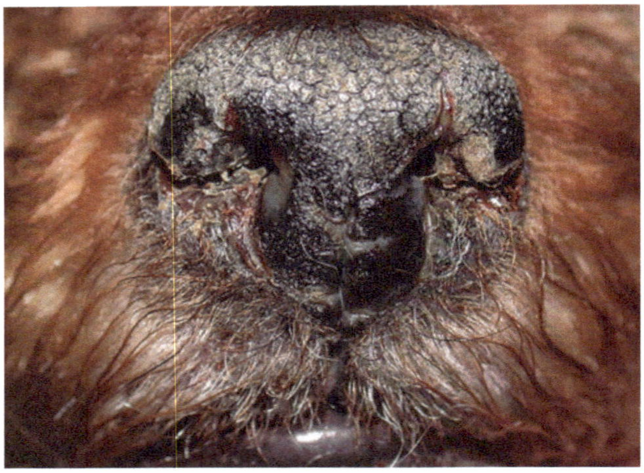

Figure 8.3B Nasal mucosal crusting and purulent exudate secondary to atopic dermatitis.

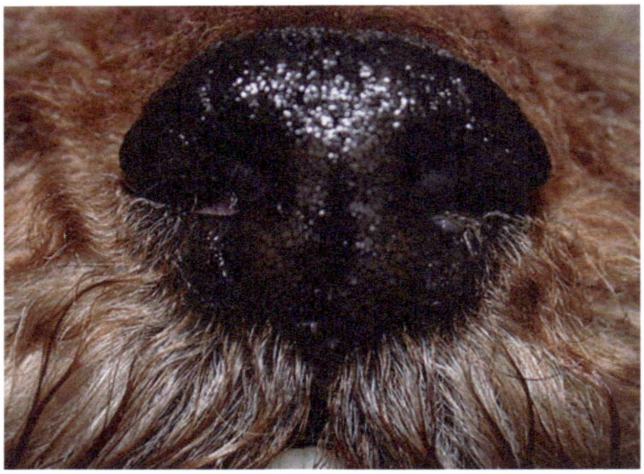

Figure 8.3C The same dog as in Figure 8.3B after a four-week course of antibiotics.

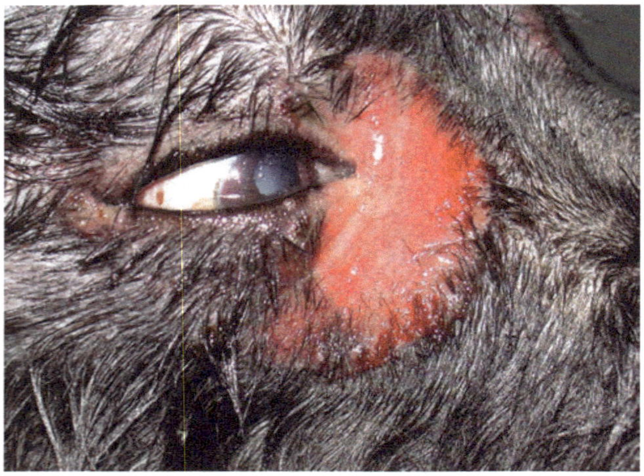

Figure 8.3D Severe ulcerative mucocutaneous pyoderma originating from the eyelids.

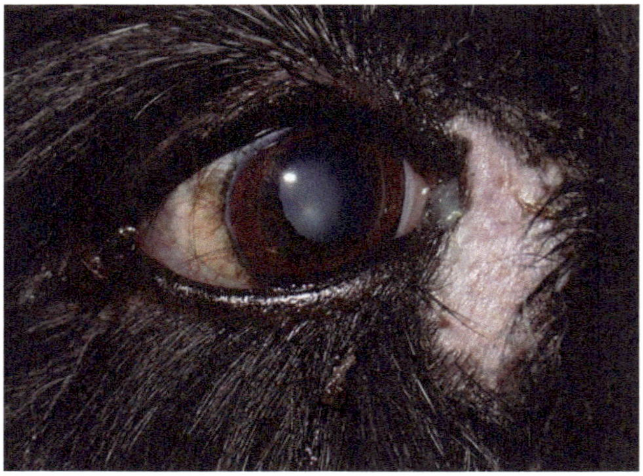

Figure 8.3E The same dog as in Figure 8.3D after a four-week course of antibiotics.

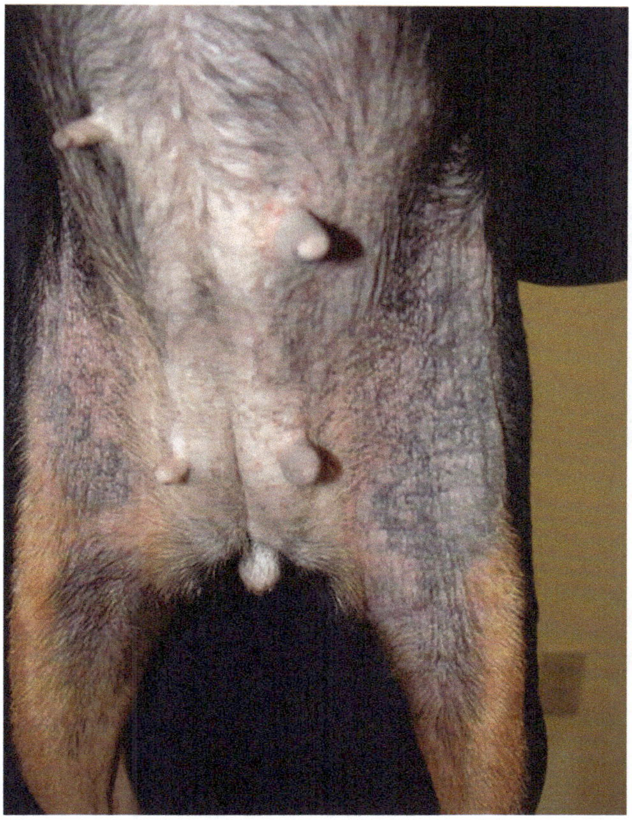

Figure 8.4A Bacterial overgrowth in an atopic Miniature Pinscher causing erythema, hyperpigmentation, and lichenification on the groin and medial thighs.

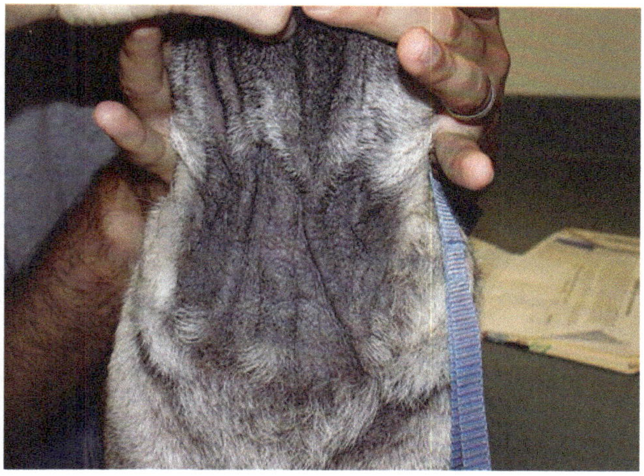

Figure 8.4B Bacterial overgrowth on the ventral neck of an allergic Pug; note the resemblance to *Malassezia* dermatitis.

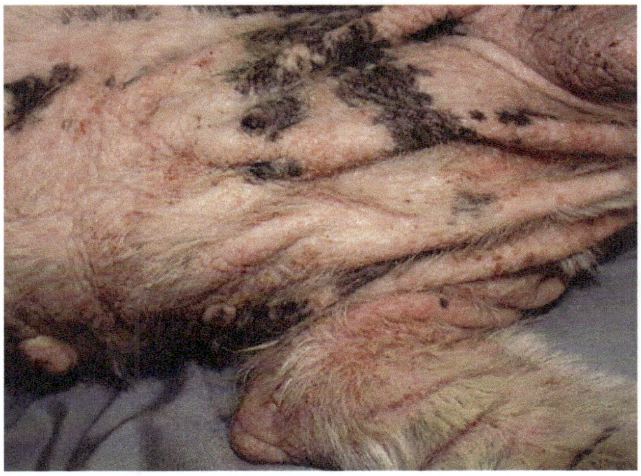

Figure 8.4C Marked erythema and lichenification in an atopic Shih Tzu due to bacterial overgrowth.

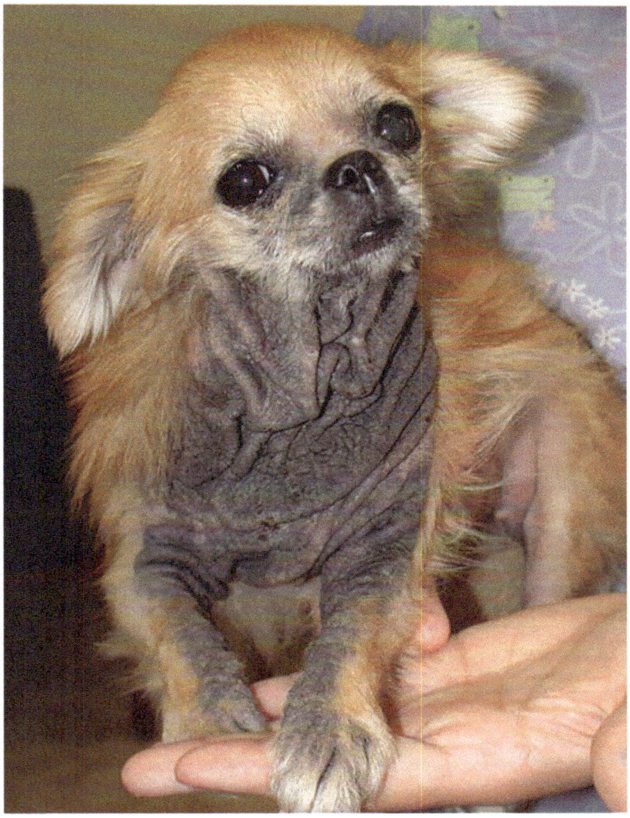

Figure 8.4D Lichenification and hyperpigmentation on the ventral neck and medial limbs of an allergic Chihuahua; despite clinical appearance only bacteria and no yeast were found on cytology.

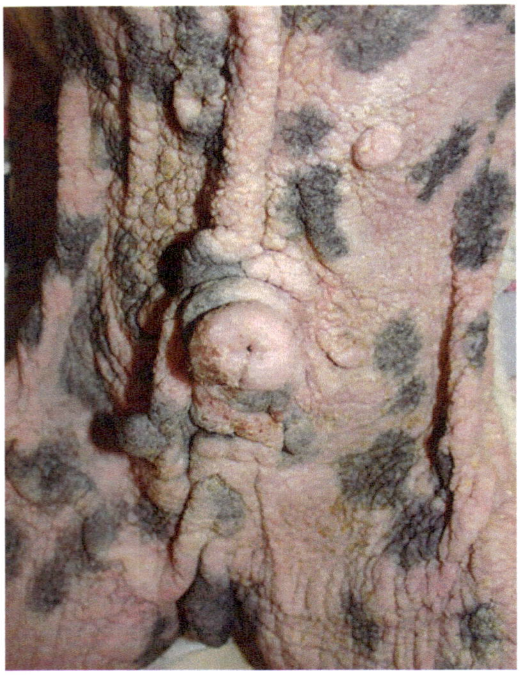

Figure 8.4E Bacterial overgrowth causing marked erythema and lichenification in an atopic Terrier.

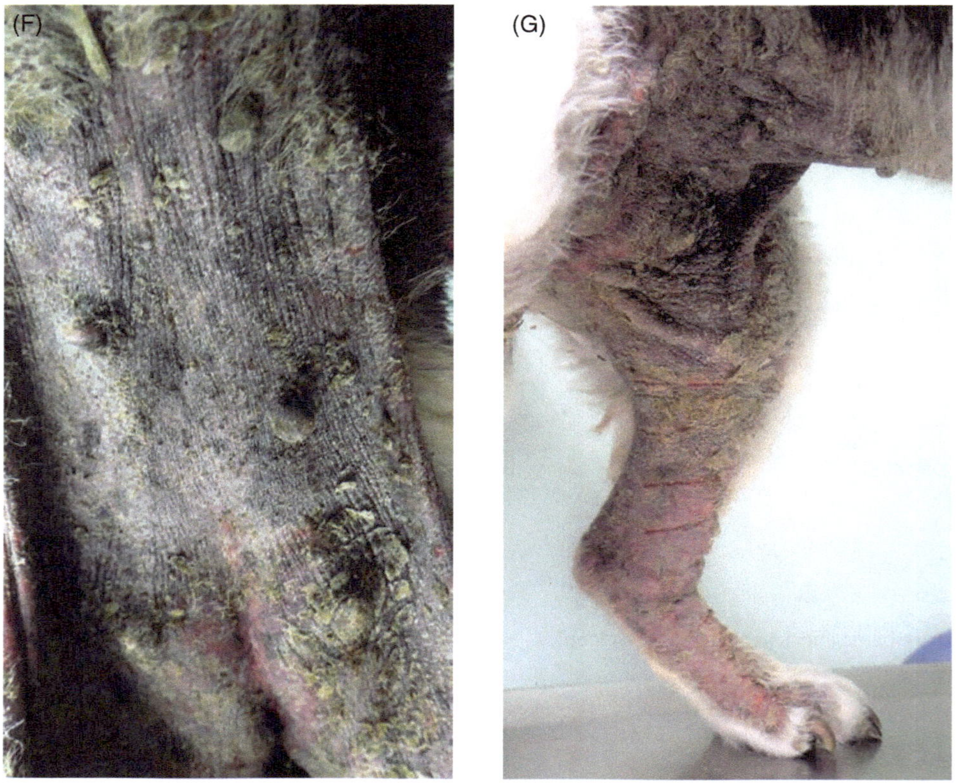

Figures 8.4F and G Lichenification, hyperpigmentation, and adherent yellowish crusting on the groin and medial limbs caused by bacterial and yeast overgrowth in a Beagle with hypothyroidism and atopic dermatitis.

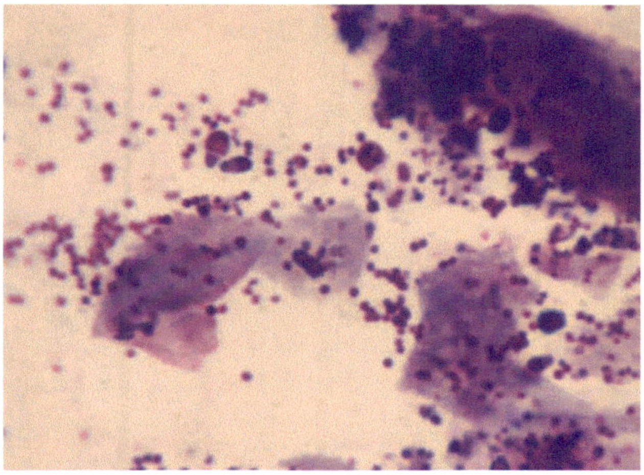

Figure 8.4H Cytology of the affected skin demonstrates numerous cocci bacteria and *Malassezia* (100×).

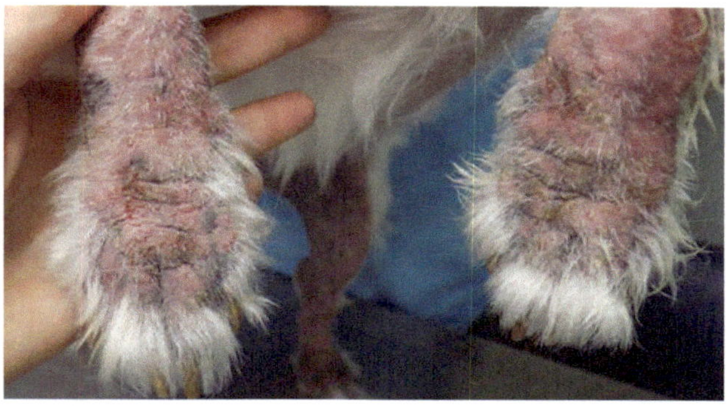

Figure 8.4I Severe lichenification and erythema of the paws due to bacterial and yeast infection caused by atopic dermatitis.

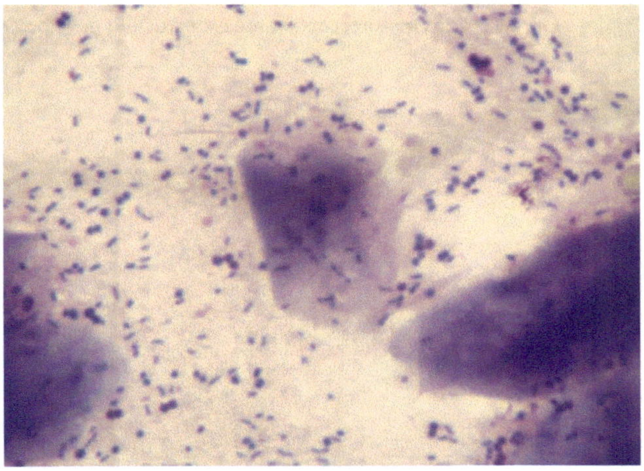

Figure 8.4J Cytology of the affected skin shows a mixed population of rod and cocci bacteria (100×).

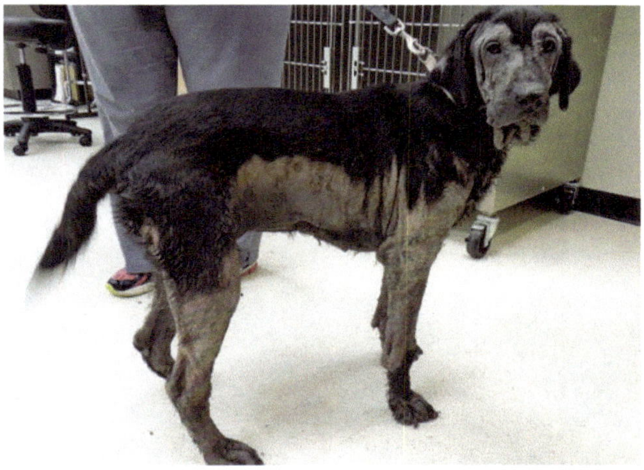

Figure 8.4K This food allergic and atopic Labrador had severe chronic methicillin resistant staphylococcal pyoderma.

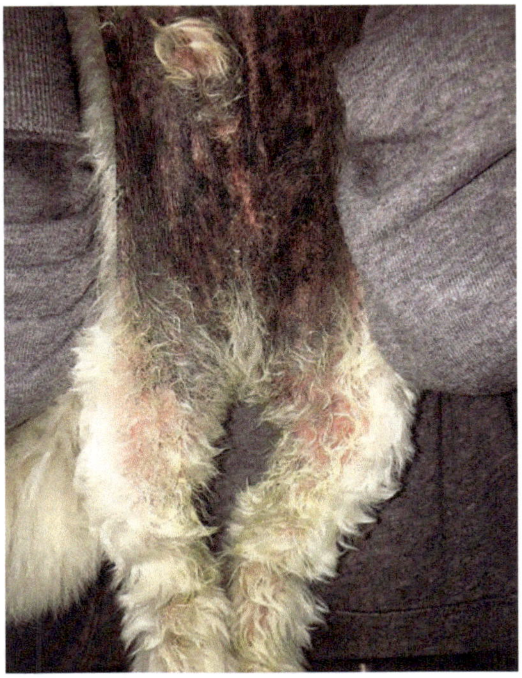

Figure 8.4L Hyperpigmentation, erythema, and mild lichenification due to bacterial overgrowth in an atopic Shih Tzu.

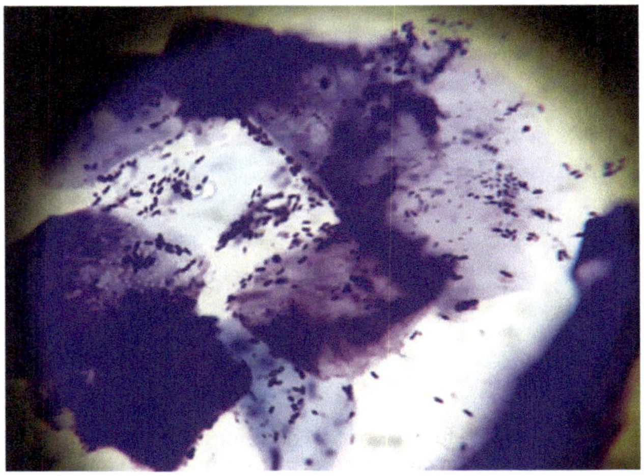

Figure 8.4M Cytology of the affected skin showed mostly rod shaped bacteria.

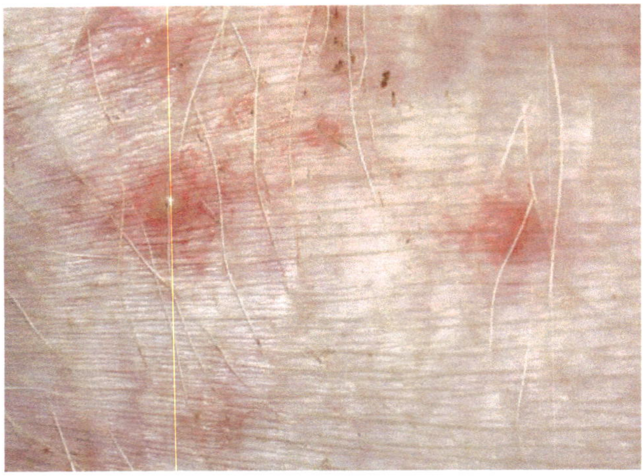

Figure 8.5A Inguinal papules and pustules in an atopic dog.

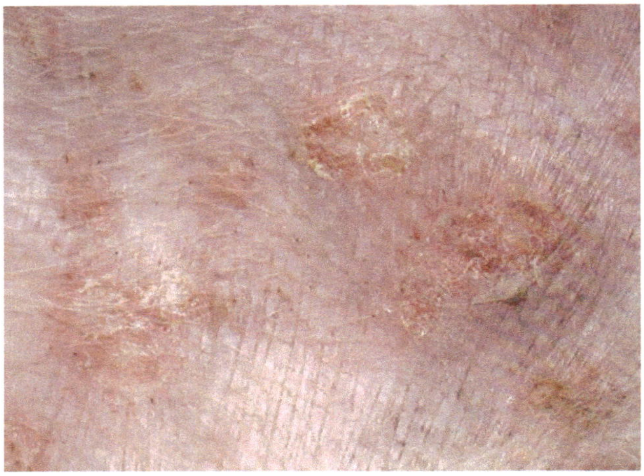

Figure 8.5B As lesions mature, circular areas of crusting develop.

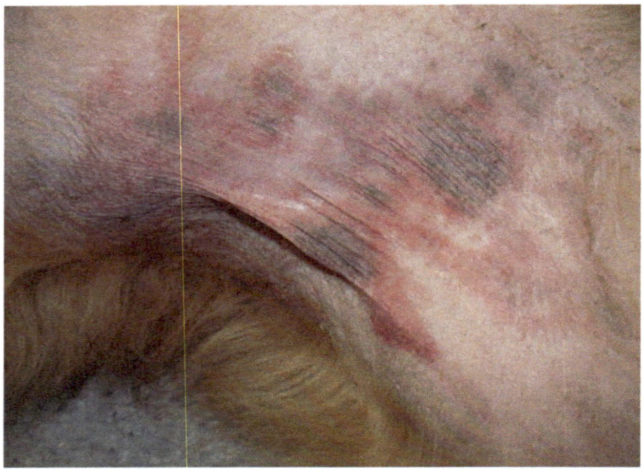

Figure 8.5C In chronic spreading pyoderma lesions often become centrally hyperpigmented, as in this hypothyroid dog.

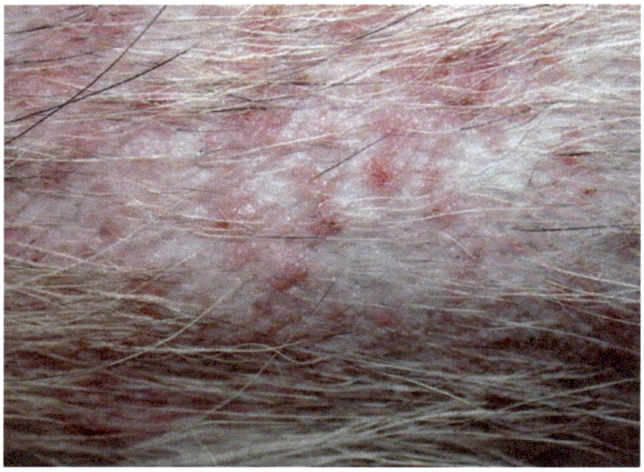

Figure 8.5D Numerous crusted papules due to bacterial folliculitis in an atopic German Shepherd.

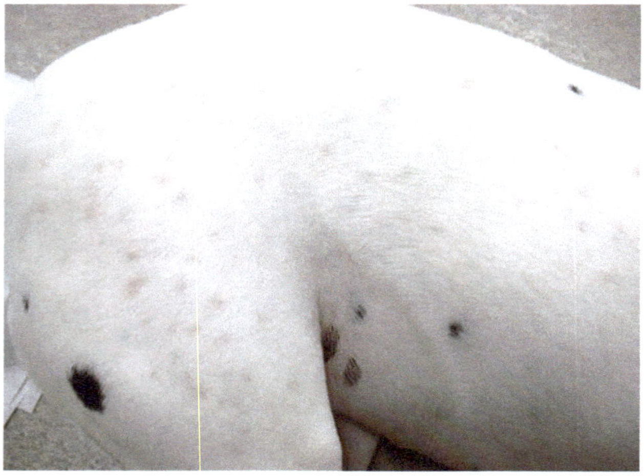

Figure 8.5E In this atopic Dalmatian, numerous small areas of brown (bronze) fur discoloration were present on the trunk and limbs.

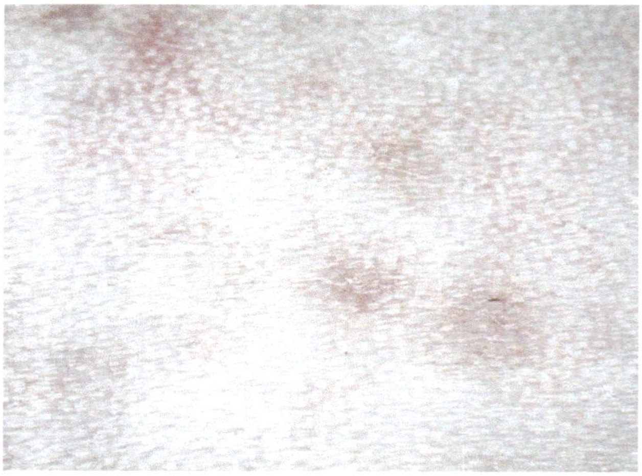

Figure 8.5F When the lesions were shaved the underlying papular dermatitis was revealed.

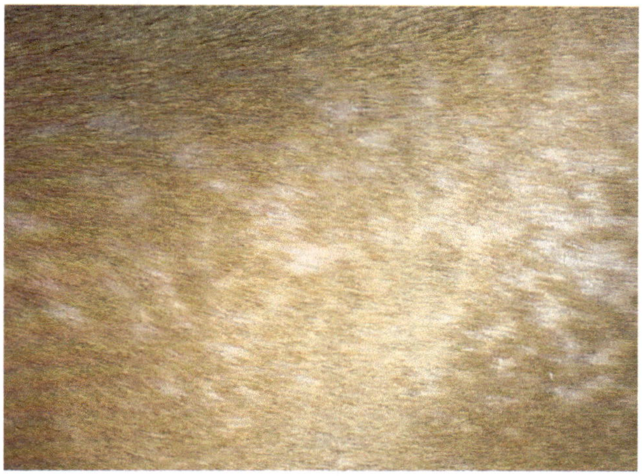

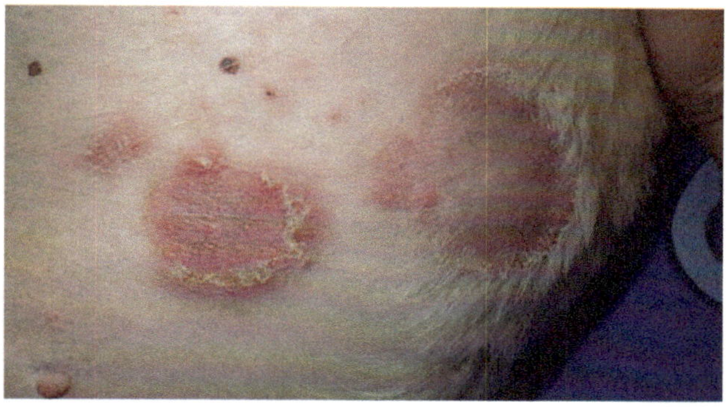

Figure 8.5H Epidermal collarettes (circular areas of alopecia, erythema, and peripheral crusting) caused by bacterial folliculitis in an atopic French Bulldog.

Figure 8.5G Patchy truncal hypotrichosis and scaling caused by bacterial folliculitis in an atopic Pitbull.

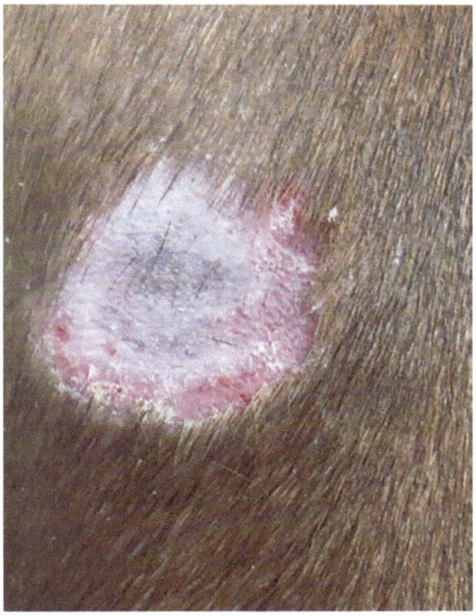

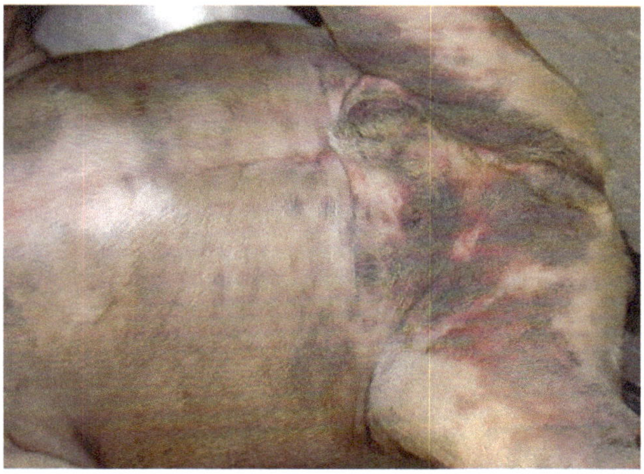

Figure 8.5J Severe chronic methicillin resistant staphylococcal pyoderma in an atopic Bulldog; hyperpigmentation and lichenification are developing.

Figure 8.5I In this epidermal collarette on a Miniature Dachshund, central post-inflammatory hyperpigmentation is developing.

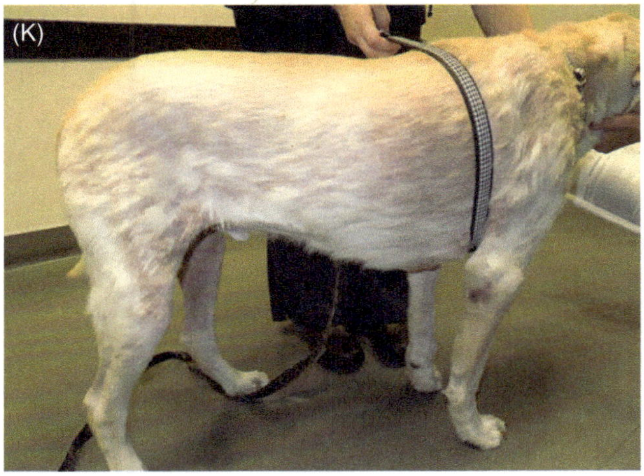

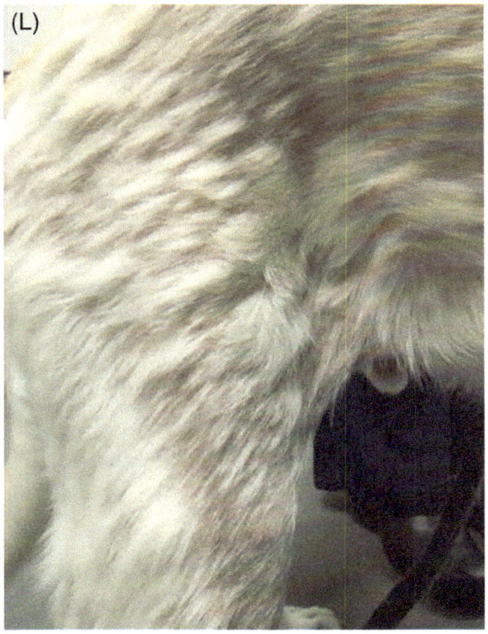

Figures 8.5K and L Patchy hypotrichosis and scaling on the trunk and limbs of an atopic Labrador with methicillin resistant staphylococcal folliculitis.

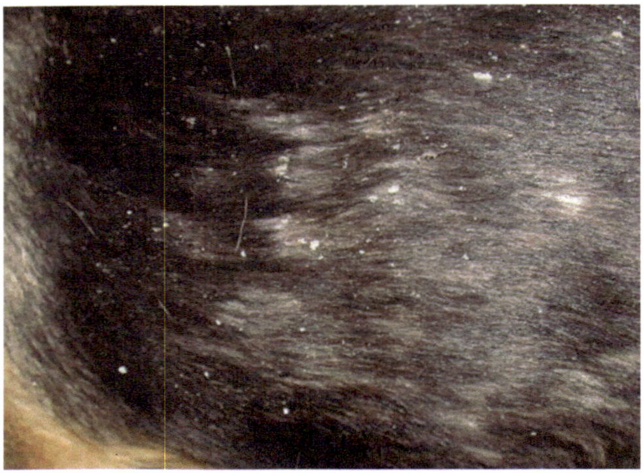

Figure 8.5M Patchy hypotrichosis and scaling with a dull coat are common symptoms of bacterial folliculitis in long coated dogs.

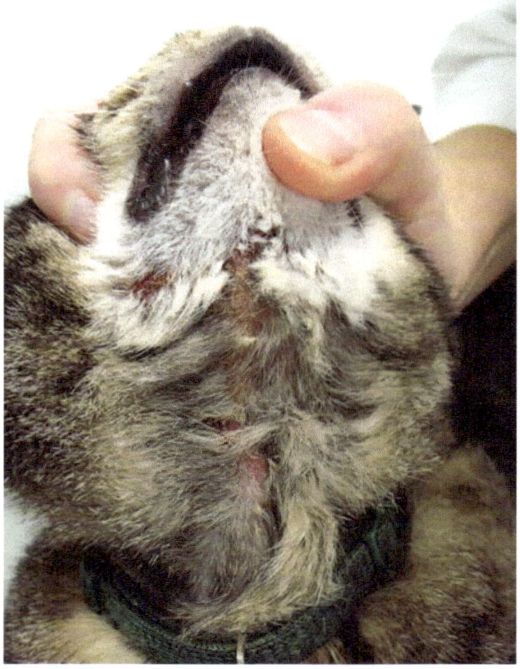

Figure 8.5N Crusting and erythema on the ventral neck of an atopic cat with secondary bacterial folliculitis.

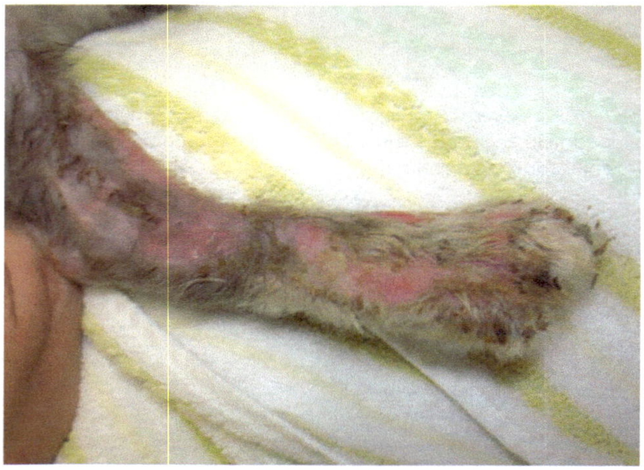

Figure 8.5O Alopecia, crusting, and erythema on the limb of an allergic cat with secondary pyoderma.

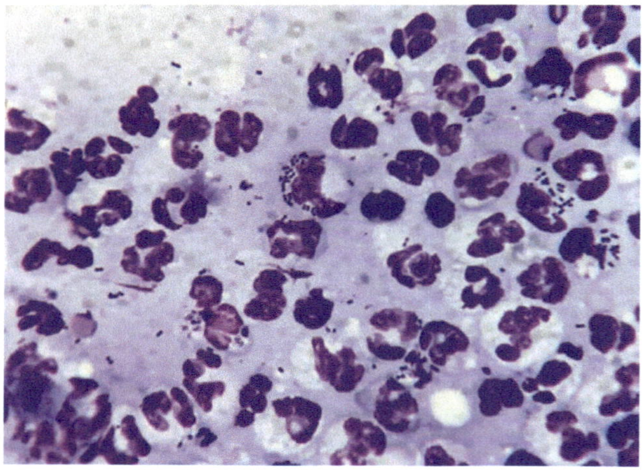

Figure 8.5P Cytology demonstrates neutrophils and numerous intra and extracellular cocci bacteria (100×).

Algorithm 8.1 Approach to chronic recurrent bacterial pyoderma.

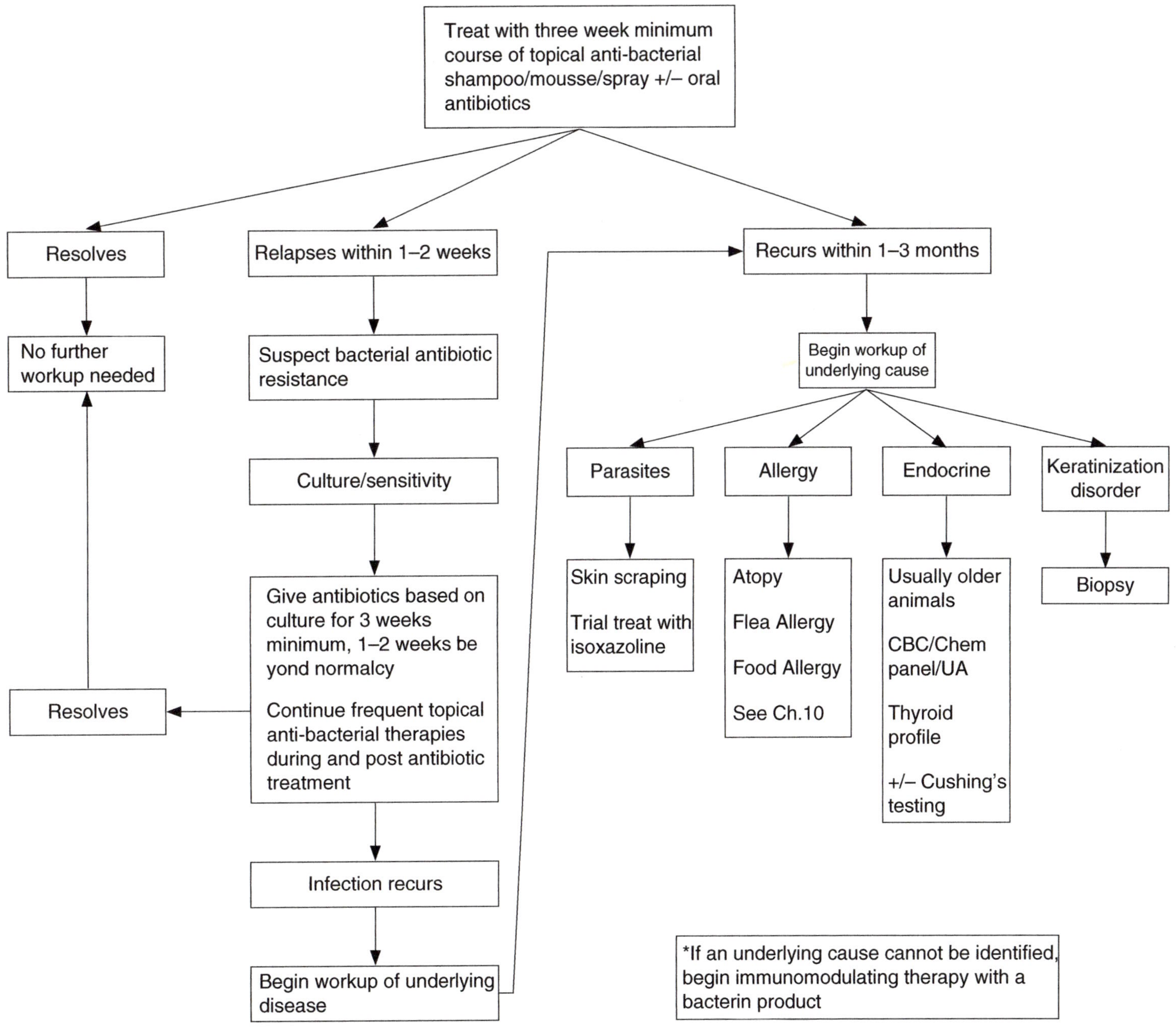

Table 8.2 Deep bacterial skin infections.

Deep pyoderma	Clinical signs	Diagnosis	Treatment
Bacterial furunculosis (Figures 8.6A–8.6J)	Focal to multifocal areas of thick crusting, alopecia, inflamed bullae, and/or ulcerative draining skin lesions, often pruritic or painful.	Clinical signs. Cytology +/− aerobic bacterial culture if bacteria are present despite prior or current antibiotics. Skin scrapings to rule out *Demodex*. +/− Dermatophyte culture.	Systemic antibiotics for 6–12 weeks (2 weeks beyond complete clinical resolution), frequent antibacterial shampoos/sprays. In recurrent cases identify and treat underlying cause (see Table 8.4 and Algorithm 8.1).
Canine acne (Figures 8.7A and 8.7B) More common in large, young, short coated dogs and may be induced by friction or trauma to the chin which pushes the short hairs under the skin.	Nonpainful, nonpruritic papules, pustules, bullae +/− draining tracts on the chin or muzzle.	Clinical signs. Cytology +/− aerobic bacterial culture if bacteria are present despite prior or current antibiotics. Skin scrapings to rule out *Demodex*. +/− Dermatophyte culture.	Mupirocin BID or benzoyl peroxide gel daily until lesions resolve then 1–2 times weekly as needed for control. For severe cases, give systemic antibiotics for 4 weeks minimum.
Callus furunculosis (Figure 8.8) Most commonly affects giant breeds.	Inflammation, swelling, ulceration, and draining tracts affecting pressure points such as lateral elbows/hocks in large breed dogs or sternal callous in deep chested breeds.	Clinical signs. Cytology +/− aerobic bacterial culture if bacteria are present despite prior or current antibiotics. Skin scrapings and hair plucks to rule out *Demodex*. +/− Dermatophyte culture.	Treat infection with mupirocin BID and systemic antibiotics based on culture for 6 weeks minimum. Hydrotherapy and bandaging needed for open lesions. Ensure dog lays on padded bedding or has padded appliances placed over wound (i.e. Dogleggs®).
Acral lick dermatitis (Figures 8.9A–8.9C) A multifactorial disorder often associated with underlying atopy, food allergy, trauma, endocrinopathy, bone pain, neuropathy, or behavioral causes, and then perpetuated by a secondary deep pyoderma.	Alopecic, firm, raised, thickened plaque or nodule which may become ulcerated, often found on the dorsal carpus, or dorsolateral metatarsus. Regional lymphadenopathy may be present. Lesion is intensely pruritic +/− painful, causing incessant licking. Other clinical lesions consistent with underlying allergic skin disease may be present, i.e. interdigital, inguinal, facial, or outer ear erythema.	Clinical signs. Cytology +/− aerobic bacterial culture if bacteria are present despite prior or current antibiotics. Skin scrapings and hair plucks to rule out *Demodex* and dermatophyte culture. Identify and treat underlying cause(s): Prescription hypoallergenic diet trial +/− allergy testing/desensitization in pruritic dogs; radiographs to screen for underlying bone or joint pathology, labwork to screen for metabolic disease in older dogs.	Antibiotics based on culture for 8 weeks minimum (2 weeks beyond complete clinical resolution). Obtain culture sample by tissue biopsy, or by firmly squeezing affected tissue to extrude deep exudate for culture (this may require the dog to be muzzled or sedated); surface culture may not reflect deep infection. Oral NSAIDs to reduce pain/inflammation. Prevent licking with E. collar or bandaging. In some cases oclacitinib or Cytopoint may be helpful to reduce licking, however oclacitinib can make infection harder to treat and should be discontinued within 2–4 weeks and antibiotics should be continued for several weeks thereafter. Some cases benefit from behavior modifying medications such as fluoxetine or clomipramine as part of combination treatment, but purely behavioral causes for acral granulomas are rare.

Pedal folliculitis/furunculosis (Figures 8.10A–8.10F) Often associated with underlying atopy, food allergy, endocrinopathy, demodicosis, etc. In some cases, isolated recurrent or chronic lesions are associated with abnormal weight bearing, elbow dysplasia, or obesity and subsequent formation of single interdigital cysts, often between P2–3 or P4–5 on front paws of large breed dogs.	Interdigital erythema, pustules, bullae, nodules, fistulas, alopecia, and swelling. Often seen in large, short coated dogs, variably painful and pruritic. May be associated with regional lymphadenopathy and/or swelling of associated metacarpus or metatarsus.	Clinical signs. Cytology +/− aerobic bacterial culture if bacteria are present despite prior or current antibiotics. Skin scrapings and hair plucks to rule out *Demodex*. +/− Dermatophyte culture.	Systemic antibiotics for 6–12 weeks (2 weeks beyond complete clinical resolution). Frequent antibacterial shampoos/sprays/wipes to help speed healing and prevent infection recurrence. Identify and address underlying cause (see Table 8.4 and Algorithm 8.1). Focal areas of scarring/interdigital cyst formation may be amenable to surgical resection or laser ablation.
Post-grooming furunculosis (Figures 8.11A and 8.11B) Contaminated shampoos or grooming apparatus, or over-zealous scrubbing of short hairs "against the grain" are implicated as causal factors. *Staphylococcus pseudintermedius, Pseudomonas, Proteus* and *E. coli* have been grown in pure or mixed culture from lesions.	Usually occurs within 24–48 hours after grooming and is manifested by areas of intense localized erythema and swelling which evolve into punctate foci of erythema, erosion, painful hemorrhagic bullae, and drainage. Lesions are usually on the dorsal trunk and occur more commonly in short coated dogs. Affected dogs may be lethargic or febrile; first sign may be difficult to localize back pain.	Clinical signs. Cytology. Aerobic bacterial culture. Skin scrapings to rule out *Demodex*. +/− Dermatophyte culture.	Pending culture, begin systemic antibiotic therapy with fluoroquinolones if rod bacteria are found on cytology, or a cephalosporin antibiotic if cocci are found on cytology. Sedation usually needed for clipping and cleaning of lesions. Pain control with opioids may be needed, +/− intravenous fluids and supportive care for severely affected or systemically ill dogs.

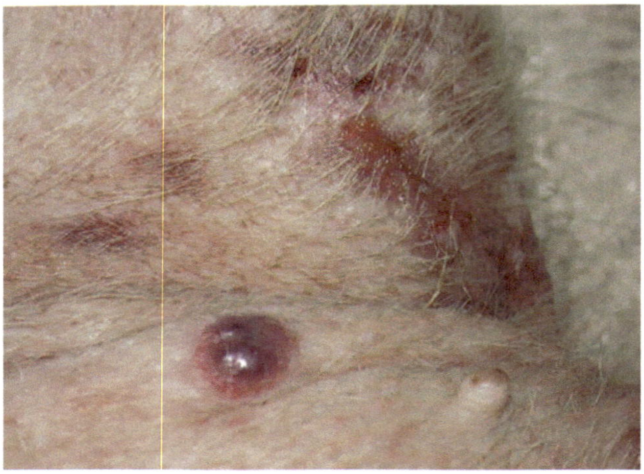

Figure 8.6A Inflamed bullae and draining tracts due to deep pyoderma in an atopic Golden Retriever.

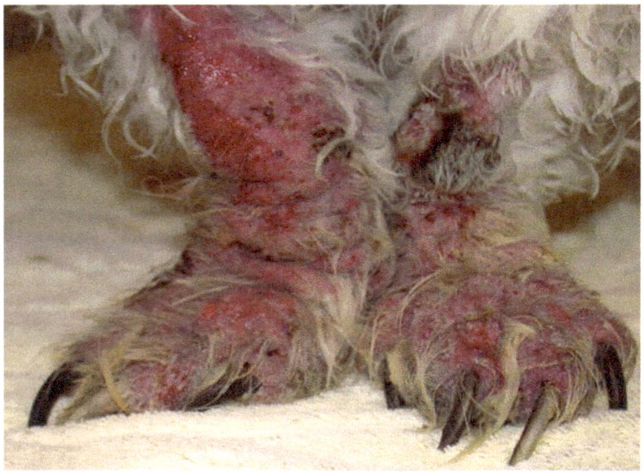

Figure 8.6B Bacterial furunculosis on the paws due to demodicosis.

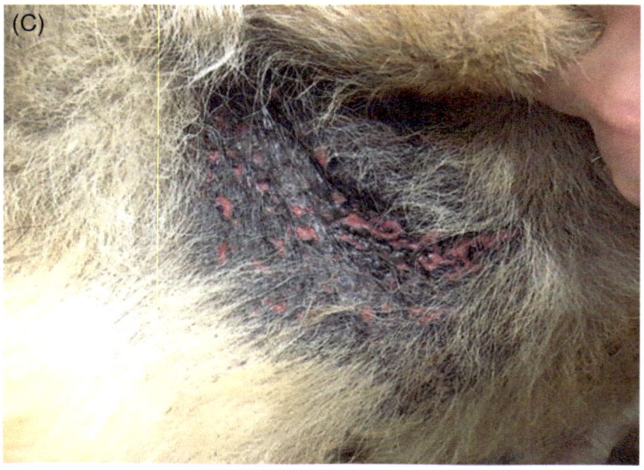

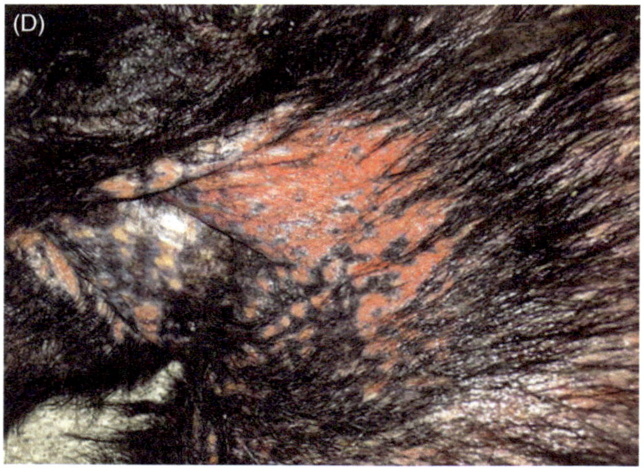

Figures 8.6C and D Inguinal and axillary deep methicillin resistant staphylococcal pyoderma causing ulcerative lesions in two atopic German Shepherds.

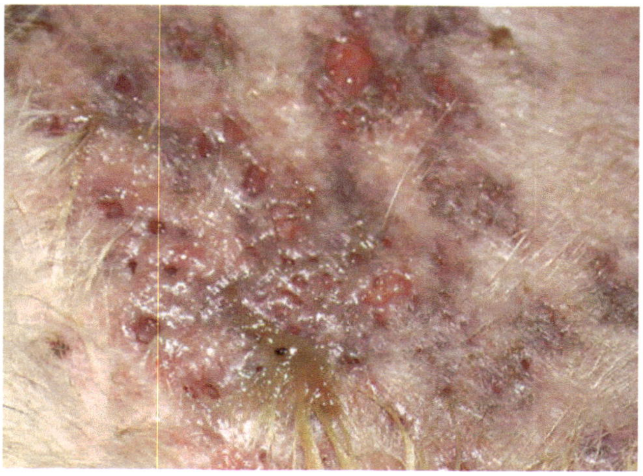

Figure 8.6E Ulcerations and draining tracts due to deep pyoderma in an atopic dog.

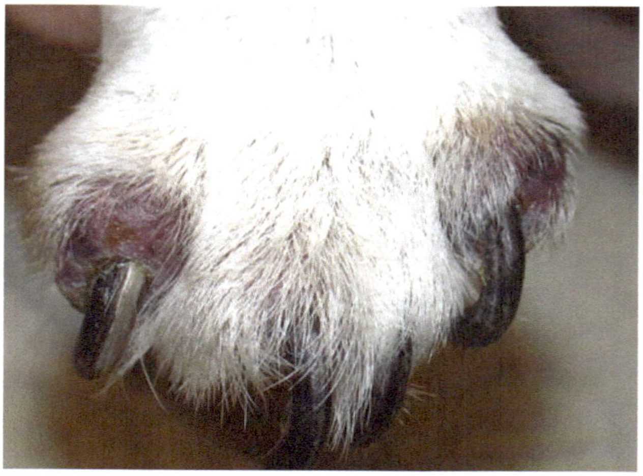

Figure 8.6F Deep bacterial paronychia causing swelling and drainage in an atopic Terrier.

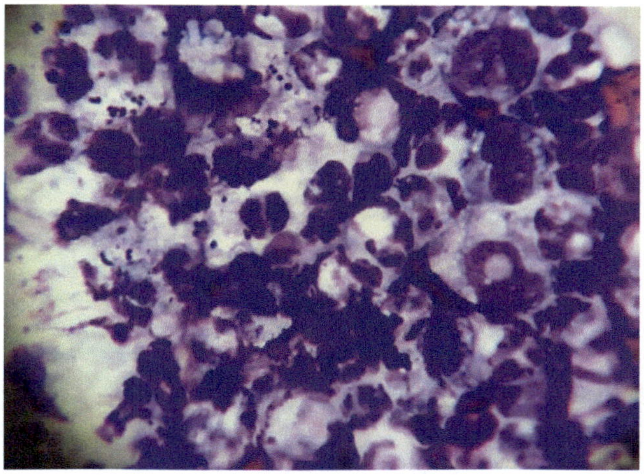

Figure 8.6G Cytology of deep pyoderma often shows pyogranulomatous inflammation; bacteria may be difficult to find (100×).

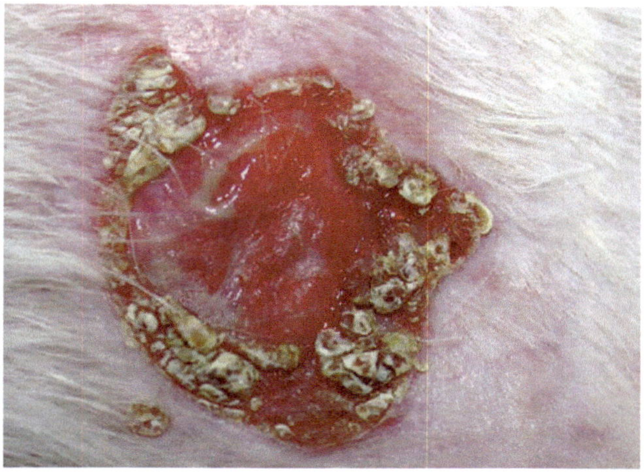

Figure 8.6H An atopic cat with secondary deep pyoderma caused by methicillin resistant *Staphylococcus aureus*.

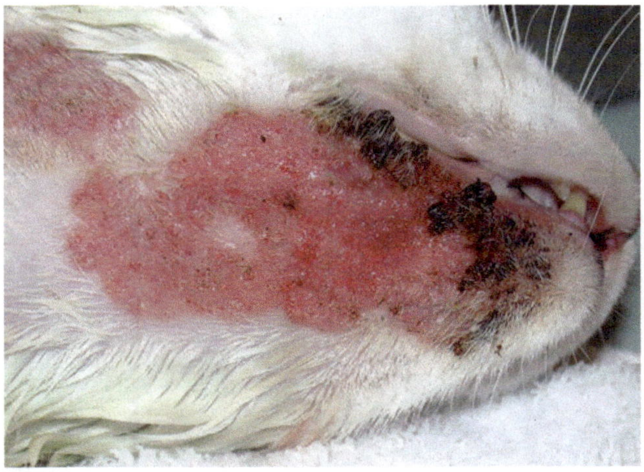

Figure 8.6I Deep bacterial pyoderma on the ventral chin of an allergic cat.

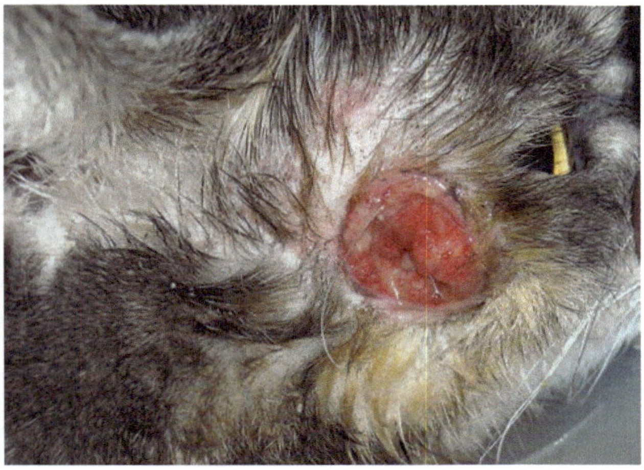

Figure 8.6J Severe ulcerative deep pyoderma caused by methicillin resistant *Staphylococcus aureus* secondary to food allergy in a cat.

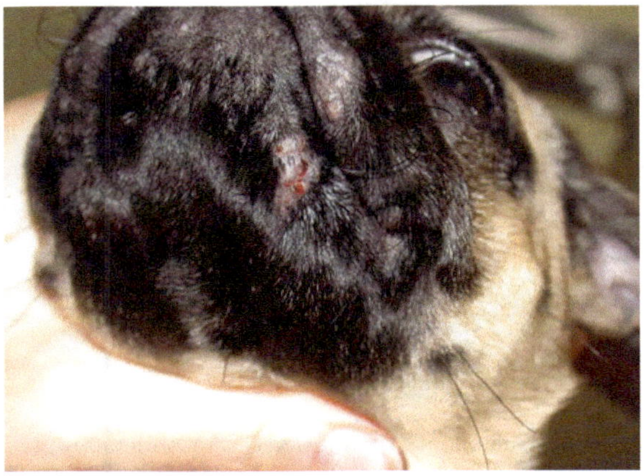

Figure 8.7A Lip and chin pustules in a Pug due to canine acne.

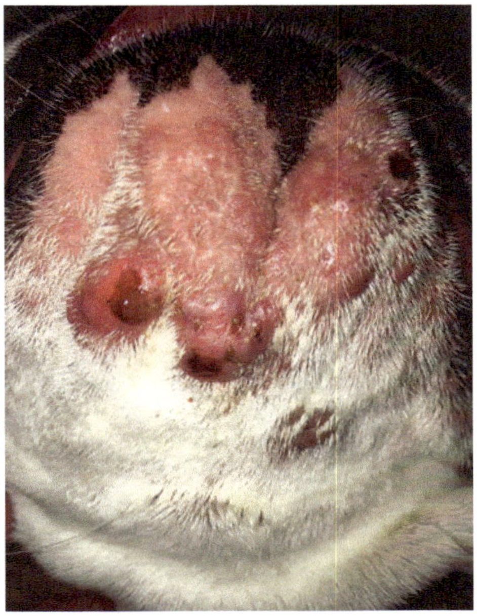

Figure 8.7B In this allergic Bulldog, severe canine acne has caused scarring and draining tracts.

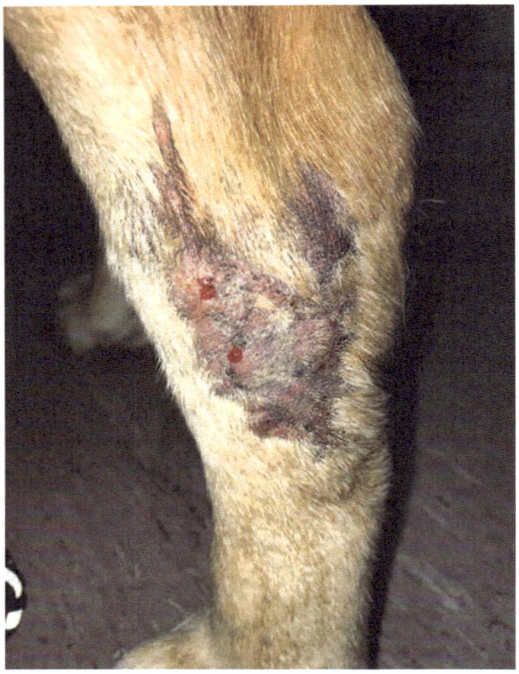

Figure 8.8 Callus furunculosis on the lateral hock on an older Labrador.

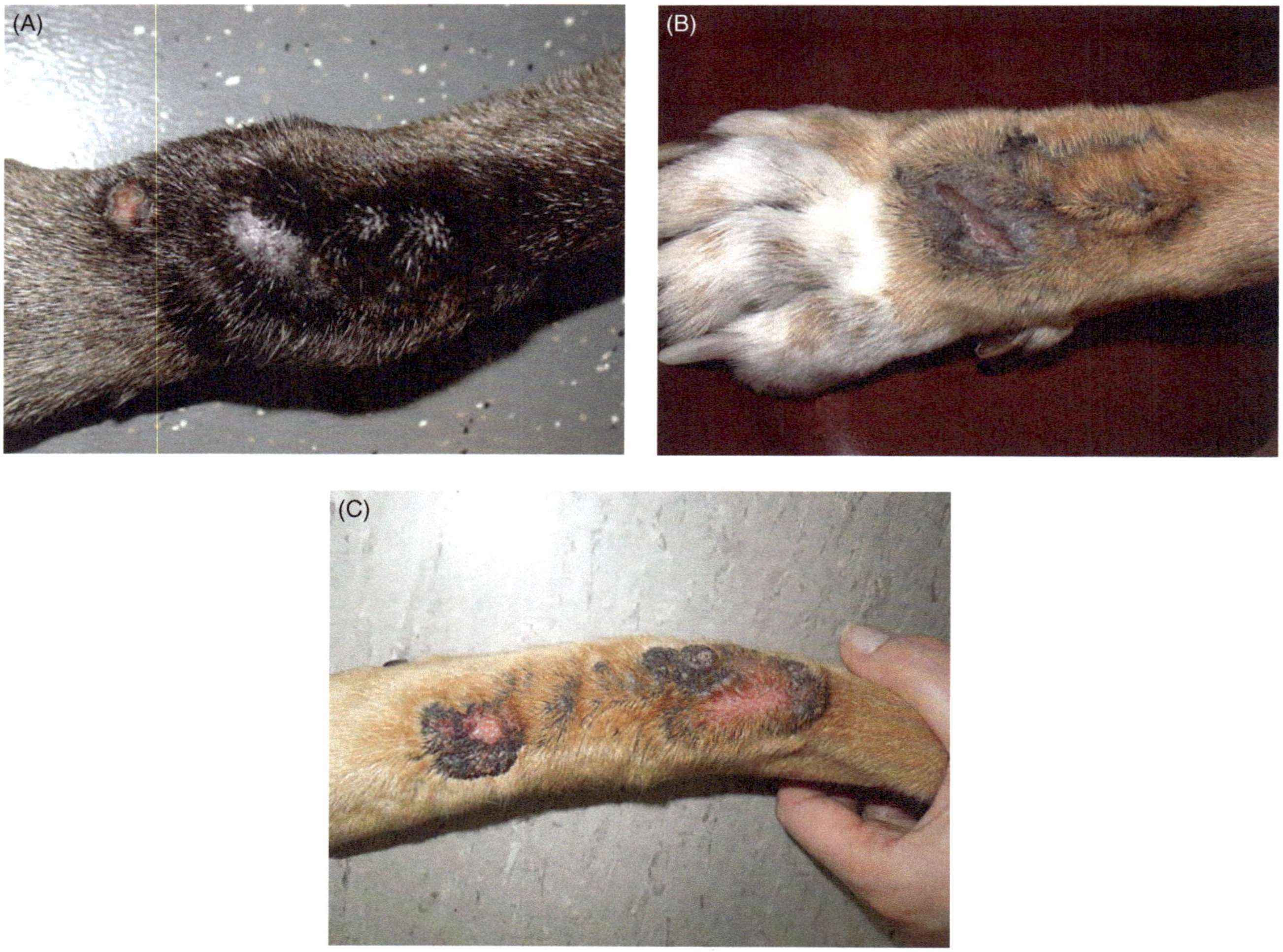

Figures 8.9A–C Patchy scarring, thickened skin, alopecia, ulceration, and crusts (acral granulomas) on the dorsal carpus/metacarpus of three atopic dogs.

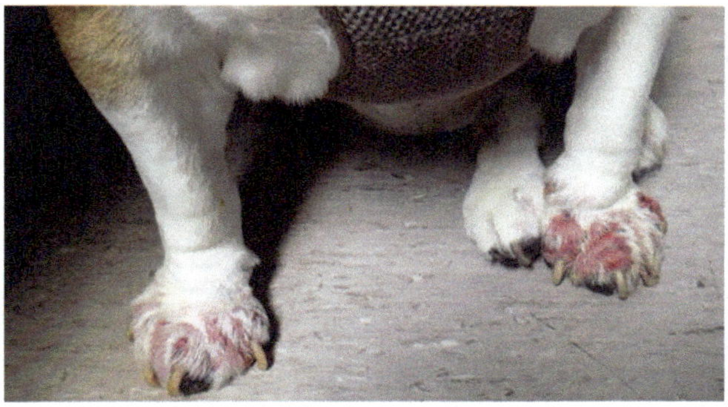

Figure 8.10A Interdigital swelling and draining tracts in an atopic Bulldog.

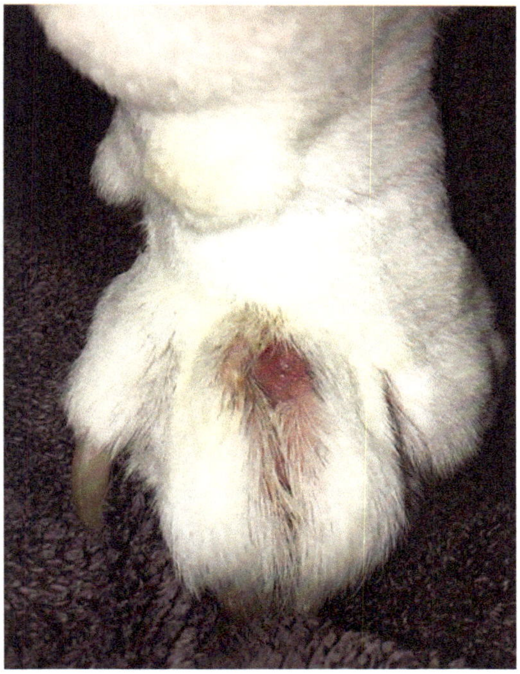

Figure 8.10B A dorsal interdigital draining granuloma in an atopic Bulldog.

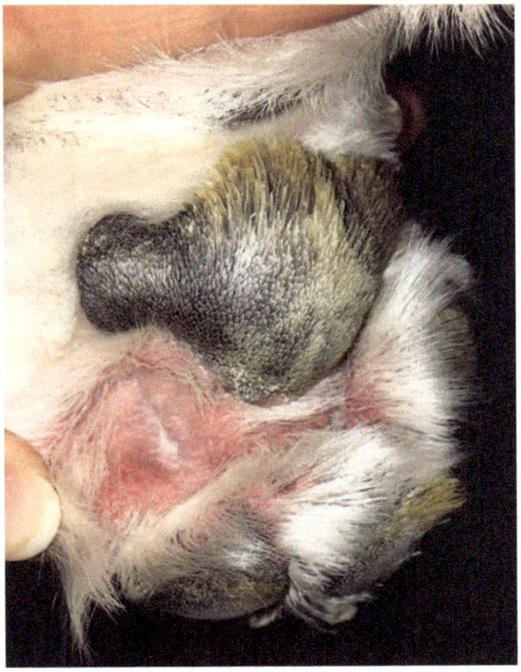

Figure 8.10C In this dog with pedal furunculosis, an inflamed follicular cyst is present between P4–5.

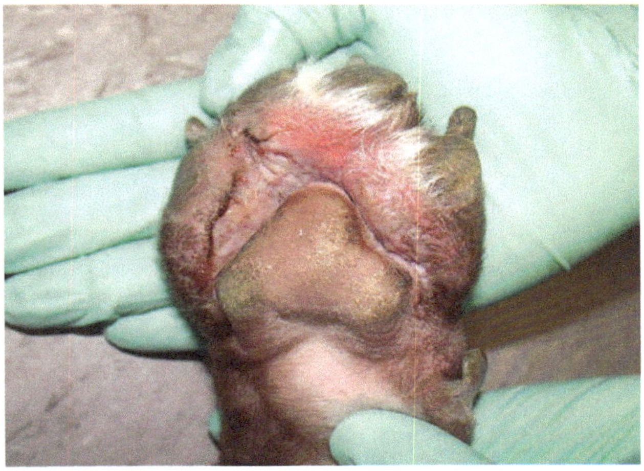

Figure 8.10D A Pitbull Terrier with bacterial pododermatitis secondary to atopy.

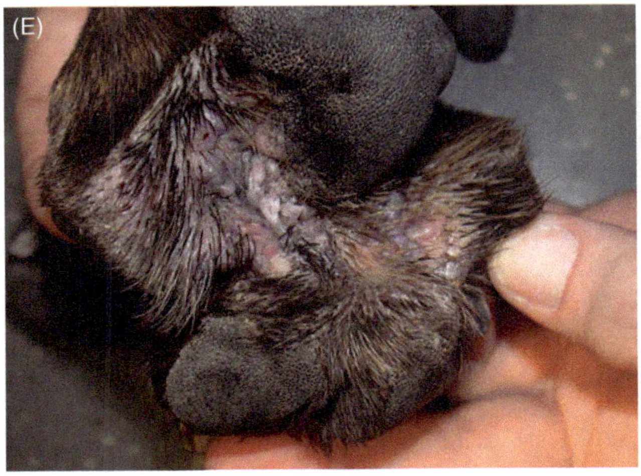

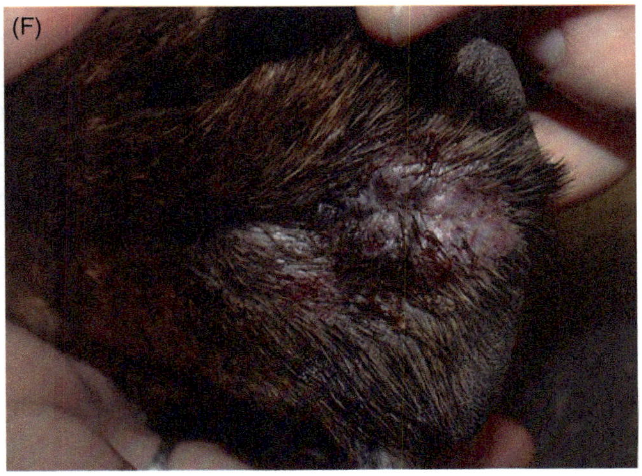

Figures 8.10E and F An atopic Labrador mix with pedal furunculosis.

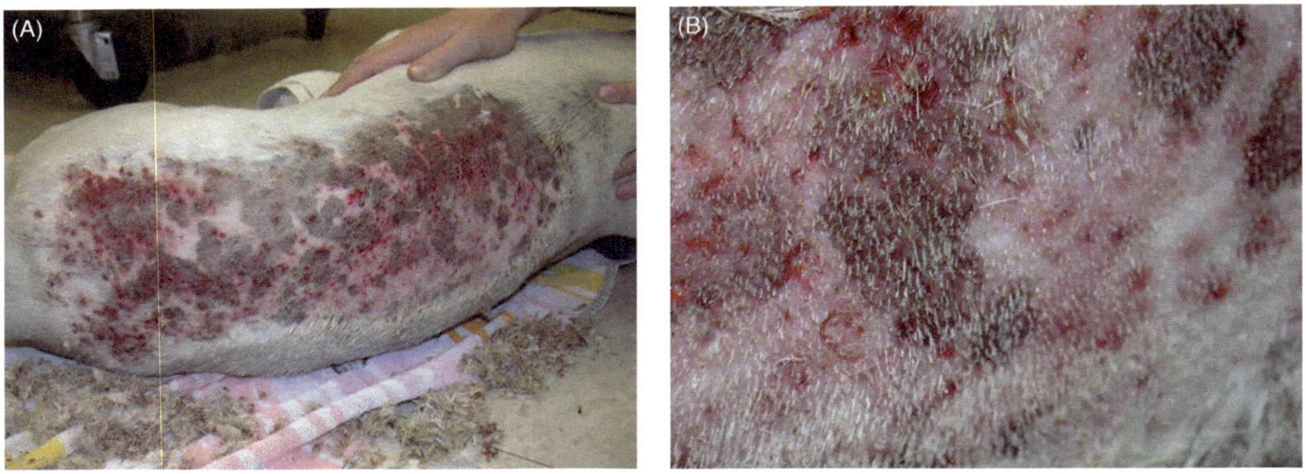

Figures 8.11A and B An American Bulldog with an acute onset of painful furunculosis, which occurred after being groomed.

Table 8.3 Meticillin resistance.

Definition what is meticillin?	• Name changed from methicillin in 2005. • A narrow spectrum beta-lactam antibiotic. • Most labs now use the more stable oxacillin for resistance testing. • Meticillin (or oxacillin) resistant *Staphylococcus* are considered resistant to *all* Beta-lactam antibiotics (penicillins and cephalosporins). • MRSP = meticillin resistant *Staphylococcus pseudintermedius* (called *Staphylococcus intermedius* in the past); this is not the same as MRSA which usually affects humans.
Multidrug resistance	Many MRSP infections in dogs have multidrug resistance: Resistant to three or more different families of antibiotics: Beta-lactams Tetracyclines Macrolides and lincosamides Chloramphenicol Aminoglycosides Trimethoprim/sulfonamides Fluoroquinolones Rifampicin Mupirocin
Most common meticillin resistant (MR) Staphylococcal species isolated in small animals	• *S. pseudintermedius* • *S. schleiferi* (coagulase negative) • *Staphylococcus aureus* (uncommon except in horses) • *Staphylococcus hyicus* (rare)
Risk factors for development of resistance	• Use of antibiotics – Especially fluoroquinolones and beta-lactams • Admission to a veterinary hospital for >1 day – Hospitalization – Surgical procedures – Comparable to "Health care-associated" MRSA in humans (HA-MRSA)
When to suspect resistance	Patient not clinically responding to appropriate dosage and duration of empiric antibiotic therapy: • Verify infection still bacterial (perform cytology). • Verify sufficient duration of treatment for improvement to have occurred. • Do *not* simply choose a different antibiotic empirically. • Remember these bacteria have genes selecting for multidrug resistance. • It is imperative to obtain culture and sensitivity.
Best practices to obtain culture	• If pustule is present use small gauge needle to puncture and collect culture from that location. • If no pustule present then lift any crust present and obtain with frequent rubbing of culture tip at that location repeatedly to create "frictional erythema". • Often there is erythema and scale at leading edge of superficial spreading pyoderma and this is a location to focus for culture. • Verify with cytology the recovery of coccoid bacteria at location of culture. • Stop topical antibacterial therapies 48 hours prior. • It is still okay to culture even if patient is on antibiotics as long as you still see bacteria on cytology.

Table 8.3 Meticillin resistance (Continued)

Antimicrobial treatment of MRSP in a patient	• Antibiotic selection based on appropriate culture. • Utilize appropriate dosage to limit development of further resistance. • Utilize appropriate duration (10–14 days beyond clinical resolution) to ensure full resolution of infection. • Identify and treat underlying cause of pyoderma simultaneously. • In cases of resistant pyoderma consultation with and/or referral to area dermatologist is recommended to identify and aggressively manage any underlying chronic primary disorder.
Additional supportive treatments of MRSP patient and ways to minimize transmission	Reduce host exposure: • Frequent bathing of pet. • Frequent hand washing and use of alcohol hand sanitizers by owners. • Cleaning of common surfaces and washing of bedding. Reduce host susceptibility: • Control underlying primary disease. • Consider underlying hypersensitivity (refer to Chapter 10 on hypersensitivity disorders) and endocrinopathies in older dogs.
What do I tell owners of patient with MRSP?	• Since the gene that confers meticillin resistance can be shared between different Staphylococcal species it is worthwhile to discuss the health status of humans in the household and, typically, standard precautions outlined above are sufficient • Concerns arise if humans in household are immunocompromised, or have medical issues such as dialysis port, feeding tube, etc. then recommend having them discuss directly with their primary physician as perhaps more intensive monitoring is necessary in their care regimen. Recommend minimized contact with the MRSP veterinary patient in these rare but special circumstances. • www.wormsandgermsblog.com is a great resource for owner reference and trustworthy internet advice.
Infection control measures within your hospital	• Staff should properly identify "at-risk" patients when possible: – Surgical patients – Wounded patients – Dermatologic patients – Hospitalized patients • Appropriate cleaning of exam rooms and common areas between patients. • Alcohol-based hand sanitizers placed in each exam room, and common treatment areas: – Should contain 70–90% alcohol – Use after contact with any/every patient – Need to be readily accessible • Frequent hand washing between patients.
Infection control program	Have a documented infection control program: • Develop protocols: – Staff handling of patient with MRSP, – How and when is cleaning performed of exam room, and common areas in these cases – Laundry and waste management • Ensure that protocols are followed. • Act as a resource for infection control questions. • Ensure proper training of new staff. • Surveillance of infections: – Active and passive surveillance methods. • Communicate with staff regarding infection control issues.
Reminder	All dogs carry *S. pseudintermedius.* Clinical infection is uncommon and requires a defect in skin barrier often caused by an underlying disease or anatomical predisposition. Opportunistic infections possible: – Hypersensitivity disorders – Otitis (often due to underlying hypersensitivity) – Urinary tract – Surgical sites – Wounds Treating MRSP is no different than treating MSSP (meticillin susceptible *Staphylococcus pseudintermedius*): • Simply have fewer systemic options • Motivated to treat more intensively with topicals • Motivated to look more diligently at underlying cause

Table 8.4 Underlying causes for recurrent pyoderma.

Hypersensitivity dermatitis
- Atopy
- Food allergy
- Flea allergy dermatitis

Parasites
- Fleas
- *Demodex*
- Scabies

Endocrinopathy
- Hypothyroidism
- Hyperadrenocorticism
- Sex hormone excess

Follicular dysplasia
- Color dilution alopecia
- Congenitally alopecic breeds

Keratinization abnormalities
- Zinc responsive dermatosis
- Sebaceous adenitis
- Ichthyosis
- Primary seborrhea

Table 8.5 Commonly used antibiotics for canine pyoderma.

- *Avoid* antibiotics to which staphylococcal bacteria are usually intrinsically resistant, including amoxicillin, ampicillin, penicillin, tetracycline, and non-potentiated sulfonamides.
- Most veterinary dermatologists use cephalosporins, clindamycin, clavulanated penicillin, or potentiated sulfonamides as first-line therapy for canine pyoderma.
- Fluoroquinolones are used as second-line therapy when indicated by culture for deep/fibrotic infections, and for *Pseudomonas* infections. Veterinary labeled fluoroquinolones are preferred over generic ciprofloxacin due to marked variability of ciprofloxacin absorption in dogs.
- Doxycycline, chloramphenicol, and aminoglycosides are used more rarely, and usually as dictated by culture results in meticillin-resistant staphylococcal infections.
- After an antibiotic has been selected, it should be dispensed at the correct dosage, administered at the correct dosing interval, and used for a sufficient period. Underdosing an antibiotic due to concern for cost savings for the client will only cost more in the long run due to increased time to cure and increased chance of inducing bacterial resistance, necessitating more expenses such as cultures and additional antibiotic courses.
- Regular rechecks are important to determine response to therapy and need for medication refills or therapy modifications.

Antibiotic	Dose
Cephalexin	22–30 mg/kg PO BID – TID
Cefadroxil	22 mg/kg PO BID
Cefpodoxime	5–10 mg/kg PO once daily
Cefovicin	8 mg/kg SC once. A second injection (same dose/route) may be administered if response to therapy is not complete 7 days later (for *Staphylococcus intermedius* infections) and 14 days later for *Staphylococcus canis* (group G) infections. Maximum treatment should not exceed two injections (adapted from label information; *Convenia*®, Pfizer.)
Amoxicillin/clavulanate	13.75–22 mg/kg PO BID – TID
Trimethoprim sulfamethoxazole	30 mg/kg PO q24 hours, or 15 mg/kg PO BID
Ormetoprim sulfadimethoxine	55 mg/kg PO Day 1, then 27.5 mg/kg PO once daily
Clindamycin	11 mg/kg PO BID
Lincomycin	15.4 mg/kg PO q8h or 22 mg/kg PO q12h
Enrofloxacin	5–20 mg/kg PO once daily; 10 mg/kg or higher preferred
Marbofloxacin	2.75–5.5 mg/kg PO once daily
Orbifloxacin	2.75–7.5 mg/kg PO once daily
Doxycycline	5 mg/kg PO q12h or 10 mg/kg PO q24h with food
Minocycline	5–10 mg/kg PO BID with small amount canned food
Chloramphenicol	30–40 mg/kg PO TID with food; tell owners to wear gloves

Table 8.6 Topical antibacterial products.

Topical product	Activity	Advantages	Disadvantages
Chlorhexidine 2–4% Available in several formulations (shampoo, conditioner, spray, flush, wipes).	Effective against most Gram-positive and Gram-negative bacteria; equivalent and excellent minimum bactericidal activities of 2, 3, and 4% chlorhexidene shampoos for *S. pseudintermedius* (both methicillin-susceptible and methicillin-resistant).	Works in the presence of organic debris, rarely sensitizing, and has good residual activity on the skin even after 29 hours. Antimicrobial activity is superior to povidone iodine and ethyl lactate, and is non-drying compared to benzoyl peroxide.	Occasional contact sensitivity; if dog is more inflamed or pruritic after use then change to different antibacterial topical.
Benzoyl peroxide 2.5–5%	Oxidizing agent to damage bacterial membranes.	Antibacterial effect can persist for 48 hours. Also, keratolytic, antipruritic, and degreasing. Increases transepidermal water loss, decreases glandular secretions, and has a follicular flushing action. Helpful in dogs with greasy seborrhea, may need to transition to milder product to prevent overdrying as skin condition improves.	Can cause cutaneous drying, erythema, and pruritus. Compared to chlorhexidene, benzoyl peroxide shampoo required a higher concentration and longer period of incubation of 30–60 minutes for bacterial killing in vitro (Loeffler, Cobb, and Bond, 2011).
Ethyl lactate 10%	Penetrates hair follicles and sebaceous glands where it is hydrolyzed by bacterial lipases into lactic acid and ethanol. This decreases skin pH, inhibits bacterial lipases, and produces a bacteriostatic and bactericidal effect.	Less likely to cause undesirable side effects compared to benzoyl peroxide.	Some studies have shown it to be less effective than chlorhexidene, or even support bacterial growth (Young et al. 2012). *In vitro*, ethyl lactate shampoo required a higher concentration and longer period of incubation of 30–60 minutes for bacterial killing.
Triclosan	Bisphenol bactericidal agent. The FDA finalized a rule, December 2017, that triclosan and 23 other active ingredients are not generally recognized as safe and effective or use in OTC health care antiseptic products.	OTC (over the counter)	Less effective than benzoyl peroxide against *S. pseudintermedius* and is not effective against *Pseudomonas*.
Iodine	Iodine is thought to damage bacterial proteins causing bacterial cell death.	Excellent antibacterial properties, and is available in shampoo, solution, and scrub forms.	Poor residual activity of 4–8 hours, higher potential for contact sensitization compared to other topicals.
Bleach/Oxychlorine compounds	Hypochlorous acid damages bacterial cellular membranes in a similar mechanism of action as the neutrophil oxidative burst. Topical diluted bleach solution at either 0.05% (500 ppm) or 0.005% (50 ppm) hypochlorite concentrations, is a well-tolerated antiseptic that also exhibits anti-inflammatory properties.	Non-irritating, water based spray, anecdotally helpful when used BID in cases of canine pyoderma, and is often used as adjunctive therapy to bathing, conditioners +/− systemic antibiotics in cases of methicillin resistant pyoderma.	Though in vitro studies have demonstrated antibacterial efficacy (Uri et al. 2016), a recent double-blind, placebo controlled study of 19 pyoderma dogs (8 treated with a commercial oxychlorine spray BID × 4 weeks, and 11 treated with saline BID × 4 weeks) showed no difference between treatment groups in lesion scores and post-treatment bacterial numbers on cytology (Udenberg et al. 2015).

(*Continued*)

Table 8.6 Topical antibacterial products (Continued)

Topical product	Activity	Advantages	Disadvantages
Bleach/Oxychlorine compounds (cont.)	A 0.05% dilution of 6% household bleach (*not* splash free variety) = approx. 30 ml bleach diluted into 1 gal of water, which is sprayed or sponged onto the entire body then allow to sit 5–10 minutes before rinsing (or some dermatologists allow the pet to dry). In humans, the typical bleach dilution is 0.005%, which equates to 120 ml (about ½ cup) of 6% bleach mixed in a full 40 gal bathtub.		
2% Mupirocin ointment	Bactericidal within 24–48 hours of application to most Gram-positive bacteria.	Helpful in treatment of localized pyodermas in dogs, such as nasal or mucocutaneous pyoderma, interdigital granulomas, canine acne, and pressure point pyoderma.	Not effective for *Pseudomonas*.
Silver sulfadiazine 1%	Binds to cell components, including DNA, thereby inhibiting transcription, interferes with bacterial metabolism.	Broad spectrum of activity, excellent vs. *Pseudomonas*. Effective in vitro at 0.1%.	Some studies have shown slower healing time in wounds treated with silver sulfadiazine.
Chloroxylenol	Halophenol; likely damages microbial membranes.	—	In vitro, chloroxylenol shampoos were ineffective for both staphylococcal and *Pseudomonas* bacteria, and viable bacteria could be isolated from all shampoo dilutions at most time points (Young et al. 2012).
2% Acetic acid/2% boric acid	A prior study of acetic acid and boric acid solution indicated synergistic activity of the ingredients and killing of *S. pseudintermedius* at a concentration of 5.0% boric acid and 0.5% acetic acid.	—	In vitro, acetic acid–boric acid shampoos were ineffective for both staphylococci and *Pseudomonas* (Young et al. 2012).

Table 8.7 Subcutaneous bacterial infections.

Infection	Clinical signs	Diagnosis	Treatment
Subcutaneous abscess (Figures 8.12A and 8.12B) Caused by penetrating wound or trauma such as interanimal aggression; abscess occurs 2–4 days post trauma.	Fluctuant swelling which often ruptures and drains septic purulent fluid. Often caused by *Pasteurella multocida* in cats (oral flora) but can also be caused by other bacteria including *S. pseudintermedius*, Streptococci, and anerobic bacteria.	Clinical signs, microscopic examination of purulent exudate +/− culture if abscess persists despite empiric antibiotics.	Lance/drain and flush abscess with dilute chlorhexidine solution, may need Penrose drain for 3–5 days. Systemic antibiotics for 7 days; select empiric antibiotic with good coverage for *P. multocida* such as a penicillin (amoxicillin +/− clavulate). Neuter intact animals. Screen cats with recurrent or refractory abscesses for retroviral infections +/− obtain tissue biopsies/cultures to screen for more unusual bacterial infections such as mycobacteria, *Actinomyces* and *Nocardia*.

Infection	Clinical signs	Diagnosis	Treatment
Botryomycosis (bacterial pseudomycetoma) Usually associated with prior penetrating wound or migrating foreign body and caused by Staphylococci, but other bacteria can also be present.	Chronically draining wounds or nodules which contain small, white, sand-like granules composed of granulomatous inflammatory debris surrounding bacteria.	Clinical signs, cytology and culture of tissue grains, biopsy for histopathology and special stains (Gram, Brown-Brenn).	Surgically excise focal lesions or if excision is not possible then debride affected tissue, prolonged (6–12 weeks) systemic antibiotics based on tissue culture; with numerous lesions, combination antibiotic therapy with rifampin may be helpful.
Cellulitis Deep infection which spreads laterally into subcutaneous (SQ) tissues. Often preceded by puncture wound or trauma or by extension of severe chronic furunculosis.	Affected areas are edematous, friable, discolored, and drain seropurulent fluid.	Clinical signs, history, cytology of exudate.	Debride devitalized tissue/ hydrotherapy, administer antibiotics based on culture for 4 weeks minimum, 2 weeks beyond clinical resolution; pending culture begin broad spectrum antibiotic with good coverage for Staphylococci and anaerobes such as clavulanated amoxicillin. Pain control is important.
Necrotizing fasciitis (Figures 8.13A and 8.13B) Usually preceded by history of puncture wound or blunt trauma; bacteria track SQ fascial planes into muscle and fat causing progressive necrosis. Concurrent shock common ("toxic shock syndrome"). Most common bacteria involved in animals are *Streptococcus* Group G (esp. *Streptococcus canis*, a commensal organism on canine skin and mucosae, facultative anaerobe), but other reported organisms include *S. pseudintermedius*, *Acinetobacter baumannii*. Tissue destruction and extension occurs due to bacterial exotoxins and proteases.	Acute, markedly painful inflammation and edema which can involve a limb or the trunk or neck; skin is discolored/devitalized and drains serohemorrhagic fluid. Affected animals are systemically ill, febrile, weak, hypotensive (canine streptococcal toxic shock syndrome), and labwork can demonstrate leukocytosis or leukopenia with left shift +/− elevated liver values, azotemia, hypoalbuminemia and/or coagulopathy.	Clinical signs, history. Positive "finger test": SQ tissue easily separated from fascia by blunt dissection. Sample (culturette or aspiration) of leading edge of necrotic area for cytology and aerobic/anaerobic bacterial cultures. Cytology: May see chains of Streptococcal bacteria and inflammatory cells; in older necrotic areas, secondary infection with other bacteria is common. Biopsy of leading edge of necrotic area for histopathology.	Aggressive debridement of affected tissue early in disease course and leaving treated area open to enable daily wound care and irrigation; surgical consultation recommended. Medical treatment alone usually not successful due to poor antibiotic penetration of affected areas and continued production of bacterial exotoxins. Antibiotics based on cultures for 4–6 weeks; pending culture results begin clindamycin 11 mg/kg BID + a beta-lactam antibiotic +/− gentamycin. Avoid NSAIDs and fluoroquinolones, as they have been associated with poorer outcomes. Supportive care essential: pain control, intravenous fluids and colloids, plasma transfusions if indicated. Hyperbaric oxygen therapy may be beneficial, if available.
Actinomycosis (Figures 8.14A and 8.14B) *Actinomyces* sp. is an oral and GI bacteria which can cause infection via bite wounds or migrating foreign bodies such as grass awns. Large breed and hunting dogs more commonly affected.	Four clinical presentations: cervicofacial, thoracic, abdominal, and subcutaneous. In dogs, often involves the head/neck, thorax, lumbar SQ fat, and epaxial muscles. Lesions in dogs and cats can present as firm and fibrous masses, chronic abscesses, draining tracts, and osteomyelitis. Pyothorax or peritonitis can occur. Purulent exudate may be odorous and may contain yellow tissue granules. In animals with severe or chronic infection, leukocytosis with left shift, anemia, hypoalbuminemia, and hyperglobulinemia may be present.	Cytology of lesion aspirate followed by biopsies for anaerobic culture of tissue and histopathology/special stains (Gram, Brown-Brenn, GMS (Gomori methenamine silver): organism is anaerobic (facultative or obligate), Gram-positive, non-acid fast, and filamentous. Isolation of *Actinomyces* sp. can be difficult, as organism is slow growing and can be overgrown by other bacteria; a negative culture does not rule out *Actinomyces*. Antimicrobial susceptibility testing may not be available due to lack of standard testing guidelines. Presurgical MRI or lesional ultrasound may be helpful to identify inciting migrating foreign body.	Surgical excision or debridement of affected tissue followed by 3–4 months minimum course of antibiotics; high dose penicillins are preferred. Amoxicillin (20–40 mg/kg PO q6–8h, give on empty stomach); other possibly effective antibiotics include clindamycin, erythromycin, doxycycline, chloramphenicol, ceftriaxone. Prognosis fair to guarded, relapse can occur in 15–42% of cases.

(*Continued*)

Table 8.7 Subcutaneous bacterial infections (Continued)

Infection	Clinical signs	Diagnosis	Treatment
Nocardiosis (Figures 8.15A and 8.15B) *Nocardia* sp. is a soil bacteria which can infect animals through a puncture or bite wound.	Three clinical forms: cutaneous/ subcutaneous, pulmonary, and disseminated. Lesions include chronically draining wounds/abscesses or ulcerated nodules and often occur on ventral abdomen in cats or on the limbs; lymphadenopathy common and pyothorax can occur. Small tissue granules may be present. Pulmonary or cutaneous disease can progress to disseminated disease. Underlying immunosuppressive disease often present. Leukocytosis with left shift, anemia, and hyperglobulinemia common.	Cytology of lesion aspirate followed by biopsies for aerobic culture of tissue and histopathology/special stains (Gram, Brown-Brenn, acid-fast): organism is aerobic, Gram-positive, partially- acid-fast, and filamentous with right angle branching. Isolation of *Nocardia* sp. can be difficult, as organism is slow growing and can be overgrown by other bacteria; a negative culture does not rule out *Nocardia*. Antimicrobial susceptibility testing may not be available due to lack of standard testing guidelines.	Drain/debride affected tissue, followed by prolonged antibiotic therapy ideally based on culture/sensitivity; treat until 1 month beyond clinical normalcy. First choice antibiotic: Potentiated sulfonamides (15–30 mg/kg PO q12h); other drugs which may be effective include erythromycin, minocycline, cefotaxime; animals with systemic infections should be treated with combination antibiotic therapy. Prognosis guarded, especially with systemic disease, but this may be due to delay in diagnosis; treatment success is better with earlier disease diagnosis and appropriate therapy.
Plague (*Yersinia pestis*) *Y. pestis is* a bacterium carried by fleas and transmitted to rodents such as prairie dogs, ground squirrels, and rats; dogs and cats are infected by contact with infected fleas or rodents. A regionally acquired disease in areas west of the Rocky Mountains in the US; present on all continents except Australia and Antarctica. Zoonotic.	Bubonic form: Abscessed draining skin lesions and lymph nodes. Pneumonic form: Lung infection after inhalation of organisms. Septicemic form: Organisms are carried in the blood and infect internal organs. Acutely draining abscesses with systemic sighs of illness: fever, lethargy, anorexia, lymphadenopathy, cough. Incubation period is 1–3 days if ingested/inhaled or 2–6 days after exposure to infected flea or exposure of skin wound. Cats are more susceptible than dogs, and mortality rate in untreated cats is up to 75%; survival rates are up to 90% with prompt treatment.	Clinical signs, cytology of purulent exudate: neutrophils and characteristic "safety pin" appearance of causative coccobacillus bacteria. Serology: *Y. pestis* antibodies (not helpful in peracute infection). Culture, direct fluorescent antibody or PCR of exudate fluid.	Wear gown, gloves, and masks to handle suspected infected animals; quarantine infected animals and double bag/incinerate cage waste. Lance/drain/flush abscess. Begin antibiotic treatment pending diagnostics, preferred drugs include gentamicin 2–4 mg/kg IM or SC q12-24h for severely ill animals; doxycycline 5–10 mg/kg PO BID may be used for milder bubonic cases. Chloramphenicol is also effective. Treat for 3 weeks minimum. Asymptomatic exposed animals: treat with doxycycline for 7 days. Apply a fast-acting flea adulticide and continue year-round flea control in endemic areas.
L-form infection Partially cell wall-deficient bacteria that can be induced by prior antibiotic exposure.	Chronically draining abscesses, often over joints. Often causes reactive bony periosteal reaction. Fever is common; polyarthritis and distant abscess formation may occur.	Clinical signs, history, characteristic radiographic findings. Cytology: Pyogranulomatous inflammation; bacteria cannot be visualized. Culture: Bacteria are difficult to culture. Labwork: Leukocytosis and hyperglobulinemia. Radiographs: Periarticular soft tissue swelling and periosteal proliferation.	Doxycycline or tetracycline given until at least 1 week beyond complete healing.

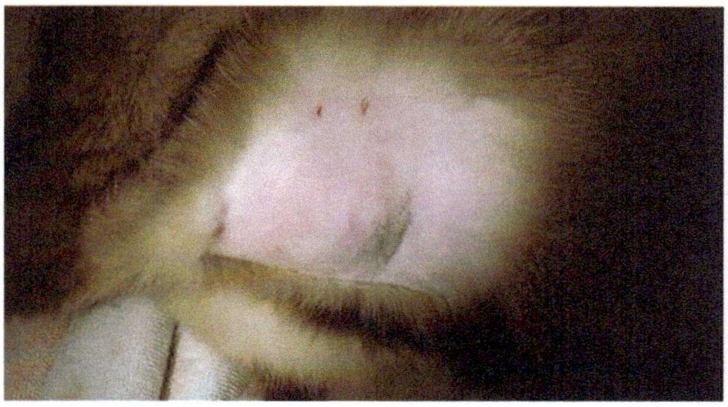

Figure 8.12A A subcutaneous abscess in a cat causing a fluctuant painful swelling.

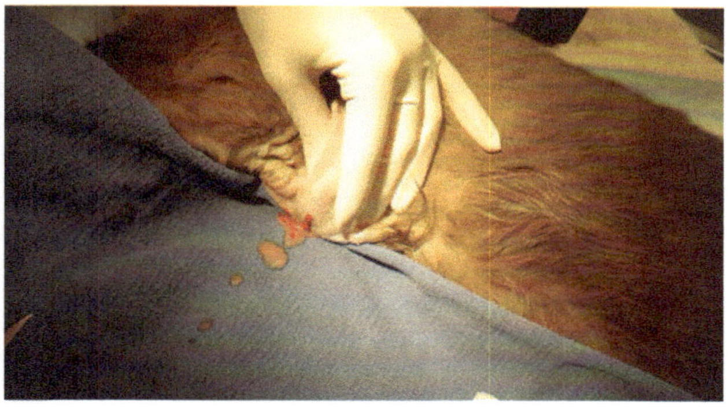

Figure 8.12B When the lesion was incised, purulent fluid emerged.

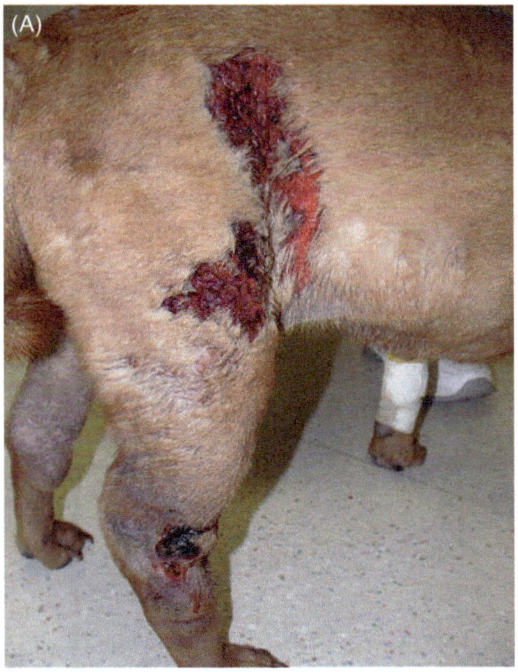

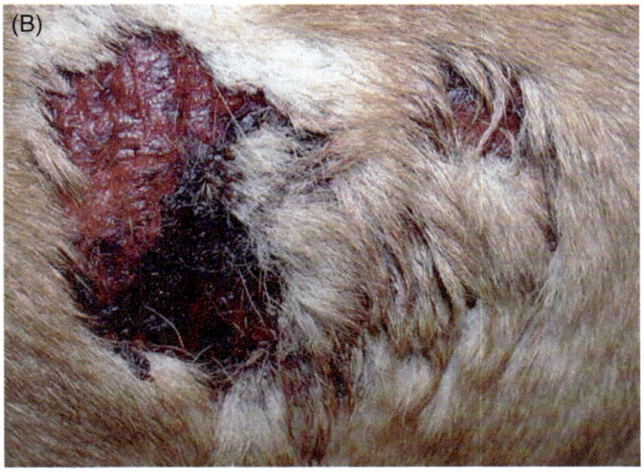

Figures 8.13A and B Deep ulcerative dermatitis and sloughing of the skin due to necrotizing fasciitis in a Shar-Pei.

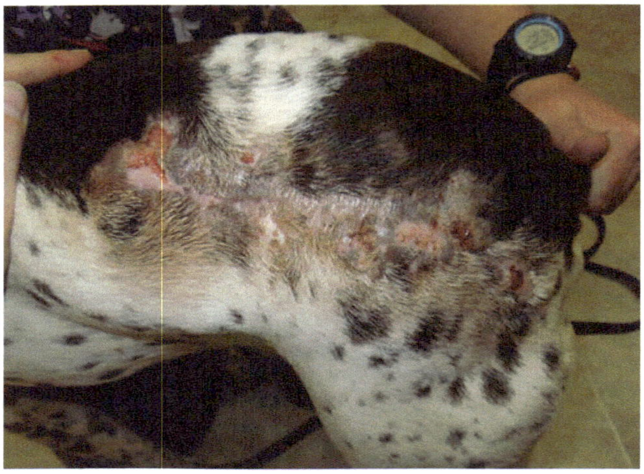

Figure 8.14A Lumbar scarring and draining tracts in a hunting dog due to actinomycosis.

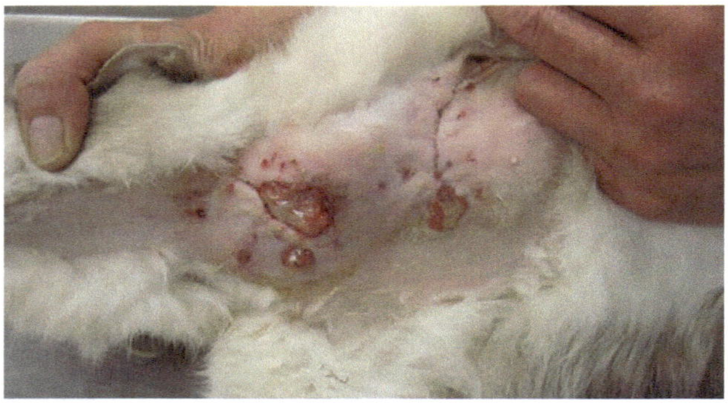

Figure 8.14B Cellulitis and draining tracts on the ventral chest of a cat due to actinomycosis. *Source:* Image courtesy of VIN and Chad Lakey, DVM.

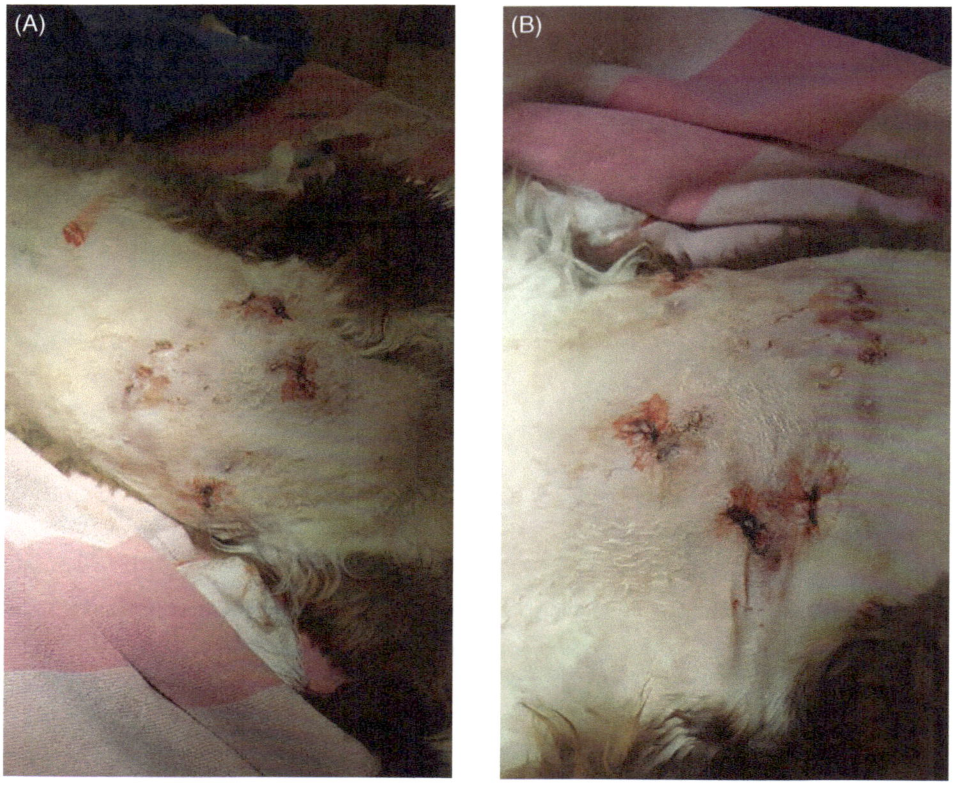

Figures 8.15A and B Firm subcutaneous masses and draining tracts on the ventral trunk of a cat caused by nocardiosis. *Source:* Images courtesy of Dr. Amy Shumaker, DACVD.

Table 8.8 Mycobacterial infections.

Mycobacterial infection	Clinical signs	Diagnosis	Treatment
Non-tuberculous (NTM) (Figures 8.16A–8.16C) Rapidly growing mycobacteria(RGM): many species. Slow growing: *Mycobacterium avium* complex. Caused by facultative pathogenic, opportunistic saprophytes in soil, water, or vegetation. Numerous species can cause infection; most common causative species in the US are *Mycobacterium fortuitum* and *Mycobacterium chelonae*. Infection is preceded by a penetrating wound, often cat fight, contaminated by dirt or soil. Obese cats predisposed to infections with RGM, as the causative bacteria prefer fat. Siamese, Abyssinian, and Somali cats predisposed to *M. avium* infection, which is a systemic infection and not usually cutaneous.	Presents as cutaneous or subcutaneous nodules which may be ulcerated or draining, chronic draining tracts with scarring (granulomatous panniculitis) often on the dorsal lumbosacral area, flanks, or ventral inguinal fat pad in cats; lesions may be painful. Less commonly causes pneumonia or rarely disseminated disease. *M. avium* is usually associated with underlying immunosuppressive disease and can cause gastrointestinal (GI), respiratory and central nervous system (CNS) disease in addition to skin disease in dogs and cats. RGM infections are rare in dogs; reported cases have had one to multiple firm to fluctuant or draining subcutaneous masses on the dorsum, flank, thorax, or neck.	Aspirate/cytology: Pyogranulomatous inflammation which may show mycobacterial organisms with special stains (Ziehl–Neesen/acid-fast); organisms can be few in number and difficult to find and are not visible with routine HE stains (though negative staining organisms may be seen). Biopsy of a non-ruptured affected SQ area for culture, histopathology, and special stains to look for mycobacterial organisms. Fine needle aspirate with large gauge needle through intact skin over mass, with direct inoculation of plate or blood culture bottle can also be used to obtain diagnostic culture. Tissue biopsy of affected subcutaneous fat should be cut in three prices; submit one piece in formalin for histopathology/special stains, place the second sample in sterile tube for macerated aerobic/anaerobic and mycobacterial tissue culture to screen for clinically similar infections such as *Actinomyces*/*Nocardia* and certain fungi (contact your reference lab to determine their preferred submission material and method); place the third sample in a sterile container in the freezer for possible further testing such as PCR. Antibiotic susceptibility of mycobacterial species ideal, but can be difficult to obtain depending on regional laboratory capabilities. Mycobacterial PCR performed on fresh tissue or exudate on slides (save non-formalin fixed tissue samples in freezer); also, may be difficult to obtain depending on regional laboratory capabilities; veterinary diagnostic laboratories at veterinary schools are increasingly offering PCR or can be contacted to obtain a recommendation of where to send samples for PCR.	Antibiotics ideally based on culture and sensitivity are given for 6–12 months, 2 months beyond complete normalcy. After 4–6 weeks of initial antibiotics, aggressive surgical removal/debridement of scarred infected SQ tissue is recommended if possible to remove sequestered infection. Pending susceptibility results, or if mycobacterial sensitivity is not possible, then begin combination antibiotic therapy with two or three of the following: 1) Pradofloxacin 3–5 mg/kg PO q24h. 2) Clarithromycin 5–15 mg/kg PO q12h. 3) Doxycycline 5–10 mg/kg PO q12–24h. Antibiotic therapy choice is guided by mycobacterial species identified on culture or PCR: *M. fortuitum* is generally treated with pradofloxacin + clarithromycin; other typically effective options include cefoxitin, amikacin, and clofazimine; 29% are sensitive to doxycycline. Generally resistant to trimethoprim. *M. chelonae-abscessus* is generally susceptible to pradofloxacin combined with amikacin, cefoxitin, or clofazimine; also often sensitive to ciprofloxacin, clarithromycin, and azithromycin. Usually resistant to doxycycline and older fluoroquinolones. DO NOT combine pradofloxacin (or moxifloxacin) with azithromycin or clarithromycin to treat this mycobacterial species. *M. smegmatis* is usually susceptible to pradofloxacin + doxycycline; other usually effective options include fluoroquinolones, trimethoprim; often resistant to clarithromycin. Avoid enrofloxacin in cats because of risk of retinal damage using high doses for long periods. *M. avium* should be treated with clarithromycin + rifampin (monitor for hepatotoxicity); other drug options to include in the multidrug protocol include doxycycline, clofazimine, pradofloxacin, amikacin; usually resistant to older fluoroquinolones. Prognosis is guarded depending on lesion severity and owner/patient compliance with need for prolonged antibiotic therapy.

(*Continued*)

Table 8.8 Mycobacterial infections (Continued)

Mycobacterial infection	Clinical signs	Diagnosis	Treatment
Feline leprosy (Figures 8.17A–8.17C) Caused by *Mycobacterium lepraemurium, Mycobacterium visible, Mycobacterium tarwinense* and *Mycobacterium lepraefelis* and other novel species depending on geographical prevalence. Infection usually occurs after rodent bites/injury and is more common in outdoor adult male cats.	Lesions are alopecic +/− ulcerated movable single to multiple movable cutaneous nodules on the head, limbs, and occasionally trunk. Regional lymph nodes may be enlarged but systemic disease is uncommon (except for *M. visible* and *M. lepraefelis*).	See NTM diagnostics above; fine needle aspirate cytology of lesions often demonstrates numerous organisms, however, bacteria cannot be cultured and PCR/molecular diagnostics are needed for definitive diagnosis of causative mycobacterial species.	Surgical removal of masses may be curative with localized lesions. Post operatively, or in cases which cannot be treated surgically, 2–3 drug combination therapy with clarithromycin, pradofloxacin, and rifampin (monitor for hepatotoxicity) or clofazimine are recommended; doxycycline, older fluoroquinolones, and aminoglycosides may be helpful. Treat 2–3 months beyond complete resolution of lesions; some cases require lifelong clarithromycin.
Canine leproid granuloma (Figures 8.17D and 8.17E) Caused by a novel mycobacterial species. Most commonly affects short coated large breeds such as Boxers which are housed outdoors in temperate or subtropical environment. Likely inoculated into the skin by biting insects.	Single to multiple well circumscribed, firm, nonpainful dermal masses which may be alopecic or ulcerated; secondary Staphylococcal infections can occur and chronic severe lesions can cause scarring. Lesions usually occur on the pinnae (especially the dorsal ear fold) and head but can occur elsewhere on the body. No systemic involvement or symptoms.	Aspirate for cytology: Numerous macrophages with variable numbers of lymphocytes, plasma cells, and neutrophils. Macrophages often contain negatively stained (clear) rod bacteria on Diff-Quik and H&E stain. Biopsy: Pyogranulomatous inflammation with intracellular ZN/acid-fast stain positive bacteria, however, bacteria cannot be cultured. PCR on tissue biopsy supports the causative bacteria is a member of the *Mycobacterium simiae*-related group.	Lesions in many cases resolve spontaneously due to host cell mediated immune response within 2–4 months of onset. In persistent cases, surgical excision can be curative. For severe cases, a 4–8 week course of combination antibiotic therapy with oral rifampin 10–15 mg/kg PO q24h (monitor for hepatotoxicity) and clarithromycin 7.5–12.5 mg/kg PO q12h or doxycycline 5–7.5 mg/kg PO q12h may be effective or pradofloxacin (or moxifloxacin).

Obligate mycobacterial infections/tuberculosis *Mycobacterium bovis* *Mycobacterium microti* *Mycobacterium tuberculosis* More common in young adult outdoor cats and dogs, infection often occurs from infected bites or fights. Zoonotic	Firm dermal nodules which may be ulcerated and/or non-healing draining wounds. In dogs, cutaneous lesions occur at site of prior penetrating injury. In cats, lesions often occur on the face, paws, tailbase, or perineum; can extend to underlying muscle or bone. Localized to generalized lymphadenopathy common. Can involve lungs, GI tract or cause disseminated disease with hepatosplenomegaly, pleural effusion, weight loss, and fever.	See NTM diagnostics above. Mycobacterial culture is the reference standard for diagnosis but can take 4–12 weeks to grow; PCR analysis of culture or tissue specimens is available and is much faster. Specialized laboratories to determine antibiotic susceptibility are ideal, such as the National Animal Disease laboratory in Ames, IA, and the National Jewish Medical and Research Center in Denver, CO. Clinical laboratory findings may include leukocytosis, hyperglobulinemia, and non-regenerative anemia. Radiography and ultrasonography may reveal pleural or pericardial fluid, enlarged tracheobronchial lymph nodes, interstitial to nodular pulmonary infiltrates, and hepatosplenomegaly. Intradermal testing can be performed using 0.1 ml purified protein derivative (PPD) from *M. tuberculosis* (supplied by US Dept. Agriculture) or Bacillus Calmette-Guerin (BCG) injected intradermally on the inner pinna or medial thigh; a positive reaction is indicated by development of a red raised indurated and eventually necrotic lesion at the injection site 48–72 hours later. Another method of tuberculin testing for dogs is to measure baseline body temperature and if normal then inject 0.75ml PPD subcutaneously and monitor rectal temperature every two hours for 12 hours; a 2 °F (1.1 °C) temperature increase is interpreted as a positive test result.	Euthanasia should be considered due to risk of zoonotic transmission. If treatment is chosen then: Dogs: Localized lesion: Give isoniazid 10–20mg/kg/day (maximum 300 mg/day) + rifampin 10mg/kg/day for 6 months (monitor labwork q 2 weeks for hepatic disease) + pyrazinamide 15–40 mg/kg/day added for first 2 months or isoniazid/rifampin alone for 9 months. Dogs: Disseminated infection: Give isoniazid and rifampin with ethambutol 10–25mg/kg/day or pyrazinamide, or both, and continue beyond 9 months. Cats: Initially use 3 drugs (rifampin, pradofloxacin, and clarithromycin or azithromycin) for 2 months, followed by 4 more months of continued 2 drug therapy with rifampin and either pradofloxacin or clarithromycin/ azithromycin. If triple therapy cannot be given then treatment with 2 drugs is continued for 6–9 months minimum, at least 3 months beyond lesion resolution.

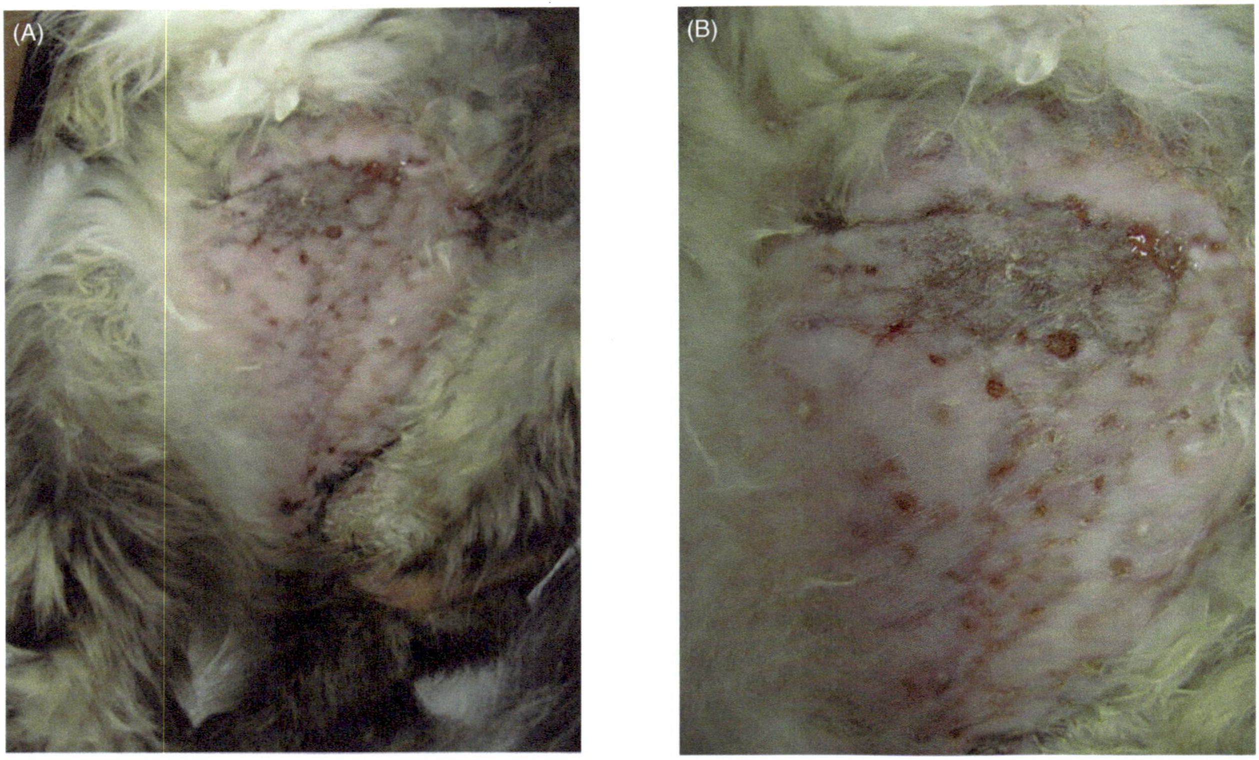

Figures 8.16A and B Scarring and draining tracts on the ventral abdomen of a cat due to mycobacterial infection. *Source:* Images courtesy of Dr. Carine Laporte, DACVD.

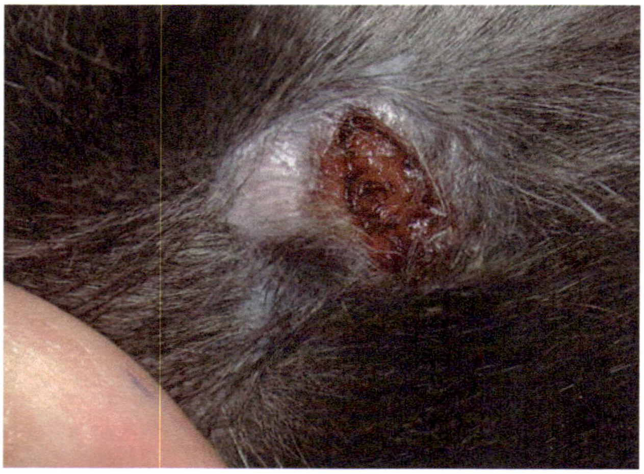

Figure 8.16C An ulcerated draining mass due to mycobacteriosis in a cat.

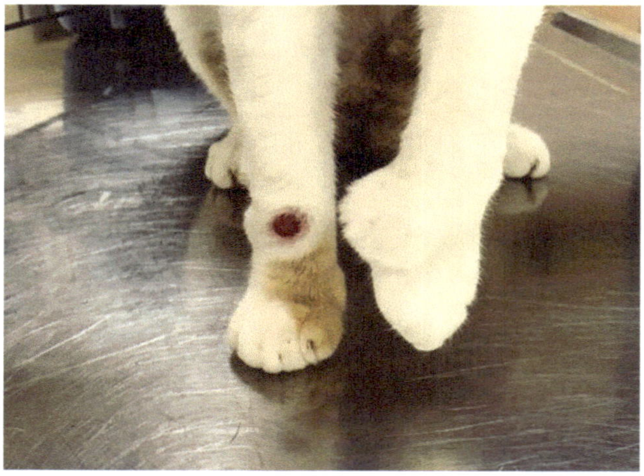

Figure 8.17A Firm subcutaneous masses with draining tracts on the paws of a cat with feline leprosy. *Source:* Image courtesy of VIN and Kevin Butler, DVM.

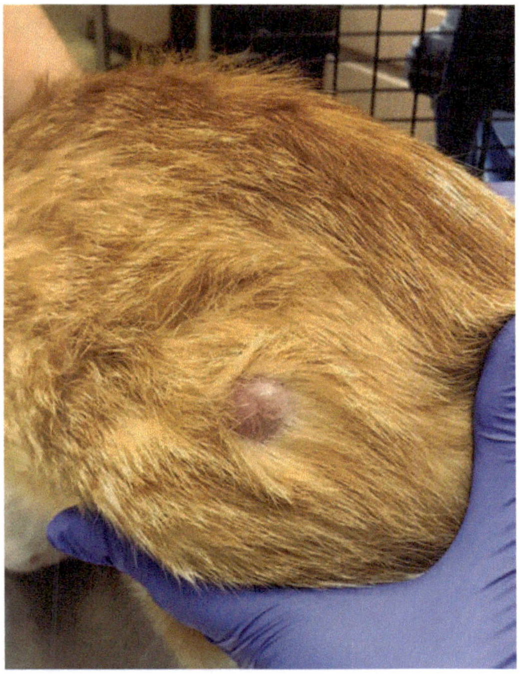

Figure 8.17B A similar non-ulcerated lesion on the lateral thigh of the cat in Figure 8.17A. *Source:* Image courtesy of VIN and Kevin Butler, DVM.

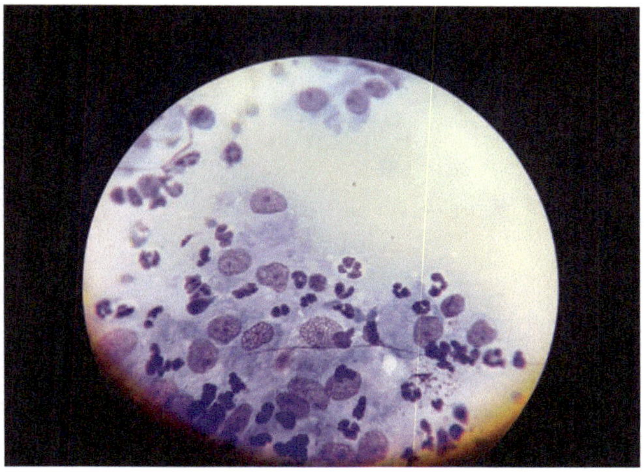

Figure 8.17C Fine needle aspirate for cytology showed pyogranulomatous inflammation with numerous negative staining rod bacteria present within macrophages (100×). *Source:* Image courtesy of VIN and Kevin Butler, DVM.

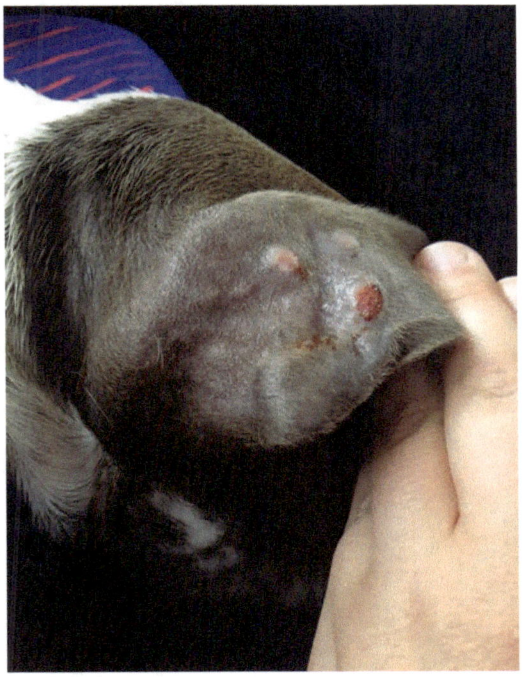

Figure 8.17D Multiple raised pink, sometimes eroded and crusted dermal masses caused by leproid granulomas on the ear of a Pitbull Terrier. *Source:* Image courtesy of Samantha Lockwood, DVM.

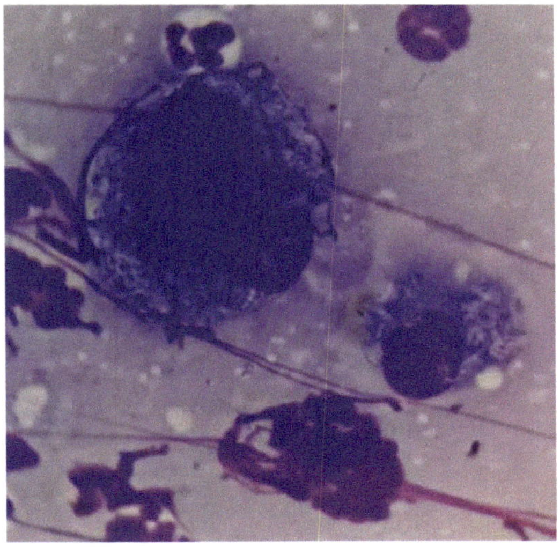

Figure 8.17E Fine needle aspirate for cytology showed macrophages engulfing numerous negative staining rod bacteria (100× with digital zoom). *Source:* Images courtesy of Samantha Lockwood, DVM.

Table 8.9 Yeast infections.

Disease	Clinical signs	Diagnosis	Treatment
Canine *Malassezia* dermatitis (*Malassezia pachydermatis*; Figures 8.18A–8.18K) Normal organism in low numbers on skin, paws, and ear canals, creates infection most commonly due to underlying hypersensitivity dermatitis (atopy, parasite, or adverse food reaction), endocrinopathy (hypothyroidism, hyperadrenocorticism), or breed related keratinization disorder. Can occur in any breed but more common in Westies, Shih Tzus, Basset Hounds, Cocker Spaniels.	Greasy scaling, lichenification, +/− alopecia and hyperpigmentation often affecting ventral neck, axilla, and inguinal areas; usually very pruritic and pruritus is poorly responsive to steroids, oclacitinib and Cytopoint. *Malassezia* pododermatitis causes interdigital erythema/pruritus and often dark brown discoloration of interdigital fur and proximal toenails +/− greasy dark keratosebaceous nailbed debris.	Cytology of affected skin may show inflammatory cells and few to many *Malassezia* organisms +/− concurrent bacteria. In animals with *Malassezia* hypersensitivity only a few organisms can cause marked pruritus.	Localized infections: Daily ketoconazole or miconazole or 4% chlorhexidene containing topical therapies (wipes/sprays/mousse) + 2–3 times weekly azole shampoos. 50 : 50 white vinegar/water sprays can be helpful astringent in intertriginous areas. Refractory cases may benefit from topical nystatin cream applied BID. Generalized infection or pododermatitis: Combine topical therapies with oral ketoconazole (dogs only), non-compounded fluconazole/itraconazole 5–10 mg/kg/day or terbinafine 30 mg/kg/day × 3 weeks. +/− pulse azole treatment 2–3 days per week for control of recurrent cases. Identify and treat underlying cause.
Feline *Malassezia* dermatitis (*M. pachydermatis, M. sympodialis;* Figures 8.19A–8.19C) Normal organism in low numbers on skin, paws, and ear canals, creates infection most commonly due to underlying hypersensitivity dermatitis (atopy, parasite, or adverse food reaction), metabolic disorder (hyperadrenocorticism, diabetes mellitus), retroviral infection, or neoplastic disorder.	Greasy dark keratosebaceous nailbed debris which may be asymptomatic in Rex and Sphynx cats. Dark greasy keratosebaceous debris on the ventral chin, axillae, and inguinal area which may be very pruritic and poorly steroid responsive (any breed).	Cytology of affected skin may show inflammatory cells and few to many *Malassezia* organisms +/− concurrent bacteria. In animals with *Malassezia* hypersensitivity only a few organisms can cause marked pruritus.	Localized infections: Daily ketoconazole or miconazole or 4% chlorhexidene containing topical therapies (wipes/sprays/mousse). Generalized infection: Combine topical therapies with oral non-compounded fluconazole or itraconazole 5–10 mg/kg/day or terbinafine 30 mg/kg/day × 3 weeks. Identify and treat (if possible) underlying cause.

***Candida* dermatitis** (*Candida albicans, C. parapsilosis* most common species; Figures 8.20A–8.20D) Normal inhabitants of the ears, nose, oral cavity, and anus which can rarely cause opportunistic infections in macerated moist areas. Predisposing causes include immunosuppressive metabolic conditions such as diabetes mellitus, hyperadrenocorticism, immunosuppressive medications, or prolonged antibiotic therapy.	Predisposed areas include mucous membranes, mucocutaneous junctions, outer ears, and interdigital areas. On mucous membranes, lesions are ulcerations covered with gray plaques. Skin lesions include papules/pustules which evolve into moist exudative plaques and ulcers. Pododermatitis may occur and affect only one or two paws. Otic infections are characterized by erythema, moist exudation, and pruritus. Creamy preputial or vaginal discharge may occur.	Cytology of affected areas shows purulent inflammation with numerous round to oblong yeast organisms. Narrow-based or multilateral budding and pseudohyphae may occur (in contrast to *Malassezia*). Biopsy: Neutrophilic inflammation with yeast organisms in surface keratin. Fungal culture.	Correct underlying cause, if possible. Avoid excessive moisture. Localized lesions are treated with clipping/drying and application of topical antifungal agents such as nystatin, azole or terbinafine cream, or amphotericin B lotion BID–TID until resolution. Oral, widespread mucocutaneous or oral lesions require systemic antifungal therapy (non-compounded itraconazole or fluconazole) for 2–4 weeks, 7–10 days beyond healing.

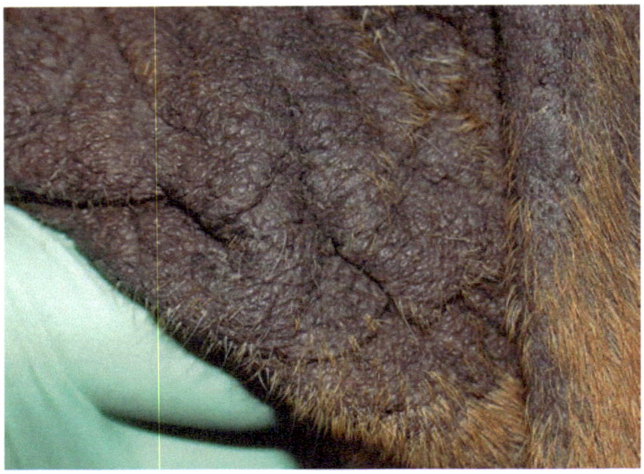

Figure 8.18A Alopecia, hyperpigmentation, and lichenification caused by *Malassezia* dermatitis in a hypothyroid Bloodhound.

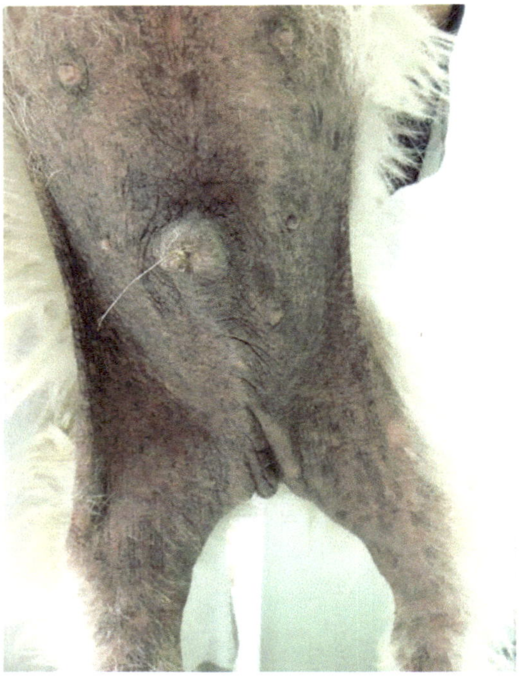

Figure 8.18B Lichenification and erythema due to *Malassezia* dermatitis secondary to atopy in a Westie.

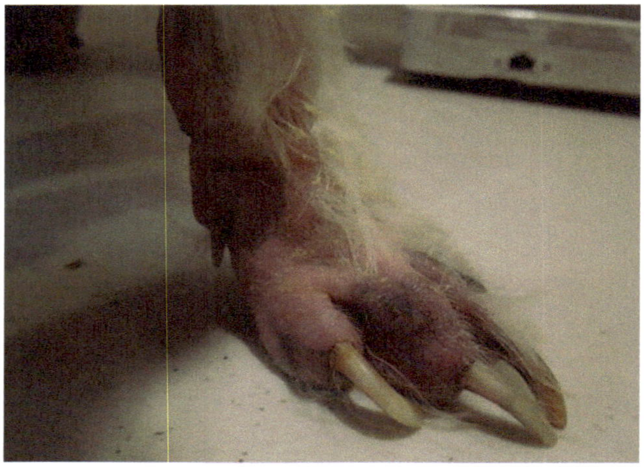

Figure 8.18C Alopecia erythema and yellowish scaling caused by *Malassezia* infection in an atopic Shih Tzu.

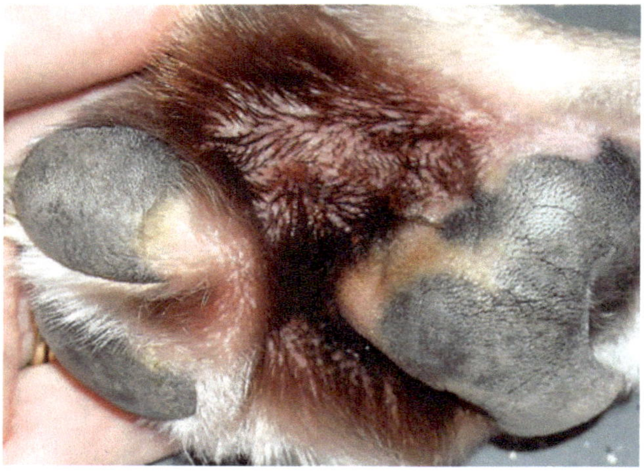

Figure 8.18D Moist, inflamed interdigital dermatitis with dark brown fur discoloration caused by *Malassezia* in an atopic Labrador.

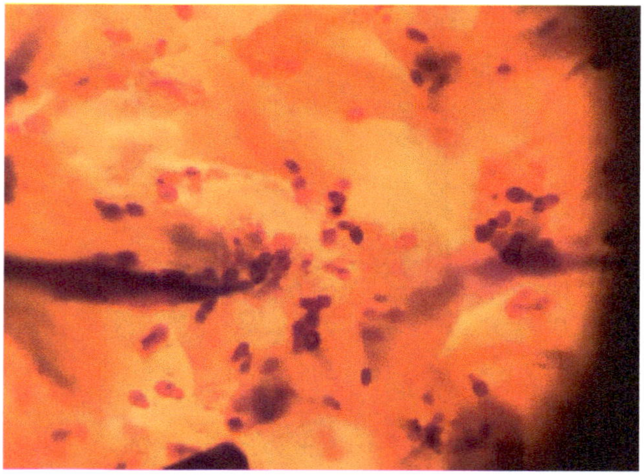

Figure 8.18E Impression smear for cytology demonstrates numerous *Malassezia* organisms (100×).

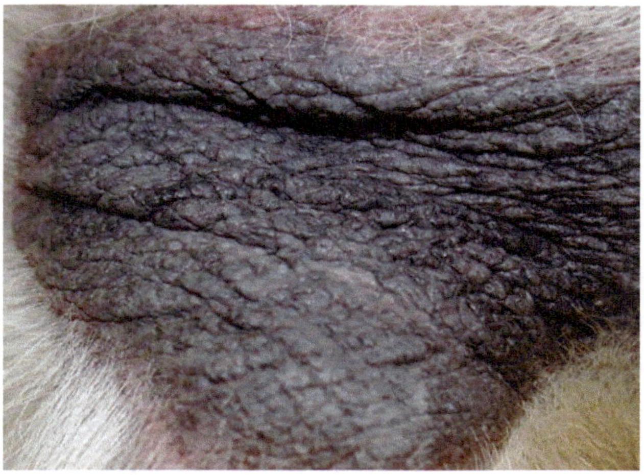

Figure 8.18F Marked inguinal lichenification and hyperpigmentation due to *Malassezia* dermatitis triggered by hypothyroidism.

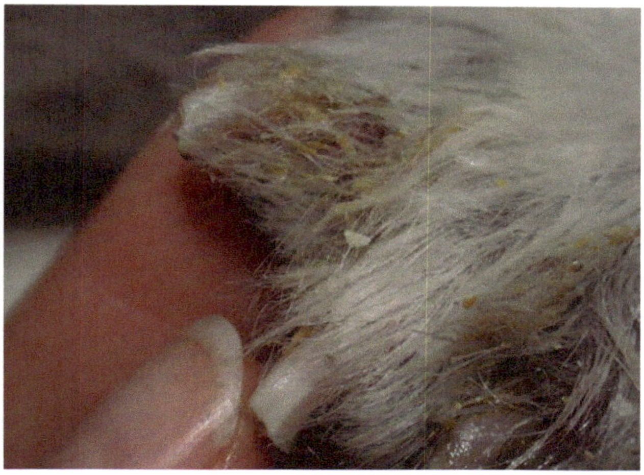

Figure 8.18G Yellowish adherent greasy crusting on the paws of an atopic Shih Tzu due to *Malassezia* pododermatitis.

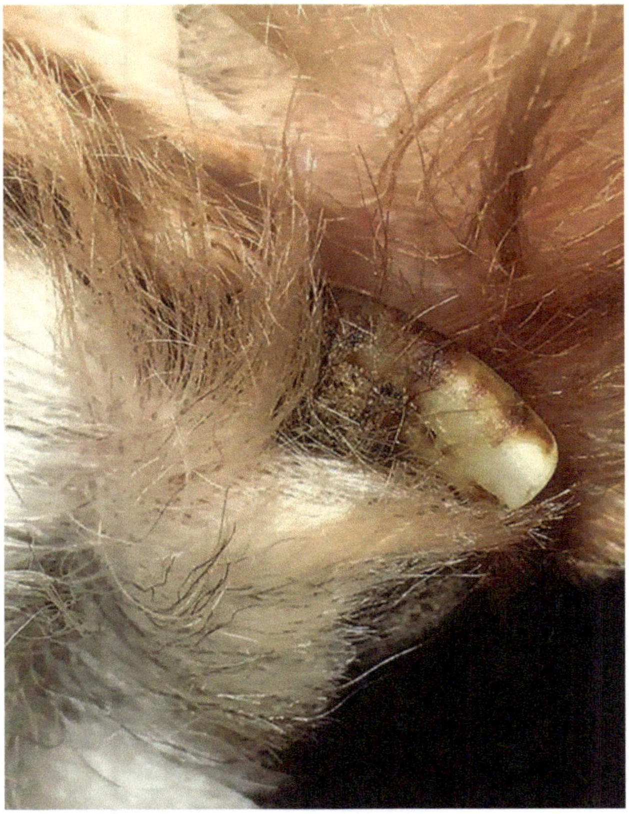

Figure 8.18H Dark brown discoloration of the proximal toenail and paw fur is caused by *Malassezia* infection.

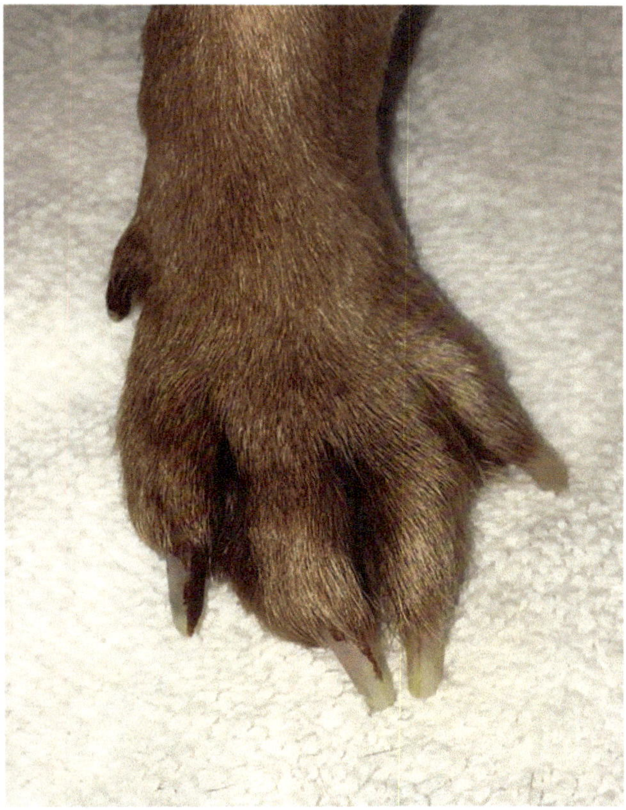

Figure 8.18I In this white dog with chronic *Malassezia* pododermatitis, the fur and toenails have turned dark brown.

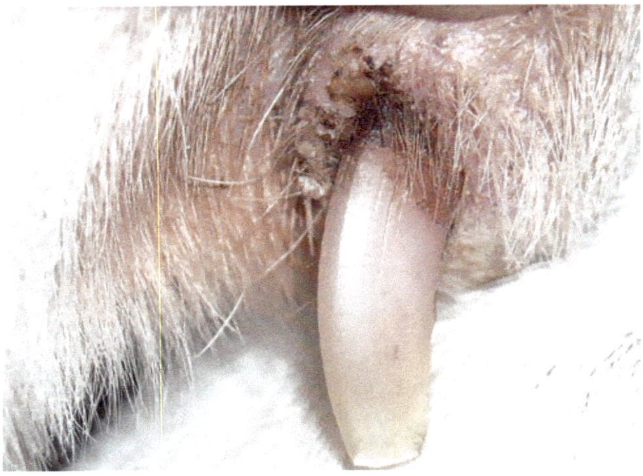

Figure 8.18J *Malassezia* paronychia demonstrating erythema, mild crusting, and dark brown nailbed debris.

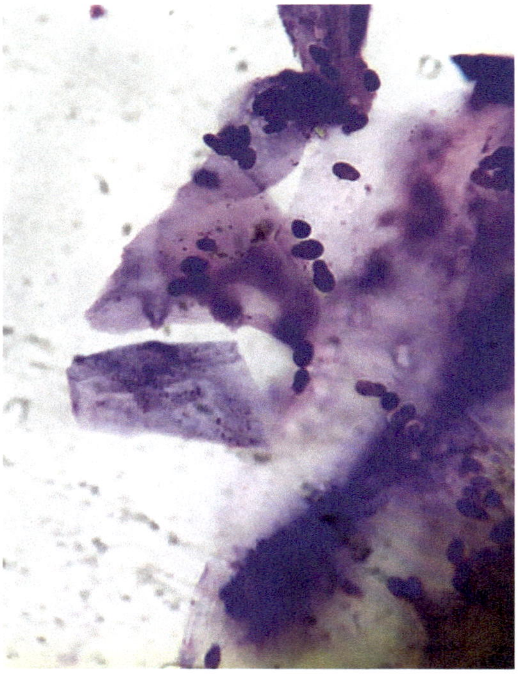

Figure 8.18K Cytology of the nailbed debris shows numerous *Malassezia* yeast (100×).

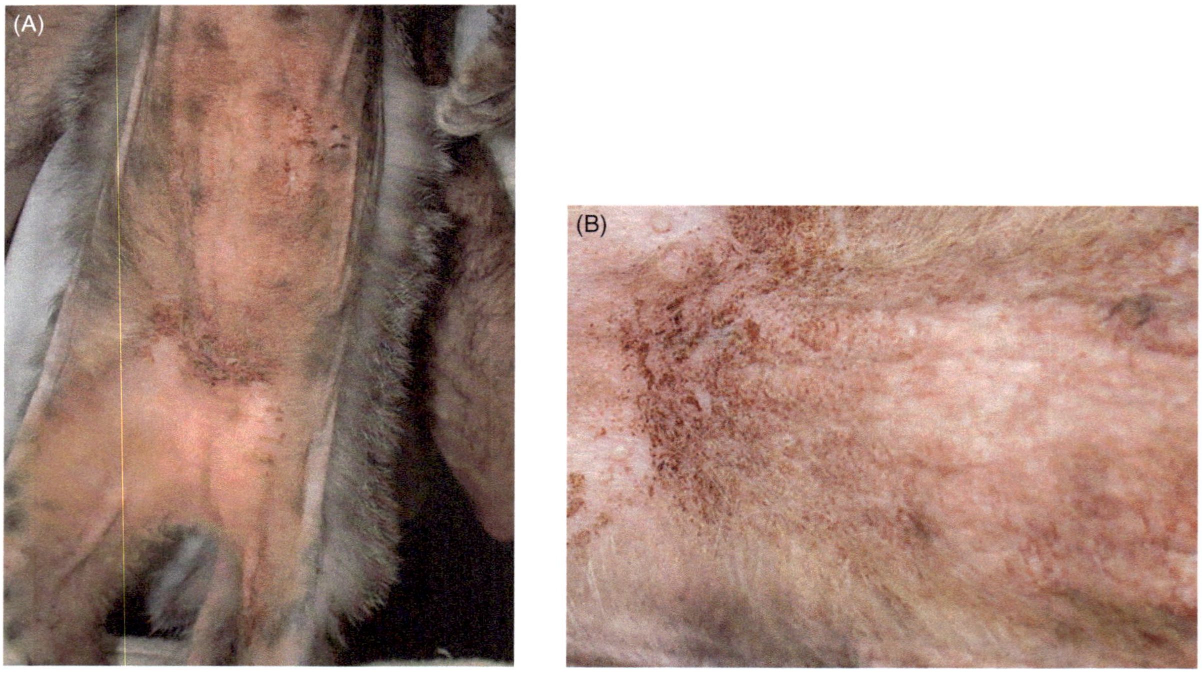

Figures 8.19A and B *Malassezia* dermatitis in an atopic cat causing inguinal erythema with brown epithelial debris; the cat was intensely pruritic.

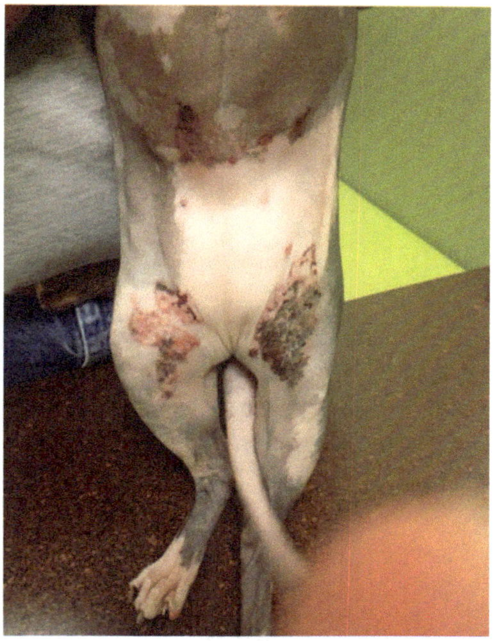

Figure 8.19C *Malassezia* dermatitis on the groin of an atopic Sphynx cat. *Source:* Images courtesy of Dr. Ann Trimmer, DACVD.

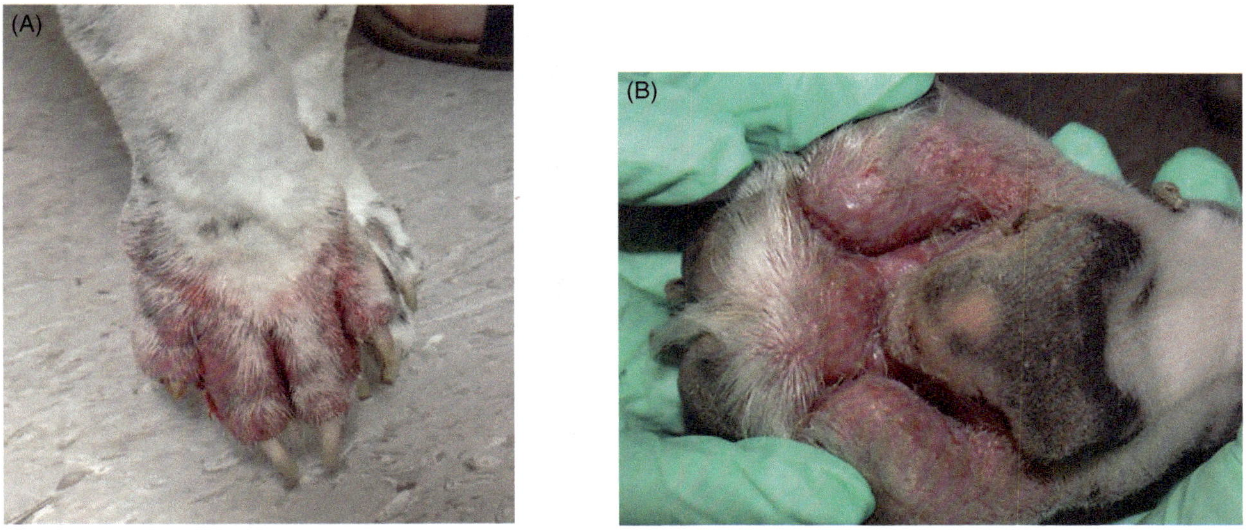

Figures 8.20A and B Marked interdigital erythema, swelling, and moist exudative dermatitis caused by *Candida* infection in a diabetic dog.

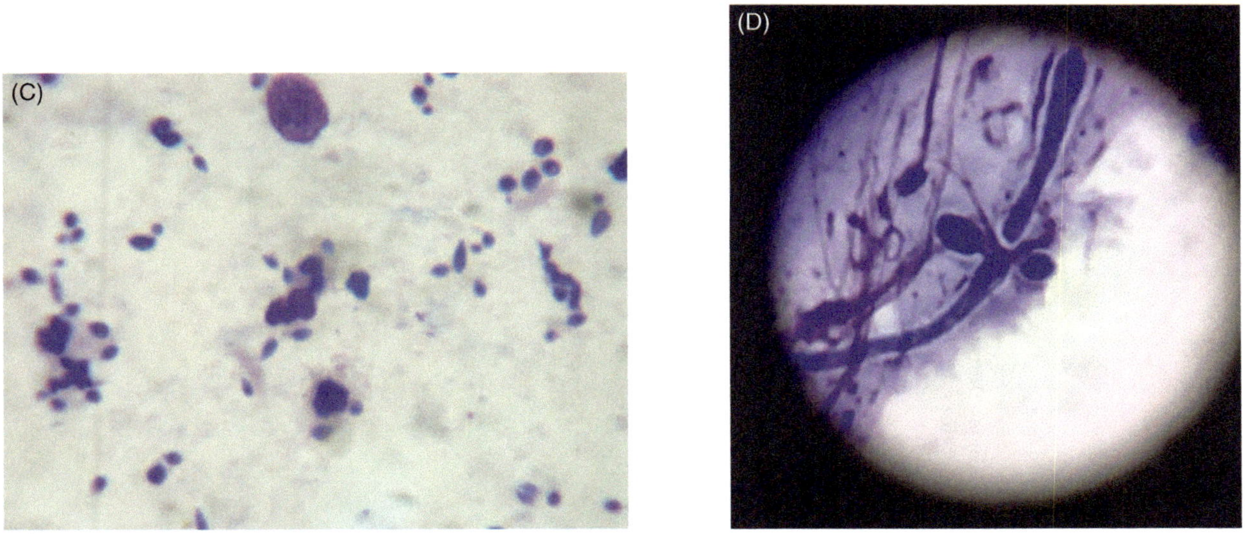

Figures 8.20C and D Cytology revealing round to teardrop shaped *Candida* organisms, which occasionally formed pseudohyphae (100×).

Table 8.10 Dermatophytosis.

Disease	Clinical signs	Diagnosis	Treatment
Canine Dermatophytosis – localized (Figures 8.21A and 8.21B) *Microsporum canis* *Microsporum gypseum* *Trichophyton mentagrophytes*	Circular to irregular alopecia with variable scaling, papules, crusts. Differentials: • Pyoderma • *Demodex* • If nodular: neoplasia, histiocytoma, acral lick dermatitis.	Initial point of care tests (see Chapter 1): • Wood's lamp examination. • Direct examination. – Trichograms of affected hair in mineral oil. – Skin scrapings and cytology of lesions. • Rule out other causes for folliculitis. – Pyoderma, *Demodex*. Further/confirmatory testing: • Dermatophyte culture (see Chapter 1). • Dermatophyte PCR. – Helpful screening test if negative (very sensitive test), as long as sufficient hair roots and skin debris are submitted for analysis. – Can have false positive results because PCR does not quantitate spores (i.e. one dermatophyte spore present on the fur is likely not significant). – Does not differentiate between live and dead fungal organisms in successfully treated animals. • Biopsy: – May be needed for fungal kerions or in cases with suspected false negative DTM. – Very specific test (no false positive results), but false negative results can occur if organisms are obscured due to inflammation, if wrong area sampled, or if specific fungal stains not performed.	Topical antifungal cream, solution or ointment BID, i.e. clotrimazole, miconazole, terbinafine, climbazole, until negative DTM.

Canine Dermatophytosis – multifocal to generalized (Figures 8.22A–8.22V) *M. canis* *M. gypseum* *T. mentagrophytes*	Clinical presentation can include • Classic: Circular to irregular alopecia with variable scaling. • Also: Papules, crusts, seborrhea, paronychia, onychodystrophy, nodules/kerions. • Lesions are typically asymmetric. • Can be non-pruritic or very pruritic. • Yorkies, Terriers and hunting dogs predisposed. Differentials: • Pyoderma • *Demodex* • Other parasites Immune-mediated disease (pemphigus foliaceus).	See Canine Dermatophytosis – localized.	See Algorithm 8.2. Combine topical and systemic therapy. Topical therapies: • 2% lime sulfur whole body dips 1–2 times weekly until 2 negative DTMs. • 2% miconazole/chlorhexidene shampoos twice weekly. Better than miconazole alone. • Chlorhexidene alone does not work. • 0.2% enilconazole dips twice weekly (available in Canada and Europe). Systemic therapies – most effective: • Itraconazole 5–10 mg/kg/day PO with food (not compounded). • Terbinafine 30 mg/kg PO q24 hours. Less effective: • Ketoconazole 5–10 mg/kg/day with food (monitor liver, has decreased effectiveness for *M. canis,* DO NOT use in cats). • Fluconazole 10 mg/kg PO q12–24 hours (do not use compounded, less effective in vitro/vivo than itraconazole and terbinafine). • Griseofulvin microsize 25 mg/kg PO BID or ultramicrosize 5–10 mg/kg/day; give with fatty meal.
Feline dermatophytosis – localized (Figures 8.23A–8.23D) *M. canis* most common; rarely *M. gypseum* or *T. mentagrophytes*	Circular to irregular alopecia with variable scaling, papules, crusts. Lesions commonly occur on face/ears/paws.	See Canine Dermatophytosis – localized.	Topical antifungal cream, solution, or ointment BID, AND 2% lime sulfur whole body dips or 2% miconazole/chlorhexidene shampoos twice weekly until two negative DTMs. If lesions persist or spread then add systemic itraconazole or terbinafine (see Feline dermatophytosis – multifocal to generalized).
Feline dermatophytosis – multifocal to generalized (Figures 8.24A–8.24J) *Microsporum canis* most common; rarely *Microsporum gypseum* or *Trichophyton mentagrophytes*	Clinical presentation can include: • Classic: Circular to irregular alopecia with variable scaling. • Lesions commonly begin on face/ears/paws. Then generalize • Also: Papules, crusts, seborrhea, paronychia, onychodystrophy, nodules. • Lesions are typically asymmetric. • Can be non-pruritic or very pruritic. • Asymptomatic carriage common in cats, esp. Persians.	See Canine Dermatophytosis – localized.	See Algorithm 8.2. Combine topical and systemic therapy, treat until 2 negative dermatophyte cultures by toothbrush technique, 1–2 weeks apart. Topical therapies: • 2% lime sulfur whole body dips 1–2 times weekly until 2 negative DTMs. • 2% miconazole/chlorhexidene shampoos twice weekly.

(*Continued*)

Table 8.10 Dermatophytosis (Continued)

Disease	Clinical signs	Diagnosis	Treatment
Feline dermatophytosis – multifocal to generalized (cont.)	Differentials: • Pyoderma • *Demodex* • Other parasites		Better than miconazole alone: • Chlorhexidene alone does not work. • 0.2% enilconazole dips twice weekly (available in Canada and Europe). • Scissor clip (blunted scissors) affected areas to aid in removal of infected fur and allow penetration of dips/shampoos. • Gently combing fur with fingers or comb prior to dips can help remove infected hairs; disinfect comb after use. Systemic therapies – most effective: • Itraconazole 5–10 mg/kg/day PO with food (not compounded). • Itrafungol® 10 mg/ml solution (Elanco) 5 mg/kg (0.5 ml/kg) PO once daily on alternating weeks for three treatment cycles. • Terbinafine 30 mg/kg PO q24 hours. • Monitor liver. Less effective and not recommended: • Fluconazole 10 mg/kg PO q12–24 hours (do not use compounded, less effective in vitro/vivo than itraconazole and terbinafine). • Griseofulvin microsize 25 mg/kg PO BID or ultramicrosize 5–10 PO mg/kg/day. Give with fatty meal, teratogenic, don't use in FIV/FeLV+ cats, monitor liver/CBC. • **Lufenuron/Program is NOT effective.** Environmental decontamination: • All bedding, brushes, combs, rugs, cages, etc. should be vacuumed, scrubbed, and washed with an effective disinfectant. • Throw out any items that cannot be thoroughly disinfected (i.e. scratching posts). • See Table 8.6 for more detailed information.

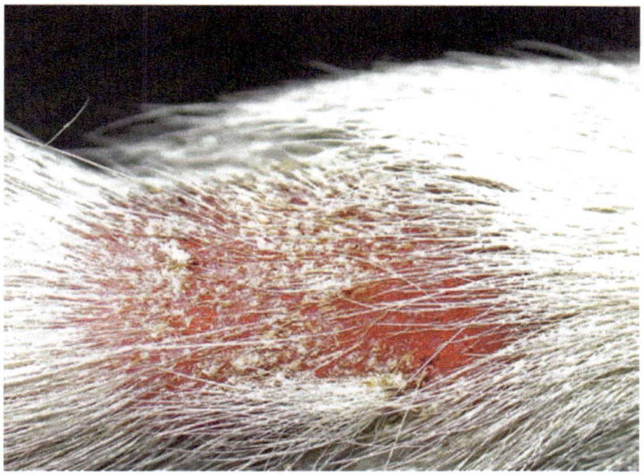

Figure 8.21A Alopecia and crusting on the tail of a dog caused by localized *Microsporum canis* infection.

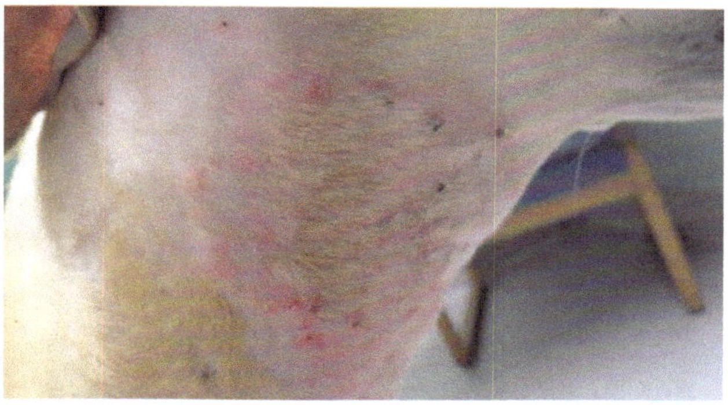

Figure 8.21B Localized hypotrichosis, papules, and crusts caused by *Microsporum gypseum* on the neck of a dog.

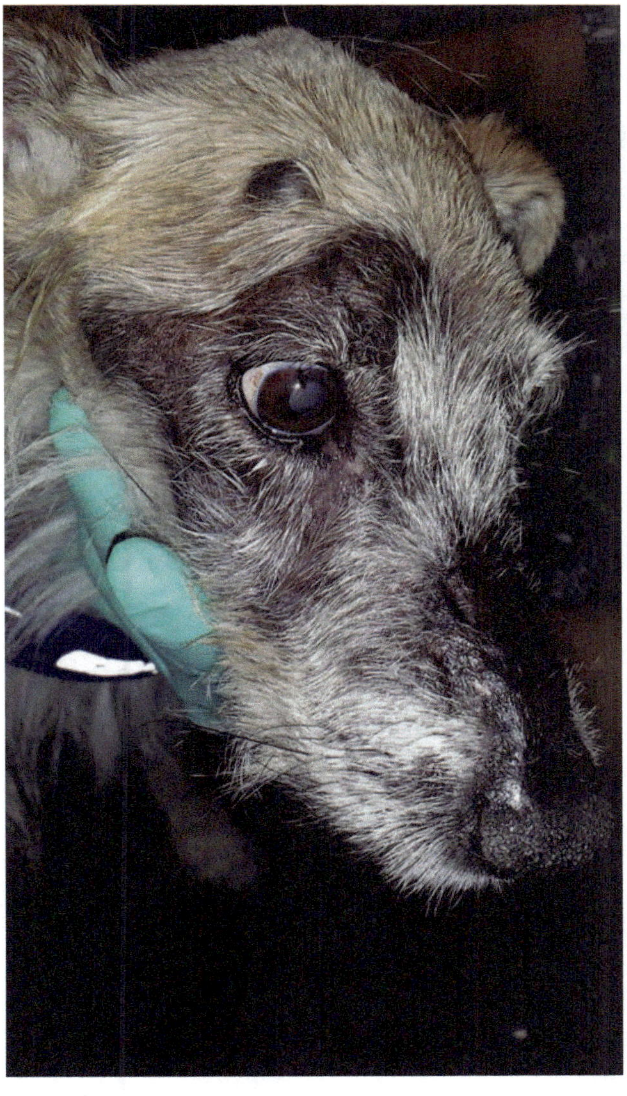

Figure 8.22A Patchy alopecia and hyperpigmentation on the face of an elderly Terrier caused by *Trichophyton mentagrophytes*.

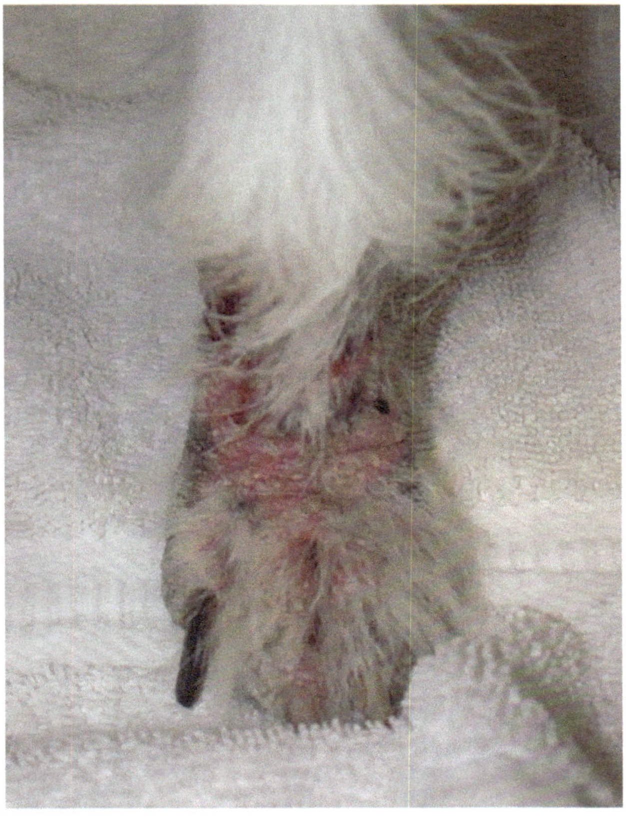

Figure 8.22B Alopecia, erythema, and crusting on the paws of the dog in Figure 8.22A.

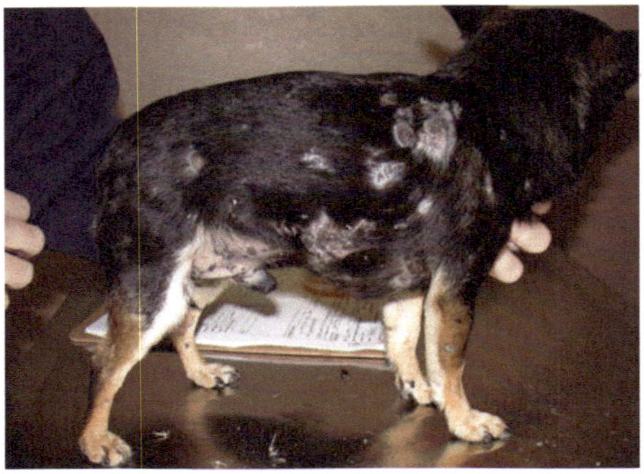

Figure 8.22C Patchy truncal alopecia, scaling, and hyperpigmentation in a Chihuahua with dermatophytosis due to *Trichophyton*.

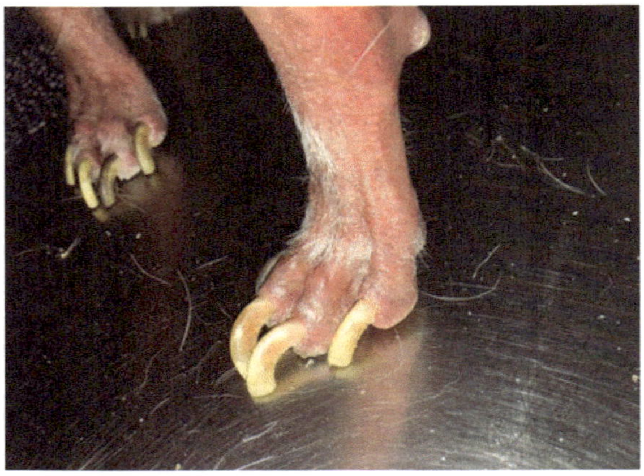

Figure 8.22D Alopecia, erythema, and thickened dystrophic toenails in a dog with an 18 month history of dermatophytosis due to *Trichophyton mentagrophytes*.

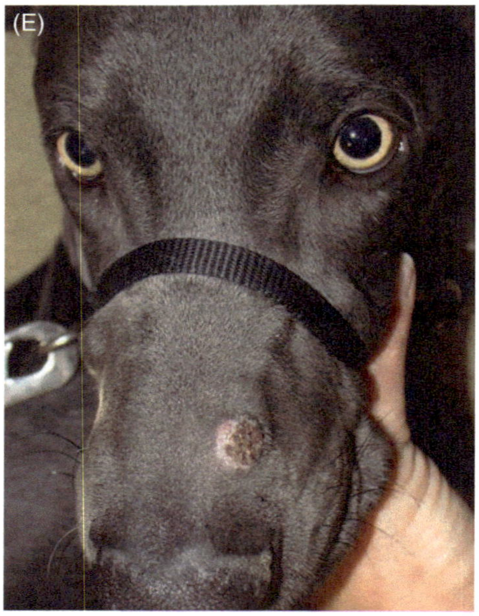

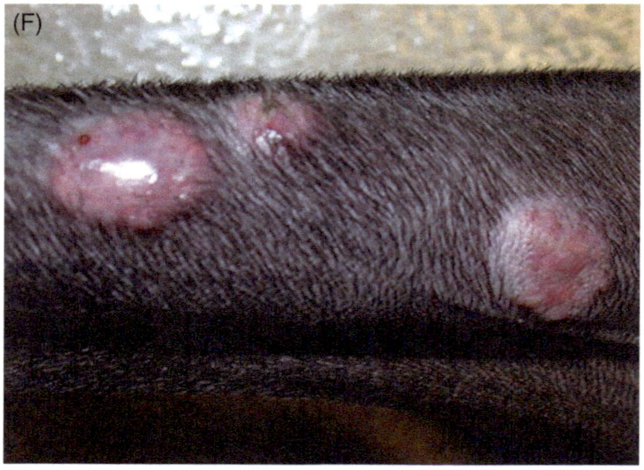

Figures 8.22E and F Raised, alopecic, pink, sometimes crusted dermal masses in young Weimaraner caused by dermatophyte kerions.

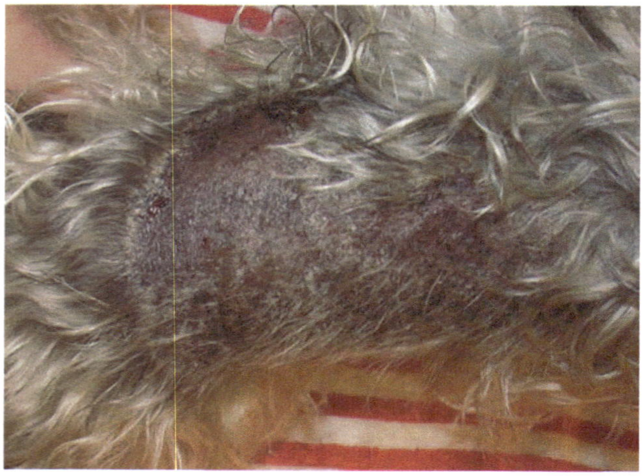

Figure 8.22G Spreading alopecia and hyperpigmentation with a crusty border caused by dermatophytosis in a Yorkie.

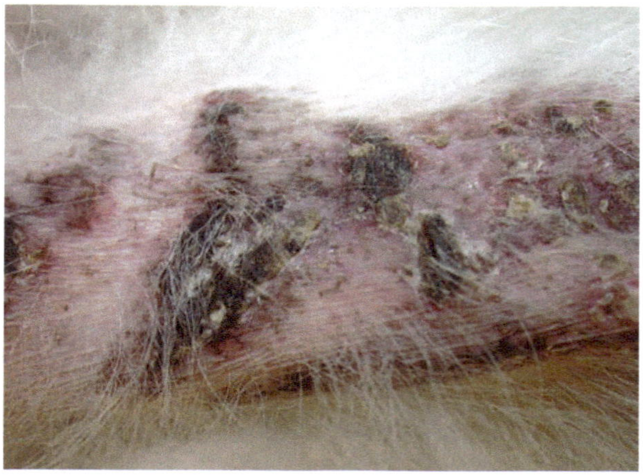

Figure 8.22H Inguinal crusts, erythema, and hyperpigmentation due to dermatophytosis in a Pomeranian receiving immunosuppressive therapy for vasculitis.

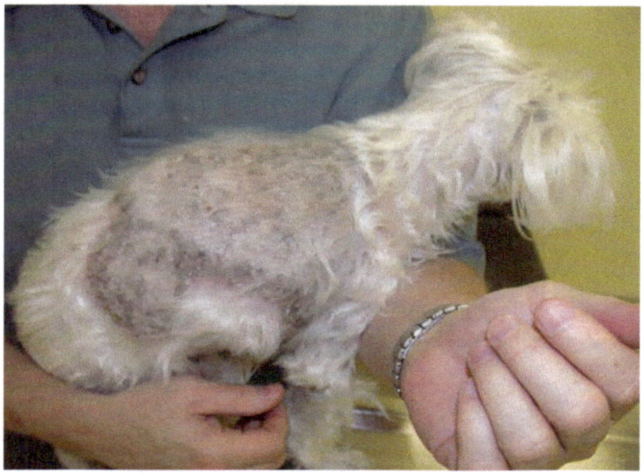

Figure 8.22I A Maltese with severe generalized dermatophytosis due to *Microsporum canis*; underlying liver cancer was suspected.

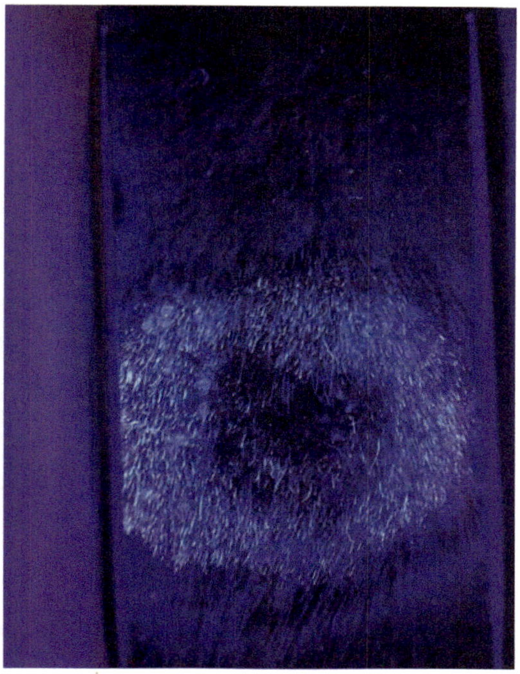

Figure 8.22J Wood's lamp examination of an alopecic skin lesion on a dog reveals apple green hair shaft fluorescence consistent with *Microsporum canis* infection. *Source:* Image courtesy of Alexandra Gould, DVM.

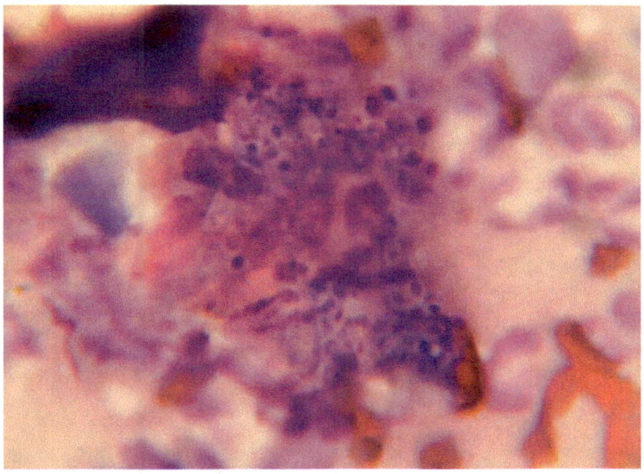

Figure 8.22K Skin surface cytology of a dog with *Microsporum canis* infection reveals numerous round to oval dermatophyte arthroconidia (100×).

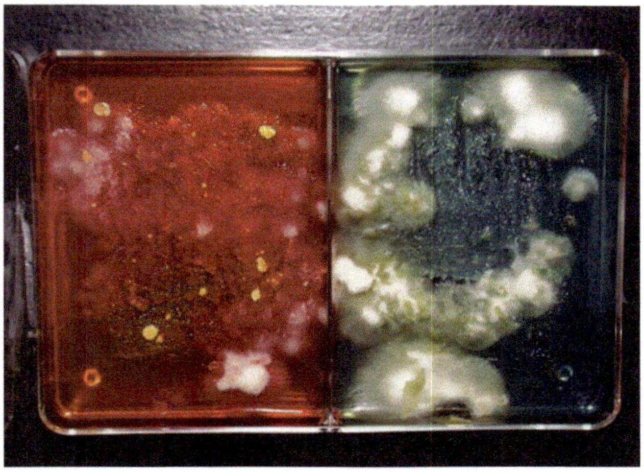

Figure 8.22L A dermatophyte culture of *Microsporum canis* showing characteristic white to light yellow fungal colonies with concurrent media color change.

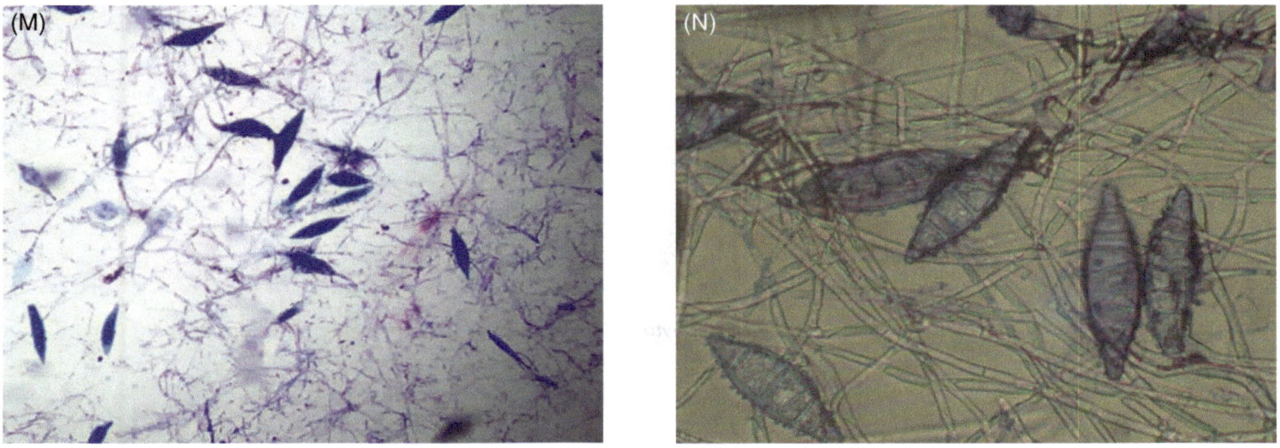

Figures 8.22M and N Tape cytology of the surface of the fungal colonies shows the characteristic large thick-walled spindle-shaped *Microsporum canis* macroconidia with six or more internal cells (8.22M is 4× and 8.22N is 10×).

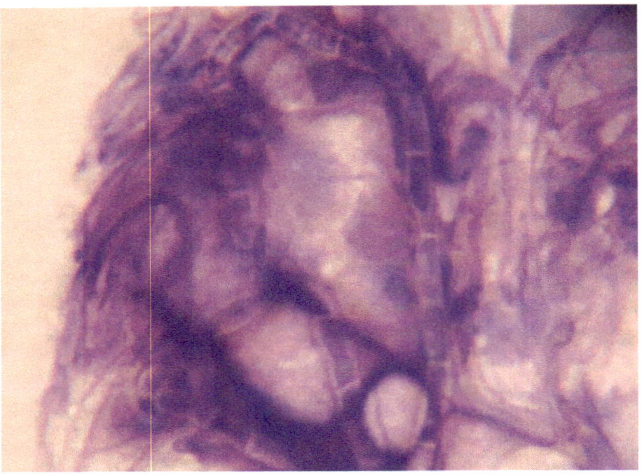

Figure 8.22O Surface skin cytology of a dog with *Microsporum gypseum* infection showing fungal hyphae and inflammatory cells (100×).

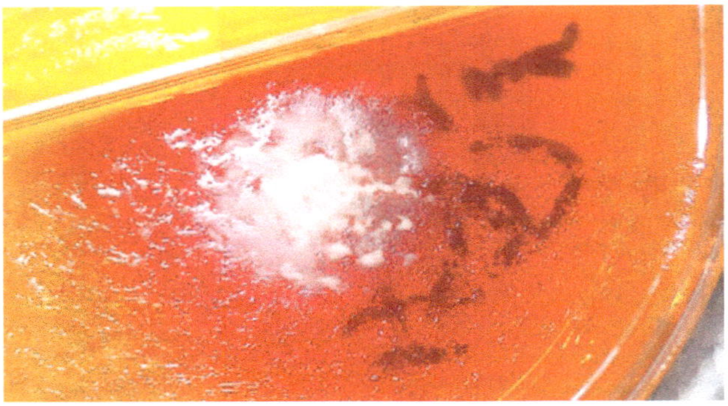

Figure 8.22P Dermatophyte culture of *Microsporum gypseum* showing a white powdery colony with concurrent media color change.

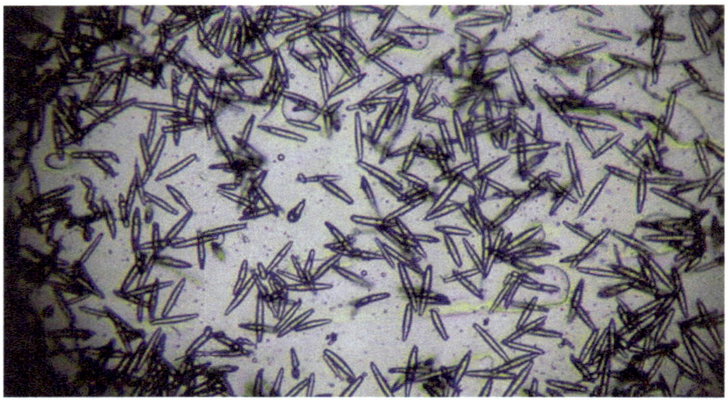

Figure 8.22Q Tape cytology of the surface of the *Microsporum gypseum* fungal colony showing numerous thin-walled macroconidia with less than six internal cells (4×).

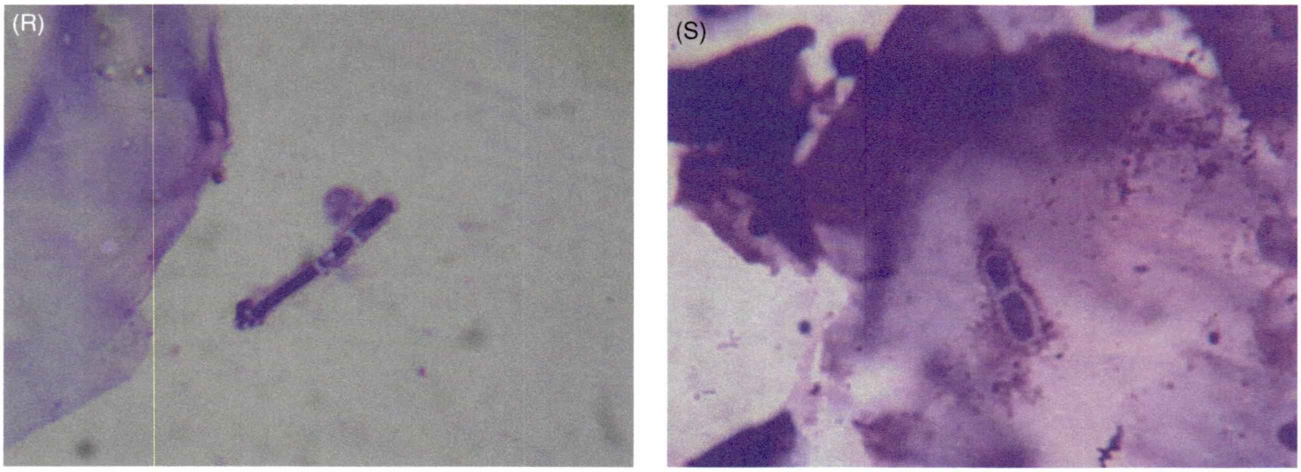

Figures 8.22R and S Skin surface cytology of a dog with *Trichophyton* infection demonstrating fragmented fungal hyphae (100×).

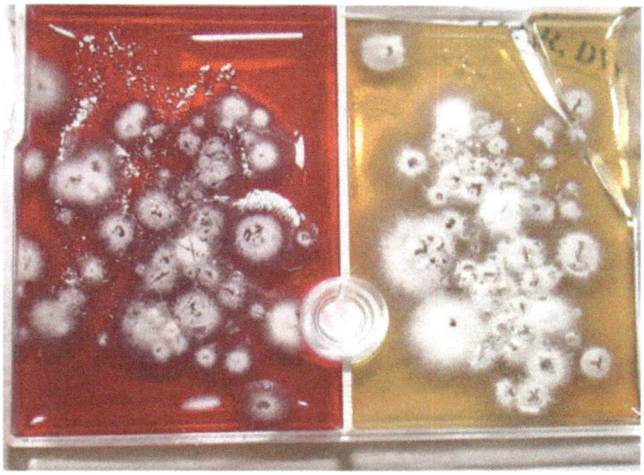

Figure 8.22T Dermatophyte culture of *Trichophyton mentagrophytes* showing white colonies with media color change occurring concurrently.

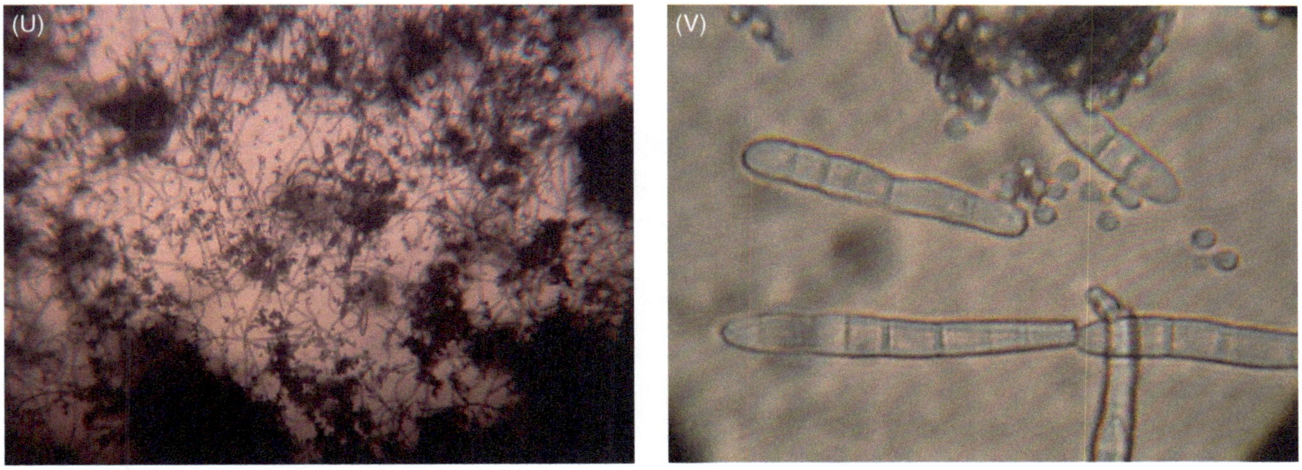

Figures 8.22U and V Tape cytology of the surface of the *Trichophyton mentagrophytes* colony showing fungal hyphae, numerous round to oval microconidia, and occasional cigar-shaped thin-walled macroconidia (8.22U is 4× and 8.22V is 10× with digital zoom).

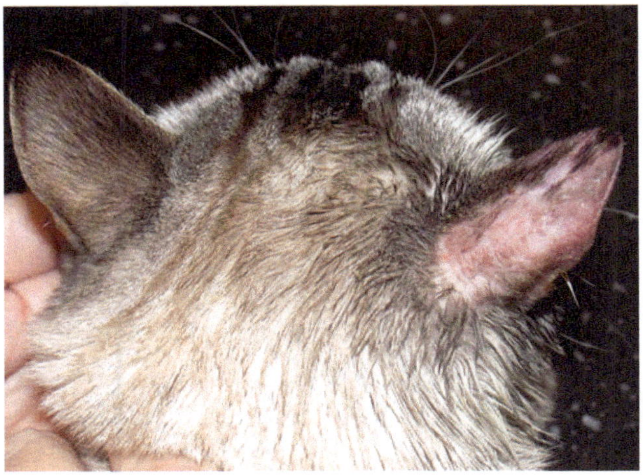

Figure 8.23A Localized dermatophytosis causing pinnal alopecia, erythema, and scaling in a cat.

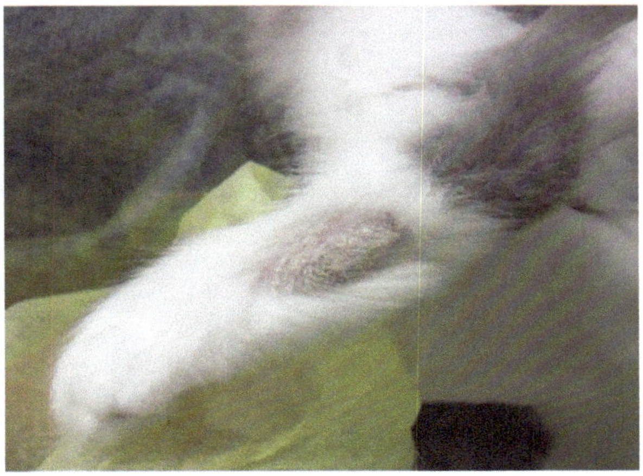

Figure 8.23B Focal alopecia and scaling on the paw of a cat with localized dermatophytosis. *Source:* Image courtesy of Dr. Karen Moriello, DACVD.

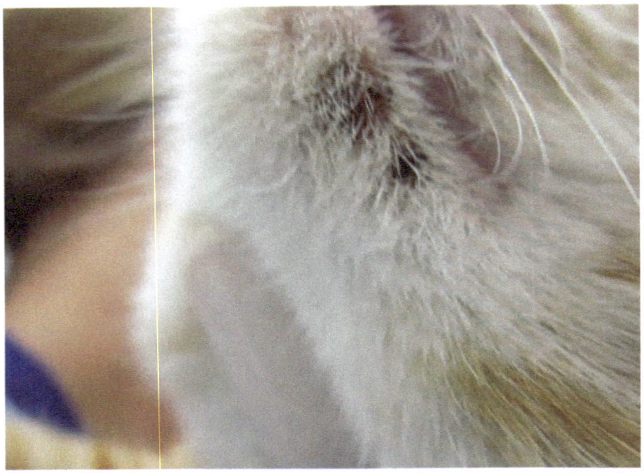

Figure 8.23C Dark keratinaceous chin debris caused by dermatophytosis in a cat. *Source:* Image courtesy of Dr. Karen Moriello, DACVD.

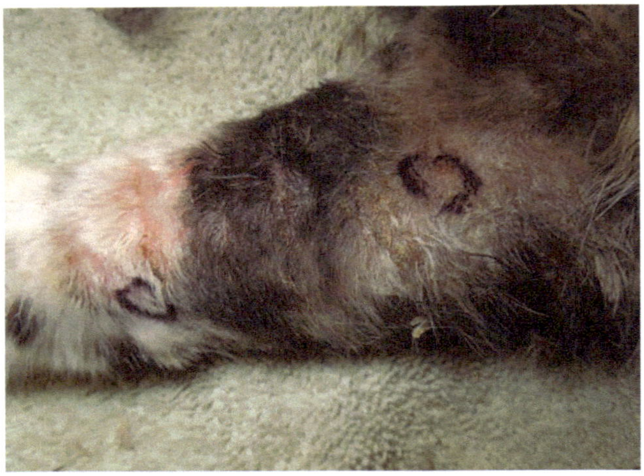

Figure 8.23D Intensely pruritic, erythematous, crusting dermatitis on one medial foreleg due to *Microsporum canis* infection in a cat.

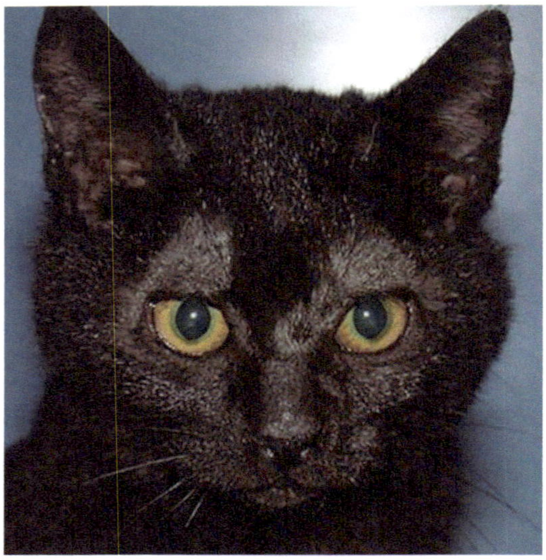

Figure 8.24A Patchy alopecia and crusting on the face of a cat with generalized dermatophytosis. *Source:* Image courtesy of Dr. Karen Moriello, DACVD.

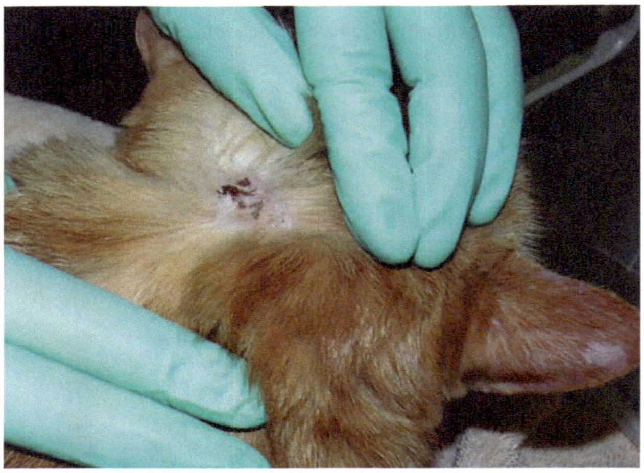

Figure 8.24B Multifocal alopecia and crusting on the neck and pinna of a cat with generalized dermatophytosis.

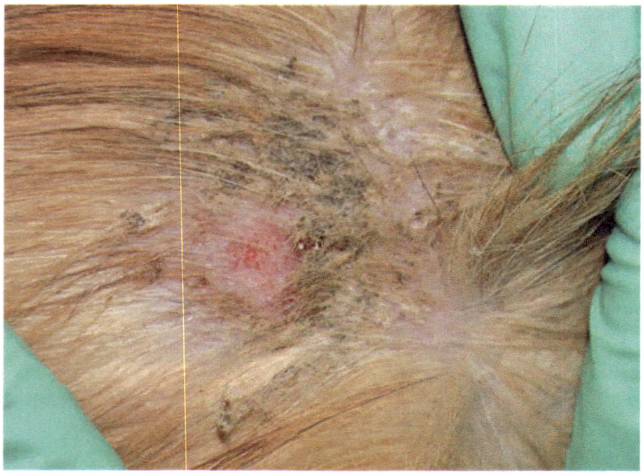

Figure 8.24C Adherent crusting due to *Microsporum canis* infection in a cat.

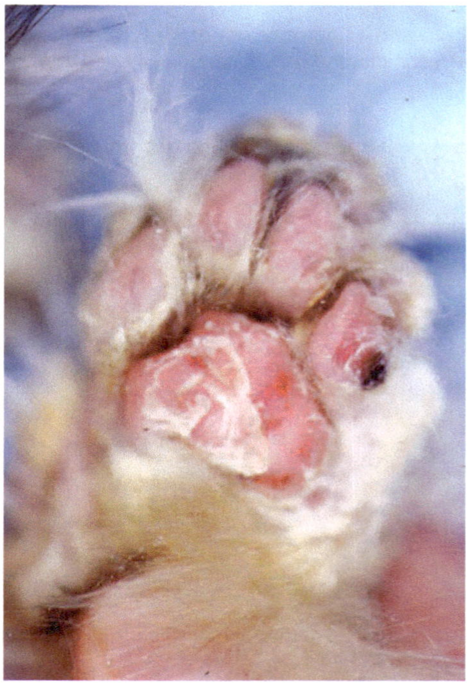

Figure 8.24D Paw pad scaling and small erosions in a cat with generalized dermatophytosis.

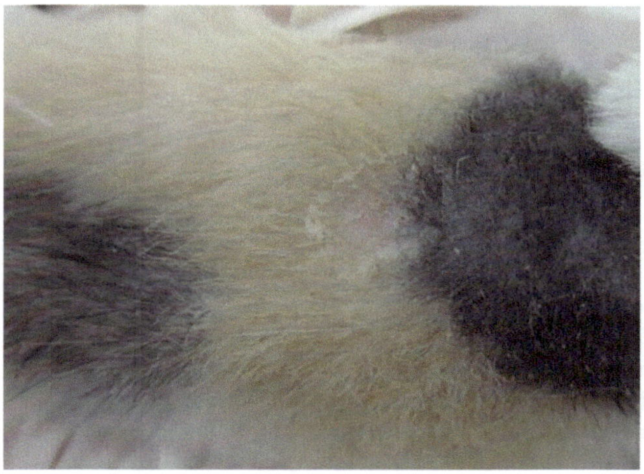

Figure 8.24E An epidermal collarette on the trunk of a cat caused by *Microsporum canis* infection. *Source:* Image courtesy of Dr. Karen Moriello, DACVD.

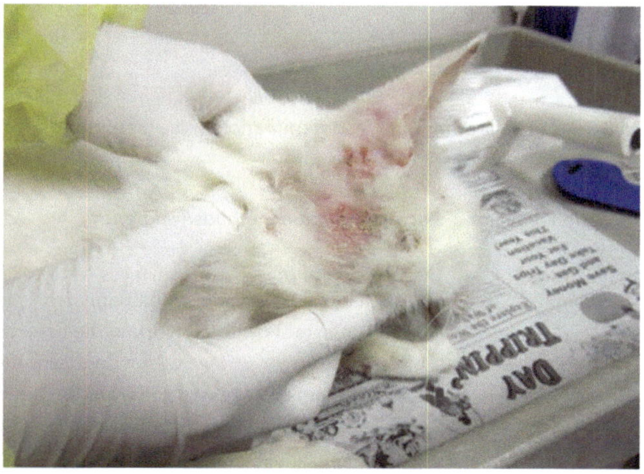

Figure 8.24F Alopecia and crusting on the caudal auricular area of a cat due to *Microsporum canis* infection. *Source:* Image courtesy of Dr. Karen Moriello, DACVD.

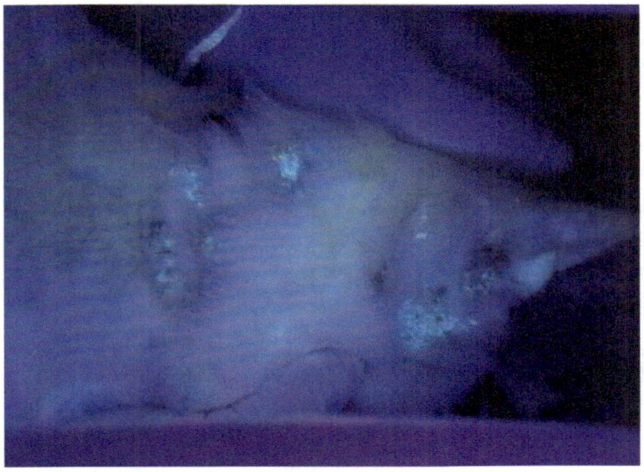

Figure 8.24G Wood's lamp examination of the cat in Figure 8.24F demonstrates strong apple green hair shaft fluorescence. *Source:* Image courtesy of Dr. Karen Moriello, DACVD.

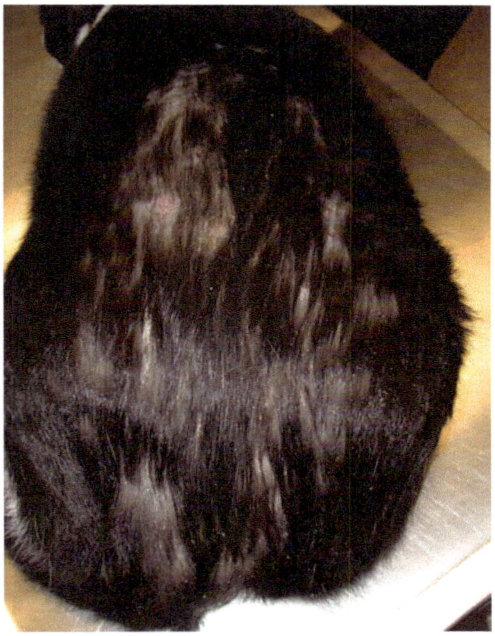

Figure 8.24H Patchy lumbar alopecia and scaling in a cat with dermatophytosis mimicking flea allergy dermatitis.

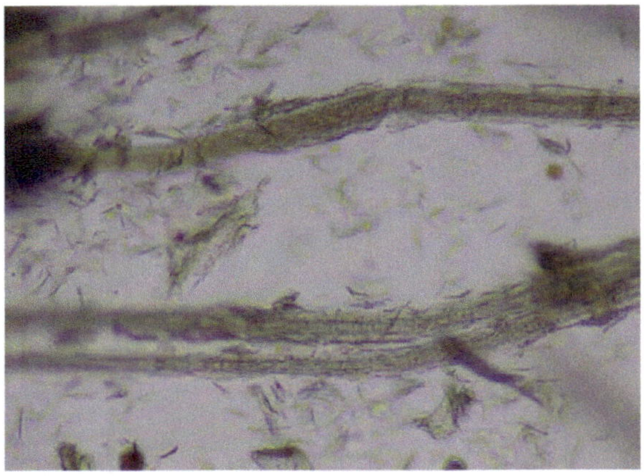

Figure 8.24I Trichogram of a cat with dermatophytosis demonstrating fuzzy infected hair shafts (4×).

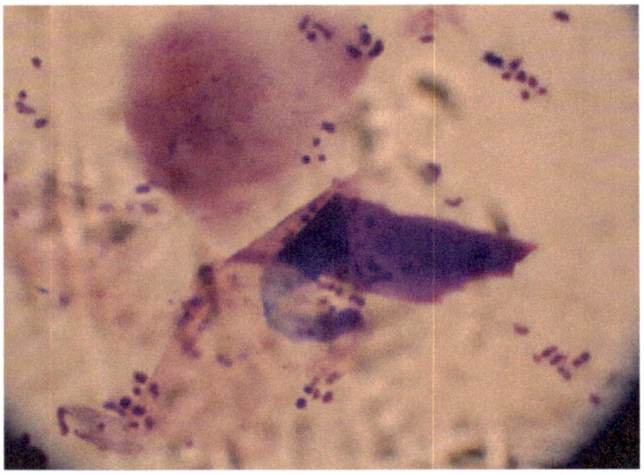

Figure 8.24J Skin surface cytology of a cat with *Microsporum canis* infection showing numerous dermatophyte arthroconidia (100×).

Table 8.11 Environmental decontamination in dermatophytosis.

Environmental location or factor	Decontamination methods/frequency
Hard floors	Disinfection of non-porous surfaces – steps: 1) Mechanical removal of all hair and debris via vacuuming or sweeping. • Disinfectants will not work in the presence of organic debris. 2) Wash the target surface with a detergent until the area is visibly clean. • Detergents must be rinsed from the target surface because some may inactivate disinfectants. 3) The final step is the application of a disinfectant to kill any residual spores. Effective disinfectants: • Preferred: Accelerated hydrogen peroxide (AHP) products (e.g. Accel, Rescue) or household cleaners with label efficacy against *Trichophyton spp.* • Potassium peroxymonosulfate (e.g. Virkon™ S). • Bleach (1 : 10 to 1 : 100 concentration). Twice weekly cleaning/disinfection is recommended. • This includes mechanical removal of hair, washing and disinfection of target areas.
Wood floors	Daily removal of pet hair using dusting clothes, flat mops, sweeping, etc.
Carpeting	Vacuuming alone does not decontaminate the surfaces but is recommended to remove gross debris including infective hairs. • Disinfect the vacuum with AHP spray and/or wipes. Carpeting can be decontaminated by washing twice with a carpet shampooer with detergent or via hot water extraction. Heavily contaminated carpets are best decontaminated by pretreatment with a disinfectant and then washed with a beater brush carpet shampooer. Household cleaners with label efficacy against *Trichophyton spp.* are effective as well as 1% potassium peroxymonosulfate. Twice weekly cleaning/disinfection is recommended: • This includes mechanical removal of hair, washing and disinfection of target areas.
Furniture	Vacuuming alone does not decontaminate the surfaces but is recommended to remove gross debris including infective hairs. • Disinfect the vacuum with AHP spray and/or wipes.
Clothing	A recent study found that washable textiles could be decontaminated via mechanical washing in any water temperature and that bleach was not needed. Two washings on the longest wash cycle were effective. It is important not to overload the machine to allow for maximum agitation. After wash, disinfect the interiors of washing machine and dryer by spraying the surfaces with an AHP product at appropriate dilution.
Kennels	Daily removal of pet hair from the room/area where the pet is being confined using dusting clothes, flat mops, sweeping, etc. A daily one-step antifungal cleaner can be used on days between more thorough cleanings.

Algorithm 8.2 Treatment of generalized dermatophytosis.

Generalized dermatophytosis with consistent clinical signs diagnosed by positive dermatophyte culture and/or PCR with microscopic confirmation of culture and/or direct examination

→ Treat topically to decontaminate fur and reduce contagion

- Anti-fungal cream (e.g. terbinafine, miconazole) to focal lesions twice daily
- 2% lime sulfur dip twice weekly
- 2% Miconazole/ 2% Chlorhexidene shampoo twice weekly
- 0.2% Enilconazole dip twice weekly (not available in US)

→ Treat systemically to kill fungus within hair follicles

- Itraconazole 5mg/kg/day (non-compounded; can pulse treat week on/week off in cats)
- Terbinafine 30mg/kg/day (in cats can pulse treat week on/week off after 21 days)

→ Decontaminate environment

Twice weekly:

- Vacuum/sweep hard surfaces
- Wash with detergent cleaner/ rinse
- Apply anti-fungal disinfectant: accelerated peroxide product or OTC bathroom disinfectant labeled as effective vs. *Trichophyton*
- Sweep wood floors daily

Clothing:

- Wash exposed clothing twice on longest cycle or until fur is not visible
- Do not overload washer
- Bleach not needed
- Disinfect interior of washer and dryer with accelerated peroxide product or OTC bathroom disinfectant labeled as effective vs. *Trichophyton*

Furniture/Carpet:

- Vacuum twice weekly
- Disinfect vacuum head with accelerated peroxide product
- Steam clean
- Disinfect twice using beater brush carpet shampooer and anti-fungal shampoo

Kennel:

- Clean daily as for hard surfaces with one step anti-fungal cleaner

→ Examine +/– culture in contact animals to determine if they may require systemic anti-fungal treatment

Either separate non-infected animals or prophylactically treat with weekly anti-fungal shampoo or dip

Table 8.12 Deep fungal, oomycete, and algal infections.

Disease	Clinical signs	Diagnosis	Treatment
Blastomycosis (*Blastomyces dermatitidis*, Figures 8.25A–8.25J) A dimorphic saprophytic soil fungus; requires moist sandy acidic soil/organic material. Animals are usually infected by inhaling mycelial spores (which convert to yeast form in the lungs and disseminates hematogenously) +/− rarely inoculation of organisms into a puncture wound. Young, large breed and hunting dogs predisposed. In the US endemic to the Mississippi, Missouri, and Ohio river valleys and Mid-Atlantic states; also reported in Canada, Africa, India, Europe, and Central America.	Skin lesions occur in 20–50% of infected dogs and include firm papules, nodules, plaques which may ulcerate or drain. Lesions can occur anyplace but most commonly occur on the nasal planum and clawbeds. Other systemic signs common, including cough, dyspnea, fever, weight loss, uveitis, and lameness. Rare in cats; clinical signs include draining skin lesions (especially on paws), dyspnea, uveitis, and weight loss.	Cytology and biopsy of draining skin lesions: pyogranulomatous inflammation with round to oval broad based budding thick- walled yeast. Organisms are best visualized with special fungal stains (GMS, PAS). Blastomyces antigen enzyme immunoassay (EIA) on urine (cross reactive with *Histoplasma*). Culture: Not recommended due to health risk of laboratory personnel. Labwork: Often leukocytosis with left shift, hyperglobulinemia, hypoalbuminemia +/− hypercalcemia.	Itraconazole (non-compounded): Dogs: 5 mg/kg PO q24h; Cats: 5 mg/kg PO q12h is the drug of choice (68–74% response rate; median duration of treatment 138 days). Fluconazole (non-compounded) 10 mg/kg/day can also be effective (and is preferred for infection involving urinary tract) but requires a longer course of treatment (median duration 183 days). Amphotericin B also effective (77% response rate). Treat for 2 months minimum (3 months minimum if severe lung disease present), until negative urine antigen (Ag) test. 20% of treated dogs relapse within 6 months −3 years and require retreatment. In dogs with severe respiratory disease, administer anti-inflammatory prednisone during initial treatment phase. Prognosis poor with severe lung or neurologic involvement.
Cryptococcosis (*Cryptococcosis neoformans, Cryptococcosis gattii* are most common species, occasionally less pathogenic species such as *Cryptococcosis laurentii*; Figures 8.26A–8.26E) *Cryptococcosis neoformans* is a ubiquitous saprophytic yeast most commonly associated with bird droppings, as it prefers a nitrogen rich, alkaline environment.	Cats: Skin or subcutaneous lesions occur in 40% of cases and can include nodules which may ulcerate or drain, most commonly present on the face, pinnae, and paws, especially at sites contiguous with the nasal cavity or planum nasale. Other common symptoms include nasal stertor/discharge +/− nasal mass occluding nare, swelling of dorsal nose or above sinuses, mandibular lymphadenopathy, uveitis, optic neuritis/retinitis, and CNS disease. Cough/lung disease is uncommon.	Cytology/Biopsy: Pyogranulomatous inflammation with numerous round to oval narrow-based budding yeasts surrounded by clear non-staining capsules; helpful special histopathologic stains include PAS, GMS, and Mayer mucicarmine. Culture of aspirates/tissue samples recommended to differentiate between fungal species.	Fluconazole (cats: 10 mg/kg PO q12h; dogs 5–15 mg/kg PO q12–24h; do not use compounded formulations) is probably the drug of choice and has superior CNS and ocular penetration compared to itraconazole. Itraconazole (non-compounded) has comparable efficacy to fluconazole for infections not involving the CNS, eye, or urinary tract.

C. neoformans has worldwide distribution. *C. gattii* is found in tropical, subtropical, and temperate climates and is commonly found in Australia, New Zealand, Southeast Asia, Mexico, Latin America, part of Europe, California, Hawaii, and recently in Vancouver Island, Canada, and the Pacific North West of the USA. The most common systemic mycosis of cats, rare in dogs. Animals are usually infected by inhaling spores causing nasal colonization followed by nasal invasion and sometimes hematogenous spread; less commonly, direct inoculation of spores or yeast cells into a puncture wound.	Dogs: Skin lesions occur in 20% of cases, and can include nodules which may ulcerate or drain, most commonly present on the nose, lips, mouth, and clawbeds. Other systemic symptoms usually present including lethargy, weight loss, nasal discharge, uveitis, and CNS disease.	Serum latex agglutination testing for cryptococcal capsular antigen are very accurate for diagnosis and to monitor therapy. Lab work: Nonregenerative anemia and leukocytosis common.	Amphotericin B + flucytosine (in cats) also very effective for CNS infection and are recommended as initial treatment in animals with severe CNS disease; anti-inflammatory doses of steroids may be needed to reduce brain inflammation during first few days of treatment. Voriconazole and posaconazole also effective but very expensive; posaconazole is useful for resistant *C. gattii* isolates. Successful treatment occurs in 75% of cats, 55% of dogs; treat until clinical and serological remission (negative titer, this may take up to 2 years), recheck titer 6 months after stopping therapy to screen for recurrence.
Histoplasmosis (*Histoplasma capsulatum*; Figures 8.27A and 8.27B) A dimorphic soilborne fungus that prefers warm, moist, nitrogen-rich soil. Endemic in the Midwest and Southern United States (most cases occur in Ohio, Missouri, and Mississippi River Valleys) but has worldwide distribution; prefers warm, moist, nitrogen-rich soil (especially soil rich in bird/bat feces). Dogs and cats are usually infected by inhaling infective microconidia then organisms convert to yeast form and infection disseminates hematogenously +/− rarely inoculation of spores into a puncture wound. Ingestion is another possible route of infection in cases with only GI disease. Young, large breed dogs predisposed; working and herding breeds often have disseminated histoplasmosis, and toy breeds often have the GI form.	Skin lesions in dogs and cats can include skin nodules, ulcers, and draining tracts which can occur anyplace on the body; in cats lesions are commonly on the face, nose, and pinnae. Systemic signs in dogs and cats are usually present and can include anorexia, weight loss, fever, lymphadenopathy, cough, chronic diarrhea, and uveitis.	Cytology or biopsy of skin lesions or rectal scrapings: Pyogranulomatous inflammation with numerous small yeast organisms usually within macrophages. For histopathology, special fungal stains (PAS/GMS) should be used to highlight fungal organisms. A urine Histoplasma EIA, which detects the fungal antigen galactomannan, is highly specific and sensitive (cross reactive with *Blastomyces*). Culture: Not recommended due to health risk of laboratory personnel. Labwork: Anemia is common +/− thrombocytopenia. Leukocyte counts are variable. Hypoalbuminemia may be present.	Drug of choice is itraconazole in dogs and cats (5–10 mg/kg PO q12–24h, non-compounded), though a recent retrospective study in dogs found fluconazole was also usually effective (clinical remission occurred in 64% of dogs receiving fluconazole and 71% of dogs receiving itraconazole); duration of treatment is usually at least 4–6 months. For severe cases, combination therapy with itraconazole and amphotericin B is recommended. In dogs with severe respiratory disease, administer anti-inflammatory prednisone during initial treatment phase. Treat until negative fungal antigen test then recheck urine Ag testing q3–6 months for 2 years to monitor for relapse. Negative prognostic factors: Severe respiratory or liver disease, anemia, thrombocytopenia, hypercalcemia, CNS disease.

(*Continued*)

Table 8.12 Deep fungal, oomycete, and algal infections (Continued)

Disease	Clinical signs	Diagnosis	Treatment
Coccidioidomycosis (*Coccidioides immitis, Coccidioides posadasii*; Figures 8.28A–8.28C) A dimorphic saprophytic soil fungus which thrives in sandy, dry, alkaline soils and warm temperatures. Animals are usually infected by inhaling arthroconidia which converts in lungs to spherules which contain endospores; infection disseminates hematogenously +/− rarely inoculation of spores into a puncture wound. Young, large breed dogs are predisposed. In the US occurs in the southwestern states including Arizona (AZ), Texas (TX), New Mexico (NM), Nevada (NV), Utah (UT) (*Coccidioides posadasii*) and the San Joaquin Valley of CA and south-central Washington (WA) (*Coccidioides immitis*); also occurs in Mexico, Central and South America.	Skin lesions include nodules which may ulcerate or drain; lesions may occur over site of infected bone, but in a recent retrospective study skin lesions occurred widely over the body including the trunk, neck, head, and limbs usually with no boney involvement. Regional lymphadenopathy may be present. Cough and lameness due to boney lesions are common in dogs, and signs of disseminated disease in both dogs and cats often include fever, weight loss, lethargy, uveitis, and CNS disease.	Cytology and biopsy: Pyogranulomatous inflammation with fungal spherules which may be few in number and difficult find; special fungal stains (PAS or GMS) are needed. Culture: Not recommended due to health risk of laboratory personnel. Serology: AGID (agar gel immunodiffusion) and ELISA (enzyme-linked immunosorbent assay) serologic tests for detection of antibodies to *Coccidioides*; titers may stay positive indefinitely and many animals in endemic areas have low titers due to exposure but do not have clinical disease. Labwork: Mild non-regenerative anemia and leukocytosis common, as well as hyperglobulinemia and hypoalbuminemia.	Fluconazole 5–10 mg/kg PO q12h (preferred for CNS infection, do not use compounded formulation), ketoconazole 5–10 mg/kg PO q12h (dogs only) or itraconazole 5 mg/kg PO q12h (non-compounded) until 3–6 months beyond remission of clinical signs and unchanging, low follow up titer, usually 8–12 months; animals with disseminated disease should be treated for a minimum of 1 year. A rising recheck titer indicates need to change treatment. Prognosis guarded to poor with bone or CNS involvement.
Sporotrichosis (*Sporothrix schenckii*; Figures 8.29A–8.29H) A ubiquitous dimorphic soil saprophyte, grows on living and decaying plant material. Occurs worldwide; in the US most commonly found in coastal regions and river valleys of the southern states. Infects animals by inoculation of mycelial organisms into puncture or fight wounds, less frequently by inhalation; organisms then covert to yeast form and cause local, regional lymphatic, or disseminated disease. Uncommon in dogs and cats; hunting dogs and outdoor, unneutered, male cats predisposed. Zoonotic	Dogs: Cutaneous lesions include nodules, ulcerated plaques, and alopecic crusted areas, most commonly on head (including nasal planum), limbs, and trunk. The cutaneolymphatic form is characterized by a dermal mass on a distal limb with ascending lymphatic involvement causing secondary nodules which may drain; lymphadenopathy is present. Disseminated disease is very rare in dogs. Cats: Lesions often present as abscesses and ulcerated crusted nodules on the head, ears, nose, distal limbs, or tail (areas of fight wounds); large areas of necrosis can occur and expose muscle/bone. Grooming behavior can spread infection to other areas on body. Most cats have disseminated disease and systemic signs may be present including fever, respiratory signs, lymphadenopathy, lethargy, and anorexia.	Cytology and biopsy: Pyogranulomatous inflammation with round, oval, or cigar shaped yeast organisms (rare in dogs but usually numerous in cats). Special fungal stains (PAS/GMS) facilitate visualization of organisms on biopsy. Fungal culture of macerated deep tissue sample. Serum antibody testing available but does not distinguish exposure from active infection.	Itraconazole 5–10 mg/kg PO q12–24h (non-compounded) is the drug of choice; other potentially effective drugs include terbinafine, potassium iodide solution, ketoconazole (dogs only), and amphotericin B. Treat minimum of 8 weeks, until 1 month beyond clinical normalcy.

Phaeohyphomycosis (a.k.a. Chromomycosis) (Figures 8.30A–8.30F) Caused by many ubiquitous saprophytic fungi living in soil and organic material; fungal species include (among others) *Alternaria, Bipolaris, Cladosporium*, and *Curvularia*. Infection occurs when fungal organism is inoculated into skin through a wound. Rare in dogs and uncommon in cats, immunosuppressive medications can predispose to infection.	Single to multifocal dermal to subcutaneous nodules which may ulcerate or develop draining tracts, in cats most commonly occur on the face, paws, and trunk. Lesions may be darkly pigmented.	Cytology and biopsy: Pyogranulomatous inflammation with pigmented fungal hyphae and yeast forms. Special fungal stains (Masson-Fontana) helpful to demonstrate organisms. Fungal tissue culture. Fungal PCR on tissue or cytology specimens: Available at select laboratories such as Texas A&M Veterinary Medical Diagnostic Laboratory. Drug susceptibility testing ideal (Fungus Testing Lab at University of Texas Health Science Center).	Reduce or taper off immunosuppressive medications if present. Wide surgical excision of isolated lesions (if possible), followed by prolonged systemic antifungal therapy ideally based on sensitivity testing, as antifungal susceptibility of the different causative organisms is unpredictable. Pending sensitivity results, or if fungal sensitivity is not possible, begin non-compounded itraconazole 10 mg/kg/day PO × 3 months minimum. Voriconazole, posaconazole, and amphoterin B should be considered for animals with recurrent or disseminated disease.
Pythiosis (*Pythium insidiosum*; Figures 8.31A–8.31C) An oomycete; a filamentous microorganism which shares many physical characteristics with fungi, however, unlike fungi the cell walls of *Pythium* contain cellulose and beta-glucan but not chitin. Classified together with diatoms and brown algae in a completely different taxonomic group, (*Stramenopila*). *P. insidiosum* colonizes aquatic plants and soil of wetlands/swamps, mycelia on plants produce mobile zoospores which move through the water with a strong tropism for mammalian injured tissue and cause infection by encysting in damaged skin or GI mucosa.	Dogs: Nonhealing wounds and ulcerated invasive cutaneous to subcutaneous masses with draining tracts. Lesions most commonly occur on the limbs, tailhead, ventrum, or perineum. Regional lymphadenopathy is often present. Cats: Invasive subcutaneous masses in the inguinal, tailhead, or face (including the nasal cavity), and draining nodular lesions or ulcerated plaques on the paws. GI involvement may cause weight loss, vomiting, diarrhea, and an abdominal mass. Cutaneous and GI lesions rarely are encountered together in the same patient.	Cytology and biopsy: Pyogranulomatous inflammation with numerous eosinophils and scattered, poorly staining hyphae; special stains (GMS) are often needed to visualize organisms on histopathology. Culture: *P. insidiosum* is highly inhibited by low temperatures; samples should be sent to the laboratory within 24 hours of collection and stored in water or saline-soaked gauze and at room temperature. If samples cannot be shipped for more than 2 days after collection then store samples in refrigerator and ship with ice packs to slow bacterial contamination. Recommended lab: University of Tennessee microbiology lab; also performs PCR ID of cultured isolate.	Skin lesions are usually progressive, invasive, and poorly responsive to medical treatment. Therapy includes radical surgery (including amputation of isolated distal limb lesions), followed by itraconazole (10 mg/kg PO q24h, do not use compounded formulations) and terbinafine (30 mg/kg PO q24h for at least 2–3 months after surgery. In vitro synergism occurs with terbinafine + azole antifungals, amphotericin B + terbinafine, and terbinafine + caspofungin.

(*Continued*)

Table 8.12 Deep fungal, oomycete, and algal infections (Continued)

Disease	Clinical signs	Diagnosis	Treatment
Pythiosis (cont.) Animal pythiosis cases occur in tropical and subtropical climatic regions of Australia, Asia, Latin America, the United States, and temperate areas of Japan, South Korea, Oceania, and Africa. In the United States, pythiosis usually occurs often in the Gulf Coast states, but it has also been diagnosed in animals in multiple other states. Occurs most commonly in young, male, large breed, working breed dogs; often with a history of frequent exposure to warm freshwater habitats. Rare in cats.		Pythiosis serum ELISA: Recommended lab: Auburn University, Alabama. PCR: Can be performed on formalin fixed or frozen samples or fresh samples preserved in 95% ethanol at room temperature. Recommended lab: Texas A&M dermatopathology service. Immunohistochemistry to demonstrate organisms on fixed tissue may be available at veterinary diagnostic laboratories; cross reactivity with *Lagenidium* and *Conidiobolus* may occur depending on antibody used. Labwork: Eosinophilia, anemia, hyperglobulinemia, and hypoalbuminemia are common.	To monitor for recurrence, ELISA serology should be performed before and 2–3 months after surgery. In successfully treated animals, serum antibody titers typically drop dramatically within 3 months of surgery, and medical therapy can be discontinued, with subsequent re-evaluation of serum antibody levels every 3 months for 1 year. If antibody levels remain elevated 2–3 months after surgery, continue treatment and recheck ELISA test q2–3 months. Pythiosis vaccines have not been helpful in most small animal pythiosis cases, possibly due to delay in diagnosis, but are worth trying. At the time of this writing, Pythiosis vaccines were available from: Pan American Veterinary Labs (www.pavlab.com), *and* Pythium Technologies, Inc. 812 NE 24th Street Newcastle, OK, USA, (405) 387–3300.
Lagenidiosis (Figures 8.32A–8.32C) Also an oomycete; the genus *Lagenidium* includes more than 50 species, most of which occur as parasites of algae, fungi, rotifers, nematodes, crustaceans, Daphne, and mosquito larvae. The lifecycle and mode of animal infection have not been definitively characterized but are likely similar to *Pythium*. Affected animals are typically young to middle-aged dogs living in the southeastern United States (especially Florida and Louisiana, though cases have been reported in multiple other states) and have frequent exposure to lakes or ponds. Not described in cats.	Progressive dermal or subcutaneous firm masses (often multifocal) which are often ulcerated/draining or necrotic involving the limbs, ventrum, trunk, or perineum. Regional lymphadenopathy is common. Hind limb edema may occur with abdominal/sublumbar lymph node involvement. Most dogs have lesions in distant sites, including great vessels, sublumbar and inguinal lymph nodes, and lung.	Cytology and biopsy: Pyogranulomatous inflammation with numerous eosinophils and scattered, poorly staining hyphae; special stains (GMS) are often needed to visualize organisms on histopathology. Culture: Tissue biopsy for culture should be collected and handled as for *Pythium*; for isolation of *Lagenidium* species, peptone-yeast-glucose (PYG) agar is optimal. Serologic testing for *Lagenidium* antibodies is not accurate. PCR: Can be performed on formalin fixed or frozen samples or fresh samples preserved in 95% ethanol at room temperature.	Skin lesions are usually progressive, invasive, and poorly responsive to medical treatment. Chest/abdominal radiographs and abdominal ultrasound recommended prior to considering surgery, as most dogs have systemic lesions and prognosis is grave. In dogs with isolated lesions and no evidence of infection elsewhere, therapy includes radical surgery (including amputation of isolated distal limb lesions), followed by itraconazole (10 mg/kg by mouth every 24 hours; non-compounded) and terbinafine (5–10 mg/kg by mouth every 24 hours) for at least 2–3 months after surgery.

Zygomycosis Rare in dogs and cats; causative organisms are in order Entomophthorales (*Conidiobolus* and *Basidiobolus*), and Mucorales (*Rhizopus, Mucor* and others). Ubiquitous fungal saprophytes in soil and decaying vegetation; worldwide distribution. *Basidiobolus* also isolated from insect, amphibian, and reptile feces. Entomophthorales typically cause chronic localized infections in subcutaneous tissue or nasal submucosa of immunocompetent patients; Mucorales tend to cause acute, rapidly progressive disease in debilitated or immunocompromised individuals. May infect via wound contamination, insect bites, or via GI or respiratory tract.	Single to multiple ulcerated draining nodules often on the limbs and paws. *Conidiobolus* often causes mucocutaneous oral lesions and sinusitis, described to cause draining skin masses and lymphadenopathy in one dog. *Basidiobolus* can cause ulcerative skin lesions on trunk and extremities. Concurrent fatal GI disease may occur.	Cytology and biopsy: Pyogranulomatous inflammation with numerous eosinophils and scattered, poorly staining hyphae; special stains (GMS) are often needed to visualize organisms on histopathology. Fungal tissue culture (punch or wedge biopsy, but not macerated). Potato flake agar (PFA) potato dextrose agar, or cornmeal agar are optimal. Once the organism has been grown, culture samples should ideally be forwarded to the Fungus Testing Laboratory in the Department of Pathology at the University of Texas Health Science Center at San Antonio for species level identification by combined phenotypic characterization and DNA sequencing, as well as antifungal drug sensitivity.	Excise solitary lesions or debulk followed by prolonged antifungal therapy guided by in vitro susceptibility testing. Pending sensitivity results, or if fungal sensitivity is not possible, begin non-compounded itraconazole 10 mg/kg/day PO × 3 months minimum or treat with amphotericin B lipid complex. Recurrence is common.
Protothecosis (*Prototheca wickerhamii;* Figures 8.33A–8.33C) Ubiquitous saprophytic, achlorophyllous algae found in soil, sewage, streams, swimming pools, and stagnant water. Can infect wounds to cause cutaneous lesions or colon to cause disseminated disease. Causes opportunistic infection in immunosuppressed animals. Rare; in the US, most cases have occurred in the Southeast states.	Cutaneous lesions include nodules or ulcerations often on pressure points, mucocutaneous junctions (including nasal planum, which may be depigmented), scrotum, and paw pads. Cutaneous disease may disseminate to lymph nodes, heart, lungs. Dogs with disseminated disease due to *Prototheca zopfii* have bloody, large bowel diarrhea and lesions which start in the GI tract then spread to kidneys, heart, brain, and eyes.	Cytology and biopsy: Pyogranulomatous inflammation with numerous intracellular round to oval non-budding spherules which may have internal septations imparting a wheel or daisy-like appearance. Culture of tissue biopsy is needed for definitive diagnosis. Immunohistochemistry for causative organisms on formalin fixed tissue may be available. Labwork: Leukocytosis and hyperglobulinemia are common; chemistry panel abnormalities may reflect site of infection.	Surgical excision of localized lesions may be curative in immunocompetent animals, however distant lesions may recur in 50% of animals. For non-resectable lesions or disseminated disease, treatment is recommended with a combination of non-compounded itraconazole and amphotericin B for 2–4 months minimum, 1 month beyond clinical cure. In vitro susceptibility to posaconazole has been documented and voriconazole has been successfully used in human infections. Ketoconazole has been curative or palliative in some dogs; fluconazole is ineffective. Tetracycline is synergistic with amphotericin B in vitro and has been used in humans as part of combination therapy. Concurrent topical application of antifungal creams containing clotrimazole or nystatin to ulcerated skin lesions is recommended. Dogs with disseminated disease have a poor prognosis.

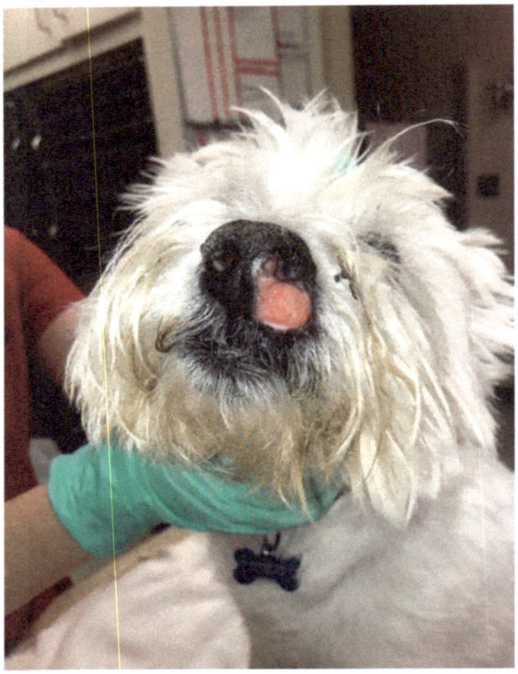

Figure 8.25A Ulcerative nasal dermatitis due to blastomycosis in a dog. *Source:* Image courtesy of Meghan Solc, DVM.

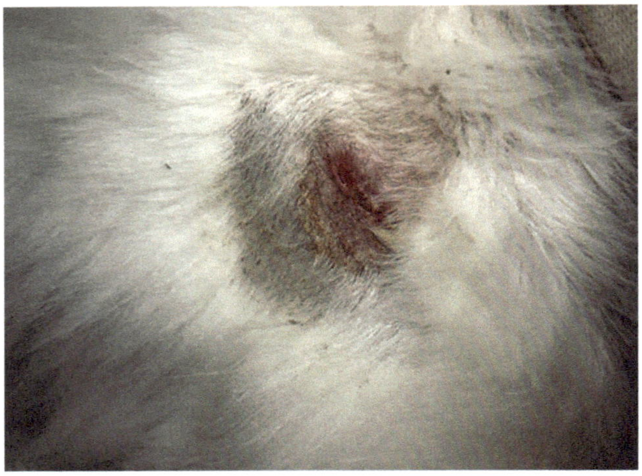

Figure 8.25B The same dog as in Figure 8.25A; ulcerative draining tracts were present on the shoulder. *Source:* Image courtesy of Meghan Solc, DVM.

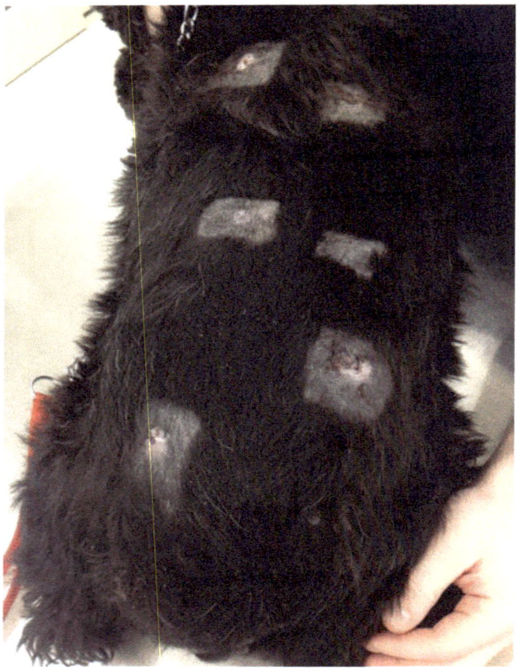

Figure 8.25C Multiple, crusted, truncal draining tracts caused by blastomycosis. *Source:* Image courtesy of Dr. Andrew Simpson, DACVD.

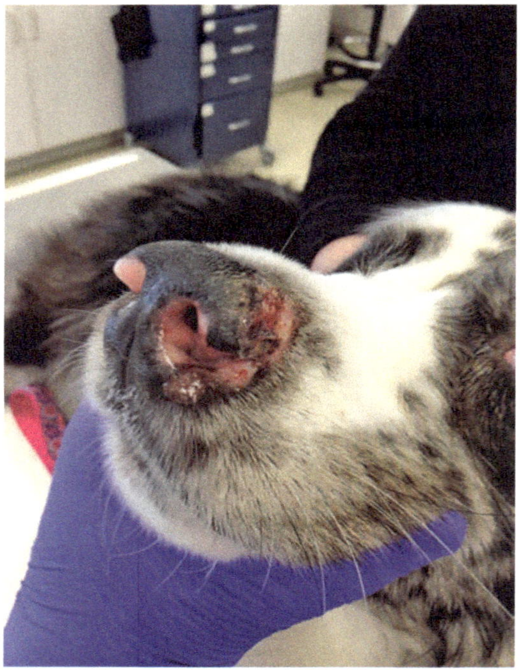

Figure 8.25D Nasal ulceration and depigmentation in a dog due to *Blastomyces* infection. *Source:* Image courtesy of Dr. Andrew Simpson, DACVD.

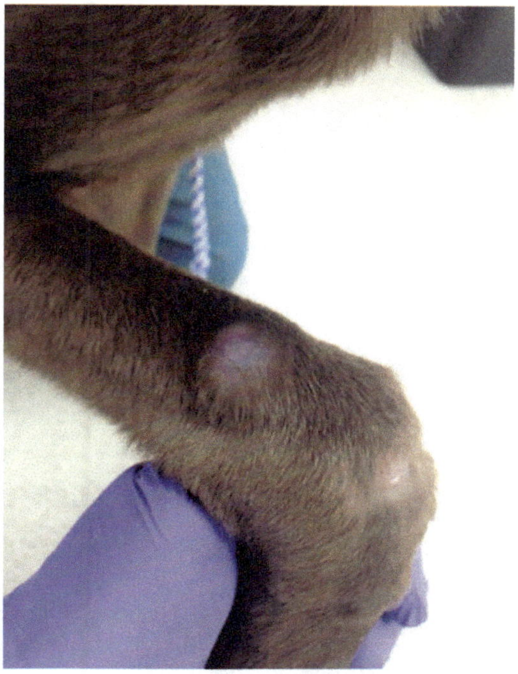

Figure 8.25E Alopecic nodules on the limb of a dog caused by blastomycosis. *Source:* Image courtesy of Dr. Andrew Simpson, DACVD.

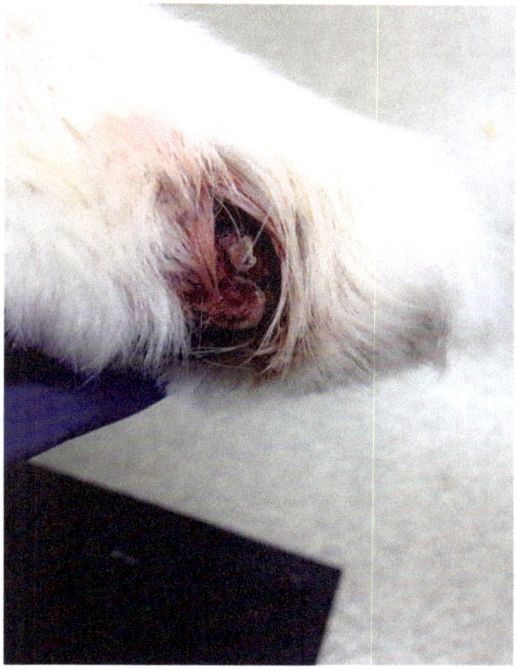

Figure 8.25F Purulent paronychia due to blastomycosis in a dog. *Source:* Image courtesy of Dr. Andrew Simpson, DACVD.

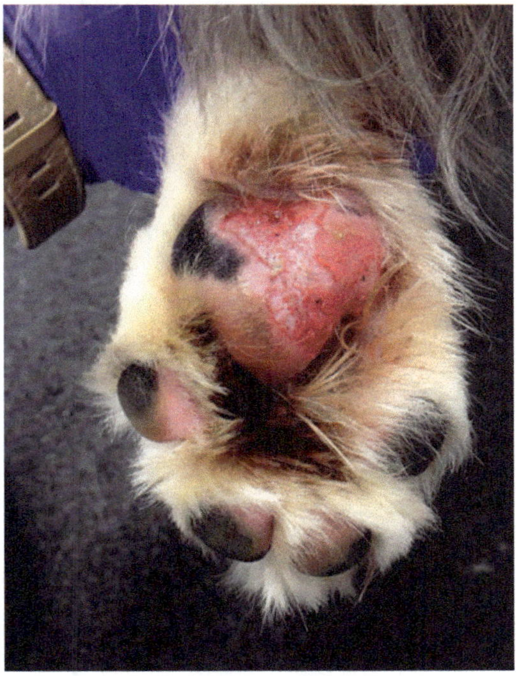

Figure 8.25G Paw pad swelling and ulceration in a dog caused by blastomycosis. *Source:* Image courtesy of Dr. Andrew Simpson, DACVD.

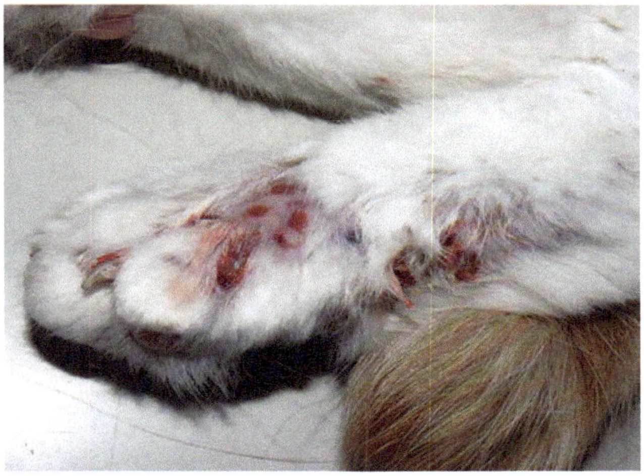

Figure 8.25H Draining tracts on the paw of a cat due to blastomycosis. *Source:* Image courtesy of Massimo Beccati, Medico Veterinario.

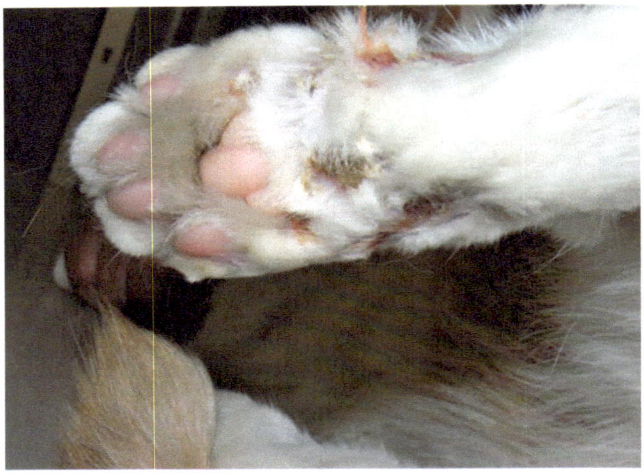

Figure 8.25I Draining tracts on the paw of a cat due to blastomycosis. *Source:* Image courtesy of Massimo Beccati, Medico Veterinario.

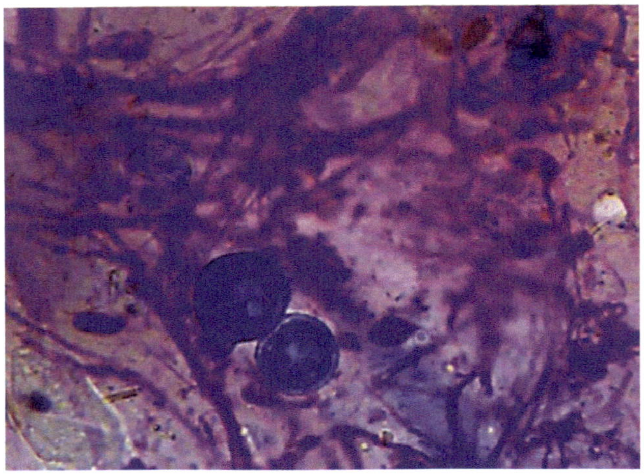

Figure 8.25J Cytology of a draining tract demonstrating inflammatory debris and a single large budding *Blastomyces* organism (100×). *Source:* Image courtesy of VIN and Drew Sullivan, DVM.

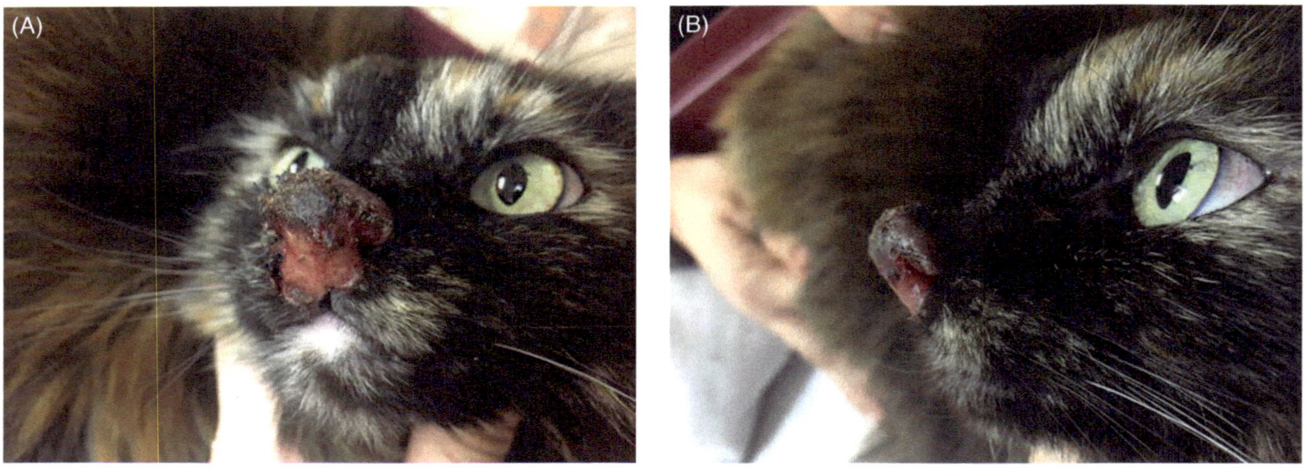

Figures 8.26A and B A cat with a swollen ulcerated nose caused by cryptococcosis. *Source:* Images courtesy of Sara Morar, DVM.

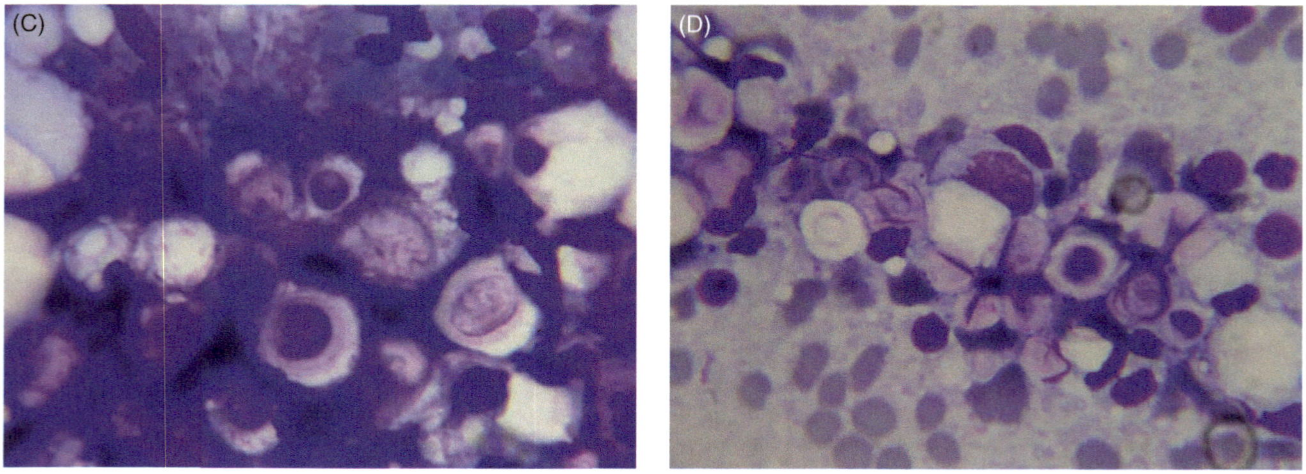

Figures 8.26C–D Cytology of a cat with cryptococcosis demonstrating round fungal organisms with thick capsules and narrow-based budding (100×).

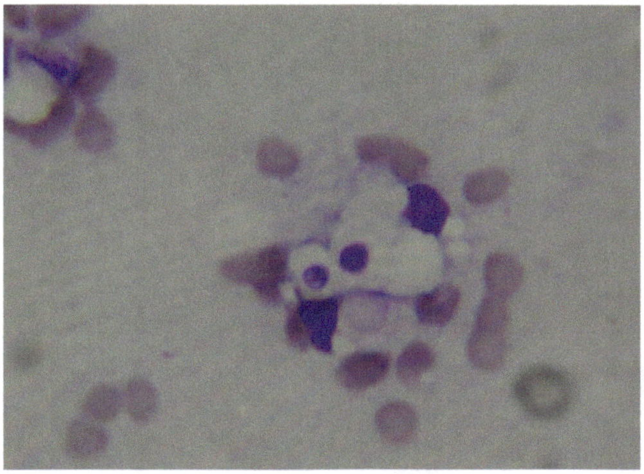

Figure 8.26E Cryptococcal yeast; red blood cells are also in the field (100×).

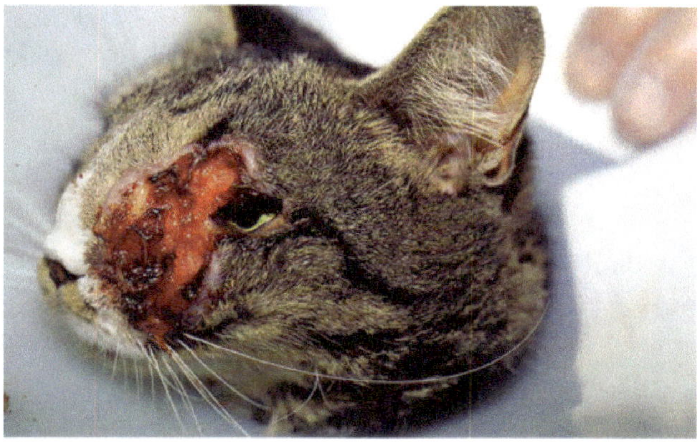

Figure 8.27A Ulcerative facial dermatitis caused by histoplasmosis. *Source:* Image courtesy of Dr. Michele Rosenbaum, DACVD.

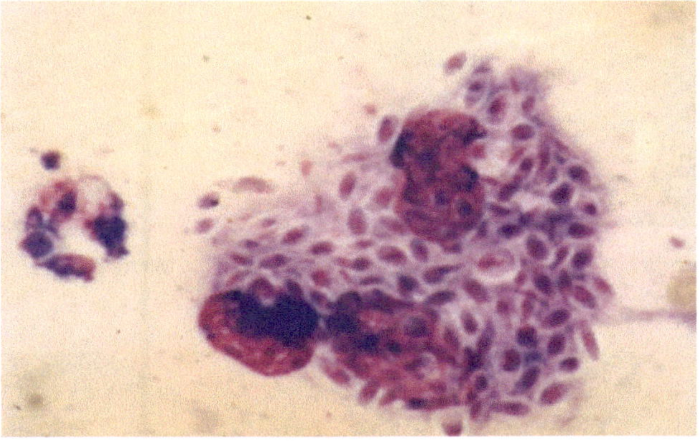

Figure 8.27B Cytology of the affected area demonstrates numerous small oval to oblong *Histoplasma* organisms within macrophage cytoplasm (100×). *Source:* Image courtesy of Dr. Michele Rosenbaum, DACVD.

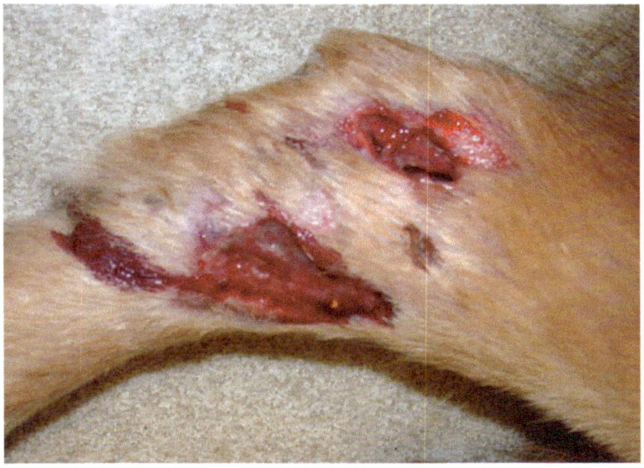

Figure 8.28A Ulcerations and draining tracts caused by coccidioidomycosis in a dog.

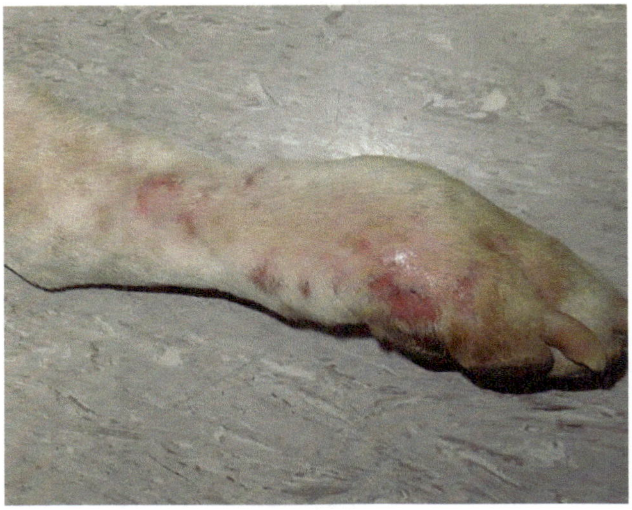

Figure 8.28B Cellulitis with small draining tracts on the paw of a dog due to coccidioidomycosis.

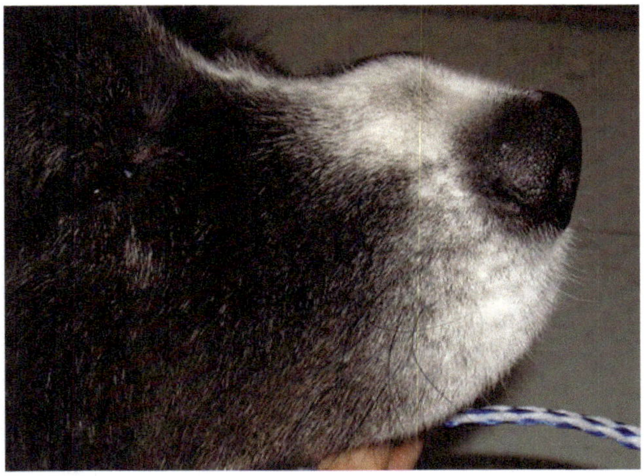

Figure 8.28C Swelling of the dorsal muzzle caused by coccidioidomycosis. *Source:* Images courtesy of Dr. Tom Lewis, DACVD.

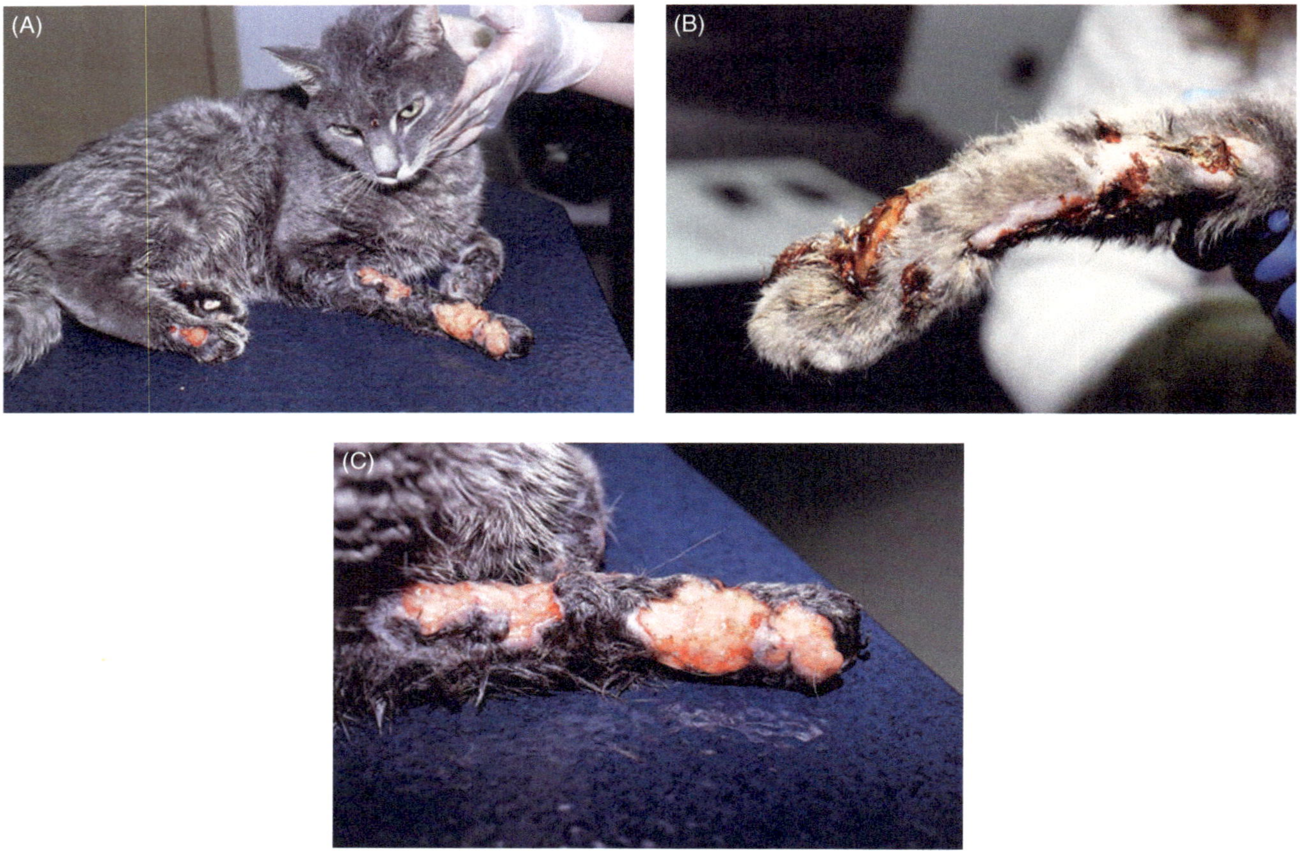

Figures 8.29A–C Ulcerated, draining lesions on the paws caused by sporotrichosis in a cat. *Source:* Images courtesy of Dr. Michele Rosenbaum, DACVD.

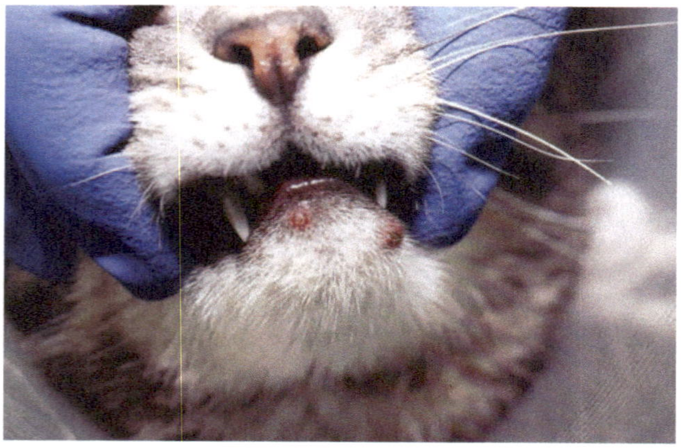

Figure 8.29D The same cat had crusted papules on the face and chin. *Source:* Image courtesy of Dr. Michele Rosenbaum, DACVD.

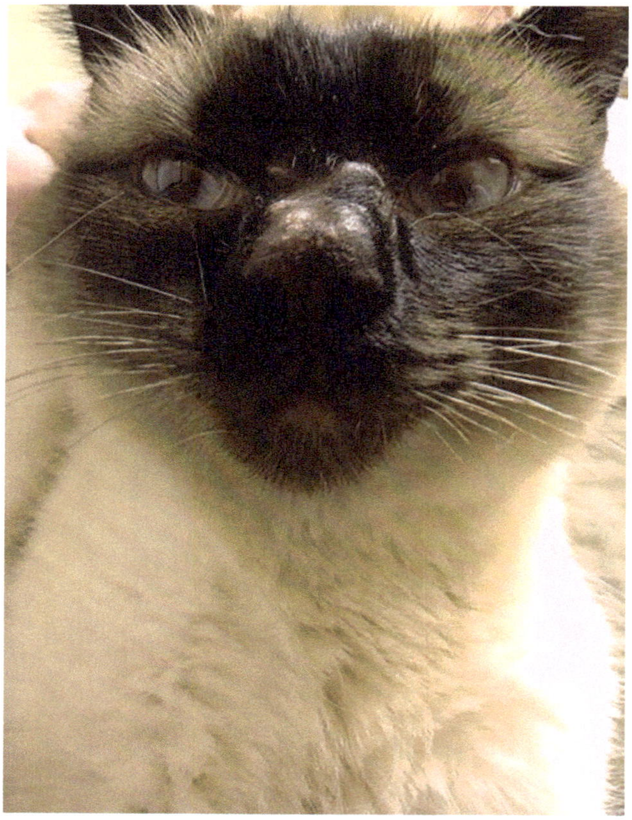

Figure 8.29E Swelling and alopecia on the dorsal nose of a cat with sporotrichosis. *Source:* Image courtesy of Dr. Jackie Campbell, DACVD.

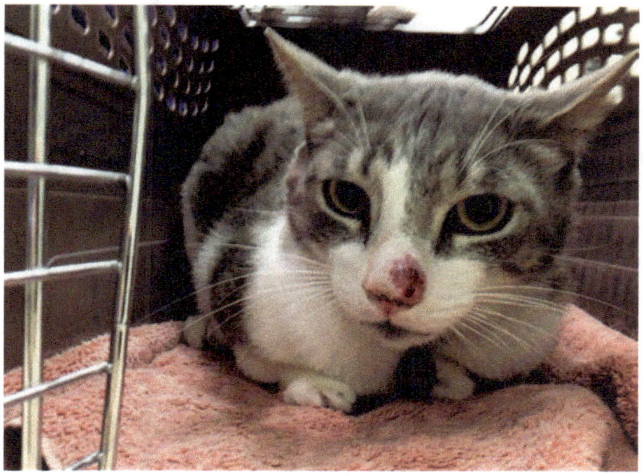

Figure 8.29F Alopecia, swelling, and draining tracts on the nose of a cat due to sporotrichosis. *Source:* Image courtesy of Dr. Heather Willis-Goulet, DACVD.

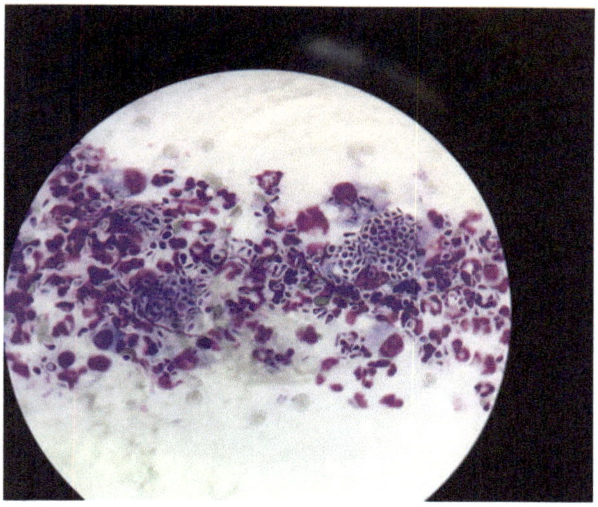

Figure 8.29G Pyogranulomatous inflammation with numerous oval to bullet-shaped *Sporothrix* organisms (100×). *Source:* Image courtesy of Dr. Jackie Campbell, DACVD.

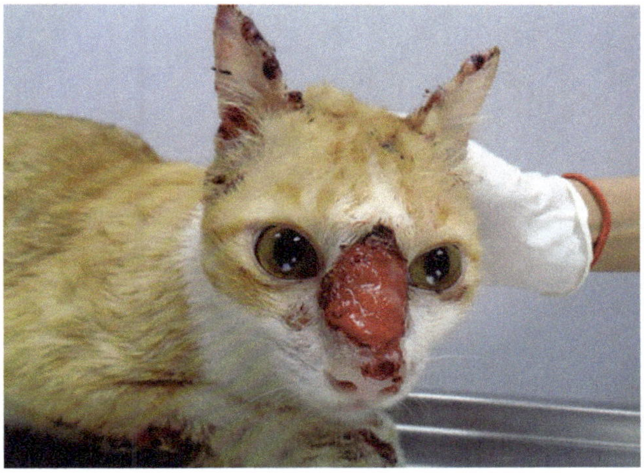

Figure 8.29H Severe facial ulceration and exudative dermatitis as well as crusted and eroded nodules on pinnae caused by sporotrichosis. *Source:* Image courtesy of Dr. Han Hock Siew.

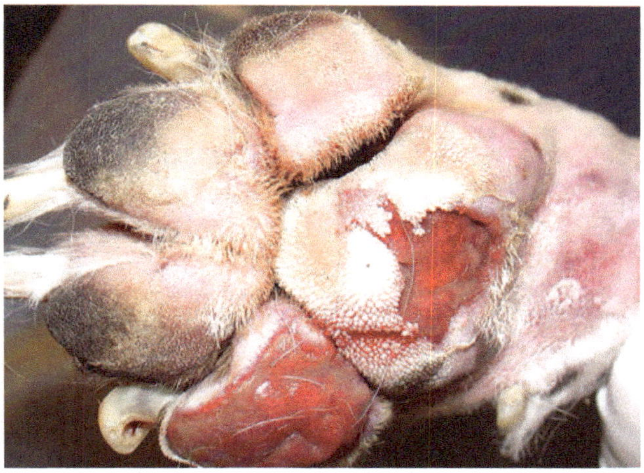

Figure 8.30A Ulcerative paw pad lesions caused by *Bipolaris* fungal infection in an immunosuppressed dog.

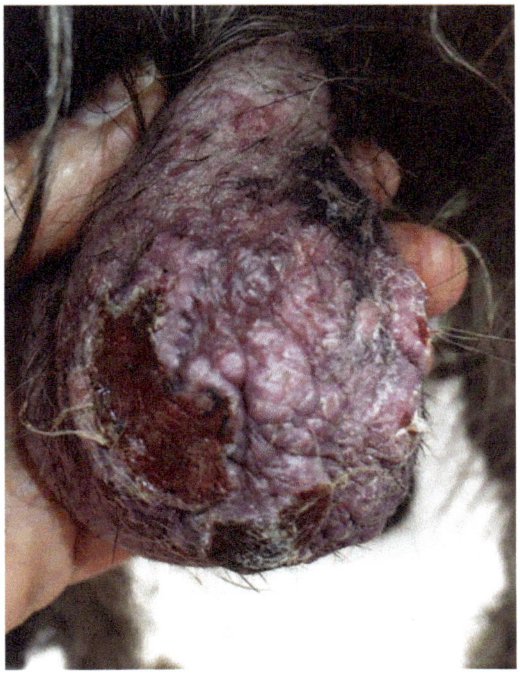

Figure 8.30B Scrotal phaeohyphomycosis in an immunosuppressed dog.

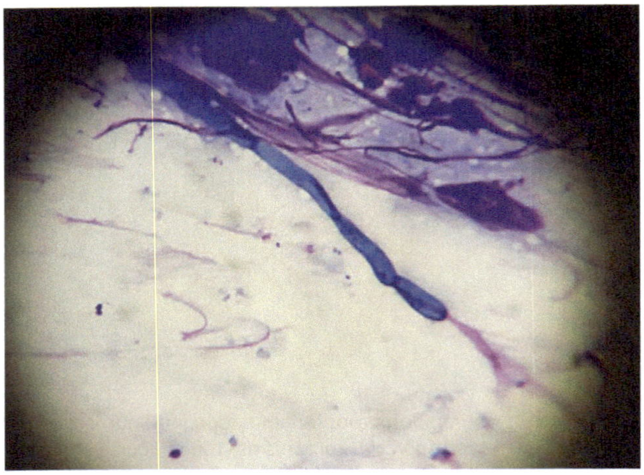

Figure 8.30C Surface cytology of the lesion in Figures 8.29B showed the pigmented fungal organism (100×).

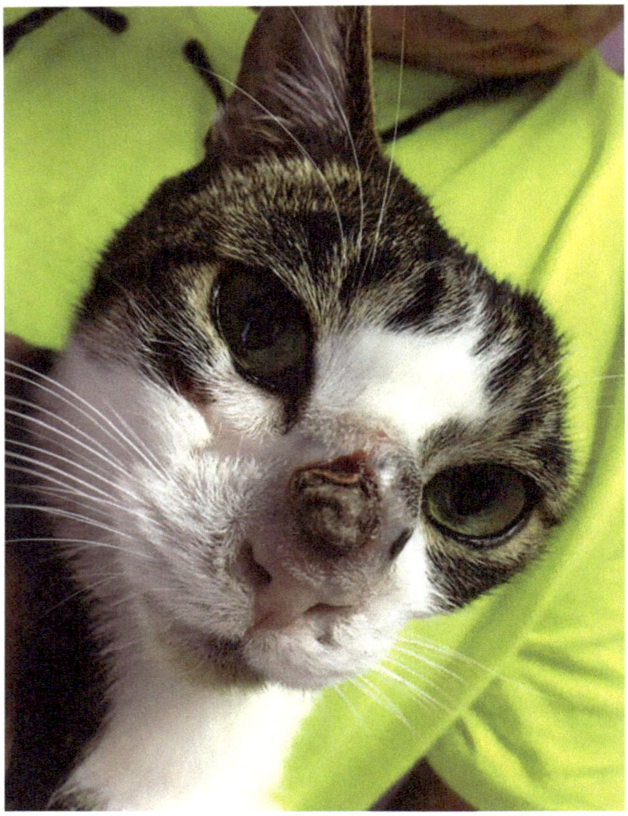

Figure 8.30D Phaeohyphomycosis causing swelling, ulceration, and crusting on the nose of a cat. *Source:* Image courtesy of VIN and Tammy Brown, DVM.

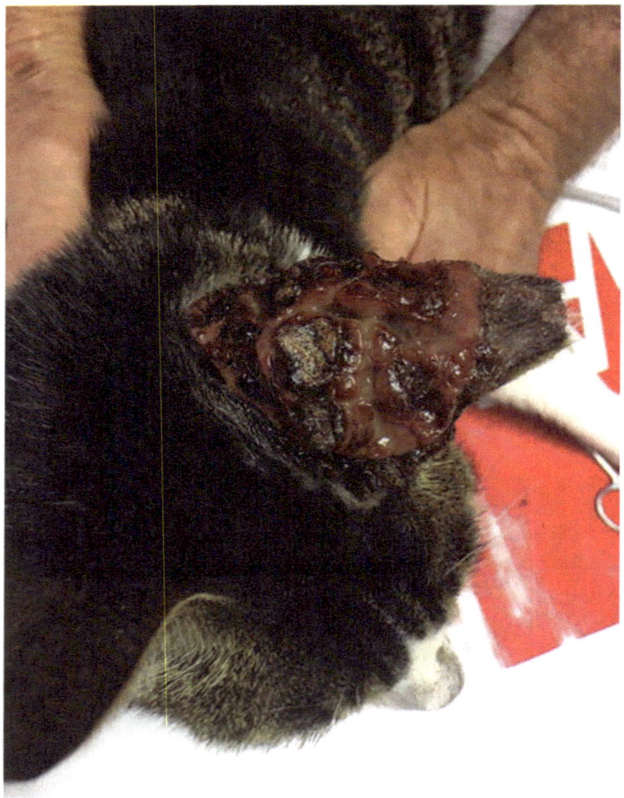

Figure 8.30E Severe ulceration and necrosis on the pinna of a cat due to phaeohyphomycosis. *Source:* Image courtesy of VIN and Tammy Brown, DVM.

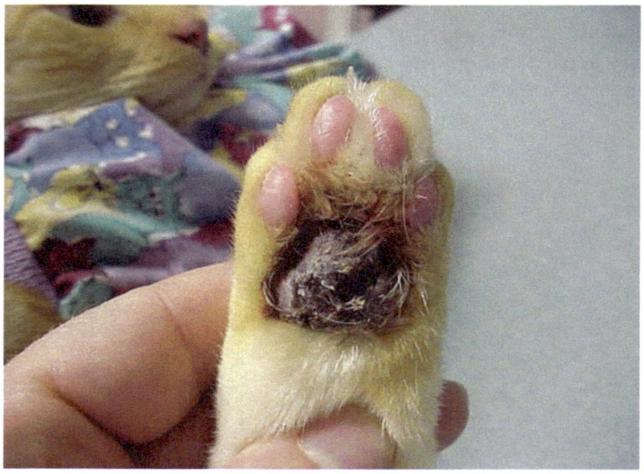

Figure 8.30F Ulceration and gray discoloration of a paw pad caused by phaeohyphomycosis. *Source:* Image courtesy of VIN and Stephen Bailey, DVM.

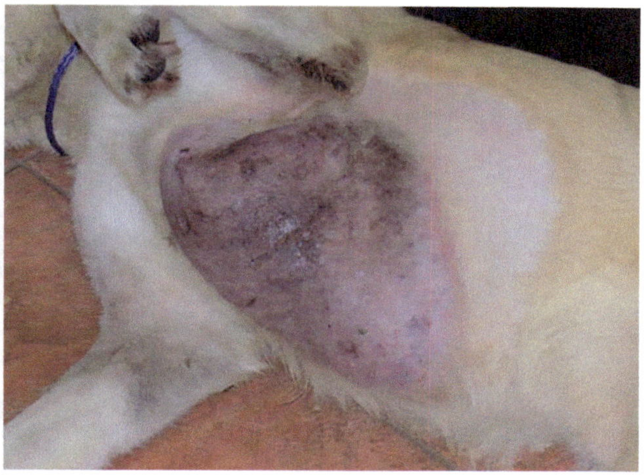

Figure 8.31A Cellulitis and draining tracts on the ventral chest of a dog caused by pythiosis. *Source:* Image courtesy of VIN and Ralph Pope, DVM.

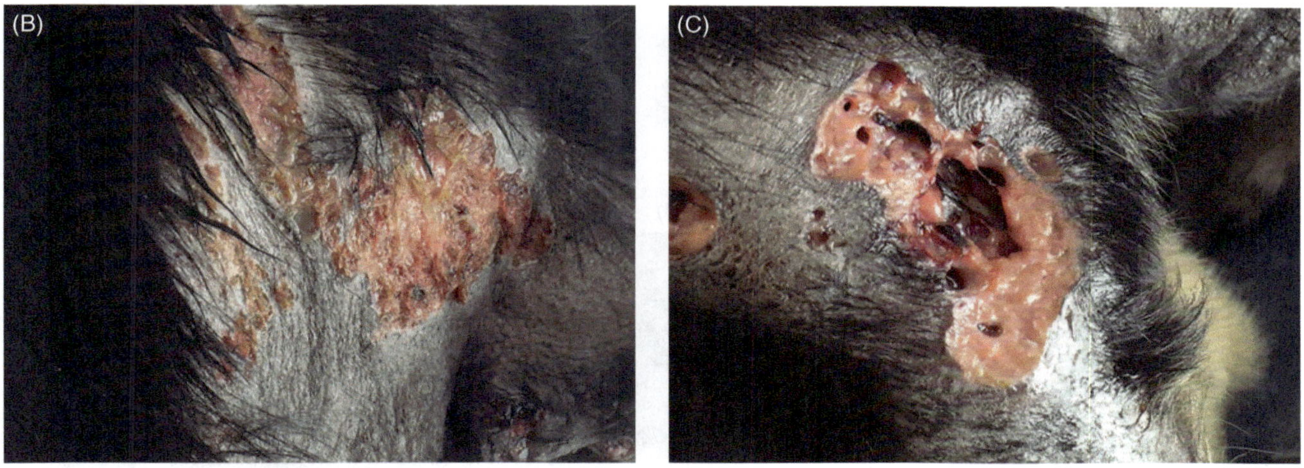

Figures 8.31B and C Ulcerative, purulent skin lesions with underlying bone exposure in a dog caused by pythiosis. *Source:* Images courtesy of Dr. Robert Schick, DACVD.

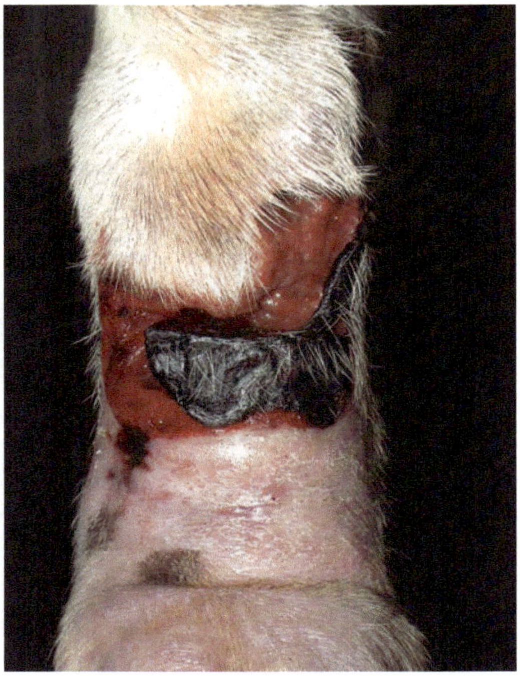

Figure 8.32A A necrotic, deeply ulcerative lesion on the metatarsus of a dog caused by lagenidiosis. *Source:* Image courtesy of Dr. Med. Vet. C. Nett-Mettler, Diplomate ACVD & ECVD.

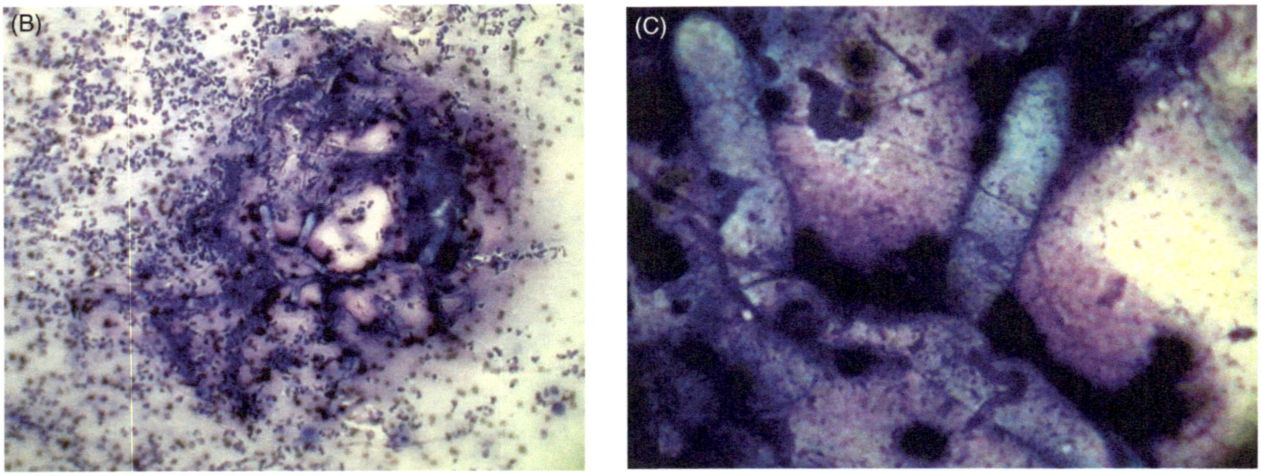

Figures 8.32B and C Cytology of the patient in Figure 8.32A demonstrating inflammatory cells and large, poorly staining hyphae with 90° branching characteristic of this organism (Fig. 8.32B is 4× and Fig. 8.32C is 100×). *Source:* Image courtesy of Dr. Med. Vet. C. Nett-Mettler, Diplomate ACVD & ECVD.

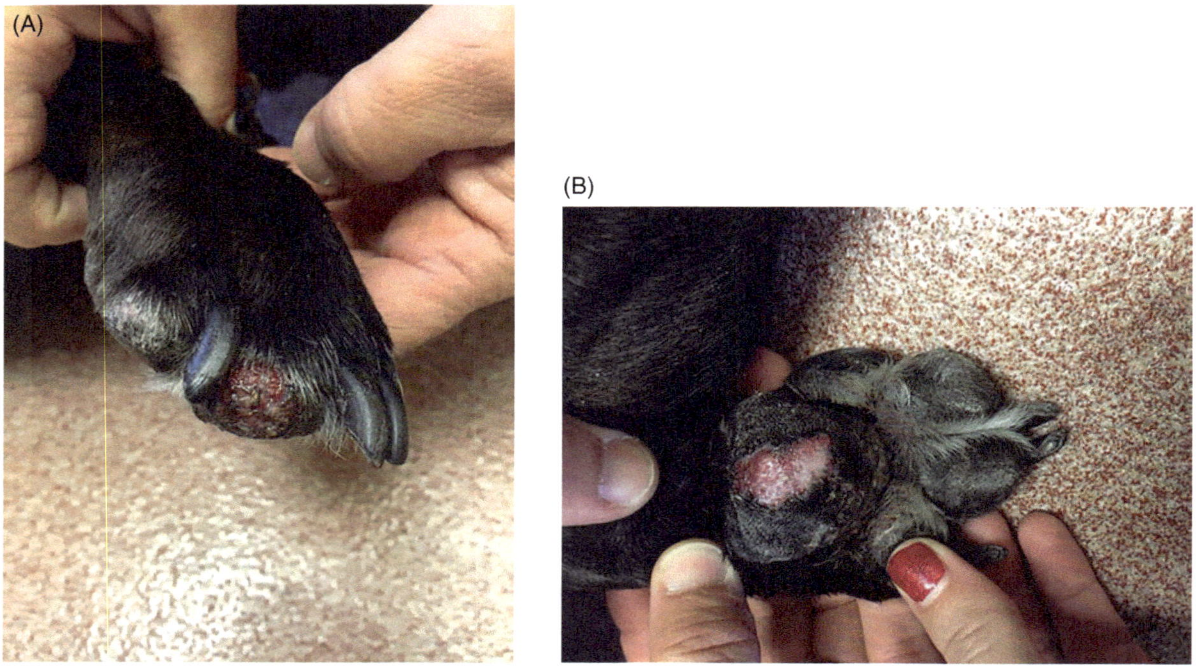

Figures 8.33A and B Ulcerative granulomas on the paw pads of a dog caused by *Prototheca* infection. *Source:* Images courtesy of Dr. Becca Mount, DACVD.

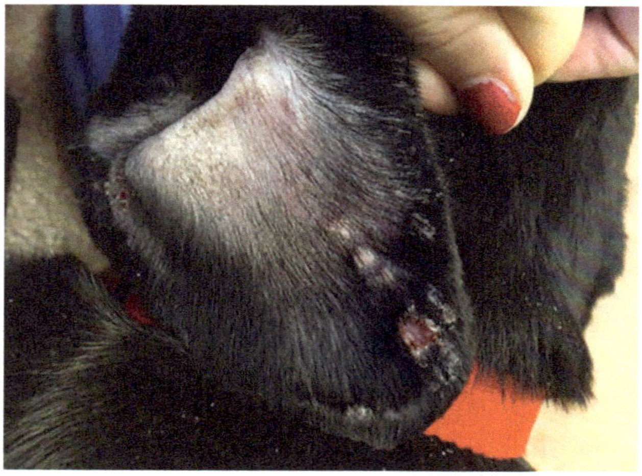

Figure 8.33C The same dog as in Figures 8.31A and 8.31B; similar crusted nodules were present on the pinna. *Source:* Image courtesy of Dr. Becca Mount, DACVD.

References/Further reading

Banovic, F., Olivry, T., Bäumer, W. et al. (2018). Diluted sodium hypochlorite (bleach) in dogs: antiseptic efficacy, local tolerability and *in vitro* effect on skin barrier function and inflammation. *Vet. Dermatol.* 29 (1): 6–e5.

Beco, L., Guaguère, E., Lorente Méndez, C. et al. (2013). Suggested guidelines for using systemic antimicrobials in bacterial skin infections (1): diagnosis based on clinical presentation, cytology and culture. *Vet. Rec.* 172 (3): 72–78.

Beco, L., Guaguère, E., Lorente Méndez, C. et al. (2013). Suggested guidelines for using systemic antimicrobials in bacterial skin infections (2): antimicrobial choice, treatment regimens and compliance. *Vet. Rec.* 172 (6): 156–160.

Connolly, P., Hage, C.A., Bariola, J.R. et al. (2012). Blastomyces dermatitidis antigen detection by quantitative enzyme immunoassay. *Clin. Vaccine Immunol.* 19: 53–56.

Coyner, K. (2011). Skills laboratory: how to perform skin scraping and skin surface cytology. *Vet. Med.* 106 (11): 554–563.

Coyner, K. (2012). The emergence and prevalence of MRSA, MRSP, and MRSS in pets and people. *Vet. Med.* 107 (12): 516–521.

Coyner, K. (2013). Managing MRSA, MRSP, and MRSS dermatologic infections in pets. *Vet. Med.* 108 (1): 32–38.

Crothers, S.L., White, S.D., Ihrke, P.J., and Affolter, V.K. (2009). Sporotrichosis: a retrospective evaluation of 23 cases seen in northern California (1987–2007). *Vet. Dermatol.* 20 (4): 249–259.

Duclos, D.D., Hargis, A.M., and Hanley, P.W. (2008). Pathogenesis of canine interdigital palmar and plantar comedones and follicular cysts, and their response to laser surgery. *Vet. Dermatol.* 19 (3): 134–141.

Ginel, P.J., Pérez, J., Molleda, J.M. et al. (1997). Cutaneous protothecosis in a dog. *Vet. Rec.* 140 (25): 651–653.

Girard, C. and Higgins, R. (1999). *Staphylococcus intermedius* cellulitis and toxic shock in a dog. *Can. Vet. J.* 40: 501–502.

Grooters, A.M. (2003). Pythiosis, lagenidiosis, and zygomycosis in small animals. *Vet. Clin. Small Anim.* 33: 695–720.

Greene, C.E. (ed.) (2012). *Infectious Diseases of the Dog and Cat.* St. Louis, MO: Elsevier Saunders.

Greene, C.E., Brockus, C.W., Currin, M.P., and Jones, C.J. (2002). Infection with *Basidiobolus ranarum* in two dogs. *J. Am. Vet. Med. Assoc.* 221 (4): 528–532.

Gremião, I.D., Menezes, R.C., Schubach, T.M. et al. (2015). Feline sporotrichosis: epidemiological and clinical aspects. *Med. Mycol.* 53 (1): 15–21.

Gremião, I., Schubach, T., Pereira, S. et al. (2011). Treatment of refractory feline sporotrichosis with a combination of intralesional amphotericin B and oral itraconazole. *Aust. Vet. J.* 89 (9): 346–351.

Gunn-Moore, D.A. (2014). Feline mycobacterial infections. *Vet. J.* 201 (2): 230–238.

Hillier, A., Alcorn, J.R., Cole, L.K. et al. (2006). Pyoderma caused by *Pseudomonas aeruginosa* infection in dogs: 20 cases. *Vet. Dermatol.* 17 (6): 432–439.

Hillier, A., Lloyd, D.H., Weese, J.S. et al. (2014). Guidelines for the diagnosis and antimicrobial therapy of canine superficial bacterial folliculitis (Antimicrobial Guidelines Working Group of the International Society for Companion Animal Infectious Diseases). *Vet. Dermatol.* 25 (3): 163–175e42–3.

Kloos, I., Straubinger, R.K., Werckenthin, C., and Mueller, R.S. (2013). Residual antibacterial activity of dog hairs after therapy with antimicrobial shampoos. *Vet. Dermatol.* 24 (2): 250–e54.

Laporte, C., Boothe, D., Cruz-Espindola, C. et al. (2016). Quality assessment of compounded fluconazole capsules and oral suspensions in the United States. *Vet. Dermatol.* 27 (Supplement S1): 6–121.

Loeffler, A., Cobb, M.A., and Bond, R. (2011). Comparison of a chlohexidine and a benzoyl peroxide shampoo as sole treatment in canine superficial pyoderma. *Vet Rec* 169 (10): 249.

Loreto, E.S., Tondolo, J.S.M., Zanette, R.A. et al. (2014). Update on pythiosis immunobiology and immunotherapy. *World J. Immunol.* 4 (2): 88–97.

Mackey, P.E., Cappe, K.G., Mani, R. et al. (2015). Disseminated *Conidiobolus incongruus* in a dog: a case report and literature review. *Med. Mycol. Case Rep.* 8: 24–28.

Magalhaes, R. and Loeffler, A. (2010). Risk factors for meticillin-resistant *Staphylococcus aureus* (MRSA) infection in dogs and cats: a case–control study. *Vet. Res.* 41: 55.

Mawby, D.I., Whittemore, J.C., Genger, S., and Papich, M.G. (2014). Bioequivalence of orally administered generic, compounded, and innovator-formulated itraconazole in healthy dogs. *J. Vet. Intern. Med.* 28 (1): 72–77.

Mendoza, L. and Newton, J.C. (2005). Immunology and immunotherapy of the infections caused by *Pythium insidiosum*. *Med. Mycol.* 43 (6): 477–486.

Miller, C., Prescott, J., Mathews, K. et al. (1996). Streptococcal toxic shock syndrome in dogs. *J. Am. Vet. Med. Assoc.* 209: 1421–1426.

Miller, W.H., Griffen, C.E., and Campbell, K.L. (2013). *Muller and Kirk's Small Animal Dermatology*, 7e. St Louis, MO: Elsevier Mosby.

Moriello, K. (2014). Feline dermatophytosis. Aspects pertinent to disease management in single and multiple cat situations. *J. Feline Med. Surg.* 16 (5): 419–431.

Moriello, K. (2016). Decontamination of laundry exposed to *Microsporum canis* hairs and spores. *J. Feline Med. Surg.* 18 (6): 457–461.

Moriello, K. (2017). Decontamination of carpet exposed to *Microsporum canis* hairs and spores. *J. Feline Med. Surg.* 19 (4): 435–439.

Moriello, K., Coyner, K., Paterson, S., and Mignon, B. (2017). Diagnosis and treatment of dermatophytosis in dogs and cats: Clinical Consensus Guidelines of the World Association for Veterinary Dermatology. *Vet. Dermatol.* 28 (3): 266–e68.

Moriello, K., Coyner, K., Trimmer, A. et al. (2013). Treatment of shelter cats with oral terbinafine and concurrent lime sulphur rinses. *Vet. Dermatol.* 26 (6): 618–620.

Morris, D.O., Loeffler, A., Davis, M.F. et al. (2017). Recommendations for approaches to meticillin-resistant staphylococcal infections of small animals: diagnosis, therapeutic considerations and preventative measures: Clinical Consensus Guidelines of the World Association for Veterinary Dermatology. *Vet. Dermatol.* 28 (3): 304–e69.

Mourning, A.C., Patterson, E.E., Kirsch, E.J. et al. (2015). Evaluation of an enzyme immunoassay for antibodies to a recombinant *Blastomyces* adhesin-1 repeat antigen as an aid in the diagnosis of blastomycosis in dogs. *JAVMA* 247 (10): 1133–1138.

Newbury, S., Moriello, K., Coyner, K. et al. (2015). Management of endemic *Microsporum canis* dermatophytosis in an open admission shelter: a field study. *J. Feline Med. Surg.* 17 (4): 342–347.

Pereira, D.I., Botton, S.A., Azevedo, M.I. et al. (2013). Canine gastrointestinal pythiosis treatment by combined antifungal and immunotherapy and review of published studies. *Mycopathologia* 176: 309–315.

Prescott, J., Miller, C., Mathews, K. et al. (1997). Update on canine streptococcal toxic shock syndrome and necrotizing fasciitis. *Can. Vet. J.* 38: 241–242.

Renschler, J., Albers, A., Sinclair-Mackling, H., and Wheat, L.J. (2018). Comparison of compounded, generic, and innovator-formulated itraconazole in dogs and cats. *J. Am. Anim. Hosp. Assoc.* 54 (4): 195–200.

Simões, D.M., Dial, S.M., Coyner, K.S. et al. (2016). Retrospective analysis of cutaneous lesions in 23 canine and 17 feline cases of coccidiodomycosis seen in Arizona, USA (2009–2015). *Vet. Dermatol.* 27 (5): 346–e87.

Spector, D., Legendre, A.M., Wheat, J. et al. (2008). Antigen and antibody testing for the diagnosis of blastomycosis in dogs. *J. Vet. Intern. Med.* 22: 839–843.

Udenberg, T., Griffin, C., Rosenkrantz, W. et al. (2015). Efficacy of 0.011% topical hypochlorous acid for the treatment of canine superficial pyoderma. *Vet. Dermatol.* 26: 133.

Uri, M., Buckley, L.M., Marriage, L. et al. (2016). A pilot study comparing in vitro efficacy of topical preparations against veterinary pathogens. *Vet. Dermatol.* 27 (3): 152–e39. https://doi.org/10.1111/vde.12306. Epub 2016 Apr 24.

Weber, S.G., Gold, H.S., Hooper, D.C. et al. (2003). Fluoroquinolones and the risk for meticillin-resistant *Staphylococcus aureus in* hospitalized patients. *Emerg. Infect. Dis.* 9 (11): 1415–1422.

Weese, J.S. and van Duijkeren, E. (2010). Meticillin-resistant *Staphylococcus aureus* and *Staphylococcus pseudintermedius* in veterinary medicine. *Vet. Microbiol.* 140: 418–429.

Weese, J.S., Faires, M.C., Frank, L.A. et al. (2012). Factors associated with meticillin-resistant versus meticillin-susceptible *Staphylococcus pseudintermedius* infection in dogs. *JAVMA* 240 (12): 1450–1455.

Wilson, A.G., KuKanich, K.S., Hanzlicek, A.S., and Payton, M.E. (2018). Clinical signs, treatment, and prognostic factors for dogs with histoplasmosis. *JAVMA* 252 (2): 201–209.

Young, R., Buckley, L., McEwan, N., and Nuttall, T. (2012). Comparative *in vitro* efficacy of antimicrobial shampoos: A pilot study. *Vet. Dermatol.* 23 (1): 36–40.

Zur, G., Gurevich, B., and Elad, D. (2016). Prior antimicrobial use as a risk factor for resistance in selected *Staphylococcus pseudintermedius* isolates from the skin and ears of dogs. *Vet. Dermatol.* 27 (6): 468.

9

Viral, rickettsial, and protozoal dermatologic diseases

Kimberly S. Coyner, DVM, DACVD

Dermatology Clinic for Animals, Lacey, WA, USA

Clinical Atlas of Canine and Feline Dermatology, First Edition. Edited by Kimberly S. Coyner.

Companion website: www.wiley.com/go/coyner/dermatology

Table 9.1 Viral dermatologic diseases.

Disease	Clinical signs	Diagnosis	Treatment
Feline herpesvirus dermatitis (A.k.a. feline rhinotracheitis virus; Figures 9.1–9.4, Chapter 3, Figure 3.11B) DNA virus. Most infected cats become chronic carriers; stress or immunosuppressive medications can cause reactivation of clinical disease.	Acute infection symptoms include sneezing, oculonasal discharge, conjunctivitis +/− corneal or lingual ulcers, fever, lethargy, and hyporexia. Cutaneous lesions can include crusting, erythema, and erosions/ulcers on the haired dorsal nose, the non-haired nasal planum, and/or the eyelids; rarely, crusting lesions on other locations such as the trunk and paws may occur. Lesions may be pruritic or non-pruritic, can be slowly progressive over several weeks and secondary bacterial infection may occur.	Clinical presentation, cytology to screen for secondary infection. Biopsy: intranuclear viral inclusion bodies may be present but can be difficult to find. Necrosis of sweat glands is a unique feature. Eosinophils are prominent and can mimic allergic dermatoses; careful evaluation by a dermatopathologist is recommended. Herpesvirus PCR testing of skin biopsy.	Supportive care for acute infection includes fluids, nutritional care, antibiotics for secondary bacterial infection (doxycycline or clavulanated amoxicillin). Steroids are contraindicated. Famciclovir: Typical dose is 125 mg PO BID in adult cats, or up to 40–90 mg/kg BID-TID; monitor renal function and reduce dose in cats with renal disease. Treat until skin disease has resolved, which can take several weeks. Topical antiviral treatment with acyclovir cold sore cream applied daily to lesions or topical imiquimod applied 2–3 consecutive days per week may be helpful (transient worsening of inflammation may occur with imiquimod). Recombinant feline interferon omega: One cat with herpes virus dermatitis responded well to 6 injections administered over 23 days of 1.5 million units (MU) kg of rFeIFN-ω, in 4 treatments; half the interferon dose was injected perilesionally and intradermally and the other half subcutaneously; the other 2 treatments were SQ (subcutaneous) only (Gutzwiller et al. 2007). Other varied interferon doses and administration protocols are in the literature for treatment of mostly respiratory and ocular herpes, including: Recombinant human IFNα at 10 000 U/kg subcutaneously once daily for 14 days or 1 million units/m2 SQ three times weekly. Recombinant feline IFNω three 5-day cycles of once-daily subcutaneous injections of 1 million units/kg on days 0, 14, and 60. Oral lysine: In one study, once-daily oral administration of 400 mg of L-lysine to cats latently infected with FHV-1 was associated with reduced viral shedding following changes in housing and husbandry but not following corticosteroid administration, however a recent meta-analysis found no demonstrable benefit for L-lysine administration for the treatment of herpes (Maggs, Nasisse, and Kass, 2003).

Feline calicivirus dermatitis RNA virus. 20–30% of infected cats become chronic carriers.	Acute symptoms: Sneezing, conjunctivitis, oculonasal discharge, oral ulcerations, fever, lethargy, anorexia. Cutaneous lesions may include ulcerations on the lips, nasal planum, and paw pads. A pustular, inguinal dermatitis has been described in 2 cats post spay. In the early 2000s a new virulent form of calicivirus emerged which causes facial and limb edema, liver disease, sepsis, and 30–50% mortality especially in adult cats; some affected cats also have cutaneous lesions including crusting and ulceration of the nose, lips, pinnae, eyelids, and paws.	Clinical signs. Biopsy: Epidermal necrosis, keratinocyte ballooning degeneration +/− edema and vasculitis. Calicivirus PCR or IHC (immunohistochemistry) on skin biopsy or PCR on conjunctival/oral swabs.	Supportive care for acute infection includes fluids, nutritional care, antibiotics for secondary bacterial infection. Traditional antiviral drugs ineffective (due to effect on only DNA or retroviruses) or toxic to cats (ribavirin). Feline interferon-ω has been shown to inhibit FCV replication in vitro (Radford et al. 2009), however, controlled studies in clinical cases have not been published.
Viral papillomas *Dogs* (Figures 9.5–9.16) DNA virus. There are at least 18 types of papillomavirus in dogs, and most animals harbor papillomaviruses on the skin without clinical infection due to immune control. Immune suppression and genetic factors contribute to development of clinical lesions. Papillomaviruses are spread by direct contact and opportunistic viral infection occurs after skin or mucosal injury exposes basal epithelial cells to the virus which then replicates in the infected epithelial cell as it differentiates then is eventually shed containing infectious virus particles at the skin surface.	Six different clinical syndromes occur due to infection of different body sites and different types of papilloma viruses: Oral papillomas (CPV1): One to multiple, initially smooth, raised, white to pink dermal masses progressing to exophytic white, pink, or gray masses on the lips and mucous membranes +/− tongue. Lesions occur acutely and progress or wax and wane over several weeks. Most cases will spontaneously resolve within 6–8 weeks, though regression may take up to one year in some dogs. Rarely, massive oral papilloma infections filling the oral cavity and esophagus can occur in dogs with presumed immunosuppression. Cutaneous papillomas (CPV 1, 2, 6, 7) exophytic form: Single to multiple, pink to gray, pedunculated, small dermal masses often on the head and paws; usually occur in older dogs. Inverted papillomas: Raised, pink to gray, smooth, round lesions with a central keratin containing cup/pore which occur most commonly on the ventral trunk in young dogs.	Clinical appearance, biopsy: Epidermal hyperplasia with characteristic koilocytes and epidermal cells with intracytoplasmic viral inclusions. Viral immunohistochemistry and PCR usually utilized in research setting.	Azithromycin 10 mg/kg PO once daily × 10 days. Surgical or laser excision, and cryosurgery can be used for persistent lesions. Interferon alpha 1 million IU SQ 3 times per week, or oral interferon 1000–20 000 IU PO daily (anecdotal). Topical 5% imiquimod applied once daily to isolated cutaneous papillomas can be helpful. Discontinue/avoid immunosuppressive medications including steroids, cyclosporine, and oclacitinib. No commercial vaccine is currently available for canine papillomaviruses. However, at the time of writing recombinant vaccines for CPV1 and CPV2 with an anecdotal response rate of 40–50% when used for the treatment of papillomavirus infection were available from Dr. Hang Yuan at the Center for Cell Reprogramming, Georgetown University, Washington, USA.

(*Continued*)

Table 9.1 Viral dermatologic diseases (Continued)

Disease	Clinical signs	Diagnosis	Treatment
Viral papilloma (*dogs*, continued) Cell mediated immunity is required for resolution of clinical infection, though antiviral IgG blocks infection of new basal cells.	Cutaneous viral pigmented plaques (Chi-papillomavirus triggered): Multiple, round to oval, black, 1–10 mm diameter macules which become raised and scaly, occur most commonly on the ventral trunk and medial limbs; Pugs and Miniature Schnauzers are predisposed. Lesions can spontaneously regress, or persist and spread; rare malignant transformation to squamous cell carcinoma can occur. Venereal papillomas: Raised, papillomatous plaques on penile or vaginal mucosa; not well described. Pedal papillomas: One to multiple, raised, exophytic masses involving the paw pads and/or interdigital areas; lesions can be painful or pruritic and secondary bacterial infection can occur; occur most commonly in young dogs.		
Viral papillomas *Cats* (Figures 9.17–9.20) There are at least 4 types of feline papillomaviruses.	Four clinical syndromes: Cutaneous papillomas: Rarely described, single, small, exophytic alopecic lesions. Oral papillomas: Rarely described; sessile to papillomatous masses on the tongue which likely spontaneously resolve. Viral plaques and Bowenoid in situ carcinomas (BISC) (usually caused by FcaPV-2): Viral plaques are multiple, oval, usually pigmented, slightly raised, scaly plaques <1 cm diameter; can progress to BISC which are larger, can be ulcerated and crusted and can eventually progress to invasive squamous cell carcinoma. Bowen's lesions are more common in older cats and on the head, neck, and limbs. Viral plaques and BISCs can variably spontaneously resolve, remain static or slowly increase in size and number, though lesions in Devon Rex and Sphynx cats tend to be more rapidly progressive and aggressive with development of invasive squamous cell carcinoma.	Clinical presentation. Biopsy	Cutaneous papillomas: Surgical excision curative. Viral plaques and BISC: Surgical or laser excision can be curative but new lesions can develop in other locations; topical 5% imiquimod cream applied q1–2 days can cause partial to complete lesion regression but can cause side effects such as local inflammation, vomiting, increased liver enzymes, and neutropenia; keep Elizabethan collar on during treatment to prevent grooming/ingestion. Sarcoids: Wide surgical excision is the treatment of choice if possible, however, lesions tend to be locally invasive and recurrence is common; other treatment considerations may include radiation therapy and topical imiquimod.

Viral papilloma (*cats*, continued)	Feline sarcoid (cutaneous fibropapillomas): Caused by cross-species infection by bovine papillomavirus BPV-14. Occur most commonly as firm, pink, smooth to exophytic, non-ulcerated masses on the nose, lips, and digits of young adult cats living in rural environments. PV DNA is localized to dermal mesenchymal tissue, not the epidermis.		
Cowpox virus Rodents are natural hosts, cats are infected though bites sustained when catching infected rodents; cat to cat transmission is uncommon. Most commonly occurs in outdoor cats living in rural environments Endemic in Europe and western Asia. Zoonotic.	Most common primary lesion is a single ulcerated nodule on the head, neck, and front leg or paw. 1–3 weeks after initial infection, widespread secondary skin lesions develop anywhere on the body and consist of small epidermal nodules which ulcerate +/− oral vesicles/ulceration. Cutaneous lesions may be pruritic. Secondary bacterial infection may occur. Some cats have systemic signs of fever, anorexia, lethargy, respiratory disease, and diarrhea. Dogs can develop infection characterized by single, ulcerated nodules which resolve spontaneously.	Clinical signs. Skin biopsy: Ballooning degeneration of epithelial cells with necrosis of epithelium and outer root sheath; eosinophilic, intracytoplasmic inclusion bodies are present within keratinocytes of epidermis and hair follicles as well as sebaceous glands. Serologic testing: Cannot differentiate cowpox from *Orthopoxviruses*. Virus isolation from fresh tissue or PCR preferred for diagnosis.	No specific therapy; in most cats, skin lesions heal spontaneously over 4–5 weeks, permanent scarring may occur. In kittens and immunosuppressed cats, severe generalized cowpox infections can be fatal. Supportive care, fluids, nutritional support, treat secondary bacterial infection if present. Steroids are contraindicated. Advise owners of zoonosis risk.
Feline infectious peritonitis (FIP) A *Coronavirus* (RNA virus) ubiquitous in domestic cats, is shed in the feces, and is particularly common where conditions are crowded.	In addition to typical systemic symptoms, occasionally described to cause raised intradermal papules which may ulcerate on the neck, legs, and trunk due to vasculitis. Skin fragility has been reported in one cat with FIP.	Biopsy: Vasculitis, granulomatous inflammation. Please refer to appropriate infectious disease texts for details on diagnosis of FIP.	Prednisolone used at anti-inflammatory to immunosuppressive doses can be temporarily palliative and helpful to reduce inflammation and stimulate appetite. Newer therapies under development include protease inhibitors and Polyprenyl Immunostimulant; please refer to appropriate infectious disease texts for details on treatment of FIP.
Canine distemper (Figure 9.21) A *Paramyxovirus* which usually affects non-vaccinated dogs <4 mo old.	Skin lesions can include an acute pustular dermatitis on the groin, or later in the disease marked nasodigital hyperkeratosis ("hard pad disease") Other symptoms include fever, purulent oculonasal discharge, cough/pneumonia, vomiting, diarrhea. In some dogs that survive the acute illness phase, later onset seizures or myoclonus can develop.	Clinical signs CBC: Lymphopenia, hypoalbuminemia, hypo or hyperglobulinemia. Serology: Elevated distemper IgM. Skin biopsies: Keratinocyte viral inclusion bodies, occasional multinucleate, syncytial giant cells in epidermis. Viral immunohistochemistry on skin biopsies or conjunctival swabs.	Supportive care: Fluids, nutritional support, antibiotics for secondary bacterial infection, anti-seizure medications. There is no specific antiviral therapy. Severe encephalitis may require euthanasia.

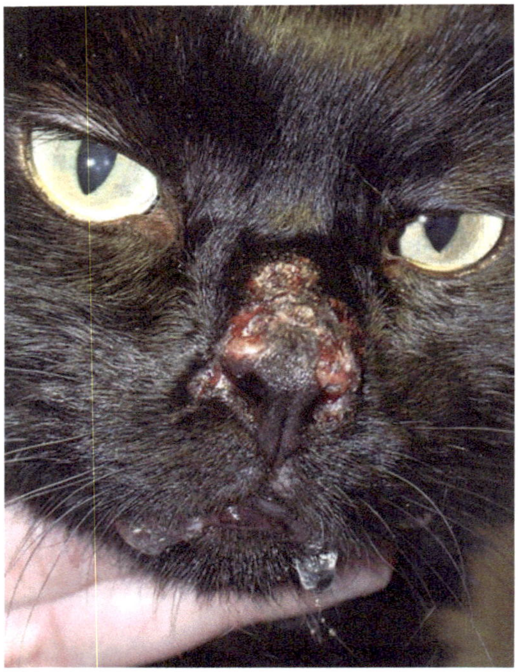

Figure 9.1 Crusting, erythema, and erosion caused by herpesvirus dermatitis on the dorsal nose of a cat.

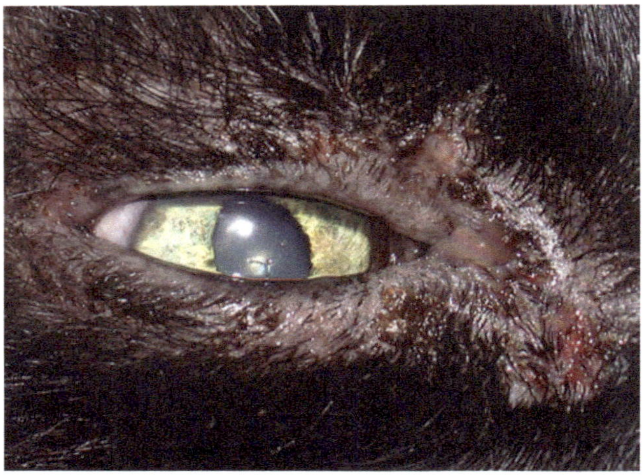

Figure 9.2 Erosive blepharitis due to herpesvirus infection.

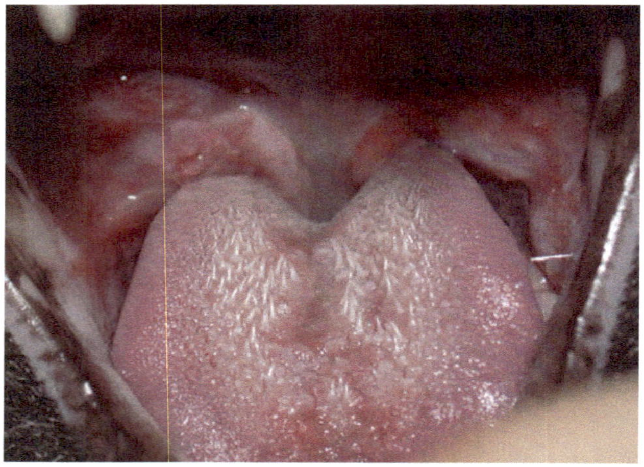

Figure 9.3 Lingual ulcers and stomatitis in a cat with herpes infection.

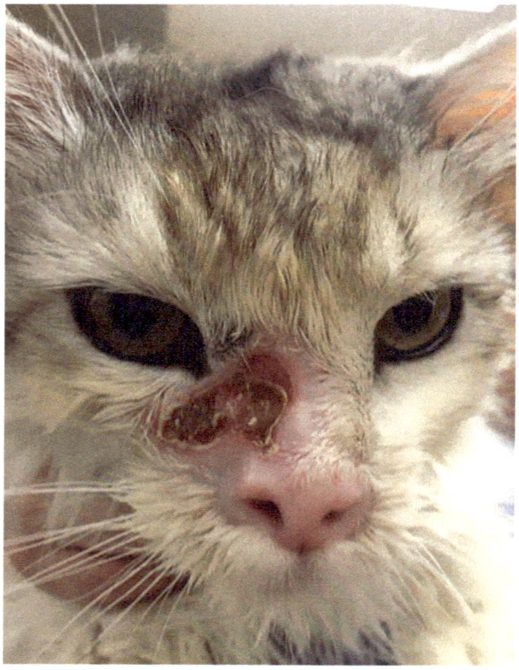

Figure 9.4 An asymmetric, alopecic, scarred, crusted facial lesion due to herpesvirus dermatitis. *Source:* Image courtesy of Dr. Ann Trimmer, DACVD.

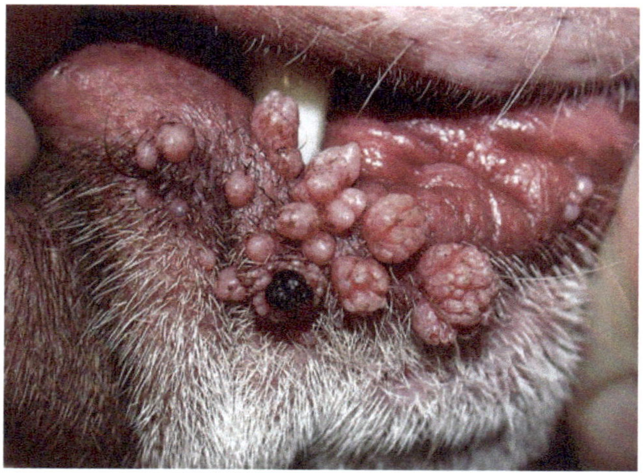

Figure 9.5 Canine oral viral papillomas on the lip of a young dog.

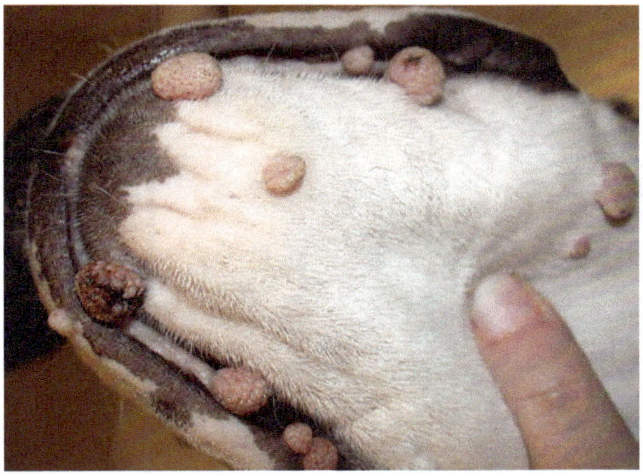

Figure 9.6 In this young Bulldog with viral papillomas, both lips and haired skin were affected.

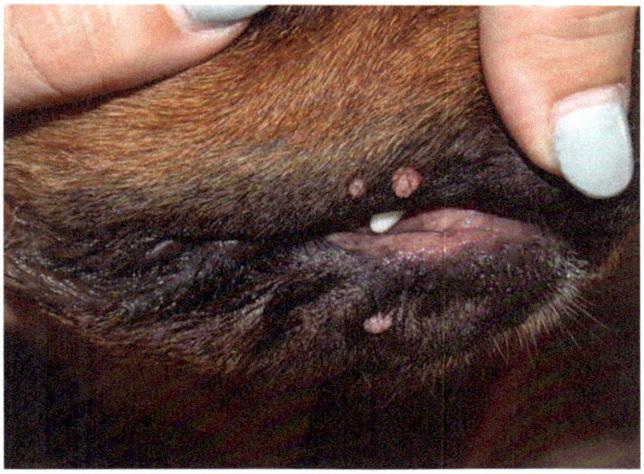

Figure 9.7 Oral viral papillomas; lesions usually begin as smooth pink papules which enlarge and become fronded.

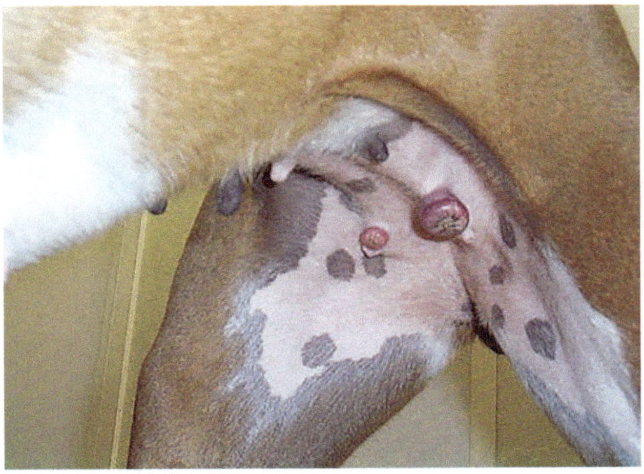

Figure 9.8 Inverted papillomas on the groin of a young Boxer.

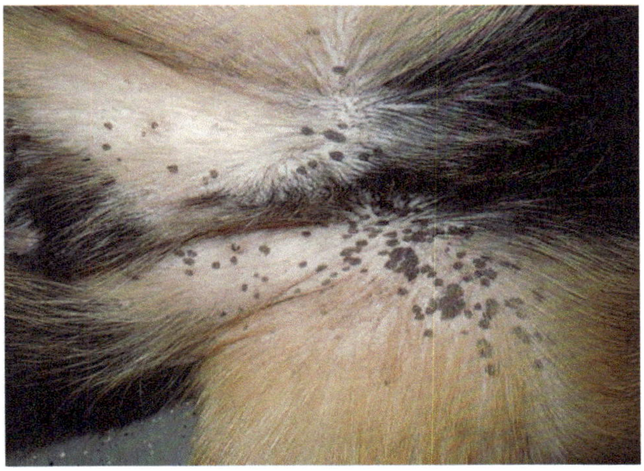

Figure 9.9 Inguinal pigmented viral plaques in a Rottweiler with immunosuppression due to lymphoma.

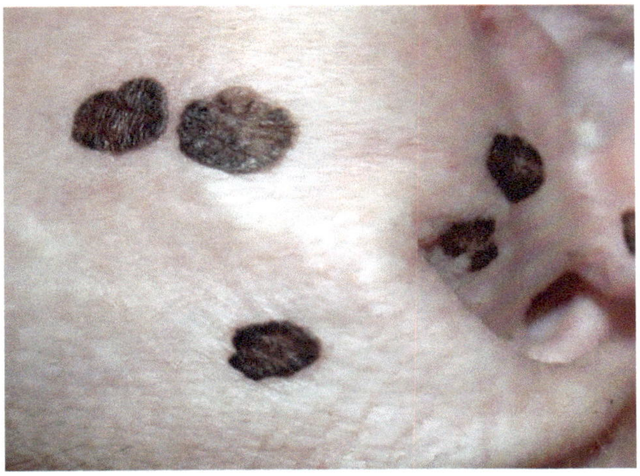

Figure 9.10 Pigmented viral plaques on the inner pinna of a young Boxer.

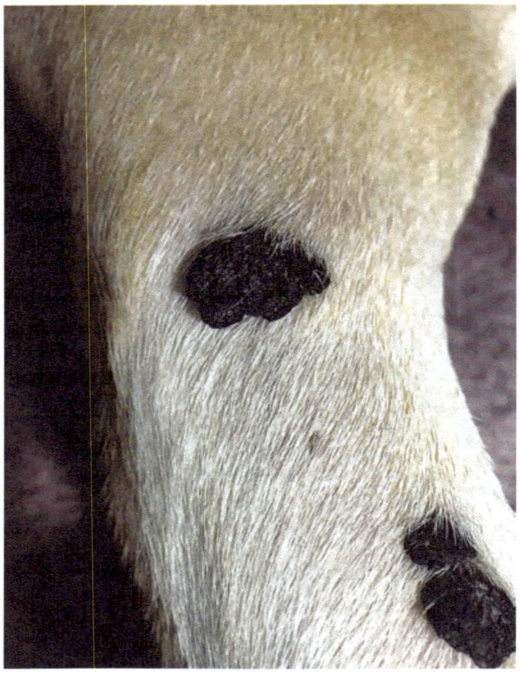

Figure 9.11 Plaque-like to pedunculated pigmented viral papillomas in a Bulldog on oclacitinib.

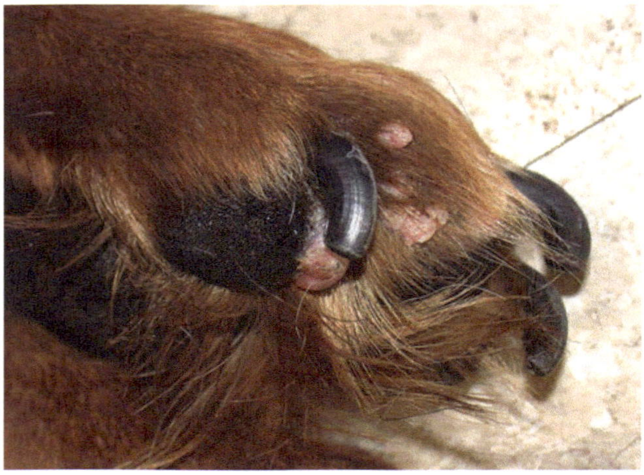

Figure 9.12 Numerous pedal papillomas in a dog with a congenital immunodeficiency disorder.

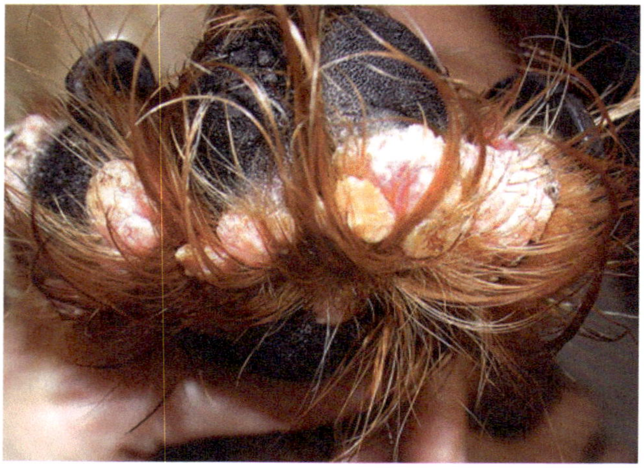

Figure 9.13 Numerous pedal papillomas in a dog with a congenital immunodeficiency disorder.

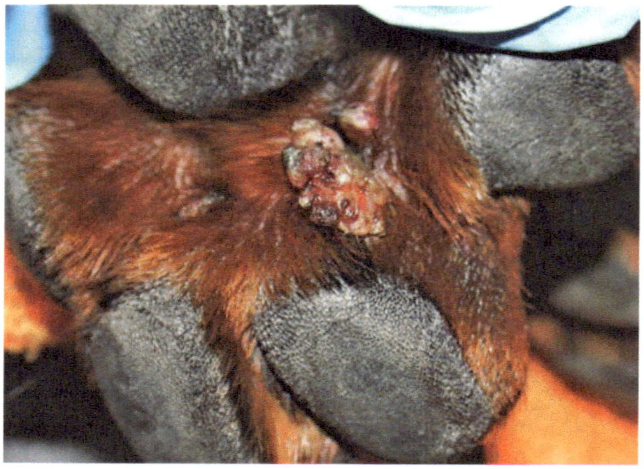

Figure 9.14 A pedal papilloma in a young Doberman.

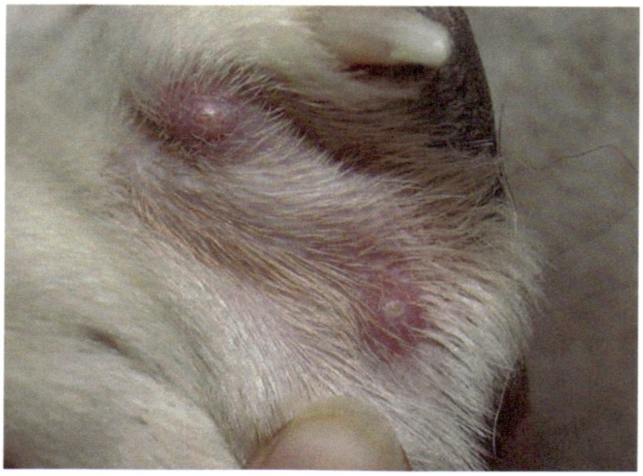

Figure 9.15 Raised firm interdigital masses which appeared acutely in a young Bulldog, biopsy revealed viral papilloma.

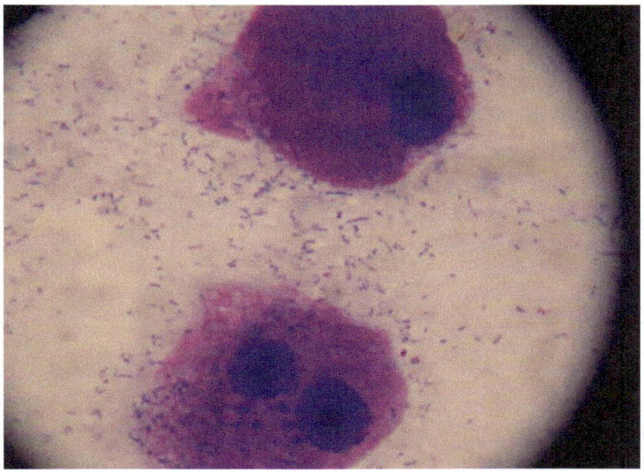

Figure 9.16 Surface cytology of one of the interdigital masses revealed large, bizarre, viral-infected epithelial cells as well as a secondary bacterial overgrowth (100×).

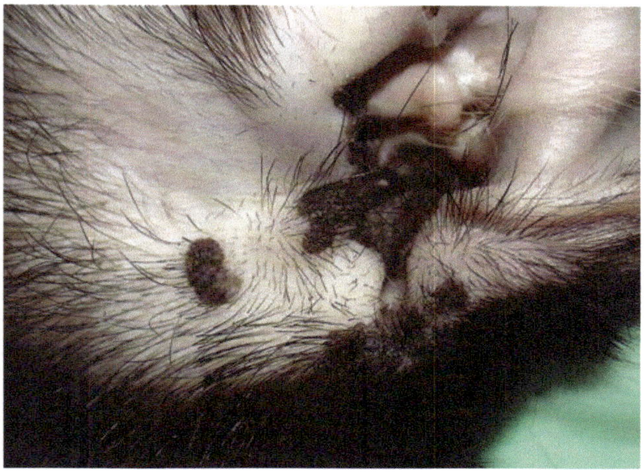

Figure 9.17 Multiple, pigmented, raised, rough dermal viral plaques on the temporal area and pinna of a cat.

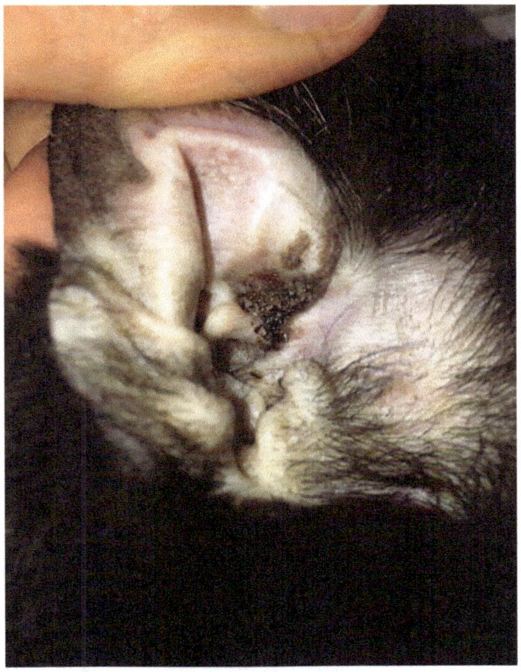

Figure 9.18 This cat's Bowenoid pinnal lesion was very hyperkeratotic.

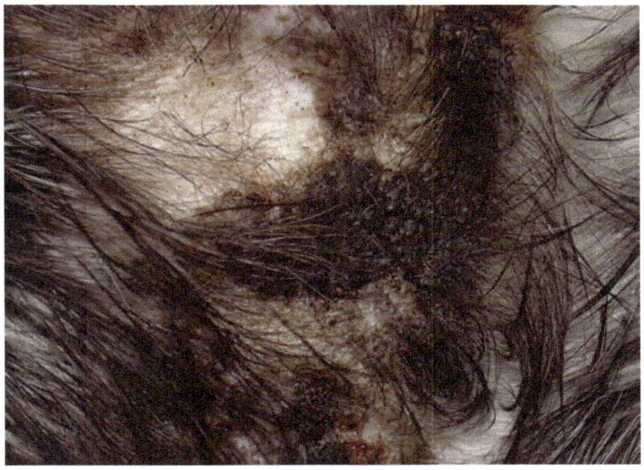

Figure 9.19 Bowen's disease on the temporal area of a cat complicated by secondary *Malassezia* infection.

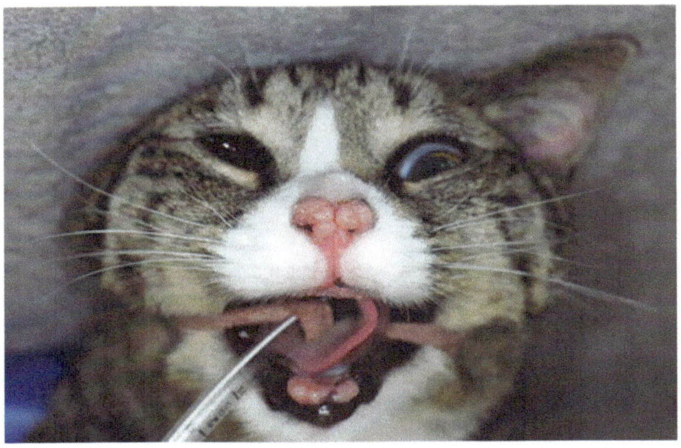

Figure 9.20 Pink, firm masses on the nasal planum and gingival mucosa of a cat with feline sarcoid.

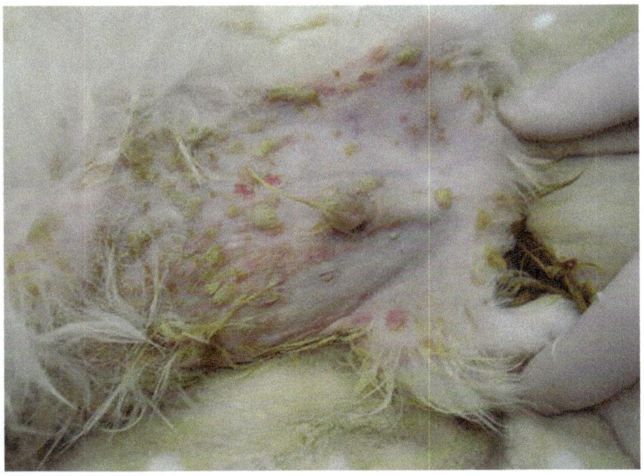

Figure 9.21 Large, inguinal pustules in a dog due to distemper virus infection. *Source:* Image courtesy of VIN and Brian Stewart, DVM.

Table 9.2 Rickettsial diseases.

Disease	Clinical signs	Diagnosis	Treatment
Rocky Mountain Spotted Fever (*Rickettsia ricketsii*, Figure 9.22) A rickettsial disease carried by *Dermacentor* ticks, occurs throughout the US, more commonly in mid-Atlantic and eastern US and mid-southern states; also reported in Canada, Mexico, Central and South America. Incubation period is 2–14 days after exposure.	Skin lesions in dogs can include petechiae/ecchymoses due to thrombocytopenia, edema, necrosis, and ulcerations on skin, paws, oral cavity, nasal planum, and scrotum. Lymphadenopathy is common. Systemic signs include fever, lethargy, epistaxis, uveitis, polyarthritis, hepatic disease/icterus, dyspnea, meningoencephalitis, renal failure.	Clinical signs. Labwork: Leukocytosis, anemia, thrombocytopenia, elevated liver enzymes, hypoalbuminemia. RMSF serology: High IgM or 4-fold increase in IgG (occurs 2–3 weeks post infection). RMSF PCR on whole blood. Skin biopsy: Necrotizing vasculitis.	Effective antibiotic options: Doxycycline 5–10 mg/kg PO or IV BID × 1 week; Tetracycline 22 mg/kg PO or IV TID × 1–2 weeks; or Enrofloxacin 3 mg/kg PO or SC BID for 1 week. Chloramphenicol 25–50 mg/kg PO TID × 1 week. Supportive care: IV fluids (use with care due to increased vascular permeability), nutritional support. Use acaricidal parasiticides to kill ticks and prevent reinfestation.
Ehrlichiosis (*Ehrlichia canis*, Figures 9.23 and 9.24) A rickettsial disease carried by ticks, most commonly the Brown Dog tick; canids are reservoir hosts. Worldwide distribution except for Australia. Incubation period 8–20 days.	Skin lesions in dogs can include petechiae/ecchymoses due to thrombocytopenia, and rarely crusting on the dorsal muzzle or a pruritic papulocrustous dermatitis. Lymphadenopathy is common. Systemic signs include fever, lethargy, epistaxis, uveitis, polyarthritis, splenomegaly.	Clinical signs. Labwork: Leukopenia, anemia, thrombocytopenia, hyperglobulinemia, hypoalbuminemia. Ehrlichia serology: IgG > 1 : 80 (15 days post infection). Ehrlichia PCR.	Effective antibiotic options: Doxycycline 10 mg/kg/day × 3–4 weeks; Tetracycline 22–30 mg/kg PO or IV TID × 3–4 weeks. Chloramphenicol 25–50 mg/kg PO TID × 3–4 weeks. Supportive care: IV fluids, nutritional support. Use acaricidal parasiticides to kill ticks and prevent reinfestation.

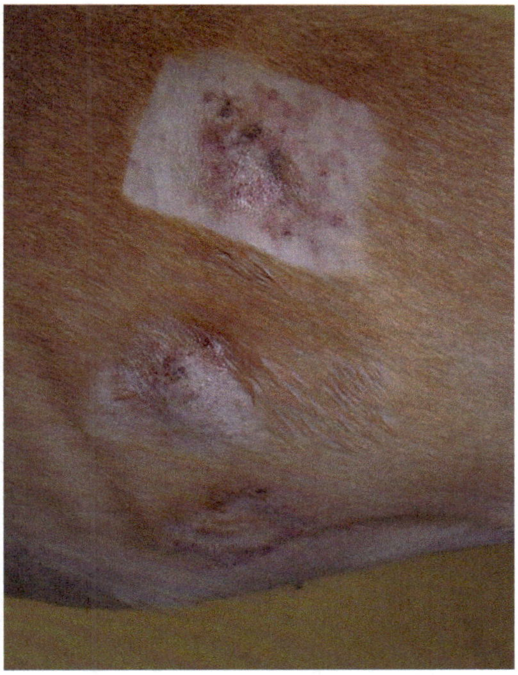

Figure 9.22 Erythematous macules, erosions, and crusts due to vasculitis on the lateral thorax of a dog infected by Rocky Mountain Spotted Fever.

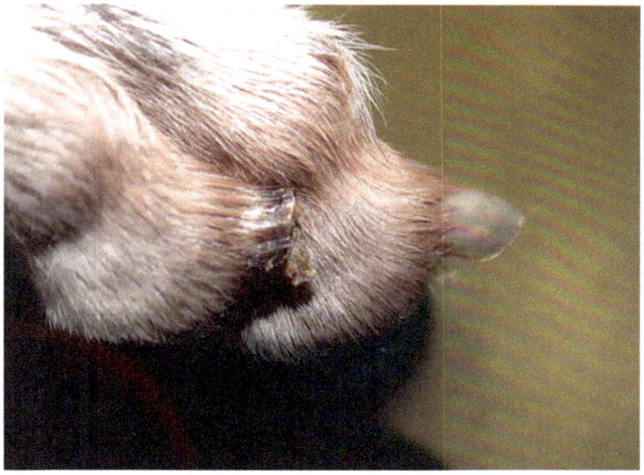

Figure 9.23 This Greyhound with ehrlichiosis and severe thrombocytopenia had vasculitis evidenced by subungual nail hemorrhage and nail loss.

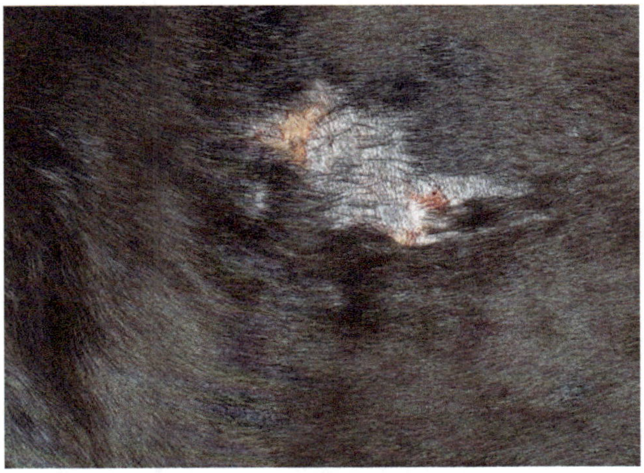

Figure 9.24 Patchy, truncal alopecia with crusts and erosions caused by *Ehrlichia canis* triggered vasculitis.

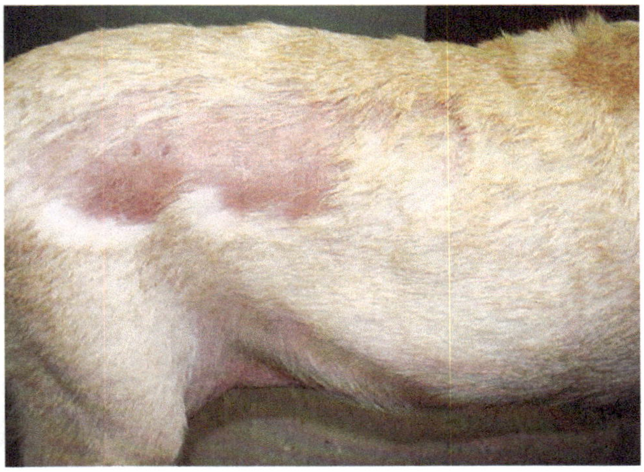

Figure 9.25 Patchy truncal alopecia, erythema and silvery scaling due to leishmaniasis.

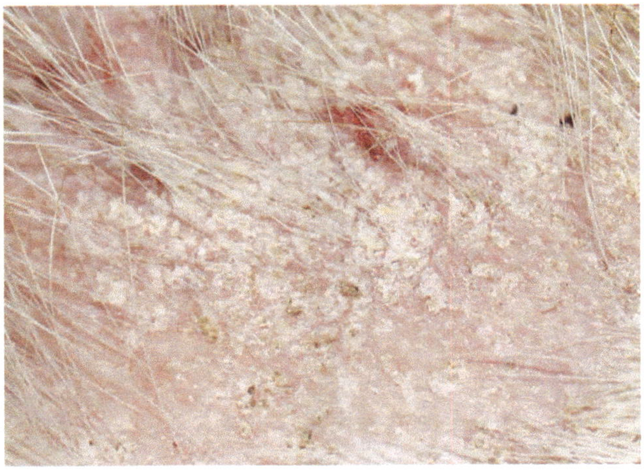

Figure 9.26 Close up view of scaling truncal lesions caused by Leishmania infection.

Table 9.3 Protozoal diseases.

Disease	Clinical signs	Diagnosis	Treatment
Leishmaniasis (*Leishmania infantum* Figures 9.25–9.29) A protozoal parasite which is transmitted by sandflies, endemic in the Mediterranean, southern Europe, Africa, Asia, and Central and South America; also endemic in Foxhounds in the eastern US and Canada, and endemic foci have been found in TX, OK, OH, MI, and AL. Cases in non-Foxhound breeds have occurred elsewhere in the US, either in dogs imported from endemic regions, or in dogs exposed to infected dogs via fighting or breeding. Vertical transmission appears to be the most common means of infection transmission in the US. A potential sandfly vector, *Lutzomyia shannoni*, is present in the southern and southeastern United States, but there is no documentation of infection transmission at this time. Most common in young adult and older dogs, Boxers and German Shepherds are predisposed.	Skin lesions are variable and include exfoliative scaling, alopecia, erythema, crusts, ulcerations of skin, nasal planum, oral cavity, or paw pads, nasal or paw pad hyperkeratosis, onychogryphosis, pustular, acantholytic or nodular dermatitis. Lymphadenopathy is common. Systemic signs include fever, weight loss, hyporexia, lethargy, vomiting, diarrhea, uveitis, lameness, hepatosplenomegaly, PU/PD, renal failure. Symptoms can occur months to years after exposure and tend to be slowly progressive. In dogs with a strong TH1 immune response, exposure can cause serologic conversion but no clinical disease. In cats, skin lesions can include a nodular or crusting dermatitis on the face, pinnae or paws +/− exfoliative scaling.	Clinical signs. Cytology of lesions and lymph node aspirate: Pyogranulomatous inflammation +/− intra or extracellular protozoal organisms/amastigotes. Skin biopsies for dermatopathology: Variable lymphoplasmacytic to pyogranulomatous dermatitis and perifolliculitis with sebaceous gland destruction and ortho to parakeratotic hyperkeratosis +/− intra or extracellular protozoal organisms/amastigotes (Giemsa stain helpful to demonstrate organisms). Lichenoid interface dermatitis, vasculitis, and acantholytic pustular dermatitis can be seen. Leishmania serology immunofluorescence antibody test (IFAT) and enzyme-linked immunosorbent assay (ELISA). Leishmania PCR (of skin biopsy, lymph node aspirate, whole blood, conjunctival scrapings; RT PCR has superior sensitivity to traditional or nested PCR). CBC/Chemistry panel may demonstrate leukocytosis, leukopenia, anemia, thrombocytopenia, hypoalbuminemia, hyperglobulinemia, azotemia, and elevated liver values.	Leishmania treatment guidelines and prognosis in dogs are based on stage of disease: Stage I Mild disease: Negative to low positive *Leishmania* titer, mild skin disease, lymphadenopathy, normal labwork: Treat with allopurinol +/− miltefosine or meglumine. Prognosis good. Stage II moderate disease: Moderate skin disease, lymphadenopathy, weight loss, fever, anemia, hyperglobulinemia Low to high *Leishmania* antibody titer, hypoalbuminemia, no to mild proteinuria with no azotemia: Treat with allopurinol + meglumine antimoniate (treatment of choice) or miltefosine, prognosis good to guarded. Stage III Severe disease: Medium to high *Leishmania* antibody titer, Stage I and II signs + renal disease; treat with allopurinol + meglumine antimoniate (treatment of choice) or miltefosine, prognosis guarded to poor. Stage IV Very severe disease: Medium to high *Leishmania* antibody titer, Stage III signs + pulmonary thromboembolic disease and/or nephrotic syndrome/end stage renal disease with marked proteinuria: treat palliatively with allopurinol alone and follow IRIS guidelines for renal failure treatment, euthanasia based on quality of life. Drug dosing: Allopurinol is given at a dose of 10 mg/kg PO BID for at least 6–18 months, and possibly lifelong to prevent relapse. Allopurinol may be discontinued if there are no clinical or labwork abnormalities and when there is a marked decrease of antibody levels (to negative or borderline by a quantitative serological assay). In addition, allopurinol might need to be discontinued if the side effect of marked xanthine crystalluria occurs and is uncontrollable by low purine diets or by drug dose reduction. Miltefosine 2 mg/kg PO once daily × 4 weeks; this is a currently available in Europe as an animal drug called Milteforan 20 mg/ml, Virbac. In the United States Miltefosine is available in human medicine as a 50 mg capsule (Impavido®, Profounda Inc.). Meglumine antimoniate 75–100 mg/kg once a day or 40–75 mg/kg twice a day for 4 weeks, S.C. (not available in the United States at the time of writing). Other promising drugs with more limited data include marbofloxacin 2.75 mg/kg PO once daily × 28 days and domperidone 1 mg/kg PO BID, a dopamine D2 receptor antagonist used as an immune stimulator. Amphotericin B in the lipid emulsion or liposomal form 0.25–0.5 mg/kg IV q48 hours or 3 times a week until a cumulative dose of 5–10 mg/kg is reached. Treatment of cats has little published information; allopurinol and meglumine antimoniate are most frequently used, however studies on pharmacokinetics and safety of these drugs in cats are lacking (Hervás et al. 1999). Allopurinol 10-20mg/kg PO q 12-24 hours is usually clinically effective (Pennisi et al. 2015). One case responded to three 4-week courses of 5 mg/kg meglumine antimoniate SQ + ketoconazole 10 mg/kg PO once daily. Monitoring: In clinically affected animals, treatment can cause clinical remission but relapse often occurs months to years later; the goal or treatment is to reduce parasite load, treat organ damage caused by the infection, and improve immune response. Response to treatment is monitored by assessing body condition/weight, skin lesions, and CBC/Chemistry panel/UA one month after starting treatment, then every 3–4 months for the first year, then every 6–12 months forever to screen for relapse of infection. Recheck *Leishmania* titer every 6 months for a year then once a year is also recommended to assess response to treatment and screen for relapse of infection. If infection relapses clinically, then retreatment is initiated.

Leishmaniasis (cont.) Can also affect cats, though they are resistant to infection and symptoms are usually milder. Zoonotic.		UA often shows proteinuria, decreased urine specific gravity, +/− casts.	Prevention: In endemic areas regular use of antiparasitic products with repellant action against sand flies is recommended, including veterinary registered products containing synthetic pyrethroids, permethrin, or deltamethrin (dogs only). Additional preventative measures include keeping dogs indoors from dusk to dawn during peak sand fly activity, removing microhabitats favorable to sand flies such as piles of wood and stones near the home and usage of indoor insecticides. There is no effective vaccine against *Leishmania* available in the United States. Two registered canine vaccines: FML-QuilA (Leishmune® in Brazil, and LiESP/QA-21 (CaniLeish® in Europe. These vaccines, consisting of parasite purified fractions with saponin derivative adjuvants, have been shown to confer significant (but not 100%) protection against disease and death under natural conditions.
Toxoplasmosis (*Toxoplasma gondii*) A multisystemic protozoal disease; cats are the primary host, are infected by ingesting rodent intermediate hosts. Zoonotic.	In additional to typical systemic signs, occasionally described to cause ulcerative skin lesions in dogs and cats. Lymphadenopathy is common.	Biopsy: Pyogranulomatous or necrotizing dermatitis and vasculitis with *Toxoplasma* organisms. Please refer to appropriate infectious disease texts for details on diagnosis of toxoplasmosis.	Clindamycin 10 mg/kg PO TID × 4 weeks. Supportive care: IV fluids, nutritional support. Advise owners of zoonosis risk.

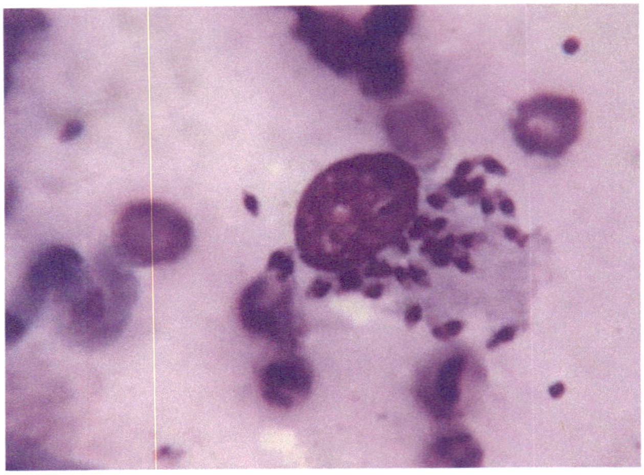

Figure 9.27 Cytology of the scaly skin lesion in Fig. 9.26 showed macrophages and numerous intra and extracellular Leishmania amastigotes (100×).

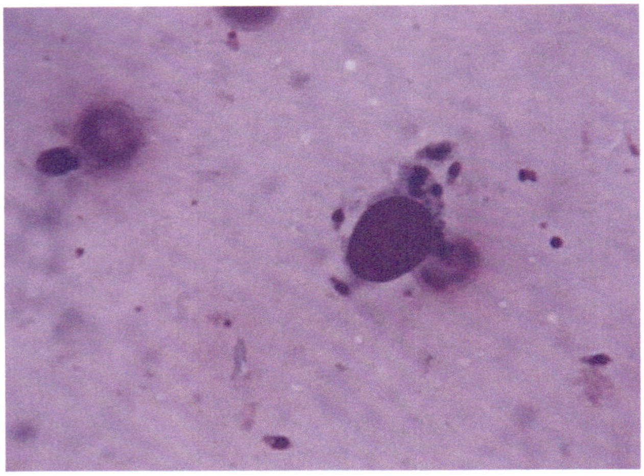

Figure 9.28 Cytology of the scaly skin lesion in Fig. 9.26 showed macrophages and numerous intra and extracellular Leishmania amastigotes (100×).

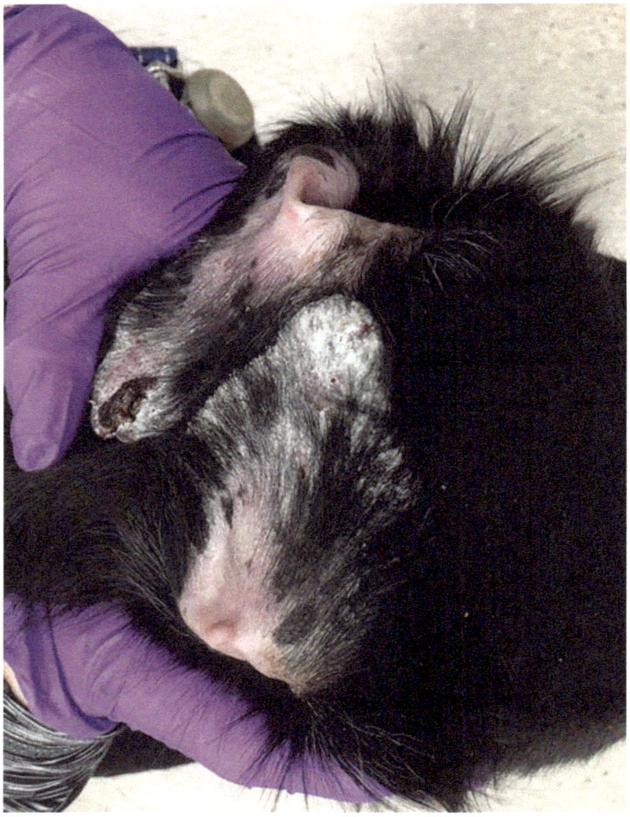

Figure 9.29 Pinnal scaling and ulceration in a dog with leishmaniasis.

References/Further reading

Bol, S. and Bunnik, E.M. (2015). Lysine supplementation is not effective for the prevention or treatment of feline herpesvirus 1 infection in cats: A systematic review. *BMC Vet. Res.* 11: 284.

Fenimore, A., Carter, K., Fankhauser, J. et al. (2016). Evaluation of intranasal vaccine administration and high-dose interferon-α2b therapy for treatment of chronic upper respiratory tract infections in shelter cats. *J. Feline Med. Surg.* 18 (8): 603–611.

Freeman, K. (2010). Update on the diagnosis and management of *Leishmania* spp. infections in dogs in the United States. *Top Companion Anim. Med.* 25 (3): 149–154.

Gill, V.L., Bergman, P.J., Baer, K.E. et al. (2008). Use of imiquimod 5% cream (Aldara) in cats with multicentric squamous cell carcinoma in situ: 12 cases (2002–2005). *Vet. Comp. Oncol.* 6 (1): 55–64.

Gradoni, L. (2015). Canine *Leishmania* vaccines: Still a long way to go. *Vet. Parasitol.* 208 (1–2): 94–100.

Greene, C.E. (2012). *Infectious Diseases of the Dog and Cat*, 4e. St Louis, MO: Elsevier Saunders.

Gutzwiller, M.E., Brachelente, C., Taglinger, K. et al. (2007). Feline herpes dermatitis treated with interferon omega. *Vet. Dermatol.* 18 (1): 50–54.

Hervás, J., Chacón-M De Lara, F., Sánchez-Isarria, M.A. et al. (1999). Two cases of feline visceral and cutaneous leishmaniosis in Spain. *J. Feline Med. Surg.* 1: 101–105.

Lange, C.E. and Favrot, C. (2011). Canine papillomaviruses. *Vet. Clin. North Am. Small Anim. Pract.* 41 (6): 1183–1195.

Legendre, A.M., Kuritz, T., Galyon, G. et al. (2017). Polyprenyl immunostimulant treatment of cats with presumptive non-effusive feline infectious peritonitis in a field study. *Front. Vet. Sci.* 4: 7.

Maggs, D.J., Nasisse, M.P., and Kass, P.H. (2003). Efficacy of oral supplementation with L-lysine in cats latently infected with feline herpesvirus. *Am. J. Vet. Res.* 64 (1): 37–42.

Malik, R., Lessels, N.S., Webb, S. et al. (2009). Treatment of feline herpesvirus-1 associated disease in cats with famciclovir and related drugs. *J. Feline Med. Surg.* 11 (1): 40–48.

Möstl, K., Addie, D., Belák, S. et al. (2013). Cowpox virus infection in cats: ABCD guidelines on prevention and management. *J. Feline Med. Surg.* 15 (7): 557–559.

Munday, J.S., Thomson, N.A., and Luff, J.A. (2017). Papillomaviruses in dogs and cats. *Vet. J.* 225: 23–31.

Oliva, G., Nieto, J., Foglia Manzillo, V. et al. (2014). A randomised, double-blind, controlled efficacy trial of the LiESP/QA-21 vaccine in Naïve dogs exposed to two *Leishmania infantum* transmission seasons. *PLoS Negl. Trop. Dis.* 8 (10): e3213.

Oliva, G., Roura, X., Crotti, A. et al. (2010). Guidelines for treatment of leishmaniasis in dogs. *J. Am. Vet. Med. Assoc.* 236 (11): 1192–1198.

Pedersen, N.C., Kim, Y., and Liu, H. (2018). Efficacy of a 3C-like protease inhibitor in treating various forms of acquired feline infectious peritonitis. *J. Feline Med. Surg.* 20 (4): 378–392.

Pennisi, M.-G., Cardoso, L., Baneth, G. et al. (2015). LeishVet update and recommendations on feline leishmaniosis. *Parasit. Vetors.* 8: 302.

Pesavento, P.A., MacLachlan, N.J., Dillard-Telm, L. et al. (2004). Pathologic, immunohistochemical, and electron microscopic findings in naturally occurring virulent systemic feline calicivirus infection in cats. *Vet. Pathol.* 41 (3): 257–263.

Peterson, C.A. and Barr, S.C. (2009). Canine Leishmaniasis in North America: Emerging or newly recognized? *Vet. Clin. North Am. Small Anim. Pract.* 39 (6): 1065–vi.

Radford, A.D., Addie, D., Belák, S. et al. (2009). Feline calcivirus infection. ABCD guidelines on prevention and management. *J. Feline Med. Surg.* 11 (7): 556–564. https://doi.org/10.1016/j.jfms.2009.05.004.

Radford, A.D., Coyne, K.P., Dawson, S. et al. (2007). Feline calicivirus. *Vet. Res.* 38 (2): 319–335.

Solano-Gallego, L., Miro, G., Koutinas, A. et al. (2011). LeishVet guidelines for the practical management of canine leishmaniosis. *Parasit. Vectors* 4: 86.

Thomasy, S.M. and Maggs, D.J. (2016). A review of antiviral drugs and other compounds with activity against feline herpesvirus-1. *Vet. Ophthalmol.* 19 (Suppl 1): 119–130.

Thomasy, S.M., Shull, O., Outerbridge, C.A. et al. (2016). Oral administration of famciclovir for treatment of spontaneous ocular, respiratory, or dermatologic disease attributed to feline herpesvirus type 1: 59 cases (2006–2013). *J. Am. Vet. Med. Assoc.* 249 (5): 526–538.

10

Allergic skin diseases in dogs and cats

Jacquelyn Campbell, DVM, DACVD

Animal Allergy and Dermatology of Colorado, Colorado Springs, CO, USA

Clinical Atlas of Canine and Feline Dermatology, First Edition. Edited by Kimberly S. Coyner.

Companion website: www.wiley.com/go/coyner/dermatology

Table 10.1 Hypersensitivity disorders and treatment of allergic skin diseases.

Disease	Clinical signs	Diagnosis	Treatment
Urticaria/ Angioedema (Figures 10.1A–10.1F) No age or sex predilection. Atopic dogs may have increased risk.	Acute or chronic onset. Variably pruritic, erythematous, flat -topped wheals ranging in diameter from 5–15 mm; lesions do not become scaly or lose fur. +/− large edematous swelling of face or body. +/− concurrent systemic anaphylactic symptoms such as vomiting, diarrhea, difficulty breathing, collapse.	History. Clinical exam: 1) May be helpful to circle some individual lesions and follow behavior over time as in true urticaria typically each lesion lasts no more than 24 hours. 2) Diascopy (Figure 10.1E): Place glass slide over erythematous lesions. If lesions blanche with the pressure of slide then lesions are due to vasodilation (urticarial). Note: If lesions persist longer than 24 hours in the same location or do not blanche on diascopy, consider pyoderma in short coated breeds which can present similarly (Figure 10.1F), or urticarial vasculitis.	Acute: 1) Glucocorticoid injection: dexamethasone SP 0.5–1 mg/kg IM. Dose dependent on severity with up to 2 mg/kg IV if life threatening angioedema. 2) If life threatening anaphylaxis give epinephrine (adrenaline) 0.01 mg/kg IM using a 1 mg/ml (1 : 1000 solution); maximum dose of 0.3 mg in patients <40 kg and 0.5 mg in patients >40 kg; intravenous fluid therapy for circulatory support. 3) Concurrent antihistamine: diphenhydramine 2–4 mg/kg PO or IM every 8 hours for 3 to 10 days. 4) If respiratory distress is present give aminophylline 5 mg/kg IV over 10 min or terbutaline 0.01 mg/kg SQ. 5) Suspected cause should be identified and avoided. Consider stinging or biting insects, drugs, vaccines, food allergens, environmental pollens, dusts or dander, intestinal parasitism. 6) Long-term antihistamines can be considered. Chronic: 1) Careful and thorough investigation for underlying trigger to include but not limited to: strict hypoallergenic diet trial, parasite treatment trial, deworming for intestinal parasites, review of drug/supplement/vitamin history, environmental exposure investigation (plants, insects, duration in sun etc.). 2) For cases with recurrent insect bite/sting induced anaphylaxis, hyposensitization to insect venoms may be considered, but availability is very limited. 3) In cases where no trigger can be identified, consider atopy/allergy testing and/or referral to area dermatologist. 4) For animals with a history of recurrent episodes of life threatening anaphylaxis, providing pet owners with epinephrine may be appropriate: • A dog greater than 20–45 kg BW can receive 0.3 mg epinephrine (EpiPen). • Dispensing the epinephrine in syringes containing the correct calculated dose should be considered for small dogs and cats, as even the EpiPen Jr. will deliver above the recommended dose of epinephrine. • Store epinephrine at 20–25° C, replace after 3 months.

Contact hypersensitivity (Figures 10.2A–10.2D) Rare compared to atopic dermatitis.	Varied degrees of macular and papular dermatitis which tend to be confined to hairless or sparsely haired areas of skin in contact areas including ventrum, muzzle, and pinnae. Ear canal may be affected if history of topical otic medications. A reaction that typically requires prolonged or repeated contact with offending allergen including but not limited to: • Plants. • Topical ointments, lotions, or otic formulations. • Home furnishings or cleansers. • Dog foods. Cases have history of slowly spreading lesions to adjacent areas. Chronic lesions are often alopecic plaques with variable pigmentation, excoriation, and lichenification. Secondary pyoderma, *Malassezia* dermatitis, or seborrheic skin disease may be present.	History, clinical signs. Rule out other differentials; if contact hypersensitivity is not immediately apparent based on history then clinician must rule out other pruritic diseases with following strategy concurrently: • Parasite treatment trial to rule out flea allergy, *Sarcoptes*, and so on. • Cytology for bacterial/yeast infections. • Otic cytology (contact otic reactions characterized by cytology showing neutrophils, lymphocytes, and absence of microbes). • *Demodex* with deep skin scrape. • Dermatophyte with DTM or PCR testing. • Food allergy with adequate diet trial (see Table 10.6). Response to confinement accomplished by thorough bathing and isolation of animal in new environment demonstrating resolution of lesions; clinical signs typically resolve within 7 to 10 days. If complete confinement not possible then barrier/protective gear may be utilized. Atopic dogs may show some improvement in clinical signs, but response is not 100%. Identification of the offending allergen may best be accomplished with the aid of a local dermatologist and patch testing.	Strategies for management: 1) Remove contact allergens with saline rinsing or bathing using a soap free, hypoallergenic shampoo. 2) Treat any secondary pyoderma or *Malassezia* infection appropriately. 3) Identify offending allergen and avoid contact. 4) Apply mechanical barriers such as t-shirt, socks, if allergen cannot be identified. 5) Topical glucocorticoids applied every 12 hours: • Low potency such as hydrocortisone. • High potency such as mometasone, betamethasone, triamcinolone (caution with long-term use as these products can cause skin atrophy and comedones). 6) Oral glucocorticoids: • Prednisone 0.5 to 1.0 mg/kg/day for 5 to 10 days. • Methylprednisolone 0.4 to 0.8 mg/kg/day for 5 to 10 days. 7) Pentoxifylline 10 to 15 mg/kg PO BID to TID prior to exposure may be helpful. If cannot identify allergenic trigger then referral to area dermatologist should be considered.

(*Continued*)

Table 10.1 Hypersensitivity disorders and treatment of allergic skin diseases (Continued)

Disease	Clinical signs	Diagnosis	Treatment
Atopy ***Dogs*** (Figures 10.3A–10.3N) Usually occurs in dogs between 6 mo-3 yr old. Can occur in any breed, but predisposed breeds include Shar-peis, Cocker Spaniels, English Bulldogs, Labradors and Golden Retrievers, Pugs, and Terriers.	Signs may be seasonal or non-seasonal. Pruritic dermatitis with or without skin changes; pruritus occurs *prior* to skin lesions in most dogs; in some dogs pruritus may not be evident until pyoderma occurs. Affected areas include front paws, concave (inner) surface of pinnae, external orifice of ears, flexor surface of metacarpi or metatarsi, axillae, ventral abdomen, inguinal, periocular, and perioral. Initially lesions present as pruritus followed by erythema, papular dermatitis, and with chronicity excoriations, crusts, hyperpigmentation, lichenification, and alopecia. Recurrent otitis externa is a common symptom. Secondary bacterial pyoderma and *Malassezia* dermatitis are common. Other symptoms can include acral lick dermatitis and allergic airway disease.	Historical and clinical criteria help support diagnosis of atopic disease, but it remains a diagnosis of exclusion. Positive clinical response (85% controlled) with 0.5 mg/kg/day of oral glucocorticoid such as prednisone is supportive of atopy diagnosis. Historical seasonality if present is helpful; for dogs with non-seasonal symptoms, atopy is a diagnosis of exclusion and ruling out concurrent hypersensitivity including: 1) Perform skin scraping for mites; if none found a diagnostic trial of isoxazoline or selamectin (Revolution®) is still recommended. 2) Perform cytology and address any concurrent secondary itch factors such as pyoderma, or *Malassezia* dermatitis. 3) Perform a DTM or dermatophyte PCR to rule out dermatophyte. 4) Perform adequate hypoallergenic diet trial for food allergy (see Table 10.6). It is important to emphasize that allergy testing is not a first-line screening test in the workup of dogs and cats with dermatologic disease. Once the clinical diagnosis of atopy has been achieved by ruling out all other possible causes for symptoms, then intradermal or serologic allergy testing is used as a management tool to determine allergens to include in immunotherapy.	An integrated approach to atopy treatment is necessary including control of secondary bacterial and yeast infections, control of concurrent parasite and/or food allergy, restoration of epidermal barrier, carefully directed use of symptomatic medications to manage remaining inflammation and pruritus, and consideration of allergy testing/desensitization to address underlying cause of pruritus/infections and try to reduce need for symptomatic drugs. See Algorithm 10.1 and Table 10.2. Therapeutic options include: 1) Oclacitinib (Apoquel®) 0.4–0.6 mg/kg PO per day (if used long-term, check CBC/Chemistry panel 4–6 weeks after starting then CBC/Chemistry panel/UA q6–12 mo). 2) Glucocorticoids at anti-inflammatory dosage: • Prednisone 0.5 mg/kg/day PO • Methylprednisolone 0.4 mg/kg/day. • Triamcinolone 0.1 to 0.2 mg/kg/day PO daily to every other day. Once clinical signs are controlled in 1–2 weeks then dosage of steroid is tapered to the lowest effective dose q2–3 days for clinical control; monitor CBC/Chemistry panel/UA q6–12 mo. Do not exceed a maximum yearly total prednisone dose of BW (kg) × 30. If prolonged steroids are required, then considerations should be made for non-steroidal drug options including oclacitinib (Apoquel®), Cytopoint®, or ciclosporin (Atopica®) to mitigate the long-term effects of chronic steroid use. 3) Lokivetmab (Cytopoint®) 2 mg/kg every 4 to 8 weeks SC. 4) Ciclosporin (Atopica®) (microemulsion/modified ciclosporin) 5 mg/kg/PO per day. • Therapy takes 4 to 6 weeks to reach steady state. • Concurrent steroid may be needed during initiation period then once pruritus is controlled steroid is tapered off. • Pet managed with lowest daily to every other day regimen of ciclosporin. • Check CBC/Chemistry panel 4–6 weeks after starting then CBC/Chemistry panel/UA q6–12 mo). 5) Allergy testing and desensitization (see Table 10.3; Tables 10.4 and 10.5 for formulation protocols). 6) Supportive therapies (helpful but not very potent): • Antihistamines. • Oral and topical fatty acids. • Topical antipruritic and/or antimicrobial therapies including bathing, conditioners, sprays, mousses.

Food allergy (Adverse food reaction) *Dogs* (Figures 10.4A–10.4E) Most common food allergens in dogs: beef, dairy, chicken, and wheat. Any age can be affected with increased index of suspicion in dogs with symptoms starting <1 or >7 yr old. Can occur in any breed but predisposed breeds include Cocker Spaniels, Labradors and Golden Retrievers, Shar-peis, Terriers, Boxers, German Shepherds. A diet change is not usually in the history and dogs can be fed the diet for 2 yr before onset of clinical signs.	Non-seasonal pruritus which may be regional or generalized; can present identically to atopic dermatitis. Variably responsive to glucocorticoids and may range from poor to good. Distribution variable but may involve face, pinnae, axillae, inguinal region, paws, perianal, and dorsolumbar region. Can present with pruritus and absence of clinical lesions. Lesions include erythema, papules progressing to alopecia, excoriations, crusts, hyperpigmentation, and lichenification. Chronic otitis may be the sole clinical sign or accompany those listed above. Secondary pyoderma, and *Malassezia* infections are common. +/− gastrointestinal symptoms including frequent normal stools, loose stools, diarrhea, vomiting, and flatulence in 10–15%.	Food allergy testing (serologic, salivary, hair, intradermal) are non-diagnostic and of no clinical value. Response to hypoallergenic diet trial confirms diagnosis (see Table 10.6). Symptoms improve within 6 to 12 weeks of restricted diet. Hypoallergenic diet options include home cooked novel protein diets or prescription novel or hydrolyzed diets. Choose ingredients with consideration of prior diets, avoid hydrolyzed chicken and soy diets in dogs which previously received chicken or soy containing diets. All treats, flavored medications, bones, flavored toys, etc. must be withdrawn. Provocative challenge will confirm diagnosis with recurrence of symptoms within 1–10 days of reintroduction of suspect allergen.	1) Maintenance of appropriate hypoallergenic diet. 2) Avoidance of dietary allergen(s). 3) Control of any secondary skin infections.

(Continued)

Table 10.1 Hypersensitivity disorders and treatment of allergic skin diseases (Continued)

Disease	Clinical signs	Diagnosis	Treatment
Canine Flea Bite Allergy (Figures 10.5A–10.5E)	Presence of adult fleas and their feces on the pet (flea feces can be confirmed by placing on moist white paper or cotton ball). It is important to note that many dogs can harbor some parasites without substantial clinical signs except mild pruritus. Acutely dogs experience intense pruritus with sudden turning, biting, scratching, rolling. Flea allergy is a common cause of pyotraumatic dermatitis ("hot spots"). Lesions typically located at dorsal lumbar area, flanks, base of tail, and hindlimbs and include hypotrichosis, papules, erythematous plaques, and wheals. Within a relatively short period, hours to days, self-induced erosions, ulcerations, excoriations, and lichenification can occur. Dogs with concurrent atopic dermatitis will experience more severe pruritus and progression. In chronic cases, secondary bacterial pyoderma, hyperpigmentation, and lichenification can develop.	History, clinical examination. If fleas/flea feces are present on examination or client confirms history of flea exposure, diagnosis is straightforward; if no fleas/flea feces are present, diagnosis can be more challenging. To determine likelihood of exposure question: • Client environmental or on-pet flea control program for all pets in household including felines. • Frequent bathing or swimming. • Dog's encounters with groomer, day care, dog park, or wildlife. Physical exam findings including dorsolumbar, tail distribution. Positive response to flea treatment trial. Skin biopsy is non-diagnostic. Note: Flea allergic dogs may have minimal flea burden which can constitute a challenge in convincing owner to initiate a treatment plan.	Control of pruritus can be accomplished with one of the following: • Apoquel® PO at 0.4–0.6 mg/kg/day. • Prednisone PO at 0.5 mg/kg/day until clinical response then taper off over 4 weeks as fleas are controlled. Control of secondary bacterial folliculitis with appropriate antibiotics. Flea control measures both within the environment *and* on the animal.[a] The importance of environmental control is often overlooked; new residual insecticides and insect growth regulators can markedly reduce if not eliminate fleas from pet and in-home premises within 2 to 3 months. Treatment plan: 1) Educate pet owners and veterinary staff on the biology of fleas infesting pets. It is important to note that due to flea life cycle fleas may continue to emerge within premises for 1 to 3 months after initiation of treatment protocol. Treatment of all in contact pets within household is a key factor. 2) Implement mechanical control measures such as frequent vacuuming and flea traps. 3) Application of insect growth regulators including but not limited to: • Juvenile hormone analogs including pyriproxyfen 1%w/v, methoprene. • Insect development inhibitor lufenuron. 4) Administration of flea adulticides including but not limited to: • Isoxazolines including fluralaner, afoxolaner, sarolaner. • Neonicotinoids including imidacloprid, nitenpyram, dinotefuran. • Spinosad. • Metaflumizone. • Oxydiazines including indoxacarb 13%. • Avermectins including selamectin, moxidectin. • Phenylpyrazoles including fipronil. • Pyrethroids, permethrin, flumethrin (NOT ON CATS). [a] Caution with pyrethroids, permethrin containing products in households with felines as these are toxic and can be fatal if feline is exposed inadvertently.

Canine eosinophilic furunculosis of face (Figures 10.6A–10.6C) Likely triggered by insect bite/sting.	Sudden onset of papules, nodules, crusts, and exudative lesions of muzzle, bridge of nose, and periocular areas; nonhaired nasal planum is spared. Lesions may be minimally to intensely pruritic and variably painful. Some appear otherwise healthy while others are systemically ill and may exhibit fever, anorexia, and malaise. Rarely generalized lesions may be noted involving extremities, and glabrous skin of ventral abdomen.	History, clinical exam, and ruling out other differentials. Cytology of lesions shows numerous eosinophils. Bacteria on cytology may be seen if secondary pyoderma present. Dermatohistopathology shows infiltrative eosinophilic perifolliculitis, folliculitis, and furunculosis. Infiltration with neutrophils, lymphocytes, and macrophages, +/− dermal hemorrhage and collagen degeneration.	1) Any secondary pyoderma should be treated with appropriate antibiotics of 3 to 4 week duration. 2) Glucocorticoids: • Prednisolone PO at 1 to 2 mg/kg BID to q24h. • Methylprednisolone PO at 1 to 2 mg/kg BID to q24h. • Once lesions are improved a gradual taper of steroids over 2 to 4 weeks is warranted. Tapering steroids too quickly may lead to recurrence of symptoms.
Canine eosinophilic granuloma (Figure 10.7) Breed predilection seen in Cavalier King Charles Spaniel, German Shepherd, Siberian Husky, and Bull Mastiff.	Affects oral mucosa, and rarely haired skin on trunk, limbs, face, or on paws. Lesions of skin characterized by nodules and plaques with variable ulceration. Oral lesions are well-demarcated yellow to green granulomatous plaques to nodules.	Clinical appearance may distinguish from other diseases, but biopsy is recommended for confirmation. Histopathology shows perivascular to diffuse inflammation composed primarily of eosinophilic and histiocytic cells, some of which surround collagen fibers and form flame figures and palisading granulomas. Variable degrees of ulceration, necrosis, edema, mucin, and fibrosis may be present.	Glucocorticoids are the most well described treatment: • Prednisone PO 0.5 to 2 mg/kg/day. • Methylprednisolone PO 0.5 to 2 mg/kg/day. • Administer until clinical resolution then steroid dose is slowly tapered over weeks to months to lowest dosage that controls symptoms. Additional treatments of consideration and for steroid sparing include: • Surgical CO_2 laser to ablate lesion. • Cyclosporine. • Chlorambucil. • Refractory or recurrent cases may benefit from referral to area specialist (dermatologist or dentist) depending on location of lesions.

(*Continued*)

Table 10.1 Hypersensitivity disorders and treatment of allergic skin diseases (Continued)

Disease	Clinical signs	Diagnosis	Treatment
Atopy ***Cats*** (Figures 10.8A–10.8O) Usually occurs between 6 and 24 months.	See Table 10.7 for extensive descriptions of the following patterns: Pruritus can manifest in a variety of reaction patterns: • Miliary dermatitis. • Head and neck pruritus. • Self-induced alopecia. • Eosinophilic dermatitides. Head, neck, ears, ventral abdomen, caudal thighs, lateral thorax, and forelegs. Other symptoms can include otitis externa, recurrent pyoderma and *Malassezia* dermatitis, and allergic airway disease.	Historical seasonality if present is helpful; for cats with non-seasonal symptoms atopy is a diagnosis of exclusion and ruling out concurrent hypersensitivity (food allergy, parasite hypersensitivity, dermatophyte). Good clinical response (85% improved) usually occurs with label dosage of Atopica® or glucocorticoids, however, response can diminish with chronicity. Dermatohistopathology is non-diagnostic. It is important to emphasize that allergy testing is not a first-line screening test in the workup of dogs and cats with dermatologic disease. Once the clinical diagnosis of atopy has been achieved by ruling out all other possible causes for symptoms, then intradermal or serologic allergy testing is used as a management tool to determine allergens to include in immunotherapy. See Table 10.3.	Therapeutic options include: 1) Management of secondary pruritic conditions including flea infestation and microbial (bacteria/*Malassezia*) overgrowth. 2) Essential fatty acids and antihistamines may be attempted but lack potency. It is important to consider the difficulty in medicating most felines when prescribing these low potency items. 3) Glucocorticoids. Oral administration preferred for consistency of control: • Prednisolone or methylprednisolone initially 1–2 mg/kg/day PO then tapered to 0.5–1 mg/kg every other day. • Dexamethasone tablets (or give injectable solution orally if liquid easier) 0.1 to 0.2 mg/kg/day taper to 0.1 mg/kg every 72 h or less. • Triamcinolone 0.1 to 0.2 mg/kg/day PO than tapered to every 48 to 72 hours for maintenance. • Generally steroid dosage is tapered in 7 to 14 days after initiation to the lowest effective dosage that controls the clinical signs. If intolerant to oral medications then repository steroid injectable formulations can be considered. • Repository steroid less desirable due to higher risk of long-term side effects including diabetes mellitus and skin fragility. • Repository steroid less desirable due to risk of recurrent flare of disease as injection efficacy can diminish at variable durations depending on patient *and* disease factors. • Triamcinolone (Kenalog) 0.11–0.22 mg/kg SC/IM: effect typically lasts 7 to 15 days. • Methylprednisolone acetate (Depo-Medrol®) 10–20 mg SC/IM per cat depending on cat size and severity of symptoms; effect typically lasts 4 to 8 weeks. In cats which require frequent or long-term steroids, then consider non-steroidal treatment options: 4) Ciclosporin modified (Atopica®) initially dosed at 7 mg/kg/day PO. • Takes 4 to 6 weeks to achieve therapeutic benefit, and steroids initially can be utilized concurrently to maintain control in the patient. • Once patient is 4 to 6 weeks into therapy concurrent steroid dosage is tapered and discontinued. • If patient well controlled on ciclosporin then dosage or frequency is lowered to the lowest dose that maintains clinical control. • Typically well tolerated with gastrointestinal upset reported and more common in the initiation phase. • Ciclosporin should not be prescribed to indoor/outdoor cats due to risk of exposure to FELV, FIV, and toxoplasmosis. • Check labs/*Toxoplasma* titer pre-treatment, then CBC/Chemistry panel 6 weeks into treatment, then CBC/Chemistry panel/UA q6–12 months.

			5) Apoquel® (extralabel) 0.4–0.6 mg/kg PO q12–24 h has been used by some dermatologists and practitioners with improvement in approx. 50% of cats; labwork should be carefully monitored, as Apoquel safety has not been studied in cats. Note Cytopoint® is not labeled or effective for cats, and may trigger reaction as it contains caninized antibody (dog specific). 6) Allergy testing and desensitization (see Tables 10.3–10.5). 7) Topical therapies including bathing, conditioners, sprays, mousse are considered but less ideal in cats due to grooming behaviors. 8) Referral to area dermatologist for comprehensive management.
Food Allergy ***Cats*** (Figures 10.9A–10.9F) Can occur at any age, but mean age of onset is 4–5 yr. Predisposed breeds: Siamese. Most common food allergens in cats: beef, fish, and chicken.	See Table 10.7. Pruritus can manifest in a variety of reaction patterns: • Miliary dermatitis. • Head and neck pruritus. • Self-induced alopecia. • Eosinophilic dermatitides. Commonly affected areas include head, neck, ears, ventral abdomen, caudal thighs, lateral thorax, and forelegs. Other symptoms can include otitis externa, recurrent pyoderma and *Malassezia* dermatitis, and allergic airway disease. Frequent normal stools, loose stools, diarrhea, vomiting, and flatulence occur in 10–15% of cases.	Food allergy testing (serologic, salivary, hair, intradermal) are non-diagnostic and of no clinical value. Response to hypoallergenic diet trial confirms diagnosis (see Table 10.6). Symptoms improve within 6 to 12 weeks of restricted diet. Hypoallergenic diet options include prescription novel protein diets, or hydrolyzed diets (see Table 10.6). All treats, flavored medications, flavored toys must be withdrawn. Provocative challenge will confirm diagnosis with recurrence of symptoms within 1 to 10 days of reintroduction of suspect allergen.	1) Maintenance of appropriate hypoallergenic diet (see Table 10.6). 2) Avoidance of dietary allergen(s). 3) Control of any secondary skin infections.

(*Continued*)

Table 10.1 Hypersensitivity disorders and treatment of allergic skin diseases (Continued)

Disease	Clinical signs	Diagnosis	Treatment
Feline Flea Bite Allergy (Figures 10.10A and 10.10B) The most common feline hypersensitivity diseases in flea endemic areas.	Presence of adult fleas and their feces on the pet (flea feces can be confirmed by placing on moist white paper or cotton ball). Unlike dogs that have a fairly typical clinical presentation, cats can have a *variety* of clinical signs including the following commonly observed presentations: • Miliary dermatitis consisting of acutely of multiple, small, crusted papules that may be easier to feel than see. Progression of lesions to larger crusted papules and plaques with excoriations and ulcerations. Lesions can be generalized. • Symmetrical alopecia of caudal dorsum and flank area is a common distribution of FAD. Ventrum, forelimbs, head, and neck are also commonly affected. Alopecia may be the only clinical sign with owners convinced that hair is falling out rather than a component of over-grooming. • Excoriations, erosions, ulcers, and crusting of face, head, and neck. • Eosinophilic granuloma complex reaction pattern as described within this chapter.	History, clinical examination. If fleas/flea feces are present on examination or client confirms history of flea exposure, diagnosis is straightforward; if no fleas/flea feces are present, diagnosis can be more challenging. To determine likelihood of exposure, question client regarding environmental or on-pet flea control program for all pets in household and lifestyle of feline. Positive response to flea treatment trial. Skin biopsy is non-diagnostic. Note: Flea allergic cats may have minimal flea burden which can constitute a diagnostic challenge.	Control of pruritus can be accomplished with any of the following: • Methylprednisolone PO 0.8 to 2 mg/kg/day. • Prednisolone PO 0.5 to 2 mg/kg/day. • Dexamethasone tablets (or give injectable solution orally if liquid easier) 0.1 to 0.2 mg/kg/day taper to 0.1 mg/kg every 72 h. Taper off over 2 to 3 weeks while fleas are controlled. Flea control measures both within the environment *and* on the animal. The importance of environmental control is often overlooked. New residual insecticides and insect growth regulators can markedly reduce if not eliminate fleas from pet and in-home premises within 2 to 3 months. Treatment plan: • Educate pet owners and veterinary staff on the biology of fleas infesting pets. It is important to note that due to flea life cycle fleas may continue to emerge within premises for 1 to 3 months after initiation of treatment protocol. Treatment of all in contact pets within household is a key factor. • Implement mechanical control measures such as frequent vacuuming and flea traps. • Application of insect growth regulators including but not limited to: – Juvenile hormone analogs including pyriproxyfen 1%w/v, methoprene. – Insect development inhibitor lufenuron. • Administration of flea adulticides including but not limited to: – Isoxazolines including fluralaner, afoxolaner, sarolaner. – Neonicotinoids including imidacloprid, nitenpyram, dinotefuran. – Spinosad. – Metaflumizone. – Oxydiazines including indoxacarb 13%. – Avermectins including selamectin, moxidectin. – Phenylpyrazoles including fipronil. * Caution with pyrethroids, permethrin containing products in households with felines as these are toxic and can be fatal if feline is exposed inadvertently.

Mosquito bite hypersensitivity ***Cats*** (Figures 10.11A–10.11D) No sex or breed predisposition observed. Cats often between 8 months of age to 6 years, but any age may be affected. Summer and outdoor lifestyle are risk factors.	Early lesions include mildly to severely pruritic wheals, papules, plaques, erosions, and crusts on bridge of nose, pinnae, and less commonly margins of foot pads. With chronicity progresses to nodules, crusts, excoriations, and pigmentary changes. Regional lymphadenopathy may be observed.	History, clinical exam, and response to confinement in mosquito free environment Cytology of lesions often demonstrates eosinophils, variable neutrophils, +/− coccoid bacteria if secondary pyoderma present. Differential diagnoses include ear mite infestation, dermatophytosis, food allergy, atopy, herpesvirus dermatitis, autoimmune disorders such as pemphigus, and solar induced dermatitis.	• Confinement indoors especially during dawn and dusk. • Insect repellents. • Plant derived essential oils including citronella, eucalyptus, peppermint, lavender, tea tree oil, neem. Due to grooming behavior of cats these various oils may cause gastric irritation. • Synthetic products including permethrin based DEET can be TOXIC to cats unless specifically formulated for cats. • Extreme caution with insect repellents including permethrins and pyrethroids which are toxic to cats. If exposure cannot be avoided then oral glucocorticoids are reliably effective: • Prednisolone 0.5 mg – 2 mg/kg PO per day. • Dexamethasone tablets (or give injectable solution orally if liquid easier) 0.1 to 0.2 mg/kg/day taper to 0.1 mg/kg every 72 h. • Methylprednisolone PO at 1 to 2 mg/kg/day. • Triamcinolone PO 0.1 to 0.5 mg/kg/day. Once disease control is achieved and patient is stable steroid dosage is tapered and discontinued; typically decrease dosage by 25 to 50% q2 weeks. Prognosis is good, but scarring may occur.
Eosinophilic granuloma complex See Table 10.8.	An inflammatory cutaneous or oral disease that develops as a result of underlying hypersensitivity such as atopy, food allergy, or parasite hypersensitivity.	Refer to Table 10.8.	Refer to Table 10.8.

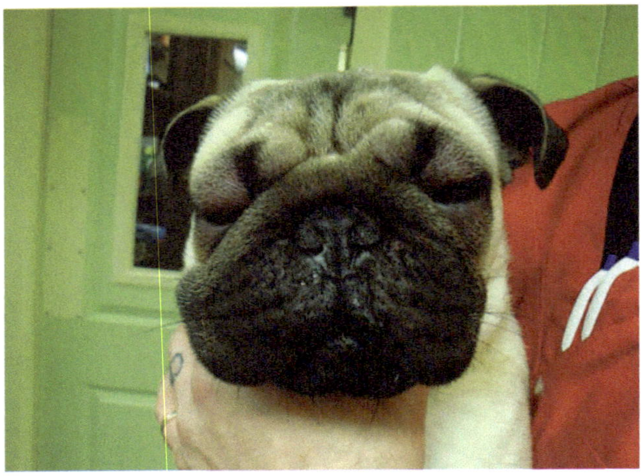

Figure 10.1A Acute angioedema in a Pug due to a vaccination reaction. *Source:* Image courtesy of VIN and Carie Wisell, DVM.

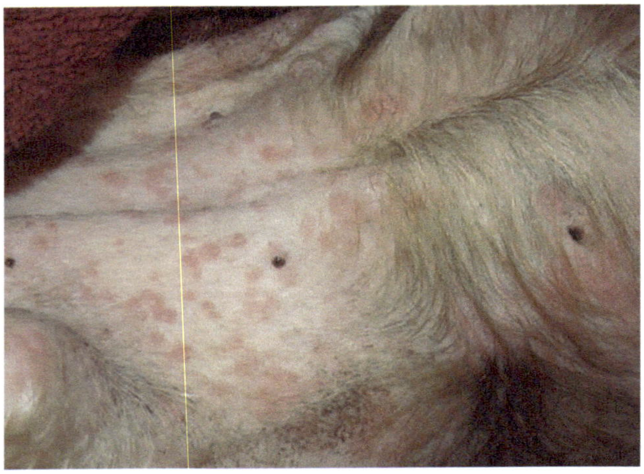

Figure 10.1C Urticaria in a Yorkie induced by an allergic reaction to a shampoo.

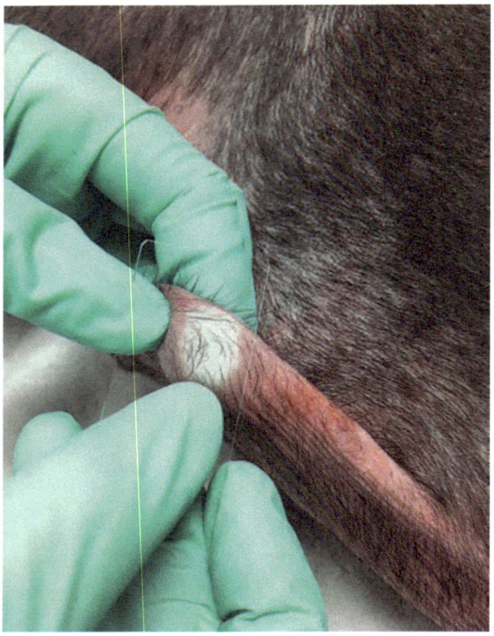

Figure 10.1E Diascopy: blanching of the skin under the pressure of the glass slide demonstrates vasodilation was the cause for the marked erythema which occurred in a dog minutes after receiving a morphine premedication.

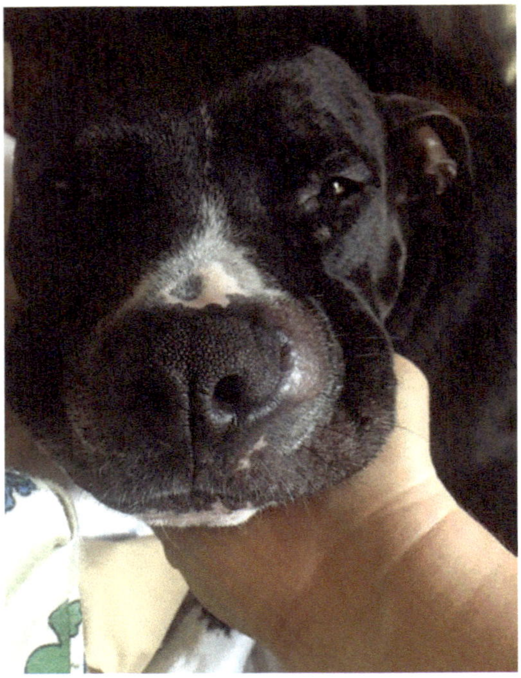

Figure 10.1B Acute urticarial wheals on the nose and eyelids of an allergic Pitbull due to a suspected insect bite reaction.

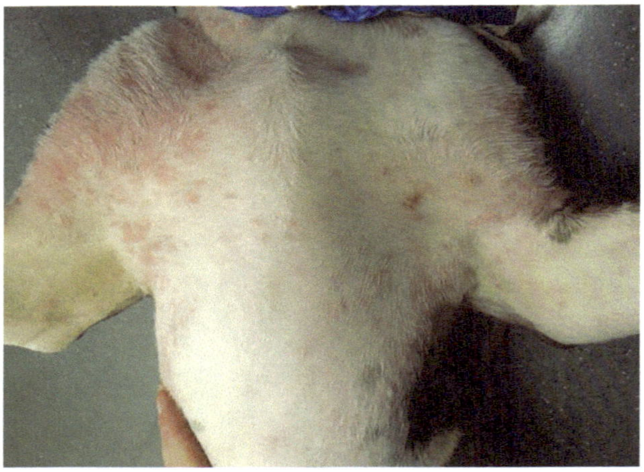

Figure 10.1D Urticarial wheals in a Pitbull which occurred during intradermal allergy testing.

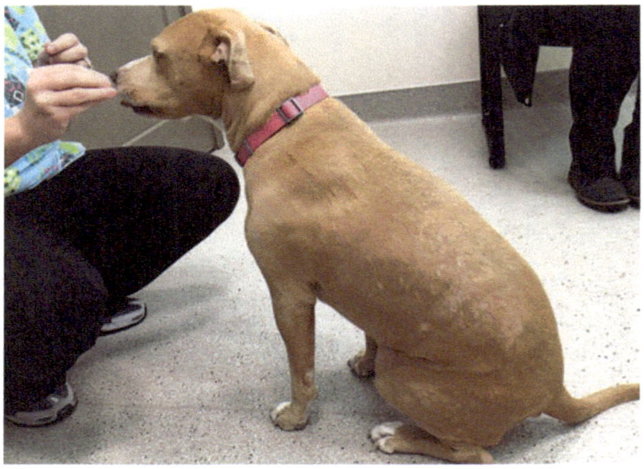

Figure 10.1F Bacterial folliculitis in an atopic Pitbull; the raised tufts of fur can mimic hives, but careful examination of the skin under the tufted fur revealed scaling and easily epilated fur due to infection.

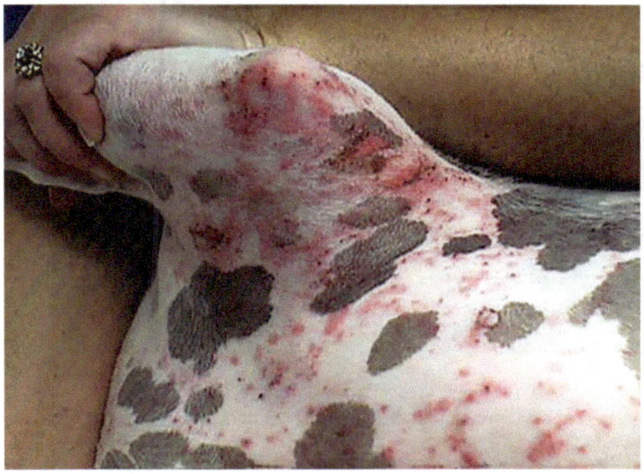

Figure 10.2A An acute papular, ventral, truncal dermatitis due to a plant induced contact dermatitis in a dog; skin lesions resolved with removal of the dog from the plants and recurred with subsequent exposure. *Source:* Image courtesy of VIN and Dr. Carol Foil, DVM DACVD.

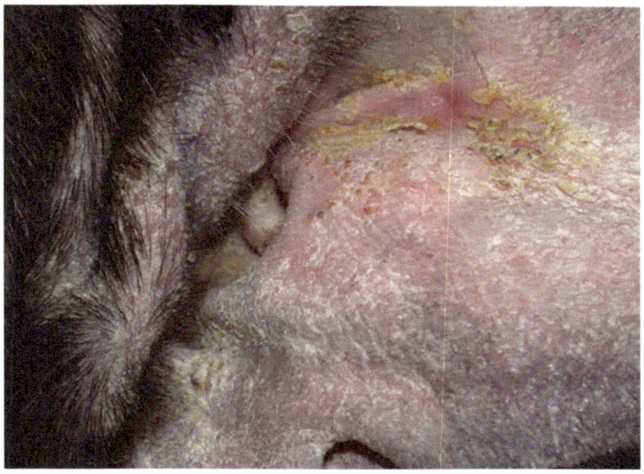

Figure 10.2B Marked pinnal inflammation and exfoliative scaling in a dog with a contact hypersensitivity reaction to eardrops containing xenodine.

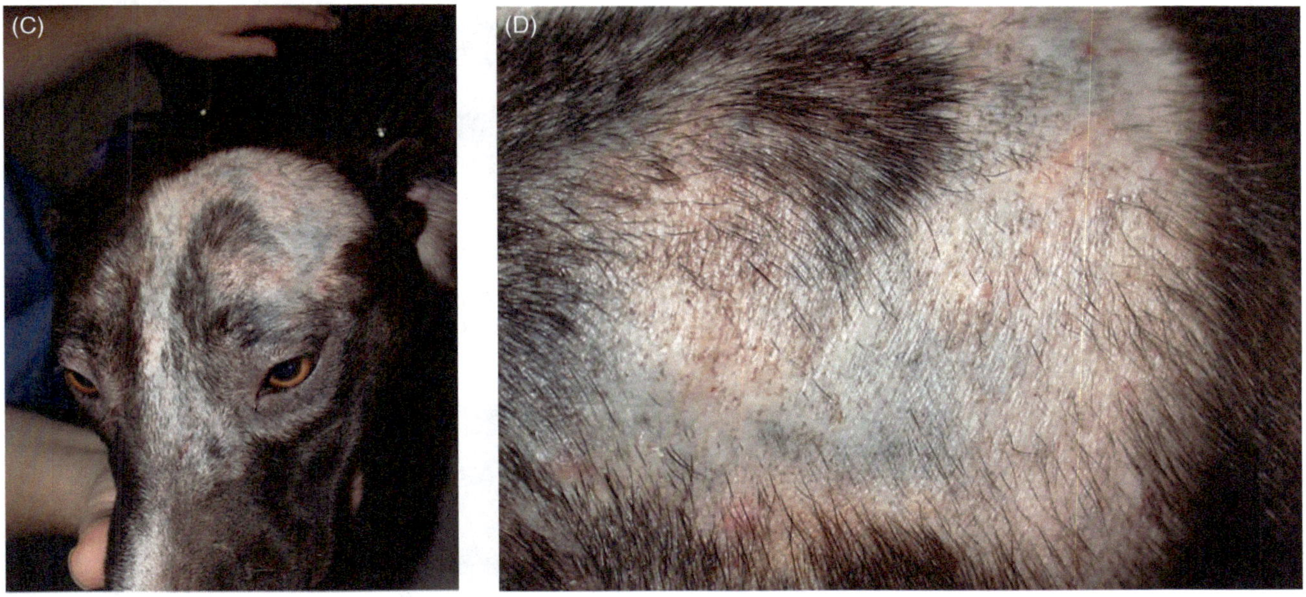

Figures 10.2C and D Spreading periocular alopecia and erythema due to a contact hypersensitivity reaction to neomycin.

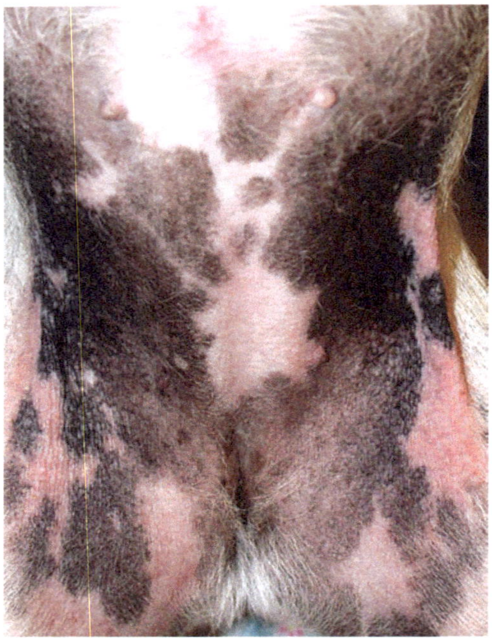

Figure 10.3A Inguinal erythema and slight lichenification due to atopic dermatitis.

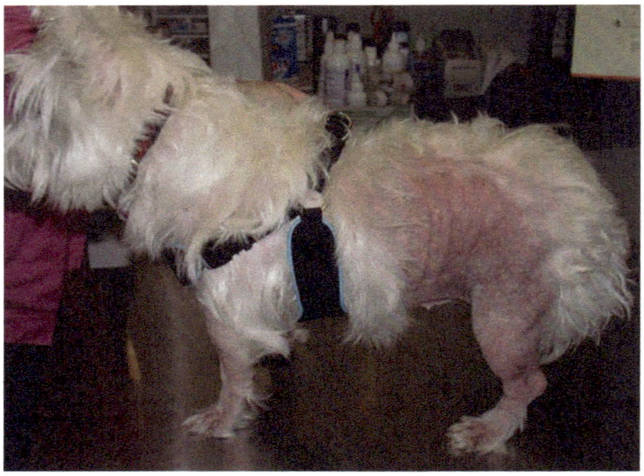

Figure 10.3B An atopic West Highland White Terrier with marked barbering/erythema and moderate lichenification on the trunk and limbs.

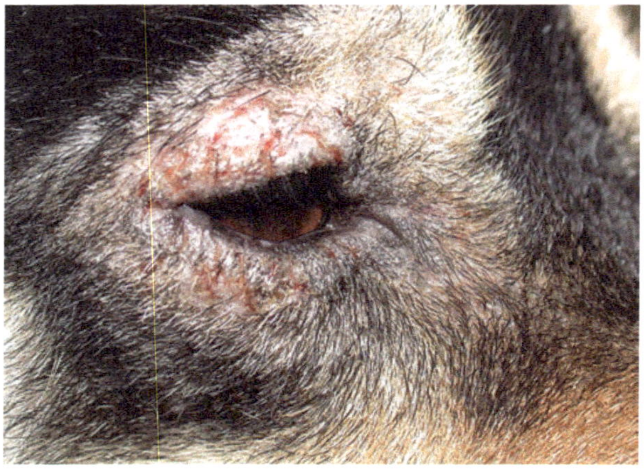

Figure 10.3C Eyelid barbering and excoriations in an atopic Shiba Inu.

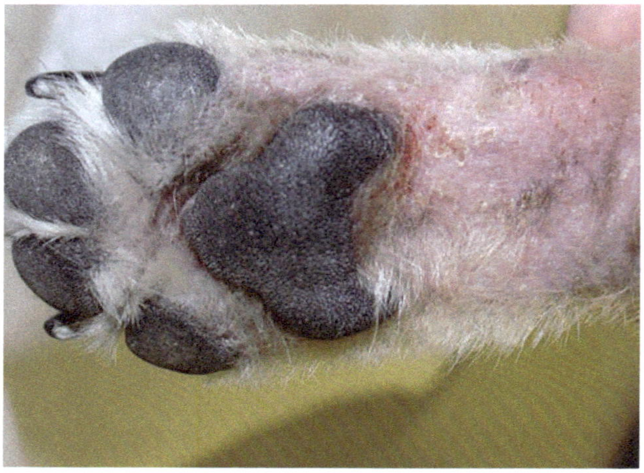

Figure 10.3D Palmar carpal barbering/erythema/excoriations typical for atopic dermatitis.

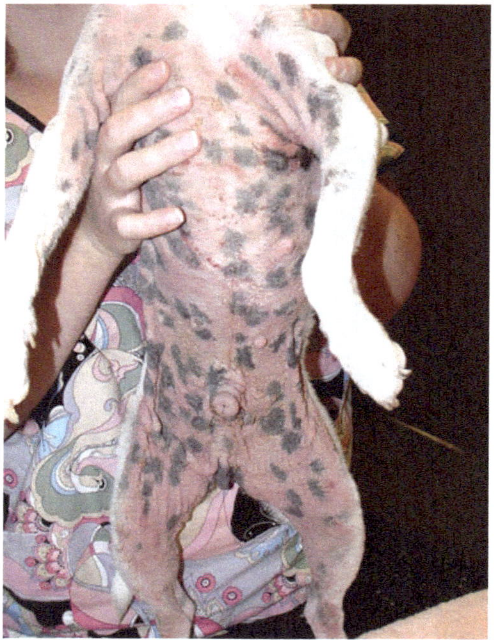

Figure 10.3E Marked ventral truncal alopecia, erythema, and lichenification in an atopic Jack Russell Terrier with secondary bacterial overgrowth.

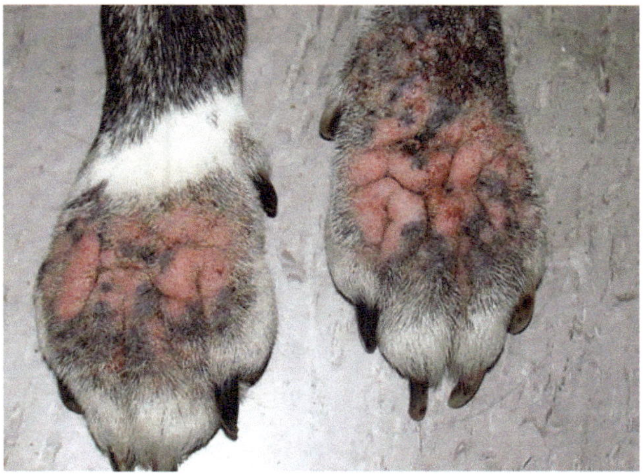

Figure 10.3F Severe pedal barbering with lichenification in an atopic dog with secondary methicillin resistant Staph infection.

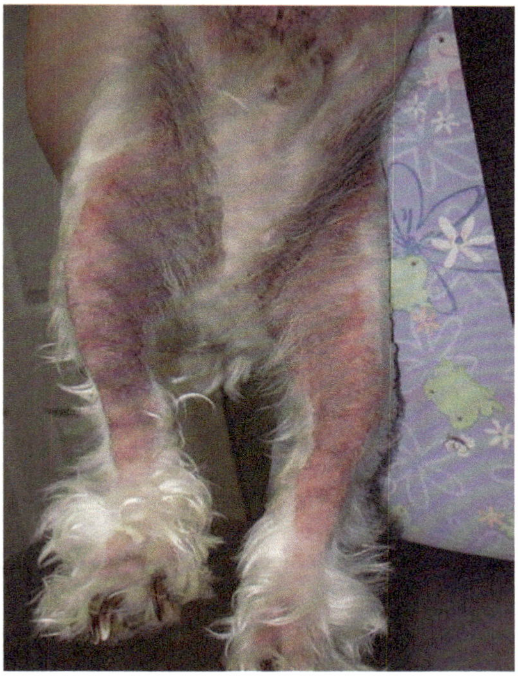

Figure 10.3G Barbering, erythema, and lichenification on the ventral trunk and limbs of an atopic Westie with secondary bacterial and yeast skin infections.

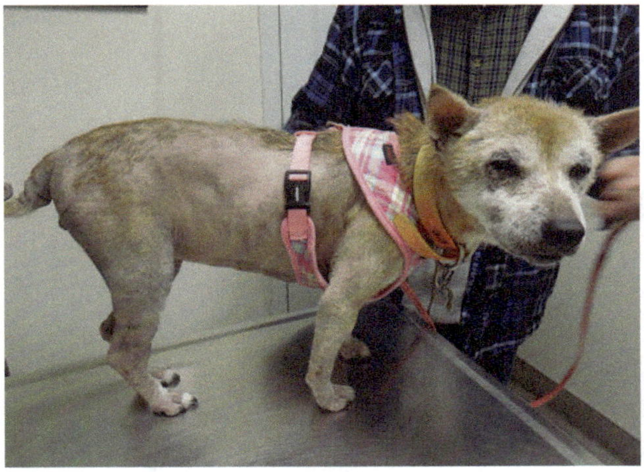

Figure 10.3H Severe truncal and limb barbering in an atopic Shiba Inu.

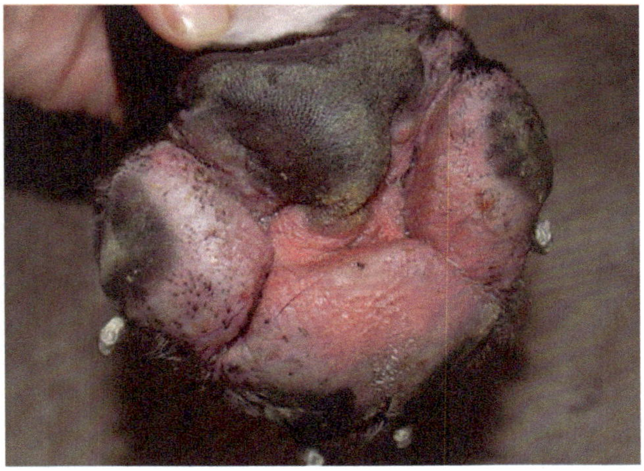

Figure 10.3I Severe interdigital inflammation, swelling, and hyperplasia in a Pitbull with atopic dermatitis.

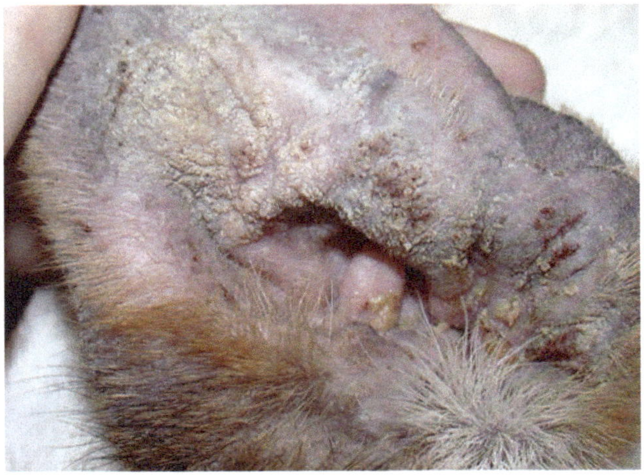

Figure 10.3J Outer ear and inner pinnal inflammation and lichenification due to atopy and secondary chronic otitis.

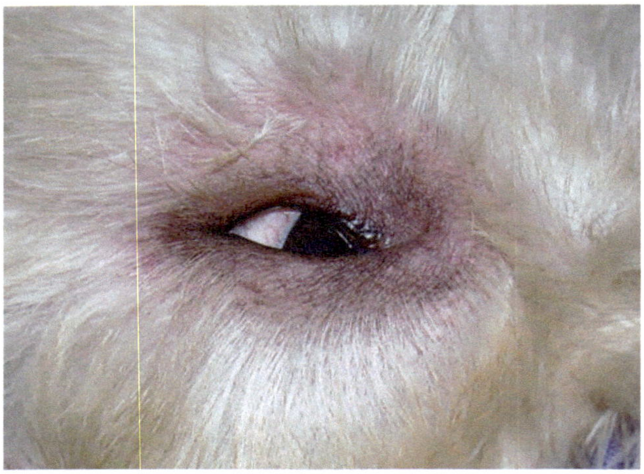

Figure 10.3K An atopic dog with eyelid barbering, erythema, and post inflammatory hyperpigmentation.

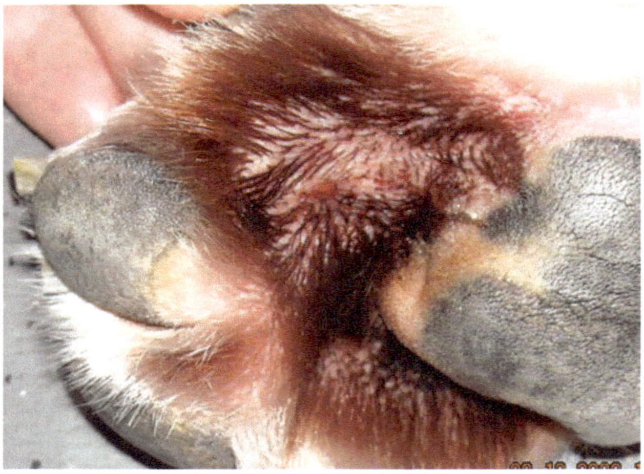

Figure 10.3L Allergic and *Malassezia* pododermatitis caused by atopy.

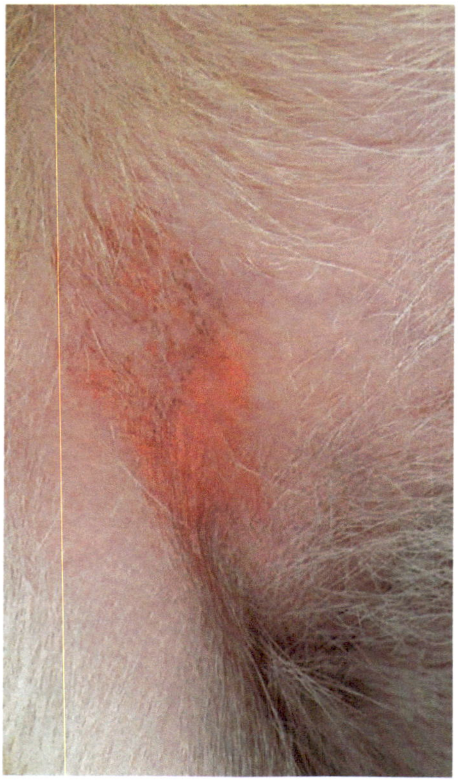

Figure 10.3M A patch of intense axillary erythema caused by atopic dermatitis; no infection was present.

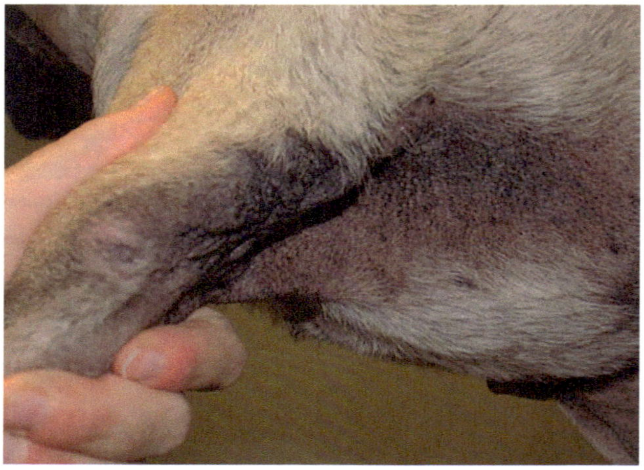

Figure 10.3N In this atopic Pug, chronicity of allergic inflammation has caused axillary post inflammatory hyperpigmentation with mild lichenification caused by mild bacterial overgrowth.

Algorithm 10.1 Canine atopic dermatitis treatment. A multipronged approach to treatment of atopic dermatitis; addressing pruritus, improving the epidermal barrier, controlling secondary infections, and using allergen specific immunotherapy are all important to optimize treatment success.

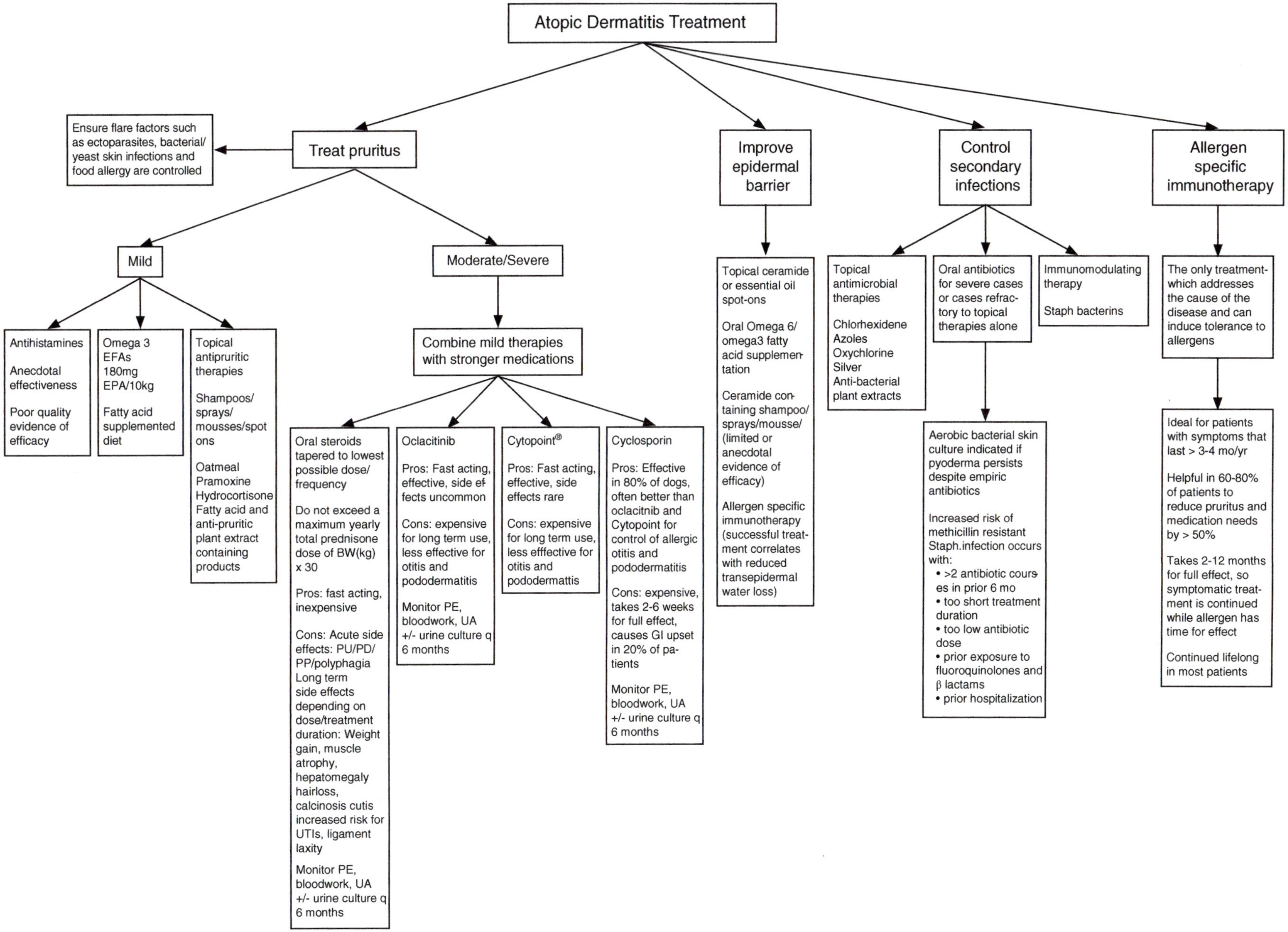

Table 10.2 Allergy treatment toolkit.

Therapeutic target	Therapy	Efficacy	Adverse effects	Dosage	Monitoring/cost
Improving epidermal barrier and minimizing allergen exposure	Bathing to remove cutaneous allergens. Topical therapies including ceramides and phytosphingosines to restore cutaneous lipid barrier.	Helpful but low potency.	Contact reaction to topicals rare but possible.	Weekly bathing generally recommended. Topical spray or mousse products to improve lipid barrier can be utilized daily. Examples: Douxo, Dermoscent products.	No specific monitoring needed. Low to moderate cost depending on product.
Inhibiting histamine release	Antihistamines	Limited evidence to support efficacy. Generally considered low potency.	Safe with rare sedation reported. Rarely some patients may experience unexpected agitation/anxiety.	Hydroxyzine 2 mg/kg PO BID. Diphenhydramine 2 mg/kg PO BID to TID. Cetirizine 1 mg/kg PO once daily. Cats: Chlorpheniramine 2–4 mg PO BID.	No specific monitoring necessary. Low cost.
Anti-pruritic/anti-inflammatory	Fatty acid supplementation.	Moderate evidence of effectiveness, but low potency. Effects are mild and may only allow dose reductions of other therapies.	None expected, although high dose may cause loose stool, avoid in patients with history of pancreatitis.	Dogs and cats: 180 mg EPA/10 lb BW. Author prefers Welactin or Nordic Naturals.	No specific monitoring needed. Low to moderate cost depending on product.
Anti-pruritic/anti-inflammatory	Oral glucocorticoids.	Typically, very effective.	Short-term PU/PD/PP/panting. Long term concerns of iatrogenic Cushing's including alopecia, pot belly, muscle atrophy, calcinosis cutis, hepatopathy, and diabetes mellitus.	Dogs: Prednisone at 0.5 mg/kg/day PO. Methylprednisolone PO at 0.4 mg/kg/day, taper to lowest effective alternate day dose, i.e. 0.25–0.5 mg/kg PO QOD. Cats: Prednisolone or methylprednisolone 1–2 mg/kg/day, taper to lowest effective alternate day dose, i.e. 0.50–1 mg/kg PO QOD.	Short-term monitoring not necessary. Long-term recommend chemistry panel, urinalysis, urine culture every 6 months. Do not exceed a maximum yearly total prednisone dose of BW (kg) × 30. If prolonged steroids are required, then considerations should be made for non-steroidal drug options including oclacitinib (Apoquel®), Cytopoint®, or ciclosporin (Atopica®) to mitigate the long-term effects of chronic steroid use. Low cost.

Anti-pruritic/ anti-inflammatory	Oclacitinib (Apoquel®).	Typically effective. Rapid onset.	Side effects uncommon. Can predispose to opportunistic infections such as *Demodex*, pyoderma, viral papillomas, pneumonia. Rare sedation, polydipsia, GI upset. Rare hepatic enzyme elevation or leukopenia.	Starting dosage at 0.4 to 0.6 mg/kg BID for up to 14 days, followed by once daily dosing. Dosing in the evening may improve control in some. Dividing once daily dosage to lower dose BID may provide more continuous control in some patients. Not labeled for use in cats nor found to be consistently effective, reported extralabel use helpful in 40% of cats.	Not for use in dogs under 1 year of age, or in dogs with serious infection, demodicosis, or neoplastic condition. Currently no specific monitoring interval is recommended, but annual Chemistry panel, CBC, and urinalysis is prudent in dogs, more frequently in cats. Monitor for development of infections including pyoderma, demodicosis, and neoplasia. Moderate to high cost.
Anti-pruritic/ anti-inflammatory	Ciclosporin modified®.	Typically effective. Maximal effect with this therapy can take 4 to 6 weeks to achieve (owners typically will not see immediate improvement, so may need concurrent oral steroids for the first 3–4 weeks of treatment).	Short-term GI upset is common (anorexia, vomiting, diarrhea), but often is mild and resolves in 1 to 3 weeks; freezing capsules helps reduce chance of GI upset. Rare but possible side effects include gingival hyperplasia, increased hair growth, and opportunistic infections such as dermatophytosis, viral papillomatosis, toxoplasmosis, deep fungal or mycobacterial infections.	Starting dosage of 5 mg/kg/day PO (dogs); 7 mg/kg (cats). If response seen dose may be tapered to lowest dose that maintains control. Typically reduce dosage by skipping 1 to 2 days per week and assessing over 2 to 4 weeks if stable then further reduction in dose frequency is considered.	Check pretreatment CBC/Chemistry panel in dogs/cats and toxoplasmosis titers in cats, then recheck CBC/Chemistry panel 4–6 weeks after starting then CBC/Chemistry panel/UA q6–12 months. Moderate to high cost; in dogs, combining with oral ketoconazole 2.5–5 mg/kg reduces cyclosporin dose (and cost). Keep cats inside to reduce risk of contracting toxoplasmosis.

(*Continued*)

Table 10.2 (Allergy treatment toolkit Continued)

Therapeutic target	Therapy	Efficacy	Adverse effects	Dosage	Monitoring/cost
Anti-pruritic	Lokivetmab (Cytopoint®). “Caninized” anti-IL31 antibody.	Very effective for most dogs. Works within 1 to 3 days. Typically lasts 4 weeks or longer in some. Initial injection may only last 2 to 3 weeks until steady state is reached. In small number of dogs ineffective or loses efficacy after 1 to 2 doses due to development of neutralizing antibodies.	Occasional injection site pruritus. Rare self-limiting, malaise, vomiting or diarrhea.	2 mg/kg of body weight subcutaneously every 4 to 8 weeks. Extra label usage of Cytopoint more frequently than every 4 weeks is not recommended. Each vial is for single use only. Not labeled or effective for cats.	No specific monitoring typically necessary, but annual Chemistry panel, CBC, and urinalysis is prudent. Moderate to high cost depending on size of patient.
Modification of immune response	Allergen immunotherapy is the only therapy able to treat the underlying cause of the pruritus and infections. Goals of therapy include: • Halting progression of disease. • Dosage reduction of symptomatic drug therapies.	Efficacy depends on multiple variables outlined elsewhere but in the hands of a board-certified dermatologist this therapy typically improves patient symptoms and reduces symptomatic drug needs by 50% or more, in 3 out of 4 patients. Many owners hoping to avoid drug therapies are excited about this therapeutic option.	Injection site pruritus. Rarely facial swelling, hives, vomiting, or diarrhea typically noted at induction of therapy and would require dosage modifications.	Dosage schedules outlined in Table 10.5.	Initial cost of testing can be significant, but long-term maintenance is typically low to moderate cost. Cost per month of allergen will typically be far less than Apoquel® or Cytopoint® in a large breed dog. Consider these variables when treating a life-long disease that typically worsens each year.

Table 10.3 Allergy testing: Intradermal and serologic methods.

Testing method	Intradermal test (Figures 10.12A–10.12C)	In vitro serum test
What is it measuring?	Detects immediate skin reactivity to intradermal injection of allergen extracts consisting of pollens, dust mites, dander, and molds. Skin reactivity is a combination of reaginic antibody, mast cells, and type I cutaneous hypersensitivity.	Detects reaginic antibody to specific allergens (pollens, dust mites, dander, molds) in serum.
Does it test for food allergy?	No	No. Many labs offer a food allergen panel, however serology for food allergy panel is *not* accurate and lacks sensitivity and specificity. Clients' funds are better spent on a prescription hypoallergenic diet trial which is diagnostic and potentially therapeutic.
Test results inhibited by glucocorticoids or antihistamines?	Yes Withdrawal times for antihistamines, oral glucocorticoids, topical/otic glucocorticoids, and ciclosporin/oclacitinib are 7, 14, 14, and 0 days, respectively. Withdrawal of long acting steroid injections for 6 to 8 weeks.	Antihistamines and cyclosporine/oclacitinib likely do not interfere, systemic steroid withdrawal recommendations vary per laboratory.
Sensitivity %	70 to 90	70 to 100
Specificity %	>90	0 to 90 (depending on laboratory technology)
False negatives possible?	Yes	Yes
Can the test be completely negative in an atopic pet?	Very unlikely.	Possible
False positives possible?	Yes	Yes
How is this test useful?	Guides selection of allergens based on patient history, seasonality, and clinical signs. Does not diagnose atopy.	Guides selection of allergens based on patient history, seasonality, and clinical signs. Does not diagnose atopy.
Interpretation of results?	Only perform this test if intention is to formulate therapeutic allergen for patient, since allergen avoidance is not possible. The expense of the test warrants careful analysis of results in combination with patient history and needs when formulating a recipe for the pet. Refer to Tables 10.4 and 10.5.	Only perform this test if you plan to formulate therapeutic allergen for patient, since allergen avoidance is not possible. The expense of the test warrants careful analysis of results in combination with patient history and needs when formulating a recipe for the pet. Refer to Tables 10.4 and 10.5.
Preferred method?	Intradermal testing is generally considered the gold standard. Test results may be paired with serology in referral setting.	With improved technology and validation of tests this method has become more reliable.
Patient with cardiac disease or sedation concerns?	Not ideal to sedate for intradermal testing.	Preferred method if sedation is not medically ideal for patient.

It is important to emphasize that allergy testing is not a first-line screening test in the workup of dogs and cats with dermatologic disease. Once the clinical diagnosis of atopy has been achieved by ruling out all other possible causes for symptoms, then intradermal or serologic allergy testing is used as a management tool to determine allergens to include in immunotherapy.

Table 10.4 Considerations in allergen formulation.

Form of allergen	Sublingual (SLIT)	Subcutaneous (ASIT)
Why choose/ frequency?	Administered once to twice daily. Relatively easy to administer. Ideal if injections are difficult for owner or pet and in small pets.	Administered every 1 to 4 weeks depending on the patient. Many owners are able to administer injections at home. Cost is typically lower than SLIT.
Allergens to include?	Based on testing undertaken to identify significant allergens for inclusion. Intradermal testing remains gold standard. Results are then correlated with patient history. Cross reactivity of allergens should be considered; there are numerous online resources or consult with allergy testing laboratory or area veterinary dermatologist. Pollen data is useful to reference during patient flare periods.	Based on testing undertaken to identify significant allergens for inclusion. Intradermal testing remains gold standard. Results are then correlated with patient history. Cross reactivity of allergens should be considered; there are numerous online resources or consult with allergy testing laboratory or area veterinary dermatologist. Pollen data is useful to reference during patient flare periods.
Can I mix molds with pollens?	Generally, avoiding pollens and molds in the same mixture is ideal, however, due to glycerinated preservative found in SLIT this may be acceptable depending which pollens and molds are in the combination.	Generally, avoiding pollens and molds in the same mixture is ideal. Often second mold vial is needed if significant mold reactions are noted.
Number of allergens in mixture?	Depends on patient reactions, and amount that can be achieved in vial. Area dermatologist may be useful in selection of allergens and formulation. Reference laboratories typically charge an additional fee for each allergen above 12 allergens.	Depends on patient reactions, and amount that can be achieved in vial. Area dermatologist may be useful in selection of allergens and formulation. Reference laboratories typically charge an additional fee for each allergen above 12 allergens.
Initiation of therapy?	Typically started at 2–50 ul pumps once or twice daily with lower concentration mixture initially, followed by higher concentration for maintenance. Some dermatologists start at 1–140 ul pump once daily of maintenance allergen concentration and reduce dose if any pruritus flare occurs (uncommon).	Various protocols exist. Allergen extract typically administered in steadily increasing volumes and concentrations during induction.
Significant adverse events?	Generally lower risk with oral allergen administration. Rare reactions include facial itching or swelling or occasional generalized itch flare. GI upset rare. Oral ulcers or injuries increase risk of adverse reaction, recommend to temporarily stop SLIT post dental procedures.	Client to monitor pet for 1 hour following injection. Significant reactions include hives, facial swelling, increased pruritus. Signs of anaphylaxis may rarely occur including vomiting, diarrhea, weakness, collapse.
Changes to make with adverse events?	Allergic reaction to allergen indicates the right mixture, but dose modifications are necessary. These patients may ultimately respond well but require careful instruction. Consultation with area dermatologist is recommended.	Allergic reaction to allergen indicates the right mixture, but dose modifications are necessary +/− pretreatment with antihistamine or a dose of oral steroid 1 hour prior to allergen. These patients may ultimately respond well but require careful instruction. Consultation with area dermatologist is recommended.

Table 10.5 Protocols for allergen specific immunotherapy (ASIT).

Hyposensitization and induction protocols with aqueous extracts.			
Concentration	**ASIT dosage**	**ASIT frequency**	**SLIT dose/frequency**
100 to 200 PNU (protein nitrogen units)	Although referenced it is the author's opinion that this concentration lacks potency and is unlikely of benefit, nor necessary.	Lower dosage working up to higher dosage every 3 to 7 days.	1 to 2–50 ul pumps once to twice daily. Unlikely of benefit, nor necessary.
1000 to 2000 PNU	This concentration also lacks potency and is not utilized in the author's practice. Starting with 0.1 ml and working up to 1.0 ml volume in 0.1 ml increments.	Lower dosage working up to higher dosage every 3 to 7 days.	1 to 2–50 ul pumps once to twice daily. Unlikely of benefit, nor necessary.
10 000 to 20 000 PNU	Starting with 0.1 ml and working up to 1.0 ml volume in 0.1 ml increments.	Lower dosage working up to higher dosage every 3 to 30 days.[a]	1 to 2–50 ul pumps once to twice daily, or 1–140 ul pump once daily.
Consider size of patient	Toy breeds and patients less than 15 lb may benefit from reduced concentration or dosage.		Toy breeds and patients less than 15 lb may benefit from reduced concentration or dosage.

Modifications in Allergen specific immunotherapy (ASIT).	
Observation	**ASIT modification**
Increased pruritus following injection?	Lower amount administered.
Increased pruritus prior to next injection?	Decrease interval between injections.
Seasonal flare?	Correlate significant pollens to timing of flare, and modify recipe if good correlation exists.
Significant reaction to allergen administration such as hives, vomiting, diarrhea, facial swelling.	Consultation with area dermatologist recommended. Concentration of allergen and dosage should be reduced. In-hospital monitoring of patient following injection during induction phase necessary. May consider alternate formulation such as SLIT.

[a] If good response is seen the interval between injections may be lengthened, but it is important to note that allergen immunotherapy is life-long in most patients. Most patients require administration of allergen every 7 to 14 days as maintenance.

It is important to note that virtually no attempts have been made to standardize hyposensitization schedules and there is no published research to support correct allergen dosage or frequency in companion animals.

Adjustments in allergen can maximize therapeutic efficacy and are the cornerstone to good dermatologic management. Every patient requires careful consideration to the variables of allergen recipe ingredients, concentration, dosage, and frequency.

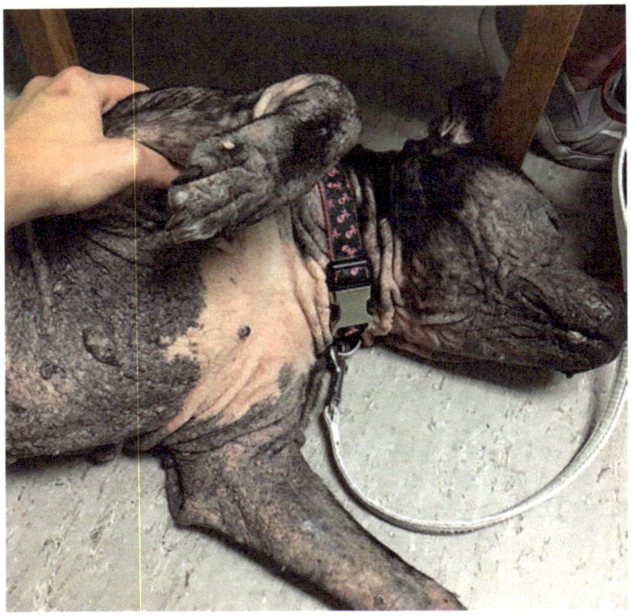

Figure 10.4A A Pitbull with severe chronic barbering, lichenification, and alopecia due to food allergy.

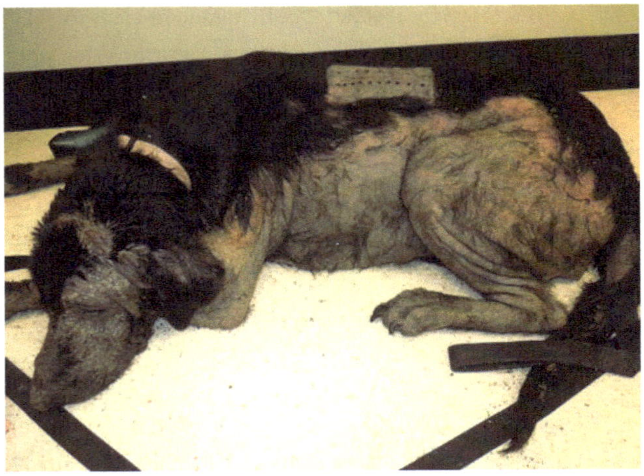

Figure 10.4B An atopic and food allergic Labrador with severe secondary MRSP pyoderma.

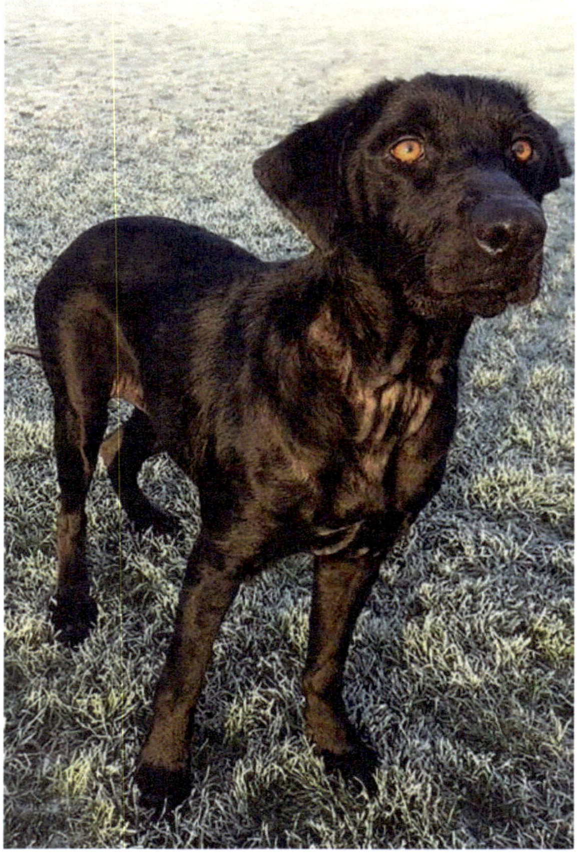

Figure 10.4C The same dog as in Figure 10.4B, six weeks later after receiving daily chlorhexidine baths and dilute bleach soaks for four weeks as well as sublingual immunotherapy and a prescription hypoallergenic diet trial.

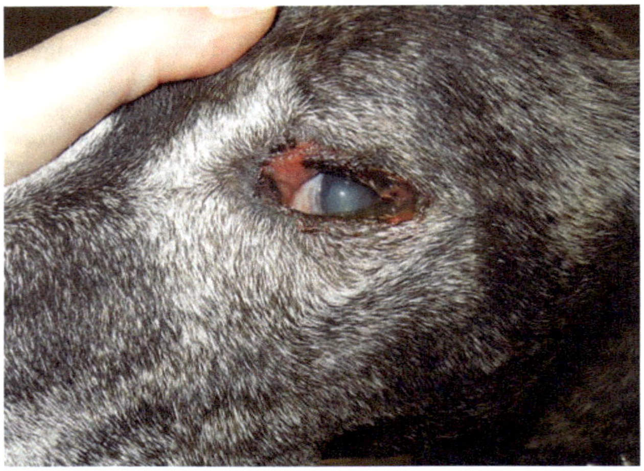

Figure 10.4D Eyelid excoriations due to food allergy in an elderly Pitbull.

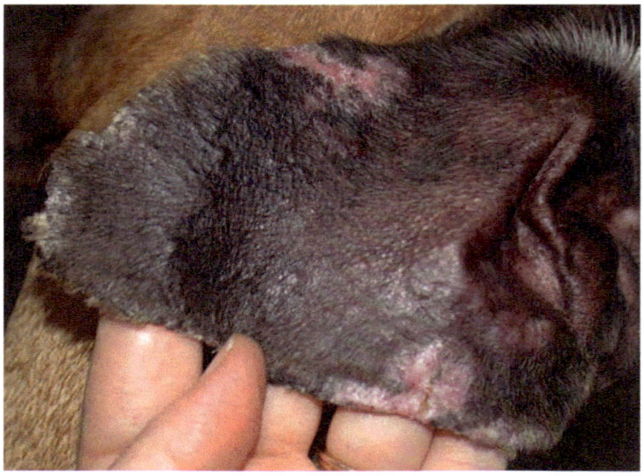

Figure 10.4E Pinnal marginal crusting, erythema, and erosions caused by food allergy in an older Great Dane.

Table 10.6 Performing an adequate diagnostic hypoallergenic diet trial.

Diet option	Sources	Pros	Cons
Home-prepared	Nutritionist formulated resource via American College of Veterinary Nutrition, or European College of Veterinary Nutrition. Alternatively, web-based service such as www.balanceit.com.	Gold standard as variables are theoretically controlled with less risk of contamination with offending allergenic proteins or carbohydrates.	Time consuming. Risk of client utilizing inadequate recipe or resource leading to nutrient deficiency. Client compliance. Should not be utilized in growing animals. May be difficult to find options in pets with concurrent urinary, renal, or hepatic disease. Not recommended in cats without direct involvement of board-certified veterinary nutritionist.
Prescription hydrolyzed protein diets[a] Protein is hydrolyzed into individual amino acids or peptides using acids or proteases.	Ensuring that hydrolysate has no peptides greater than 1 to 3 kDa would give greatest chance of eliminating residual allergens. Avoid hydrolyzed chicken and soy diets in dogs which previously received chicken or soy containing diets.	Variety of commercially available prescription diets. Convenient Cost of diets may be a factor for some pet owners.	Palatability may be diminished depending on the product, but most manufacturers offer full refunds and guarantee their product. Some pet owners may not find hydrolysate an attractive option. Some hydrolyzed diets also labeled for control of urolithiasis, renal disease, or growth.
Prescription novel protein diets[a]	As over the counter (OTC) diets extend options in marketing achieving novel proteins has become challenging. Rabbit, crocodile, alligator, kangaroo are currently the most ideal options.	Convenient Generally have good palatability. Variety of options. Cost of diets may be a factor for some pet owners.	May be difficult to find a novel protein for some patients due to prior exposure to OTC novel protein diets. May be difficult to find options in pets with concurrent urinary, renal, or hepatic disease, or those with growth needs.

[a] Prescription diets typically perform contamination control testing at certain time points in manufacturing to ensure that the diets are not contaminated with alternate proteins. Cross contamination of OTC commercial diets in processing is of concern and thus theoretically prescription diets are less likely to contain offending food allergens as contaminants are not listed on the label.

Caveats/considerations:
- Owner compliance with any of these diets is an inevitable and consistent challenge.
- Owners often do not comprehend the strict nature of a diet trial or believe that small indiscretions will not affect disease control.
- Owners begin to drift from original instruction and will begin to layer in what they believe the pet needs.
- Training staff to assist in education and follow-up with these patients is useful.
- Consideration of flavored monthly preventatives or daily supplements is critical.
- Ideally, all non-essential oral medications, vitamins, toys, treats, and supplements are discontinued. If medications are necessary during diet trial then utilize non-flavored options.

Tips for improved diet trial compliance include:
- Specific written instructions.
- Comparison of the need for a strict diet trial to well recognized peanut allergy in humans highlights the small amount of exposure necessary to trigger an intense reaction in the patient.
- Sending home prescription diet approved treat options.
- Send home canned food appropriate for diet trial for owners to use to administer medications.
- Having owners list all flea/heartworm preventatives, supplements, vitamins, and toys is helpful in identifying areas that need attention.
- Having knowledgeable support staff to follow up with client at two and four weeks into the diet trial to address concerns.
- Having owners provide packages of OTC products that they believe may be acceptable allows the practitioner to educate client and help guide judgment.
- Remind owners the food trial duration is finite.
- Comparison of a diabetic child wanting candy to a possibly food allergic dog wanting chicken or other non-hypoallergenic treat can be helpful, as many pet owners view their pets as children and understand that "parents have to know what's best for their children."
- Have several hypoallergenic diet options and brands to fit with individual clients' lifestyles and personal beliefs.

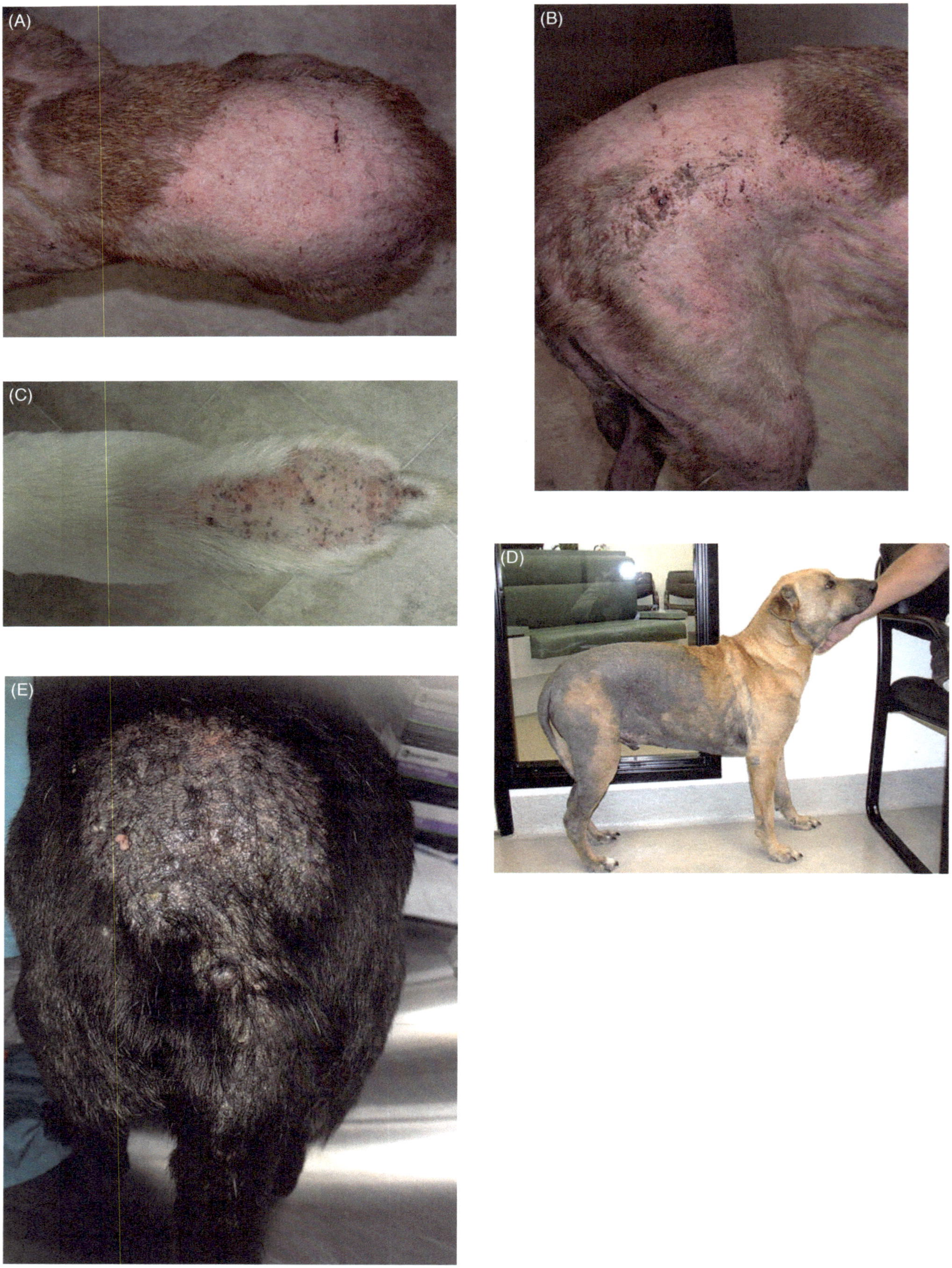

Figures 10.5A–E Lumbar barbering and excoriations due to flea bite hypersensitivity.

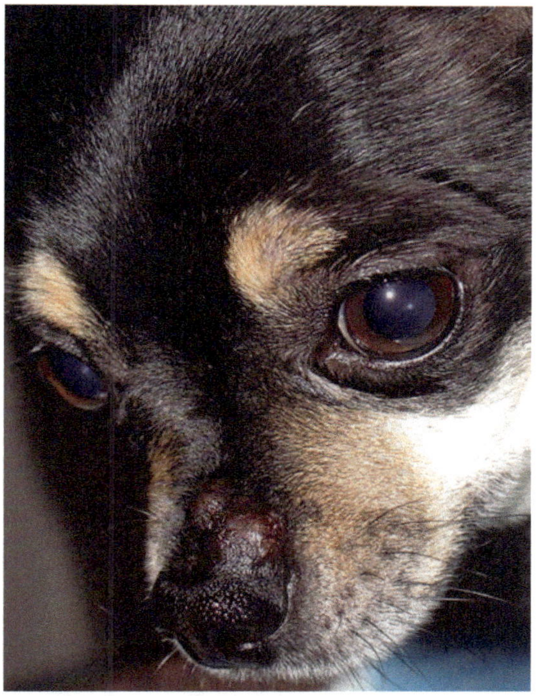

Figure 10.6A Acute raised crusted masses on the dorsal distal muzzle of a Chihuahua due to canine eosinophilic facial furunculosis.

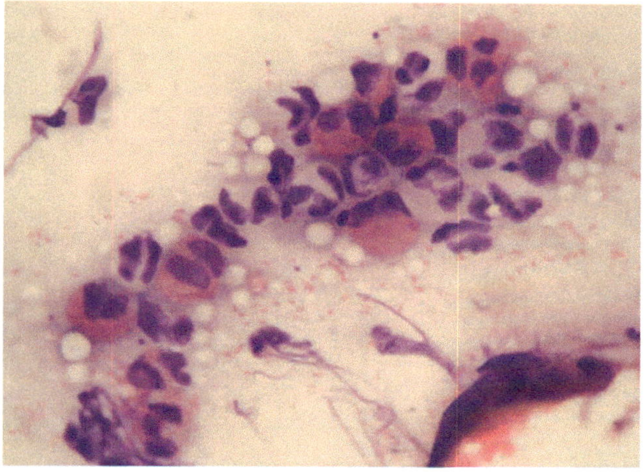

Figure 10.6B Surface cytology demonstrating numerous eosinophils. 100×

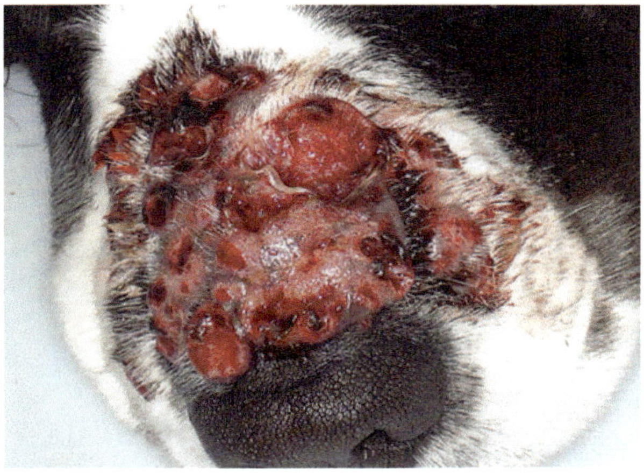

Figure 10.6C Severe exudative nasal dermatitis due to canine eosinophilic facial furunculosis; a secondary bacterial infection contributed to exudate. Source: Image courtesy of VIN and Jennifer Smallwood, DVM.

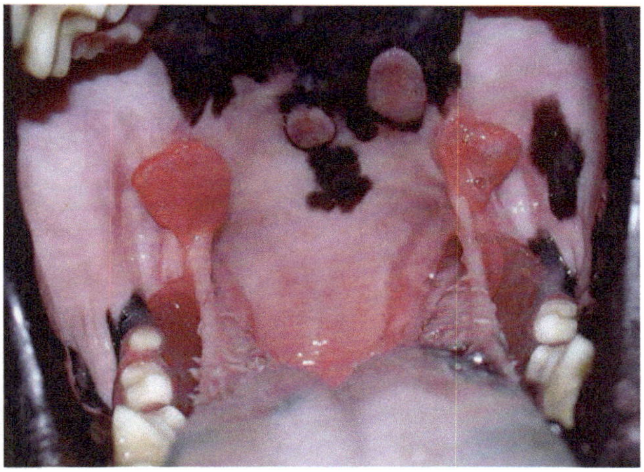

Figure 10.7 Raised erythematous oral plaques in a Cavalier King Charles Spaniel with oral eosinophilic granulomas.

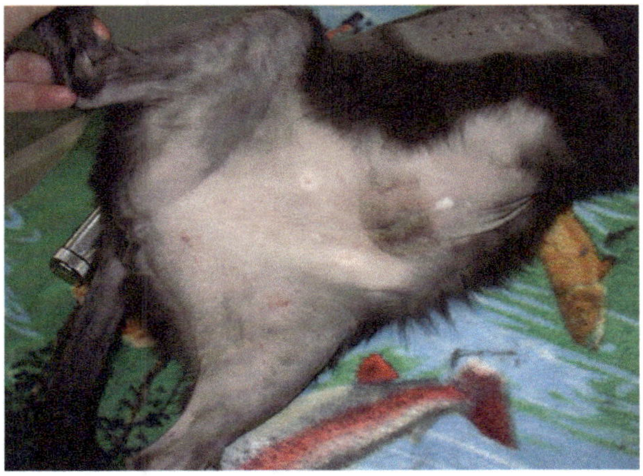

Figure 10.8A Extensive barbering of the ventral trunk and medial thighs in an atopic cat.

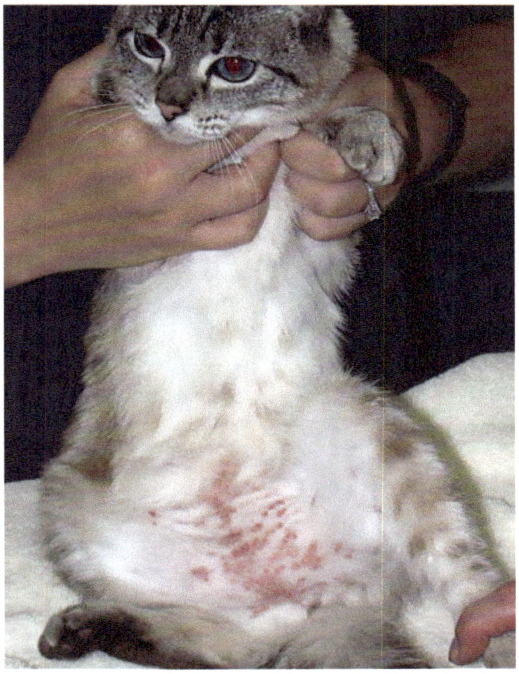

Figure 10.8B Inguinal barbering and small crusted eosinophilic plaques due to atopic dermatitis in a cat.

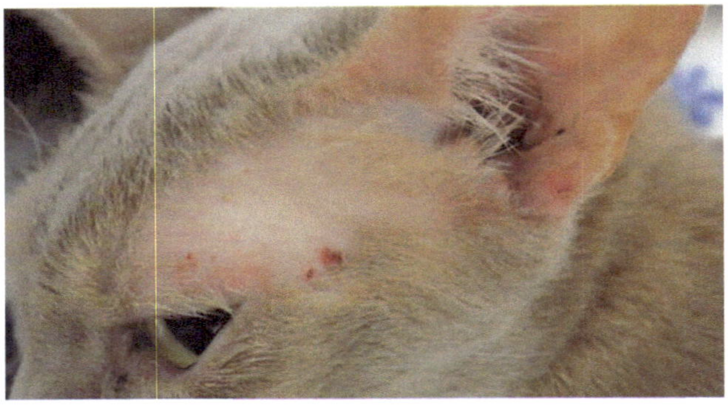

Figure 10.8C An Abyssinian cat with atopy; temporal and outer ear canal erythema, barbering, and small excoriations are present.

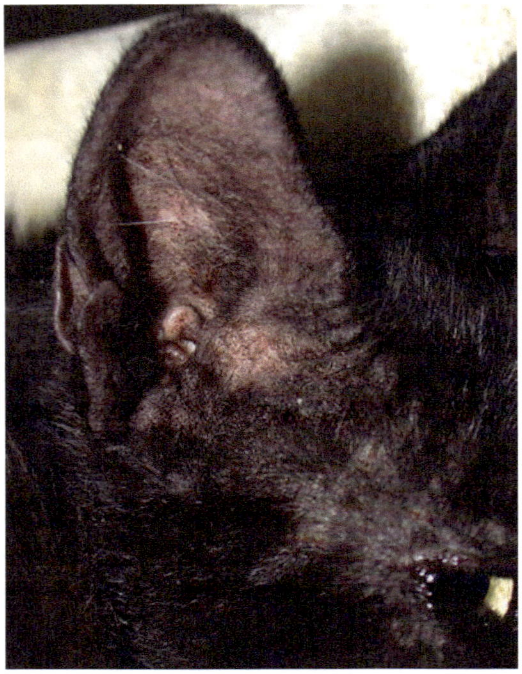

Figure 10.8D Pinnal and temporal barbering and excoriations in an atopic cat.

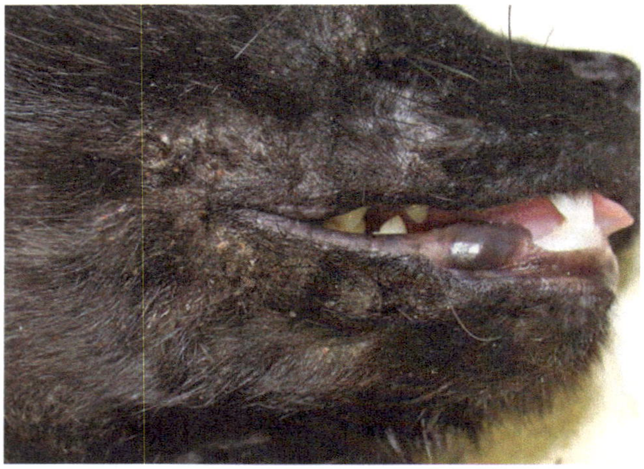

Figure 10.8E The same cat had extensive barbering and excoriations on the lateral face and lips; cytology demonstrated secondary bacterial pyoderma.

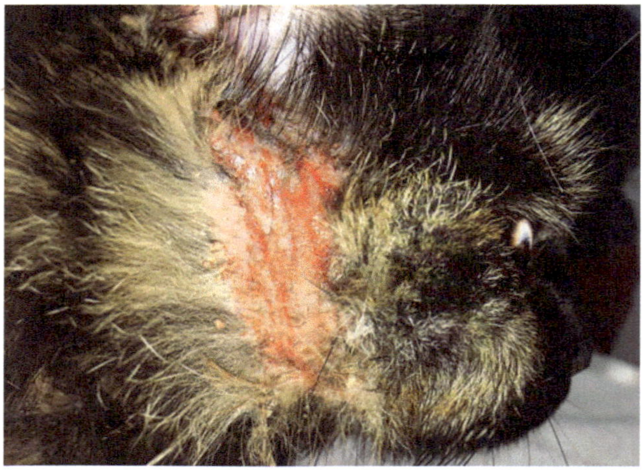

Figure 10.8F Facial excoriations in an atopic cat.

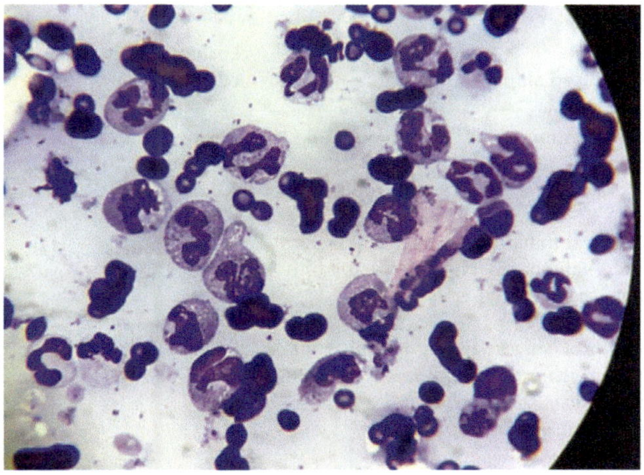

Figure 10.8G Cytology of the affected skin in the cat pictured in figure 10.8F showed marked allergic inflammation. 100x

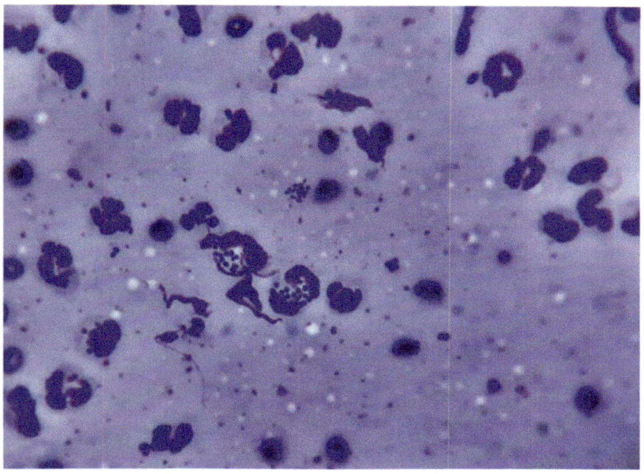

Figure 10.8H In addition, further careful examination of cytology showed neutrophils with intracellular cocci bacteria indicating a secondary bacterial pyoderma. 100x

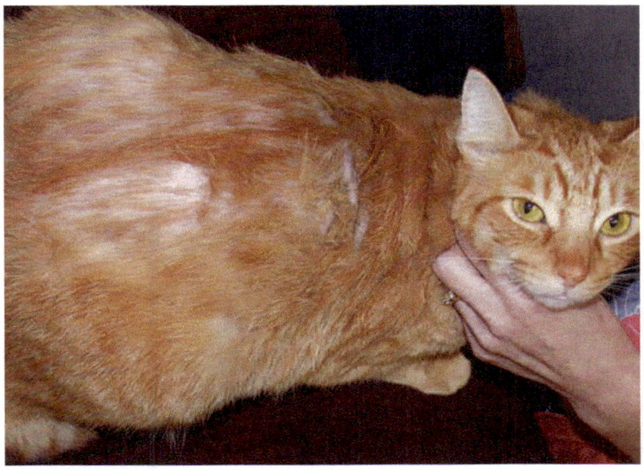

Figure 10.8I Patchy dorsal truncal barbering in an atopic cat mimicking flea bite hypersensitivity.

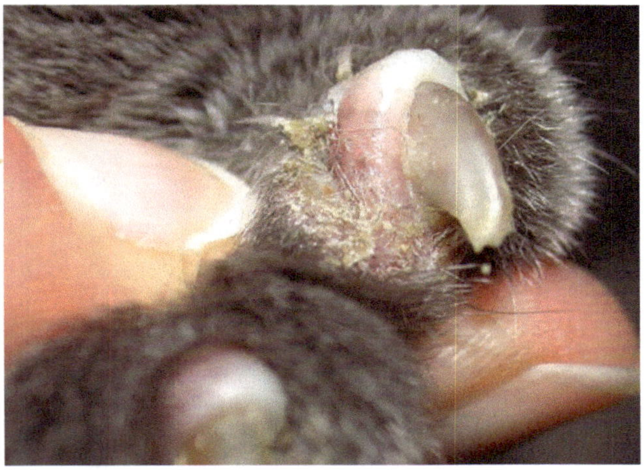

Figure 10.8J Crusted, bacterial paronychia secondary to atopy in a cat.

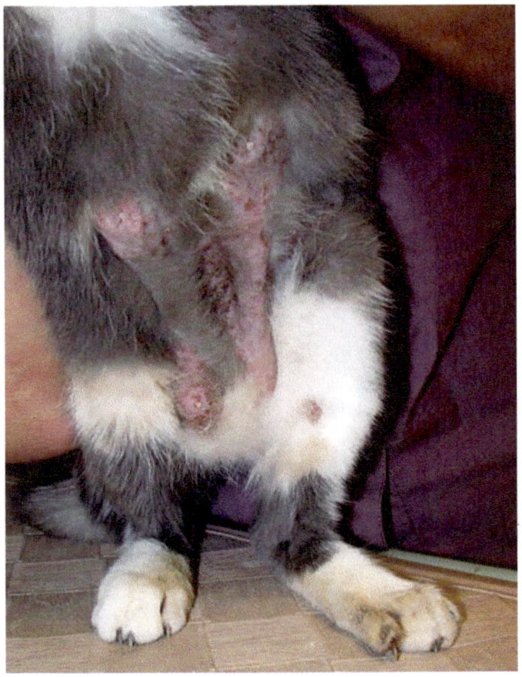

Figure 10.8K Inguinal barbering and excoriations in an atopic cat.

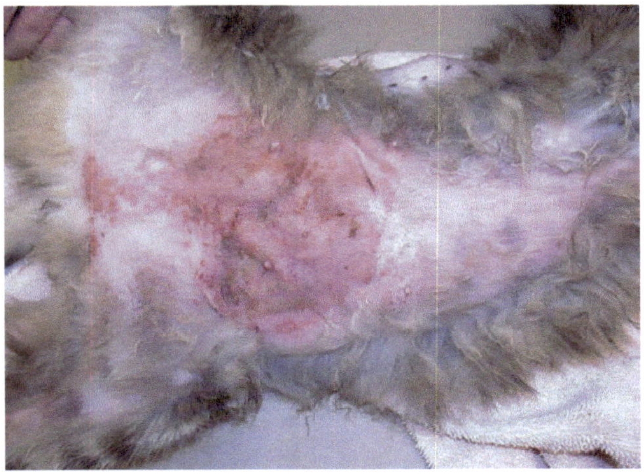

Figure 10.8L Marked inguinal barbering with moist dermatitis due to atopic dermatitis and secondary pyoderma.

Table 10.7 Feline manifestations of cutaneous allergy.

Manifestation	Miliary dermatitis	Head/neck pruritus	Self-induced alopecia	Eosinophilic granuloma complex
Clinical signs	Papulocrustous dermatitis that usually is seen on the face and dorsal aspects of the body. Lesions are small papules topped by yellow crust. Lesions may be difficult to visualize but are palpable. May be associated with facial lesions or alopecia.	Papular and erythematous dermatitis with secondary excoriations occurring on face and neck.	Usually symmetrical alopecia on flanks, abdomen, and dorsum caused by over-grooming. Trichogram of affected areas will show broken hair shafts. This may be the only clinical sign in a hypersensitivity. *Behavioral causes of overgrooming cannot be presumed until comprehensive workup for allergic, parasitic, and infectious diseases has been completed.*	Eosinophilic dermatoses consist of: • Eosinophilic plaques • Eosinophilic granulomas • Indolent ulcers Refer to Table 10.8 for further detail.
Testing/ treatment	Flea combing, DTM, dermatophyte PCR, trichography, skin scrapings for parasites, skin cytology and appropriate antimicrobials for secondary infections, parasite treatment trial (isoxazoline parasiticide), hypoallergenic diet trial, therapeutic steroid trial (prednisolone 0.5–1 mg/kg/day PO).			

Feline hypersensitivity disorders include flea bite hypersensitivity, atopic-like disease, and adverse reaction to food. Most cats with cutaneous hypersensitivity disorders present with one or more of these distinct cutaneous reaction patterns.
Recheck in 4 weeks to assess control. Addressing all variables simultaneously restores comfort to the patient in rapid manner and allows strategic observation of control as variables are changed. For example, if pet is well controlled can begin to taper steroids and if flare of disease is seen despite hypoallergenic diet and parasite treatment then atopic dermatitis is likely. Referral to area dermatologist warranted if patient is not well controlled within 4 to 6 weeks of evaluation, or to assist in diagnostic workup and management.

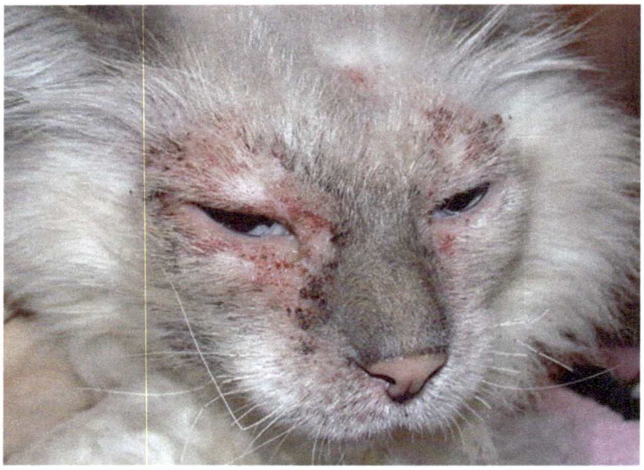

Figure 10.8M Atopic dermatitis caused periocular barbering, excoriation, and secondary bacterial infection in this cat.

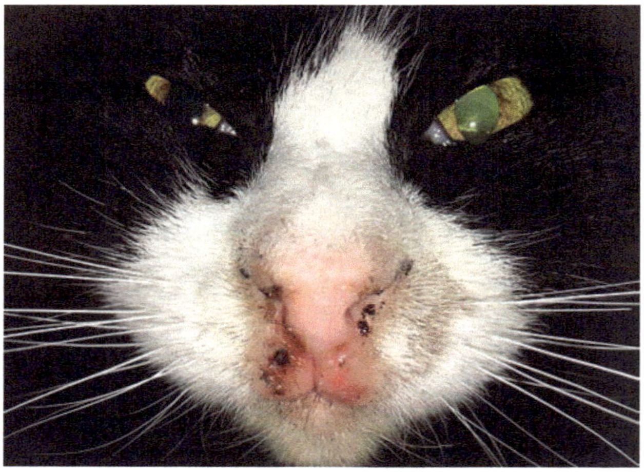

Figure 10.8N A seasonal atopic flare in a cat caused muzzle rubbing, barbering, and excoriations.

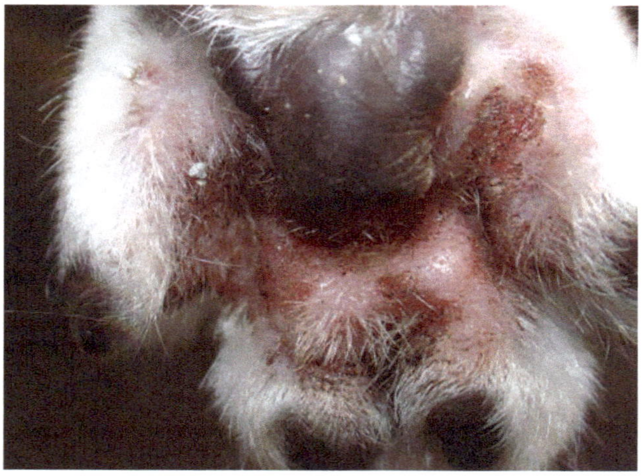

Figure 10.8O Interdigital erythema and crusted excoriations in a cat due to atopy; a secondary bacterial infection was also present.

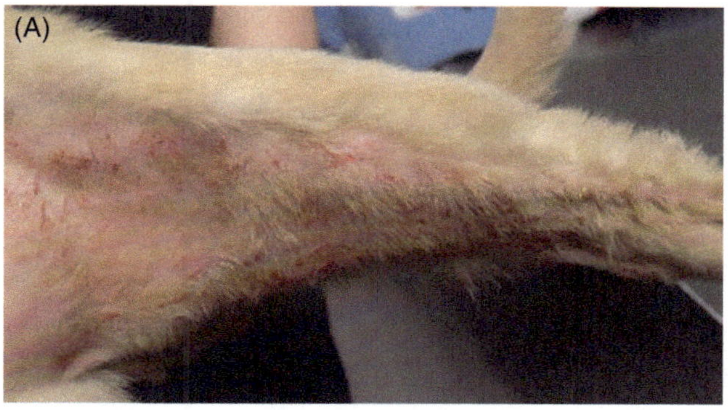

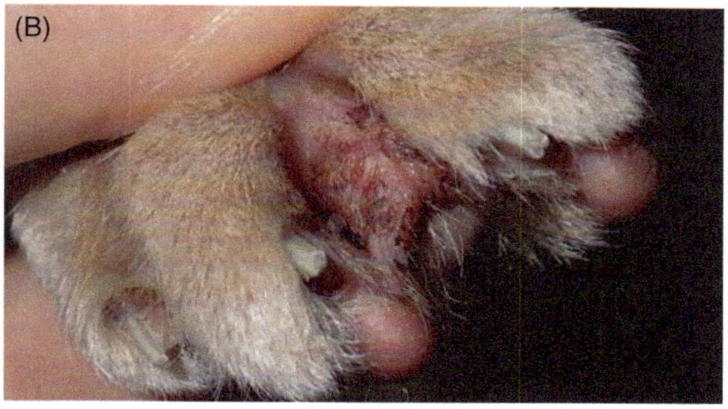

Figures 10.9A–B Food allergy in this cat caused barbering, excoriations, and secondary bacterial pyoderma/pododermatitis.

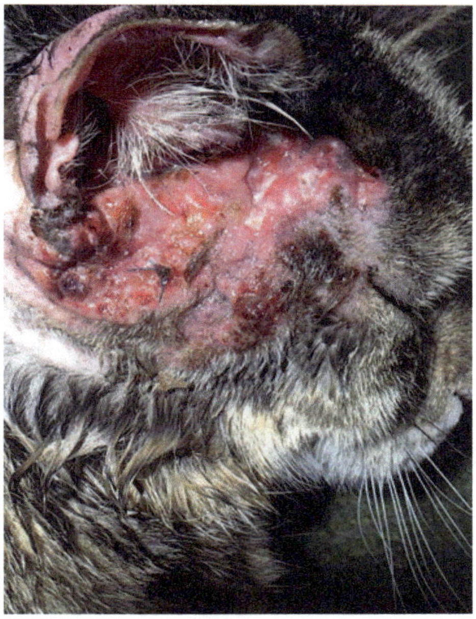

Figure 10.9C Severe ulcerative, purulent, temporal dermatitis in a food allergic cat with severe secondary deep pyoderma caused by methicillin resistant *Staphylococcus aureus*; the cat had failed to respond to steroid injections.

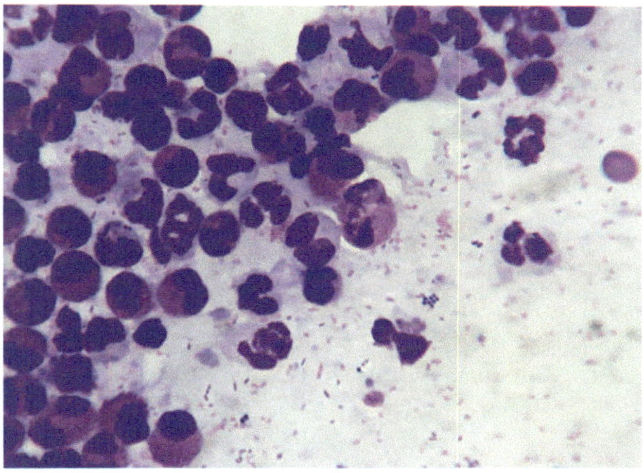

Figure 10.9D Cytology of the exudate in the cat showed marked neutrophilic and eosinophilic inflammation with numerous intra and extracellular cocci and rod bacteria. Culture grew MRSA. 100x

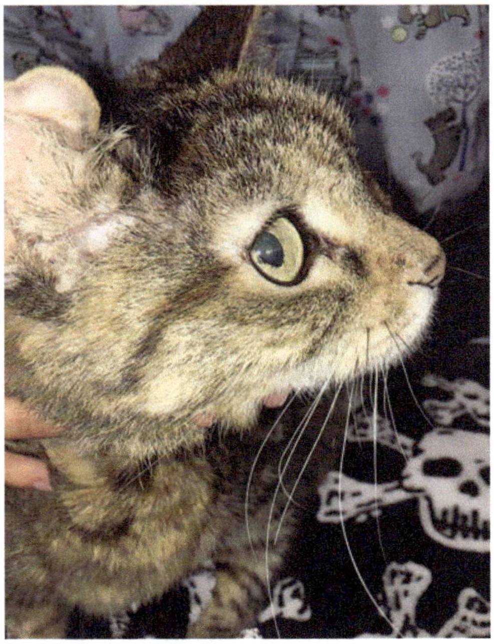

Figure 10.9E The same cat after topical and oral antibiotic treatment based on culture and a hypoallergenic diet trial.

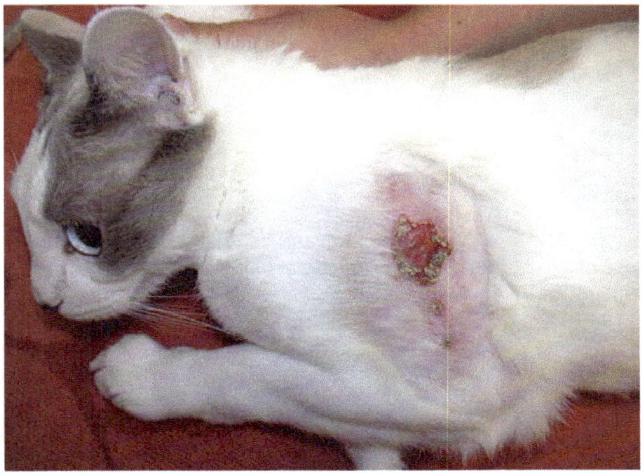

Figure 10.9F A food allergic cat with secondary deep pyoderma due to MRSA.

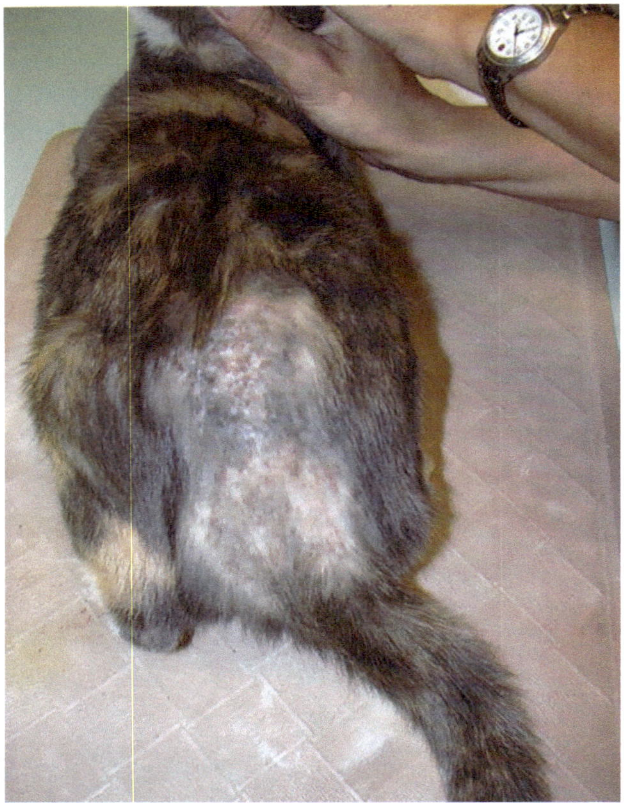

Figure 10.10A Lumbar barbering in a cat with flea bite hypersensitivity.

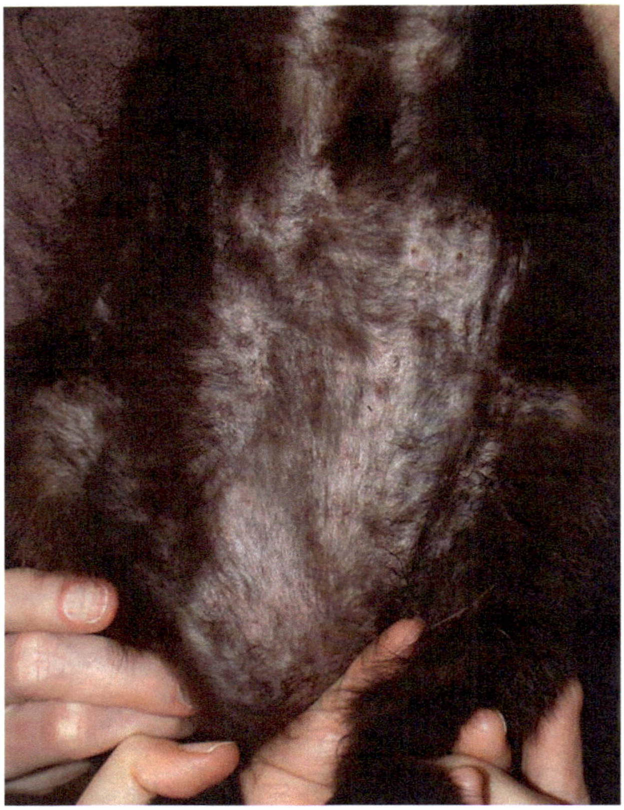

Figure 10.10B Patchy inguinal barbering and miliary dermatitis due to flea bite hypersensitivity.

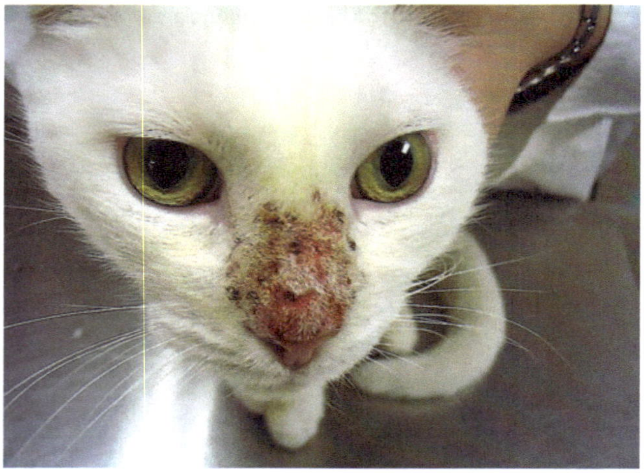

Figure 10.11A Alopecia, crusting, and papular dermatitis on the nose of a cat with mosquito bite hypersensitivity. Source: Image courtesy of Dr. Amy Shumaker DACVD.

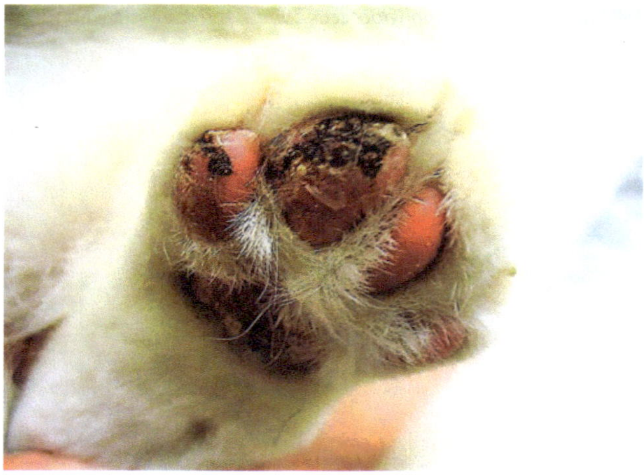

Figure 10.11B The same cat as in Figure 10.11A: Crusted lesions caused by mosquito bite hypersensitivity are present on the paw pads. Source: Image courtesy of Dr. Amy Shumaker DACVD.

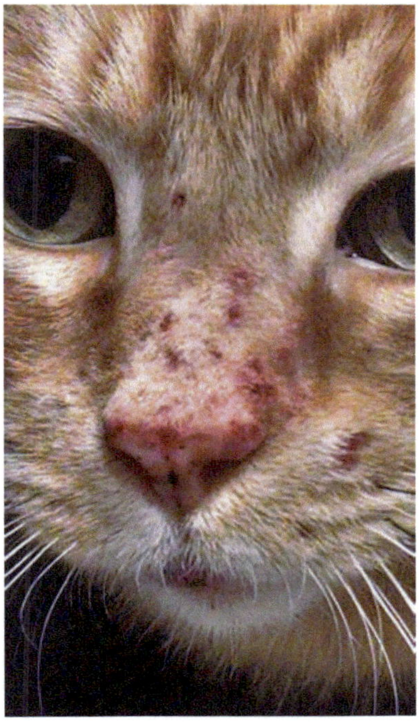

Figure 10.11C Multiple crusted papules on the dorsal nose of cat due to mosquito bite hypersensitivity. Source: Image courtesy of Dr. Thomas P. Lewis II DACVD.

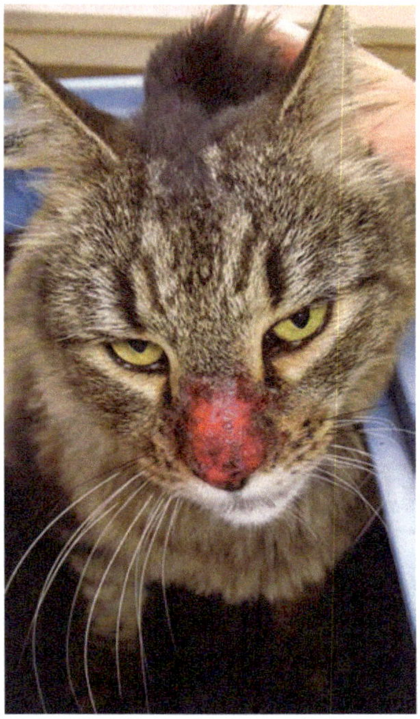

Figure 10.11D Inflamed erosions on the dorsal nose of cat due to mosquito bite hypersensitivity. Source: Image courtesy of Dr. Thomas P. Lewis II DACVD.

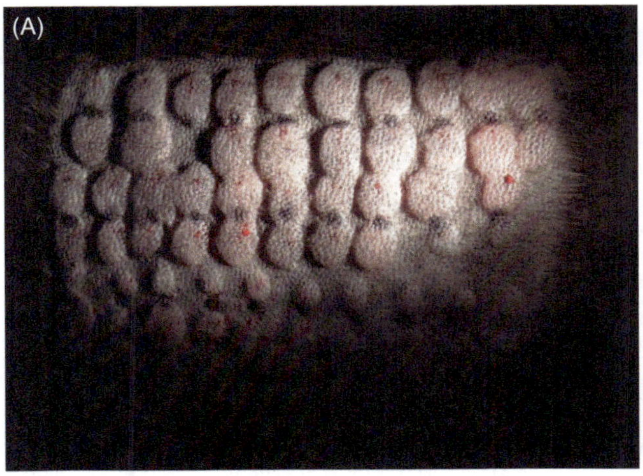

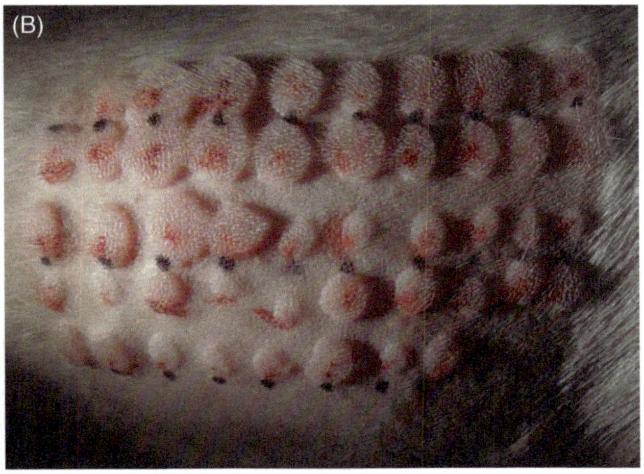

Figures 10.12A and B Intradermal allergy tests in two dogs; positive reactions are raised, red wheals.

Table 10.8 Eosinophilic granuloma complex.

Eosinophilic disease	Eosinophilic granuloma (Figures 10.13A–10.13H)	Eosinophilic plaque (Figures 10.14A–10.14F)	Indolent ulcer (Figures 10.15A and 10.15B)
Clinical presentation	Single to multifocal, raised to nodular, erythematous, firm swellings. +/− crusting +/− ulceration +/− alopecia +/− pruritus Lesions can occur anywhere on body. Oral cavity can be affected including hard palate which may hemorrhage.	Single to multifocal raised, firm, papular erythematous elevations of the skin. +/− crusting +/− ulceration Lesions are intensely pruritic. Lesions can occur anywhere on body including oral cavity.	Unilateral or bilateral lesions of the upper lip at mucocutaneous junctions at the philtrum or adjacent to upper canine tooth. Well demarcated, variably sized ulcers. +/− induration and swelling. Typically not painful or pruritic. Ulcer can be progressive and enlarge and become disfiguring.
Diagnostic testing during examination	• Clinical exam and history. • Physical exam: Evaluate for other concurrent signs of allergy including miliary dermatitis, pruritus of head and neck, symmetrical alopecia. • Cytology for secondary infections and presence of eosinophils, +/− neutrophils. • Culture if infection persists cytologically despite empiric antibiotics. • Trichography and skin scraping for parasites. • Flea combing/parasite treatment trial with isoxazoline parasiticide. • Dermatophyte culture or PCR. • If refractory to treatment consider referral to area dermatologist. • Biopsy for histopathology.		
Histopathology	<u>Granuloma:</u> Nodular to diffuse granulomatous dermatitis with multifocal areas of collagen surrounded by cytolytic eosinophils, and extruded granular material referred to as flame figures. <u>Plaque:</u> Varied degrees of epidermal hyperplasia, erosion, ulceration, and a prominent eosinophilic dermal infiltrate. <u>Indolent ulcer:</u> Hyperplastic, ulcerative, superficial perivascular to interstitial dermatitis and fibrosis. Inflammatory cells are predominantly neutrophils, and mononuclear cells; eosinophils are not typically found.		
Diagnostic workup for underlying disease	Important to pursue underlying etiology which include: <u>Hypersensitivity disorders:</u> • Flea hypersensitivity: Rule out with appropriate flea treatments (see Table 10.1). • Food allergy requires diagnostic hypoallergenic diet trial (see Table 10.6). • Environmental allergy (atopy) which is a diagnosis of exclusion and/or response to anti-inflammatory glucocorticoid therapy. <u>Infectious:</u> • Bacterial infection: Administer appropriate antibiotic treatment for 3–4 weeks. • Parasite (*Otodectes, Cheyletiella, Demodex, Notoedres*): Perform appropriate parasite treatment trial (isoxazoline parasiticide/fluralaner). • Dermatophytosis: Perform dermatophyte culture or PCR. • Herpes dermatitis can mimic eosinophilic granulomas: Look for other clinical signs (ocular/respiratory) to support +/− lesions that worsen with anti-inflammatory/ immune-suppressive therapies.		

Management	1) Treat infection with a 3–4 week course of systemic antibiotic.
	  • In one small study (Wildermuth, Griffin, and Rosenkrantz, 2012), a 3 week course of clavulanated amoxicillin caused a 96% reduction in size of eosinophilic plaques and a 43% reduction in size of lip ulcers.
	2) Typically responds well to systemic glucocorticoids, although some lesions require high dosages.
	  • Prednisolone or methylprednisolone 1 to 2 mg/kg/day PO initially, reassess at 14 to 21 days.
	  • Dexamethasone PO tablets (or give injectable solution orally if liquid easier) 0.1 to 0.2 mg/kg/day taper to 0.1 mg/kg every 72 h.
	  • Triamcinolone PO at 0.1 to 0.2 mg/kg/day initially.
	  • Once disease control is achieved and patient is stable steroid dosage is tapered. Typically decrease steroid dosage by 25 to 50% initially and observe for 2 to 4 weeks, then continue to taper dose by 25 to 50% q2 weeks to ideally alternate day therapy or lowest effective dosage. Speed of taper depends on patient factors such as side effects of steroid therapy, and severity of disease.
	  • Intralesional steroids can be helpful for some eosinophilic granulomas:
	    – Triamcinolone: Usual dose is 1.2–1.8 mg; inject around lesion at 0.5–2.5 cm intervals. Do not exceed 0.6 mg at any one site or 6 mg total dose.
	    – Methylprednisolone acetate: 10 to 20 mg total dose infused around lesion.
	3) If unable to taper steroids or disease is severe or chronic then add modified ciclosporin PO 7 mg/kg/day.
	4) In cases with underlying atopy referral to area dermatologist and consideration for allergy testing and desensitization (see Table 10.3).		

Additional therapies	• Twice-weekly or weekly subcutaneous injections of 2.5 MU interferon omega. • Oclacitinib* 0.6 mg/kg PO BID × 14 then once daily to effect anecdotally used in some cases; this is extralabel and labwork should be carefully monitored. • Progestagens such as megestrol acetate should be avoided due to risk of severe adverse effects and availability of safer treatment modalities. • Additional therapeutic considerations include surgical excision or CO_2 laser ablation of granuloma lesions.		

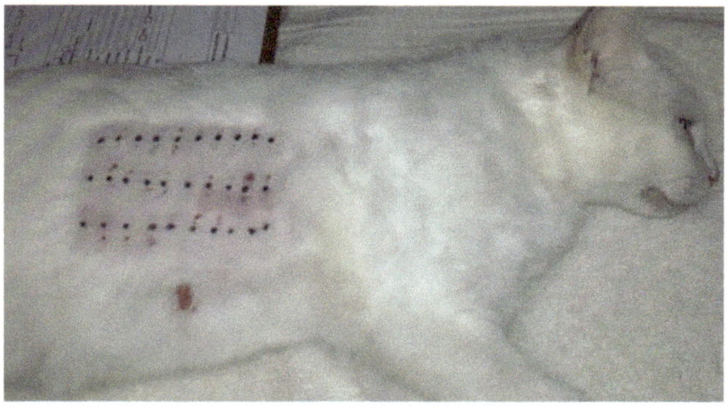

Figure 10.12C Intradermal allergy testing in a cat; positive test reactions in cats are subtler than in dogs.

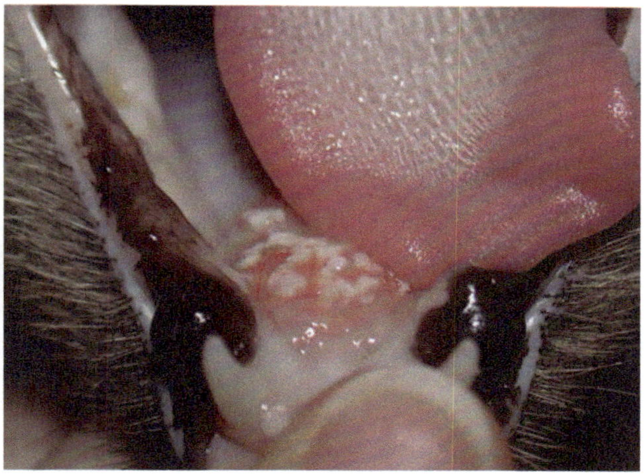

Figure 10.13A A red, raised, granular mass caused by an eosinophilic granuloma under the tongue of an atopic cat.

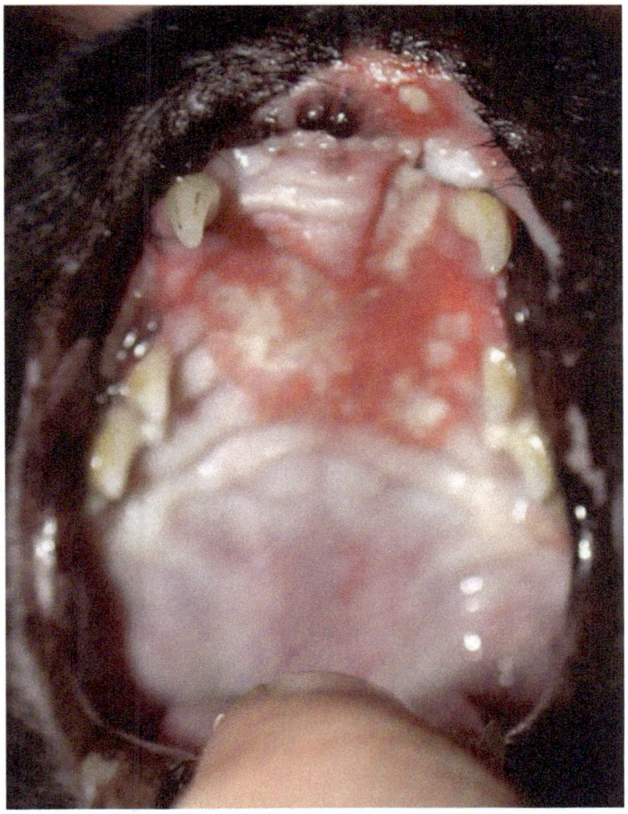

Figure 10.13B The same cat had ulcerative eosinophilic granulomas on the hard palate and upper lip.

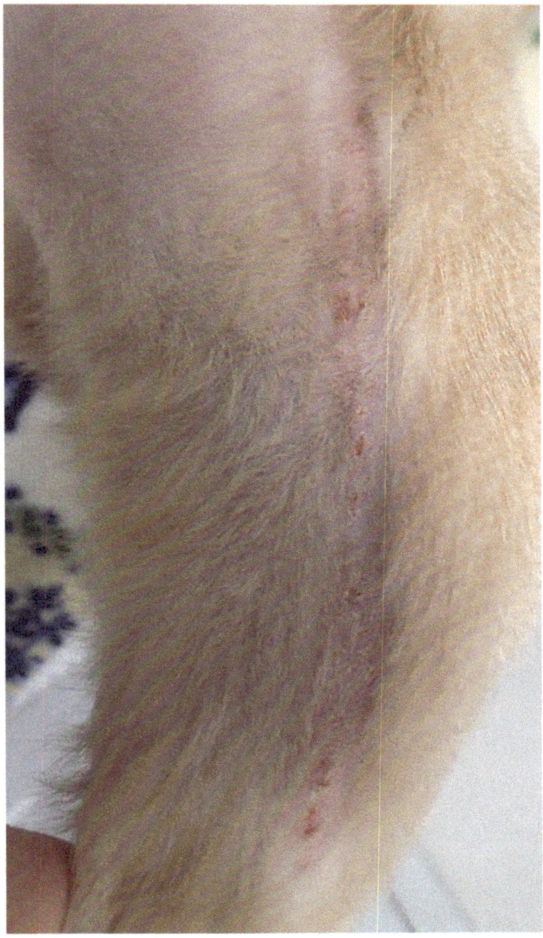

Figure 10.13C Barbering and a raised, linear eosinophilic granuloma on the medial thigh of an atopic cat.

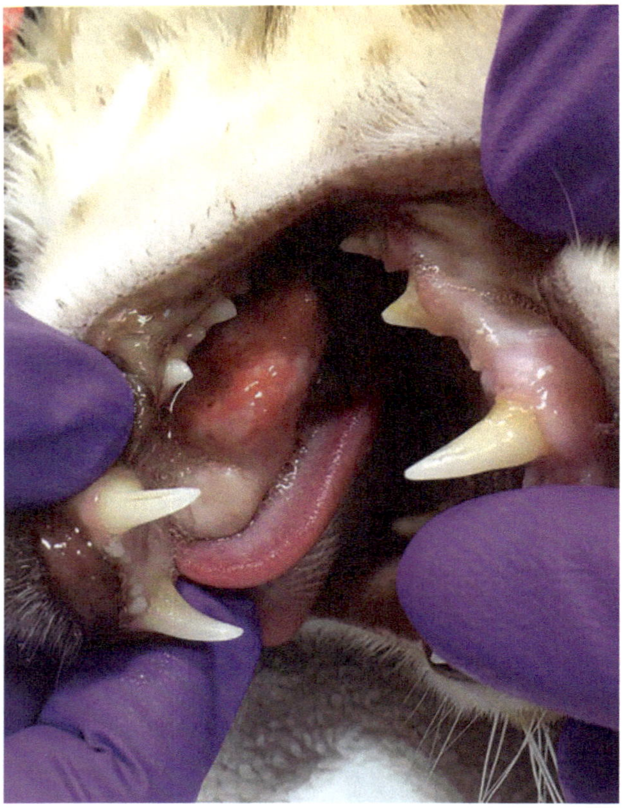

Figure 10.13D A large, sublingual eosinophilic granuloma in a Bengal cat with food allergy.

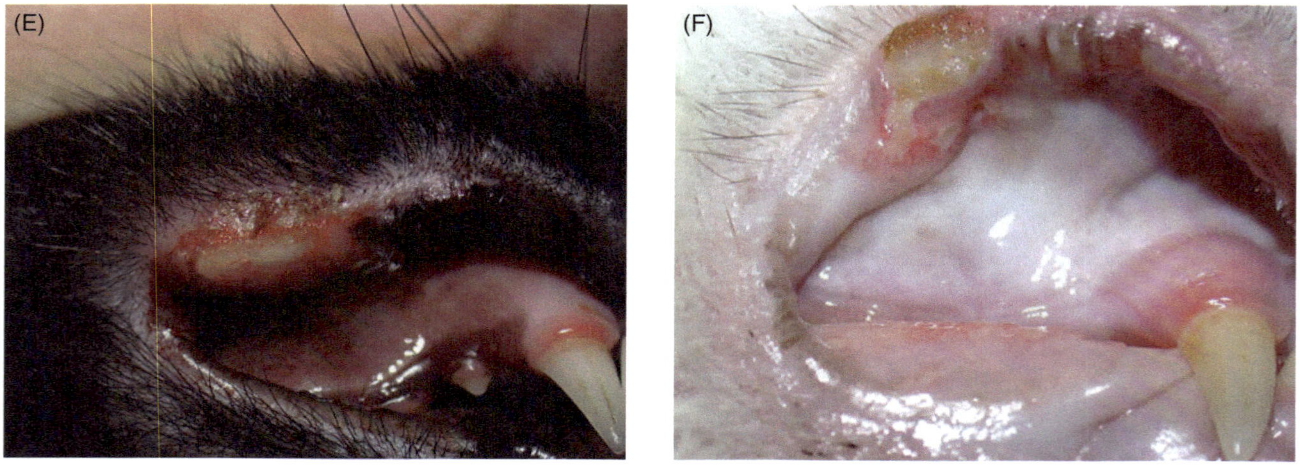

Figures 10.13E–F Eosinophilic granulomas on the lip of two atopic cats.

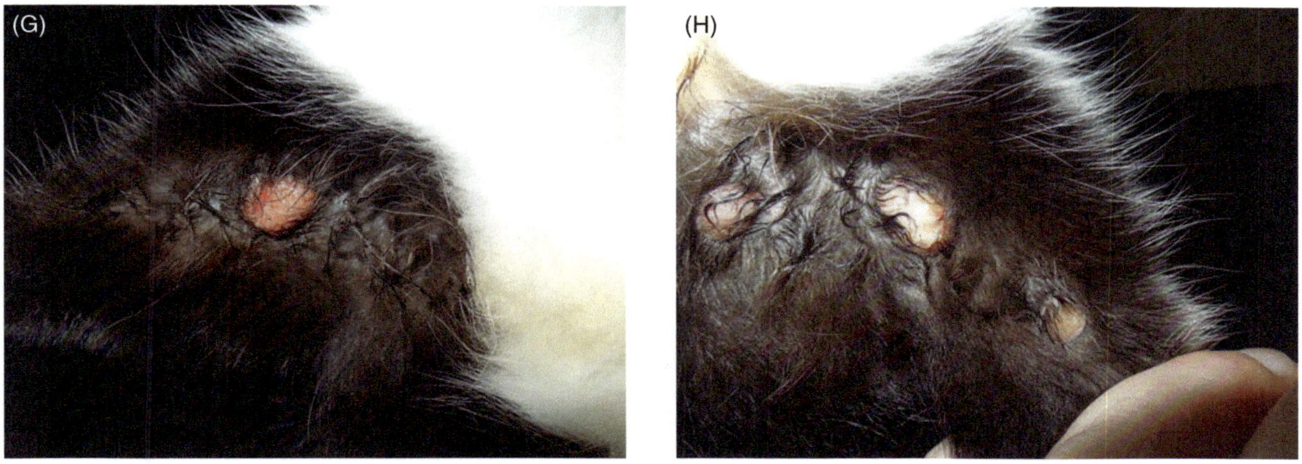

Figures 10.13G–H Raised, moist, inflamed, medial thigh masses due to eosinophilic granulomas in an atopic cat.

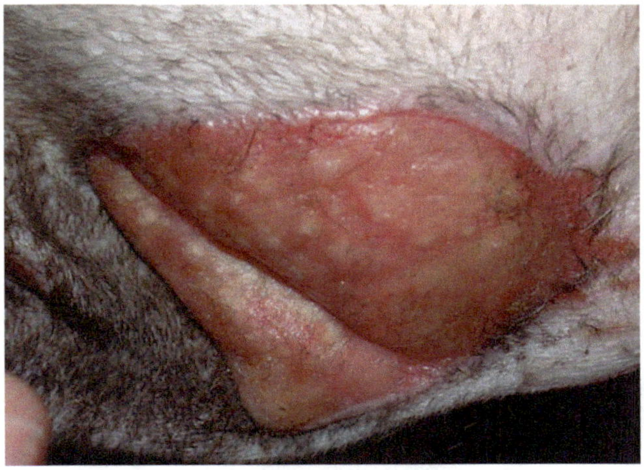

Figure 10.14A A large, inguinal eosinophilic plaque in an atopic cat.

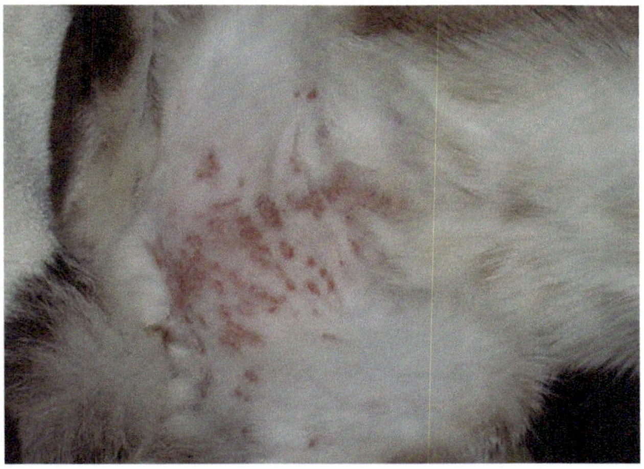

Figure 10.14B Numerous small crusted eosinophilic inguinal plaques in an atopic cat.

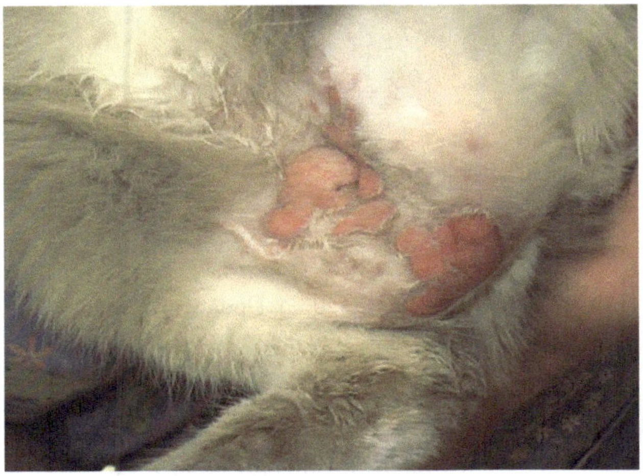

Figure 10.14C Raised moist inguinal eosinophilic plaques in an atopic cat; cytology showed inflammation with numerous bacteria.

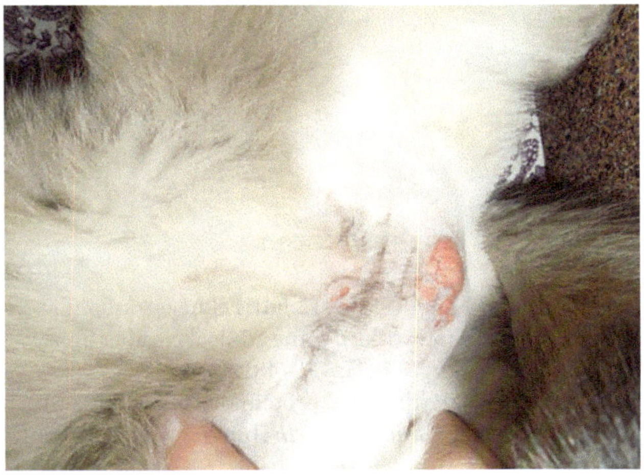

Figure 10.14D The same cat as in Figure 10.14C after a course of antibiotics once infection was resolved, a 2 week prescription of oral prednisolone resolved small residual eosinophilic plaques.

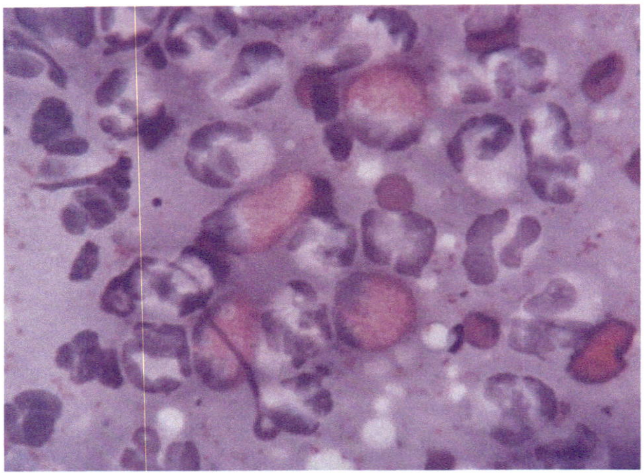

Figure 10.14E Impression cytology of an eosinophilic plaque demonstrating numerous eosinophils and neutrophils. 100x

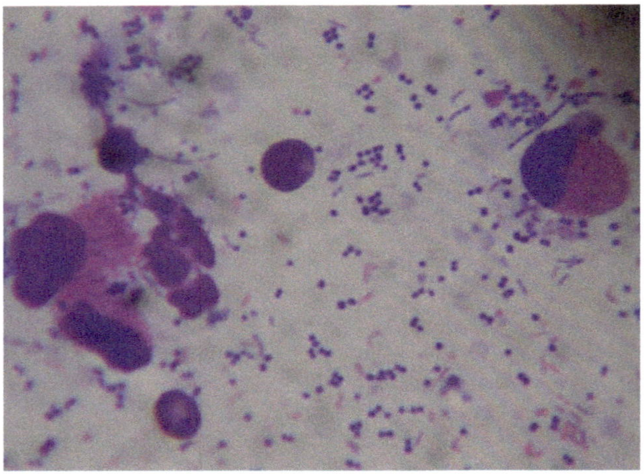

Figure 10.14F Cytology of a different eosinophilic plaque case showed there was significant secondary bacterial pyoderma. 100x

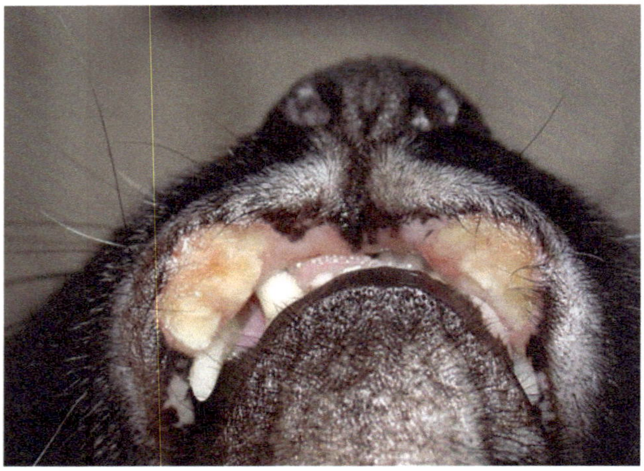

Figure 10.15A Lip swelling and ulceration due to indolent ulcers in an atopic cat.

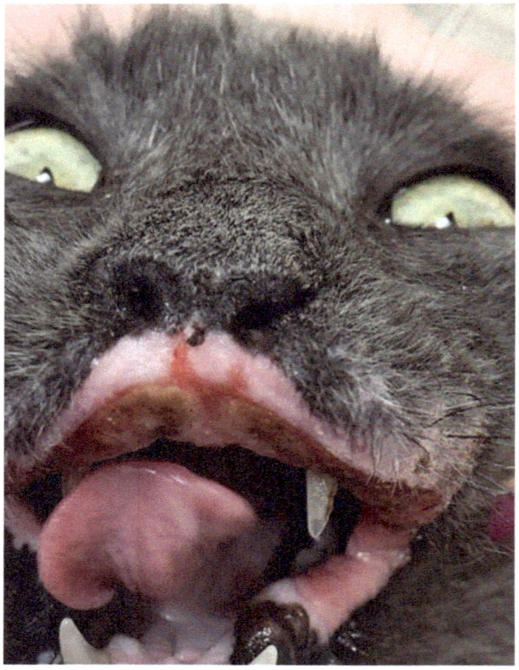

Figure 10.15B Severe, chronic indolent ulcers causing lip deformation and scarring.

References/Further reading

Buckley, L. and Nuttall, T. (2012 Jul). Feline eosinophilic granuloma complex(ities): some clinical clarification. *J. Feline Med. Surg.* 14 (7): 471–481.

Cave, N.J. (2006). Hydrolyzed protein diets for dogs and cats. *Veterinary Clinics of North America Small Animal Practice* 36: 1251–1268.

Foster, A.P. (2002). Diagnosing and treating feline atopy. *Vet. Med.* 97: 226–240.

Foster, A.P. and Roosje, P.J. (2005). Update on feline immunoglobulin E (IgE) and diagnostic recommendations for atopy. In: *Consultations in Feline Internal Medicine*, vol. 5 (ed. J.R. August), 229–238. Philadelphia: Saunders WB.

Gaschen, F.P. and Merchant, S.R. (2011 Mar). Adverse food reactions in dogs and cats. *Vet. Clin. North Am. Small Anim. Pract.* 41 (2): 361–379.

Kennis, R.A. (2006 Jan). Food allergies: update of pathogenesis, diagnoses, and management. *Vet. Clin. North Am Small Anim. Pract.* 36 (1): 175–184.

Loewenstein, C. and Mueller, R.S. (2009). A review of allergen-specific immunotherapy in human and veterinary medicine. *Vet. Dermatol.* 20: 84–98.

Mueller, R.S., Fieseler, K.V., Zabel, S. et al. (2005). Conventional and rush immunotherapy in the treatment of canine atopic dermatitis. In: *Advances in Veterinary Dermatology*, vol. 5 (ed. A. Hillier, A.P. Foster and K.W. Kwochka), 61–69. Oxford: Blackwell Publishing.

Mueller, R.S. and Olivry, T. (2017 Aug). Critically appraised topic on adverse food reactions of companion animals (4): can we diagnose adverse food reactions in dogs and cats with in vivo or in vitro tests? *BMC Vet. Res.* 13 (1): 275.

Mueller, R.S., Olivry, T., and Prelaud, P. (2015 Aug). Critically appraised topic on adverse food reactions of companion animals (1): duration of elimination diets. *BMC Vet. Res.* 11: 225.

Mueller, R.S., Olivry, T., and Prelaud, P. (2016 Jan). Critically appraised topic on adverse food reactions of companion animals (2): common food allergen sources in dogs and cats. *BMC Vet. Res.* 12: 9.

Noli, C., Foster, A., and Rosenkrantz, W. (2014). *Veterinary Allergy*. UK: Wiley.

Olivry, T. (2001). *The American College of Veterinary Dermatology. Task Force on Canine Atopic Dermatitis*, Veterinary Immunology and Immunopathology, vol. 81: 3/4. New York: Elsevier.

Olivry, T., DeBoer, D.J., Favrot, C. et al. (2010). Treatment of canine atopic dermatitis: 2010 clinical practice guidelines from the international task force on canine atopic dermatitis. *Vet. Dermatol.* 21: 233–248.

Olivry, T., Foster, A.P., Mueller, R.S. et al. (2010). Interventions for atopic dermatitis in dogs: a systematic review of randomized control trials. *Vet. Dermatol.* 21: 4–22.

Olivry, T. and Mueller, R.S. (2003). International task force on canine atopic dermatitis. Evidence-based veterinary dermatology: a systematic review of the pharmacotherapy of canine atopic dermatitis. *Vet. Dermatol.* 14: 121–146.

Olivry, T. and Mueller, R.S. (2017 Feb). Critically appraised topic on adverse food reactions of companion animals (3): prevalence of cutaneous adverse food reactions in dogs and cats. *BMC Vet. Res.* 13 (1): 51.

Olivry, T. and Mueller, R.S. (2018 Jan). Critically appraised topic on adverse food reactions of companion animals (5): discrepancies between ingredients and labeling in commercial pet foods. *BMC Vet. Res.* 14 (1): 24.

Scott, D.W., Miller, W.H., and Griffin, C.E. (2013). *Muller & Kirk's Small Animal Dermatology*, 7e. Philadelphia: Elsevier.

Wildermuth, B.E., Griffin, C.E., and Rosenkrantz, W.S. (2012). Response of feline eosinophilic plaques and lip ulcers to amoxicillin trihydrate-clavulanate potassium therapy: a randomized, double-blind placebo-controlled prospective study. *Vet. Dermatol.* 23 (2): 110–118, e24-5.

11

Autoimmune and immune-mediated dermatologic disorders

Amy Shumaker, DVM, DACVD

VCA Southshore (Weymouth) Animal Hospital, South Weymouth, MA, USA

Clinical Atlas of Canine and Feline Dermatology, First Edition. Edited by Kimberly S. Coyner.

Companion website: www.wiley.com/go/coyner/dermatology

Table 11.1 Autoimmune and immune-mediated dermatologic disorders.

Disease	Clinical signs	Diagnosis	Special considerations	Treatment
Discoid lupus erythematosus (DLE) (Figures 11.1A–11.1C; Chapter 2, Figure 2.50; Chapter 3, Figure 3.6; Chapter 6, Figure 6.28)	Nasal planum depigmentation progressing to loss of normal cobblestone architecture, erythema, scaling, crusting, and ulceration. Lesions may also affect exposed portions of the pinnae and periocular regions. Rarely can affect remote sites such as digital pads, perianal region.	Cytology to evaluate for presence of bacteria; treat infection prior to biopsy, as mucocutaneous pyoderma can appear identical to DLE on biopsy. Biopsy early areas of depigmentation, avoid ulcers. Histopathology: Basal cell apoptosis and degeneration, lichenoid-interface dermatitis.	Rule out mucocutaneous pyoderma (may need a 4–6 week treatment with systemic or topical antibiotics). Sunlight may exacerbate clinical disease; recommend sun avoidance.	Immunomodulation: Doxycycline and niacinamide; Combine with topical steroids and/or topical 0.1% tacrolimus. If severe may need to immunosuppress with corticosteroids +/– adjunctive azathioprine or cyclosporine; see Tables 11.2 and 11.3.
Pemphigus foliaceus (PF) (Figures 11.2A–11.2K; Chapter 2, Figures 2.8, 2.10, 2.39; Chapter 3, Figures 3.3, 3.19, 3.31, 3.42A and B, 3.64, 3.125; Chapter 6, Figure 6.13) Breed predispositions: Akitas, Chow chows, with Cocker Spaniels, Dachshunds, and Labrador Retrievers also listed in studies. Age of onset is typically middle age.	Pustular disease but pustules often are transient, resulting in erosions and yellow crusts. Alopecia often present and extensive. Crusting often affects head, face, and ears, including nasal planum. Paw pads often involved, with fissuring often noted. Variable pruritus. Disease can wax and wane and can often be complicated with secondary bacterial infections. May have constitutional signs, especially if disease is more acute in nature. A facially restricted form of pemphigus is sometimes termed pemphigus erythematosus.	Cytology: Numerous neutrophils (generally nondegenerate) surrounding acantholytic keratinocytes; screen for and treat bacterial infection as severe infection can cause acantholysis and alter biopsy findings. Biopsy intact pustules and center of crusts; take 4–6 mm punch biopsy samples, no prep, preserve crusts with underlying tissue. Histopathology: Crusts and intraepidermal pustules with neutrophils and acantholytic keratinocytes; eosinophils can be present in varying degrees.	Should rule out dermatophytosis, especially *Trichophyton* spp. Sunlight may exacerbate clinical disease; recommend sun avoidance.	Canine PF: Immunosuppressive medications, combine oral steroids with adjunctive non-steroidal immunosuppressive medications; see pemphigus treatment Algorithms 11.1 and 11.2 and Tables 11.2 and 11.3. Canine pemphigus erythematosus may respond to doxycycline/niacinamide and topical 0.1% tacrolimus ointment. Feline PF: Oral immunosuppressive steroids may be effective as monotherapy, in refractory cases add adjunctive non-steroidal immunosuppressive medications; see Algorithms 11.1 and 11.1 and Tables 11.2 and 11.3.
Pemphigus vulgaris (Figures 11.3A–11.3C; Chapter 3, Figure 3.139) Age of onset is typically middle age.	Initial lesions are vesicles and bullae that rapidly progress to erosions and ulcers. Primarily affects oral cavity and mucocutaneous junctions but can involve other areas. May also have pawpad and clawbed involvement with onychomadesis. Systemic signs (fever, anorexia) often present.	Biopsy intact vesicles or margins of ulcers. Histopathology: Suprabasilar cleft due to acantholysis, resulting in a "row of tombstone" appearance.	Should workup for possible neoplastic conditions to rule out paraneoplastic pemphigus. Obtain thorough drug history to rule out drug-induced pemphigus.	Immunosuppressive medications, combine oral steroids with adjunctive non-steroidal immunosuppressive medications; see Tables 11.2 and 11.3. Treat secondary infections with antibiotics.

Vesicular cutaneous lupus erythematosus (Figure 11.4; Chapter 3, Figure 3.130B; Chapter 6, Figure 6.16) Breed predispositions: Shetland Sheepdogs and Rough Coated Collies.	Focal to coalescing serpiginous erosions and ulcerations affecting primarily the ventral abdomen, groin, and medial thighs. Mucocutaneous junctions, buccal mucosa, and concave pinnae may also be involved.	Biopsy/Histopathology: Interface dermatitis with vesiculation at the dermoepidermal junction. Apoptotic keratinocytes often present.	May be exacerbated by sunlight exposure.	Immunosuppressive medications, combine oral steroids with adjunctive non-steroidal immunosuppressive medications; see Tables 11.2 and 11.3.
Mucocutaneous lupus erythematosus (Figures 11.5A–11.5C; Chapter 3, Figure 3.77; Chapter 6, Figure 6.29) Breed predispositions: German Shepherds.	Well-demarcated erosions/ulcerations of genital/perigenital, anal/perianal, perioral, or periocular regions. Nasal planum may also be involved. Lesions generally symmetric. Hyperpigmentation often present surrounding ulcerated regions or in previously affected areas.	Biopsy after resolving secondary infections as histopathologic features overlap those of mucocutaneous pyoderma.	Secondary infection often present.	Doxycycline and niacinamide +/− oral and/or topical steroids or topical tacrolimus.
Alopecia areata (Figures 11.6A–C; Chapter 2, Figure 2.33A; Chapter 6, Figure 6.17) Breed predispositions: German Shepherds, Dachshunds, and Beagles may be predisposed.	Patchy noninflammatory alopecia primarily involving head or face. May become more generalized and may affect the more darkly colored areas. Leukotrichia often results.	Trichogram may reveal dysplastic, "exclamation" point hairs. Biopsy/Histopathology: Lymphocytes surrounding and invading the anagen bulb (bulbitis).	Hair regrowth may be a lighter color or white.	Cyclosporine 5 mg/kg/day.
Uveodermatologic syndrome (a.k.a. Vogt-Koyanagi-Harada-like syndrome, (Figure 11.7; Chapter 6, Figures 6.1A and 6.1B) Breed predispositions: Akita and arctic breeds most often, described in many other breeds.	Acute uveitis often present (often bilateral, may be unilateral). Depigmentation of nose, lips, eyelids, and hair (often of the face), and less so of the footpads, scrotum, and hard palate often noted following onset of uveitis, but can precede uveitis. Occasionally oral ulcerations present. Majority of skin lesions are mild: Well-demarcated depigmentation +/− erythema, scaling, but can progress to more marked lesions with variable degrees of erosion, ulceration, and crusting. Patchy leukotrichia often surrounds areas of cutaneous depigmentation but more generalized leukotrichia/leukoderma may be present in some cases. Clinical signs of uveitis include: photophobia, blepharospasm, lacrimation, corneal edema, glaucoma, retinal detachment, cataract development, blindness.	Biopsy/Histopathology: Decreased or absent melanin in basal layer in chronic lesions; in early lesions, lichenoid dermatitis containing macrophages with engulfed melanin granules. Requires extensive ophthalmic workup and monitoring as uveitis is often severe and can rapidly progress to blindness.	Sunlight may exacerbate clinical disease, recommend sun avoidance.	Immunosuppressive medications, combine oral steroids with adjunctive non-steroidal immunosuppressive medications; see Tables 11.2 and 11.3. Aggressively treat uveitis with appropriate therapies, recommend ophthalmology consultation. Require routine eye monitoring and treatment for uveitis and sequela.

(*Continued*)

Table 11.1 Autoimmune and immune-mediated dermatologic disorders (Continued)

Disease	Clinical signs	Diagnosis	Special considerations	Treatment
Autoimmune subepidermal blistering diseases Bullous Pemphigoid (BP) Epidermolysis Bullosa Acquisita (EBA) (Figures 11.8A–11.8C) Junctional Epidermolysis Bullosa Acquisita (JEBA) Linear IgA Disease (LAD) Mucous Membrane Pemphigoid (MMP; Figure 11.8D)	Complex of diseases characterized by vesicles or blisters often filled by transudates or serum that frequently erupt, resulting in erosions and ulcerations. BP: Initial lesions are often erythematous macules, patches, or plaques that progress to vesicles with subsequent ulceration. Primary sites affected include skin, oral cavity, and mucocutaneous junctions. Typically lacks footpad involvement. Oral involvement rarely plays a role or occurs later in disease process EBA: Great Danes predisposed. Male predisposition. Occurs primarily in young dogs. Lesions: Erythema, urticarial plaques, vesicles, pustules, ulcers. Lesions typically affect face, oral cavity, pinna, axilla and groin. In most cases, footpads are affected, with sloughing and ulceration (distinguishes this disease from many of the other AISBD). Constitutional signs often present. MMP: German Shepherd dogs predisposed. Lesions: Tense vesicles, hypopigmentation, erythema. Lesions often begin in oral cavity, perinasal region, paragenital region, lips, periocular region. Lesions are often very symmetric. Slowly progressive disease. Footpads rarely affected.	Biopsy/Histopathology: Subepidermal vesiculation. Salt-split skin indirect immunofluorescence and collagen IV immunostaining can help differentiate which AISBD is present (only available at selected veterinary schools such as North Carolina State).	With a histopathology report supporting an AISBD, need to take age of patient, breed, and clinical presentation into account as this can aid in distinguishing which type of AISBD.	Majority of these diseases often have poor prognoses and often difficult to treat (MMP is the exception), and consultation with a veterinary dermatologist is recommended. Glucocorticoids +/– azathioprine or doxycycline with niacinamide, see Tables 11.2 and 11.3.

Vasculitis (Figures 11.9A–11.9J; Chapter 2, Figures 2.58, 2.64; Chapter 3, Figures 3.14, 3.37B, 3.40, 3.42C, 3.68; Chapter 6, Figures 6.8, 6.18, 6.36A and 6.36B)	Disease of the cutaneous vasculature that can result in various clinical presentations and is the potential result of multiple causes. Lesions predominantly affect pinnae, tail tip, footpads, elbows, limbs, lips, oral mucosa, claws. Lesions often present as erythematous to purpuric plaques, bullae, eschar, and ulcers. Additional lesions include erythemic papules, pustules, and urticaria or ischemic dermatopathy characterized by non-inflammatory alopecia, scale, and scarring. May have areas of pitting edema. Affected claws may exhibit onychodystrophy, petechiation within the claw and have exudate. Claws may slough (onychomadesis). Affected pads may have ulcers (often central portion of pad), hyperkeratotic plaques, or develop leukoderma.	Biopsy/Histopathology: Degree of inflammation can vary from marked to mild (cell-poor) with differing types of inflammatory cells. Inflammation is generally centered around vessels. Many cases have thrombus formation within vessels. CBC/Chemistry panel: Tick titers or PCR should be performed.	Obtain thorough drug and vaccination history.	Correct/eliminate any underlying triggers. For milder presentations, recommend immunomodulation with doxycycline, niacinamide, and/or pentoxifylline. For more affected patients, combine immunomodulating therapy with immunosuppressive medications including oral steroids, cyclosporin, or azathioprine, see Tables 11.2 and 11.3.
Post-vaccination injection site alopecia (Figures 11.10A and 11.10B; Chapter 6, Figures 6.42, 6.43, 6.58) Breed predispositions for vaccine-induced vasculitis: Jack Russell Terriers, Chihuahuas, Miniature Poodles, Bichons, Maltese, Yorkies.	Complete alopecia +/− scaling, hyperpigmentation, fat atrophy at injection site; appearance depends upon stage of the lesion. Distant lesions may occur at the same time or develop later: Paw pad ulcers, pinnal +/− pressure point crusts/ulcers.	Consider history, signalment, lesion appearance/location. Biopsy both center and periphery of lesion and include SQ (subcutaneous) fat. Histopathology: Changes consistent with cell-poor vasculitis; pale-staining collagen and atrophied hair follicles. Basophilic material surrounded by macrophages can be found consistent with vaccine product.	Lesions often occur 1–6 months following vaccination; rabies vaccination most commonly implicated.	Pentoxifylline; topical tacrolimus to focal lesions; treatment response may take several months; can self-resolve; some never resolve. Subsequent vaccinations risk recurrence of alopecia or development of generalized lesions, consider vaccine titers instead of boosters if possible or using different vaccine manufacturer.

(*Continued*)

Table 11.1 Autoimmune and immune-mediated dermatologic disorders (Continued)

Disease	Clinical signs	Diagnosis	Special considerations	Treatment
Drug eruption (a.k.a. cutaneous adverse drug reaction) (Figures 11.11A–11.11F, Chapter 3, Figure 3.32) Breed predilections: Dobermans (sulfonamides); Miniature Schnauzers (sulfonamides, shampoo).	Variable presentation and can mimic many diseases, or can occur during treatment of a prior disease, such as a drug reaction to an antibiotic used for pyoderma. Lesions can include macular and papular eruptions, sterile pustules, nodules, vesicles or bulla, ulcers, erythema multiforme, vasculitis, toxic epidermal necrolysis. Systemic symptoms such as fever, lethargy, anorexia may occur, in severe cases labwork abnormalities including leukocytosis, thrombocytopenia, elevated liver enzymes may occur.	Thorough drug history is essential in diagnosis as clinical signs and histopathology can overlap those of other diseases. Cytology of lesions to rule out infection. Biopsy/Histopathology: Varies and features often overlap those of other immune-mediated diseases.	Any drug (oral, topical, injectable, or inhalant) can cause an eruption. Antibiotics tend to be the more commonly associated causes of drug eruptions, with sulfonamides, penicillins, and cephalosporins being the more commonly implicated antibiotics. A drug reaction may occur shortly after initial exposure, after subsequent exposures, or even after being on a drug for chronic periods of time.	Discontinue the suspected inciting drug. Implement supportive therapies as needed (topical and systemic meds). Can treat with immunosuppressive doses of glucocorticoids (although often poorly responsive), CSA (cyclosporine) or pentoxifylline. Human IVIG (intravenous immunoglobulin) may be helpful in severe cases.
Erythema multiforme (EM, Figures 11.12A–11.12C; Chapter 3, Figures 3.46, 3.50, 3.130A, 3.137)	Lesions are generally symmetrical and most commonly affect the ventrum (axillae, groin), mucocutaneous junctions, oral cavity, pinnae, and pawpads. Variable lesion presentation, but often erythematous macules or elevated papules that can spread peripherally resulting in central clearance and producing annular or arciform lesions. Additional lesions include urticarial plaques and vesicles/bullae that may ulcerate as well as adherent crust overlying erythemic macules. Erythematous mucosal lesions may be present. Oral vesicles and bullae may form and result in ulcerative lesions. In cats, the trunk and mucocutaneous junctions are predominantly affected with ulcerative and crusted lesions. More severely affected animals on presentation may be systemically ill.	Obtain thorough drug history. Biopsy/Histopathology: Panepidermal keratinocyte apoptosis with lymphocytic satellitosis. Interface dermatitis may be present.	Should investigate underlying triggers, including drug exposure (primarily antibiotics), infections, especially viral infections, or neoplasia.	Correct underlying cause. Some mild cases may spontaneously regress. For idiopathic and more severe cases, immunosuppressive drugs are recommended: (glucocorticoids, azathioprine, CSA, see Tables 11.2 and 11.3). Pentoxifylline may also be of benefit. Human IVIG may be helpful in severe cases. In persistent or refractory cases a food elimination diet trial should be performed as food allergy has been reported as a possible cause.

Toxic epidermal necrolysis (Figures 11.13A and 11.13B) (Stevens-Johnson syndrome is considered a form of TEN, although milder in presentation.)	Often have acute onset of constitutional signs (pyrexia, lethargy, depression, hyporexia/anorexia) along with eruption of multifocal to generalized erythematous macules or patches of the body and mucosa, progressing to vesiculobullous lesions that can become necrotic and ulcerate. Frequently positive Nikolsky sign (epidermis sloughs with minor lateral pressure). Oral mucosa and pawpads are often involved. May also have involvement of rectal, esophageal, conjunctival, and tracheal mucosa. Often painful.	Consider drug history. Biopsy: Avoid ulcers/biopsy at margins of ulcers. Histopathology: Full-thickness necrosis of the epidermis with sparse inflammatory changes. In chronic lesions, the epidermis separates from the dermis.	Often underlying triggers, including drugs, vaccinations, neoplasia, infections.	Discontinue any suspected trigger (drug) or correct underlying cause, replace fluids (often requires hospitalization), wound management to prevent sepsis. Cyclosporine (5–7 mg/kg/d IV or PO) reportedly effective. IVIG administration can be effective. Use of glucocorticoids controversial and may increase risk of sepsis.
Sterile panniculitis (Figures 11.14A–11.14D; Chapter 2, Figures 2.59 and 2.65; Chapter 3, Figures 3.115–3.118; Chapter 6, Figures 6.9, 6.19)	Deep-seated cutaneous nodules. Nodules may be single or multiple and vary in size. Can be soft to firm on palpation. Nodules can be fixed to overlying epidermis, but often there are ulcerative lesions with draining tracts producing an oily, yellowish brown to hemorrhagic discharge. Pain may be associated with lesions. Constitutional signs may be present, especially vomiting and abdominal pain if pancreatitis is associated.	Cytologic evaluation often reveals suppurative, pyogranulomatous or granulomatous inflammation with lipid or fat cells. There is an absence of microorganisms. Biopsy of intact nodule and submit for tissue cultures (aerobic/anaerobic, +/− fungal or mycobacterial) and histopathology including special stains for organisms (acid fast, PAS, GMS) should be performed to rule out underlying infectious causes. Histopathology: Pyogranulomatous inflammation of subcutaneous fat with no microorganisms on special stains.	Pancreatitis and pancreatic tumors should be ruled out as these can be causes of panniculitis.	Immunosuppressive medications, combine oral steroids with adjunctive non-steroidal immunosuppressive medications; see Tables 11.2 and 11.3. Immunomodulating therapy with doxycycline and niacinamide may be helpful or steroid sparing.
Sterile granuloma/ pyogranuloma (Figures 11.15A–11.15E; Chapter 3, Figure 3.10) Breed predispositions: Dachshunds, Collies, Doberman Pinschers, English Bulldogs, Great Danes, Boxers, Weimaraners, Golden Retrievers.	Dogs: Nonpruritic papules, plaques, nodules that are firm and often painless. Lesions may be "donut-shaped." Lesions often alopecic, can ulcerate and become secondarily infected. Can have solitary lesions, but usually multiple. Lesions primarily affect bridge of nose, muzzle, and periocular region, pinnae, and paws.	Biopsy for histopathology and cultures (aerobic/anaerobic/fungal/ mycobacterial) performed to rule out infectious causes. Biopsy/Histopathology: Nodular to diffuse granulomatous to pyogranulomatous dermatitis with no organisms on special stains (acid fast, PAS/GMS).	Consider PCR testing for Leishmania in endemic areas.	May respond to doxycycline and niacinamide. For severe or refractory cases: Immunosuppressive medications, combine oral steroids with adjunctive non-steroidal immunosuppressive medications; see Tables 11.2 and 11.3.

(*Continued*)

Table 11.1 Autoimmune and immune-mediated dermatologic disorders (Continued)

Disease	Clinical signs	Diagnosis	Special considerations	Treatment
Sterile granuloma/ pyogranuloma (cont.)	Cats: Erythemic to violaceous papules and nodules that can coalesce into plaques. Lesions often affect head, muzzle, pinnae, paws. Rare.	Same as for dogs.		Same as for dogs.
Juvenile cellulitis (a.k.a puppy strangles) (Figures 11.16A–11.16C; Chapter 3, Figure 3.18) Breed predispositions: Golden Retriever, Dachshund, Gordon Setter. Age; generally young puppies 3 wk to 4 mo, however some older dogs have been reported.	Acute facial swelling, especially lips, eyelids, muzzle. Marked submandibular lymphadenopathy present. Initial lesions are papules and pustules, which may be transient. Edema often present. Progression of lesions often results in ulceration and crusting, occasionally fistulation and draining tracts. Pinnae are often edematous and otitis externa is often present. Can have more generalized lesions with subcutaneous nodules affecting the trunk, preputial, or perianal regions. Lethargy and depression may be present.	Skin scrapings and plucks to rule out demodicosis, cytology for bacterial pyoderma. Biopsy/Histopathology: Dermal granulomas and pyogranulomas, often centered around follicles and obliterating sebaceous glands.	Disease can be recurrent if treatment course is not long enough or suboptimal doses of steroids are used.	Immunosuppressive therapy with prednisone 2 mg/kg/day until lesions resolve then slowly taper off over 4–6 weeks. Doxycycline can be helpful steroid sparing therapy.
Plasma cell pododermatitis (Figures 11.17A–11.17C; Chapter 3, Figures 3.70C and 3.70D) Occurs in cats, very rare in dogs.	Soft swelling of multiple footpads ("mushy" on palpation), with the central metacarpal/metatarsal pads being the primarily affected pads. Digital pads may be affected but to a lesser degree. Rarely only one pad affected. Often mild scaling of affected pads noted. Ulceration and lameness may occur. Affected cats may rarely have concurrent plasmacytic nasal swelling.	Aspiration cytological evaluation may reveal numerous plasma cells. Biopsy/Histopathology: Marked dermal and often pannicular infiltration of plasma cells.	Concurrent diseases may be present including FIV and renal disease; labwork including retroviral screening is indicated.	Doxycycline 5–10 mg/kg PO once daily (hide in pill pocket or follow pill with 5 cc water to reduce risk of esophageal ulceration). In refractory cases, oral immunosuppressive steroids or cyclosporine 7 mg/kg/day until lesion resolution then taper.
Pseudopelade (Figures 11.18A and 11.18B)	Variably-sized, grossly non-inflammatory, often well-circumscribed patches of alopecia affecting one or multiple areas of the body.	Biopsy with histopathology to rule out other conditions such as alopecia areata and lymphocytic mural folliculitis.		Generally poorly responsive to treatment but anecdotal reports of improvement with cyclosporine or cyclosporine combined with triamcinolone.

	Alopecia can become diffuse, sparing only the head and neck. Occasionally scaling and hyperpigmentation may be present but pruritus is absent. In cats, a symmetrical alopecia may initially be noted involving the face, progressing to the ventrum, legs, paws. Nail disease (onychorrhexis and onychomadesis) may also be present.	Biopsy/Histopathology: Pleocellular mural inflammation primarily directed toward the isthmus.		
Symmetric lupoid onychitis (SLO) (Figures 11.19A and 11.19B; Chapter 3, Figure 3.75; Chapter 6, Figure 6.52) Breed predispositions: German Shepherds, Gordon Setters.	Variable combinations of onychoschizia (splitting of the claw), onycholysis (separation of the claw), and onychomadesis (sloughing of the claw) affecting one to multiple claws. Lameness may be first sign noted. Can initially affect one paw, but will progress to affect all paws within weeks.	CBC/Chemistry panel +/− tick titers. Rule out *Leishmania* in endemic areas. Perform hypoallergenic diet trial. Biopsy of distal phalange ideal but often not needed, as clinical presentation, normal labwork, and lack of other skin lesions are all consistent with diagnosis of SLO. Biopsy/Histopathology: Interface dermatitis, often lichenoid, between the clawbed epithelium and dermis.	Secondary infection sometimes present. May need to manually remove separating claws to prevent sequestration of infection under claws; this requires general anesthesia.	First attempt with immunomodulation: Sole treatment with pentoxifylline 25 mg/kg BID or combine with doxycycline/ tetracycline and niacinamide. Nutritional support with fatty acids. For refractory or severe cases, oral immunosuppressive steroids, cyclosporin 5 mg/kg/day.
Nasal arteritis (Figures 11.20A–11.20C; Chapter 6, Figure 6.55) Occurs most commonly in St. Bernards and Standard Schnauzers, but can occur in other breeds as well.	An ulcerative disease of the center of the nasal planum in dogs, caused by immune-mediated inflammation of the walls of the nasal arteries. There is a chronic, deep, often triangular shaped, ulceration in the center of the nose/nasal planum which can become crusty and inflamed due to secondary bacterial infection. Not usually painful or pruritic, though dogs may rub at the nose if secondary infection is present. In some dogs, acute arterial bleeding can occur which can be severe enough to cause anemia and surgery to ligate the artery may be needed.	Clinical signs often pathognomonic. Cytology of exudate to rule out secondary infections. Biopsy/Histopathology: Necrosis, hemorrhage; deep dermal arteries/ arterioles beneath ulcer exhibit proliferation of spindle cells.	Significant hemorrhage may be present in more affected cases, requiring surgery to tie off the artery. Scarring is often noted following remission.	Initially oral immunosuppressive steroids are helpful for quicker results, then long-term immunomodulating treatment with doxycycline/ niacinamide; see Tables 11.2 and 11.3. Once initial hemorrhage/infection has resolved, topical anti-inflammatory therapy with 0.1% tacrolimus ointment applied 1–2 times daily to the nose is often helpful. Cyclosporin 5mg/kg/day PO can be helpful for refractory cases.

(*Continued*)

Table 11.1 Autoimmune and immune-mediated dermatologic disorders (Continued)

Disease	Clinical signs	Diagnosis	Special considerations	Treatment
Metacarpal/metatarsal fistulas (Figures 11.21A–11.21C; Chapter 6, Figure 6.26) Most commonly affects German Shepherd dogs; rarely affects other breeds including Weimaraners.	Fistula with serosanguinous exudate at central plantar metatarsus just proximal to metatarsal pad, often bilateral and sometimes affecting metacarpus in similar fashion.	Clinical signs often pathognomonic. Cytology of exudate to rule out secondary infections. Biopsy/Histopathology: Marked inflammation involving panniculus; pyogranulomas may be present. Fibrosis is often present.	Surgical removal of fistulation usually only results in temporary resolution	First-line treatment: Control secondary bacterial infections with localized bathing with chlorhexidine shampoos 1–2 times weekly or sprays/mousse/wipes every 1–2 days on affected areas; topical corticosteroids or 0.1% tacrolimus ointment to affected areas q24h until resolution. Second-line or refractory cases: Immunomodulating treatment with doxycycline and niacinamide +/− oral prednisolone 1 mg/kg/d × 2–3 weeks, tapered to lowest effective dose, ideally 0.25–0.5 mg/kg q48h or lower; for steroid-sparing effect, add cyclosporine 5 mg/kg PO q24h × 4–8 weeks then taper to q48h.
Canine sterile neutrophilic dermatitis (a.k.a. Sweet's-like syndrome). (Figure 11.22) Rare disease occurring only in dogs. Many cases occur following drug administration, upper respiratory, or GI infections or associated with paraneoplastic syndrome.	Marked erythematous macules, papules, or plaques that may have pustules associated within them. May have edema or ulceration. Extracutaneous signs are often present and can include leukocytosis, fever, lethargy, lameness, possibly from a polyarthropathy, pneumonia.	Obtain thorough drug history. Biopsy with histopathology: Moderate to marked dermal neutrophilic infiltrate, with some clustering of inflammation around follicles. Edema often present. Vasculitis should not be present.		Discontinue any drug that may be the inciting trigger. Response to glucocorticoids is a hallmark of this disease.
Canine acute eosinophilic dermatitis with edema (a.k.a. Eosinophilic Dermatitis, Well's-like syndrome) Occurs rarely in dogs.	Acute onset of erythematous macules, progressing to serpiginous plaques and wheals. Lesions predominantly located on the ventral abdomen, pinnae, and thorax. Edema may be present, affecting the face or becoming generalized and often pitting. In several reported cases, GI symptoms (vomiting, diarrhea) preceded the cutaneous signs by 1–10 days.	Obtain thorough drug and GI history. Biopsy/Histopathology: Marked dermal edema with marked eosinophilic infiltrate. Flame figures may be present.		Drug withdrawal. Systemic immunosuppressive glucocorticoids.

Superficial suppurative necrolytic dermatitis (Figures 11.23A–11.23D) (a.k.a. sterile pustular erythroderma of Miniature Schnauzers). Breed predispositions: Miniature Schnauzers. Often occurs within 48–72 hours of shampooing often with an insecticidal shampoo.	Erythematous papules with edema, coalescing into plaques. Suppurative crusts present. Pustules are often transient. Lesions can progress to ulceration and exfoliation. Lesions may occur anywhere, but predominate on the trunk. Extracutaneous signs may be present, including fever, depression, leukocytosis. Some reported deaths.	Biopsy/Histopathology: Epidermal pustulation (subcorneal to panepidermal), often forming crusts.	Obtain grooming history as many Schnauzers have a history of recent shampooing. Reactions are more commonly implicated with insecticidal shampoos. Signs often occur within 48–72 hours of grooming.	Symptomatic therapy (fluids, antibiotics). Pentoxifylline 15–10 mg/kg q8–12h. Cyclosporine 5–8 mg/kg/day. Immunosuppressive glucocorticoids.
Systemic lupus erythematosus (SLE) (Figures 11.24A and 11.24B) Breed predisposition: German Shepherd dogs. Rare disease.	Skin lesions present in 40–50% of cases, high degree of variability. Lesions range from mild scarring to widespread ulcerations. Mucocutaneous involvement may be present. Depigmentation of nasal planum and eyelids may be present, with concurrent erythema, erosions, ulceration, and crusting. Focal ulcerations of the paw pads may be present. Joint disease is often most common clinical sign. Additional systemic signs include fever, anemia, glomerulonephritis, ulcerative stomatitis, pleuritis or pericarditis, neurologic abnormalities.	SLE is a complex diagnosis to have to make, and the diagnosis is made based on presence of a combination of consistent clinical and clinicopathologic abnormalities. Patients with 4 of the following criteria justifies a diagnosis of SLE; SLE is probable when 3 criteria are present or in cases of polyarthritis with a positive ANA. Criteria: Skin lesions/consistent histopathology, photosensitivity, oral ulcers, polyarthritis, serositis, renal disease (proteinuria, casts), neurologic disorders, hematologic disorders (hemolytic anemia, thrombocytopenia), positive ANA. Biopsy (sample margins of ulcers or erosions). Histopathology: Vacuolation and apoptosis of basal cells; dermal–epidermal separation and ulceration.	ANA can be positive with many inflammatory diseases and so cannot be used by itself for diagnosis of SLE.	Immunosuppressive medications, combine oral steroids with adjunctive non-steroidal immunosuppressive medications; see Tables 11.2 and 11.3.
Histiocytic disorders	See Chapter 19			

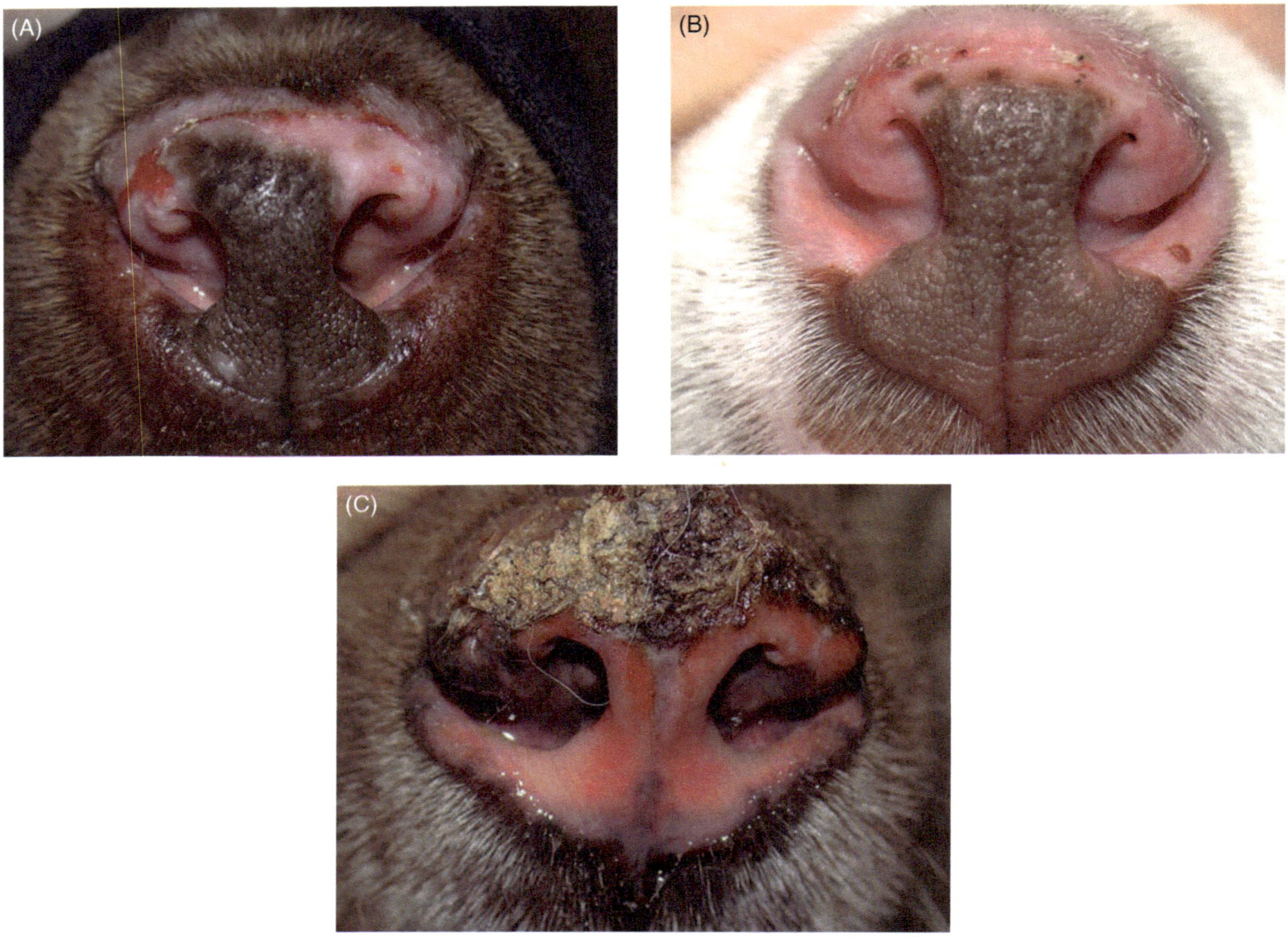

Figures 11.1A–C Variable degrees of nasal planum depigmentation, erosion, and crusting due to discoid lupus erythematosus; Figures A and B also show cartilage loss.

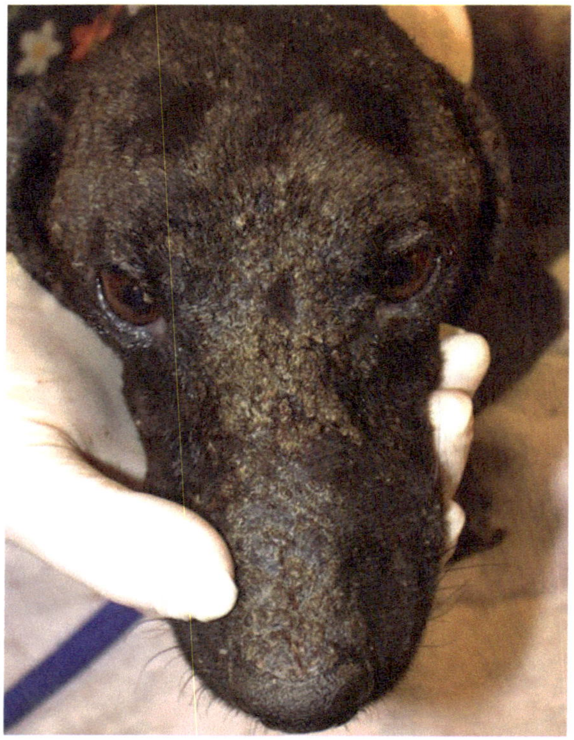

Figure 11.2A Marked facial crusting due to pemphigus foliaceus.

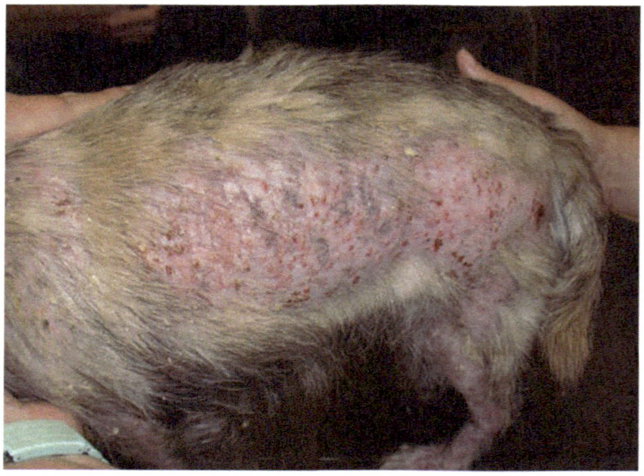

Figure 11.2B Truncal erythema, alopecia, and crusts in a dog with pemphigus foliaceus; marked pruritus mimicking allergic dermatitis was present.

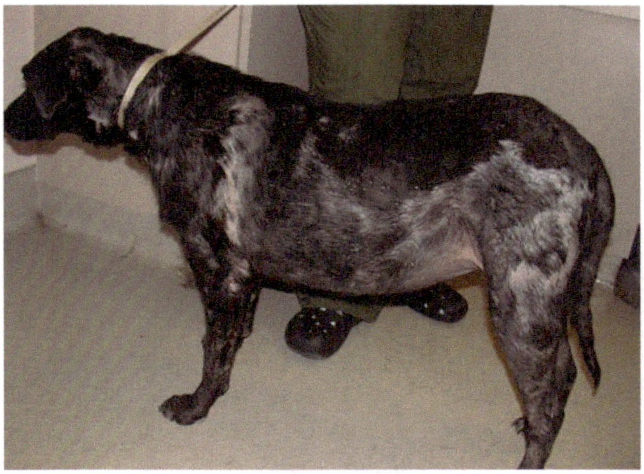

Figure 11.2C Patchy truncal alopecia. Scaling and crusting due to pemphigus foliaceus.

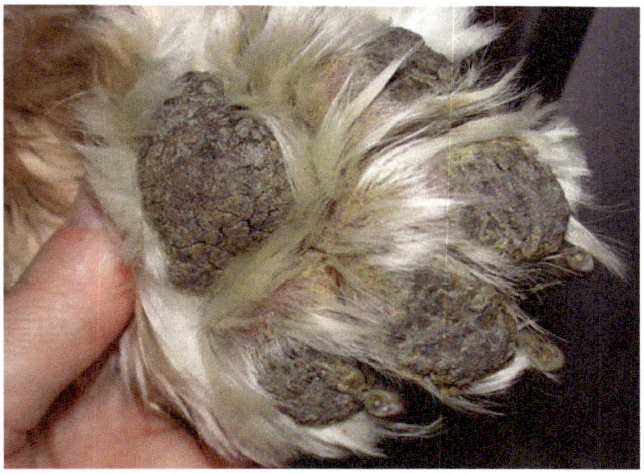

Figure 11.2D Marked paw pad hyperkeratosis due to pemphigus foliaceus.

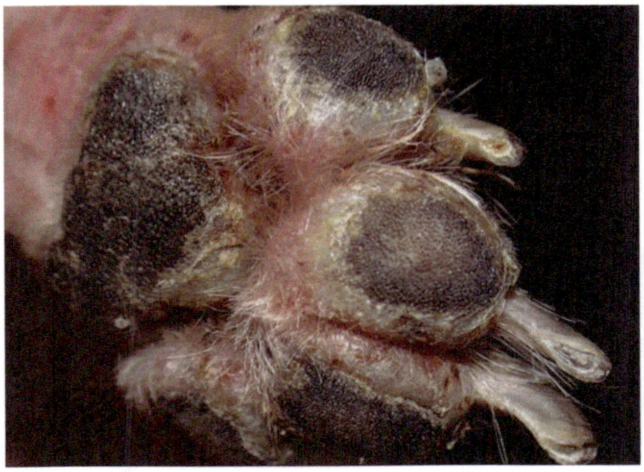

Figure 11.2E Pemphigus foliaceus induced peripheral paw pad inflammation and hyperkeratosis.

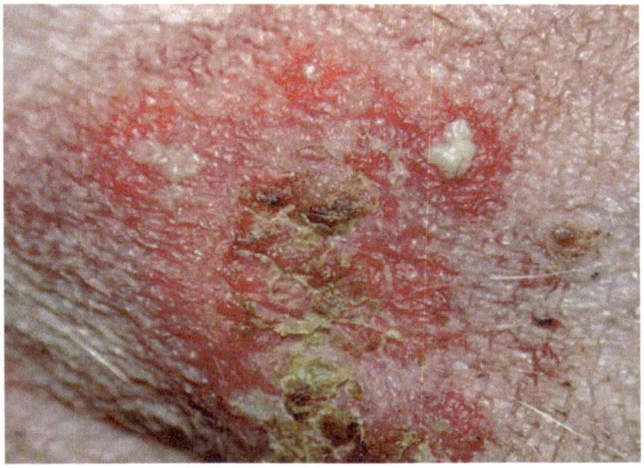

Figure 11.2F Large non-follicular pustules caused by pemphigus foliaceus.

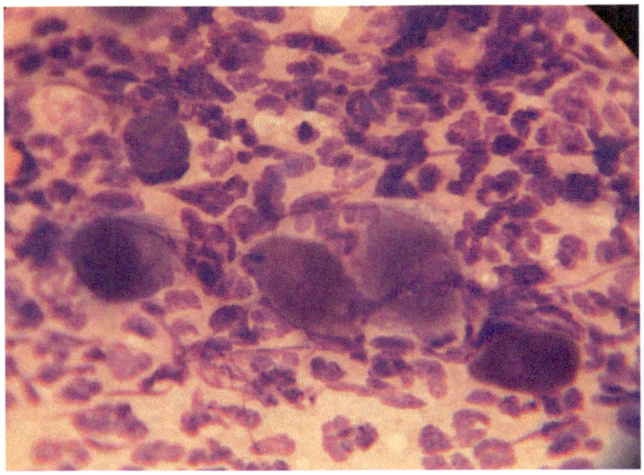

Figure 11.2G Pustule cytology demonstrating sterile neutrophilic inflammation with large, round acantholytic cells (100×).

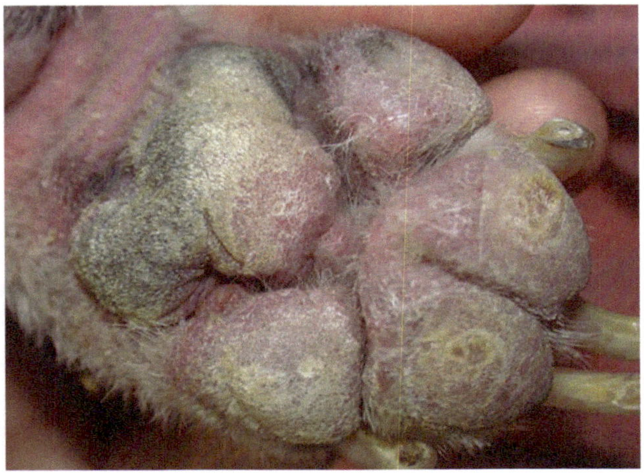

Figure 11.2H Milder, yellowish, paw pad crusting due to pemphigus foliaceus.

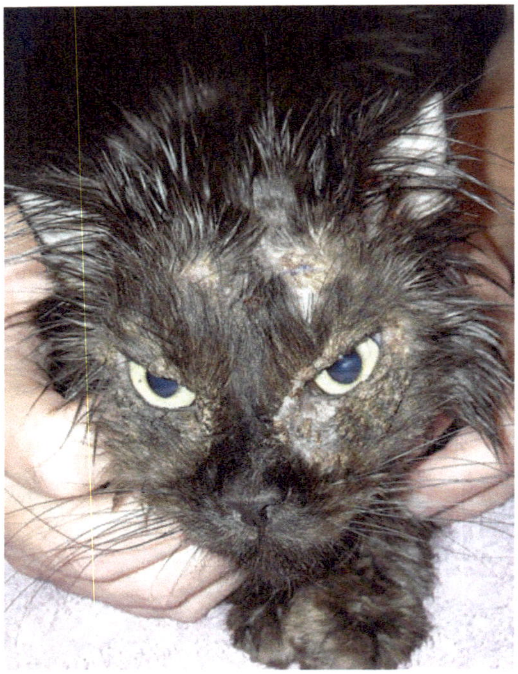

Figure 11.2I Marked facial crusting in a cat due to pemphigus foliaceus.

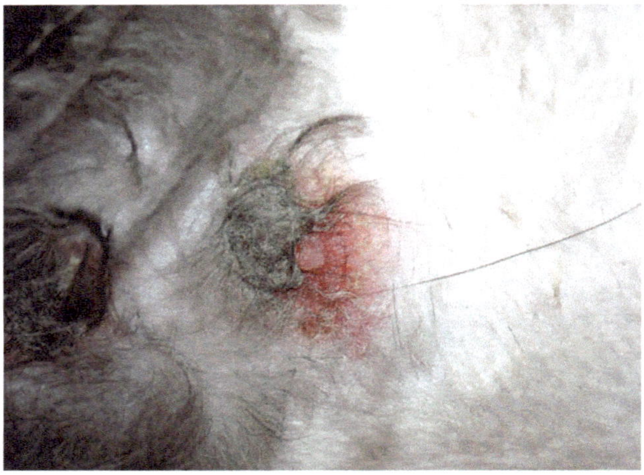

Figure 11.2J Pemphigus foliaceus often causes periaureolar crusting in cats.

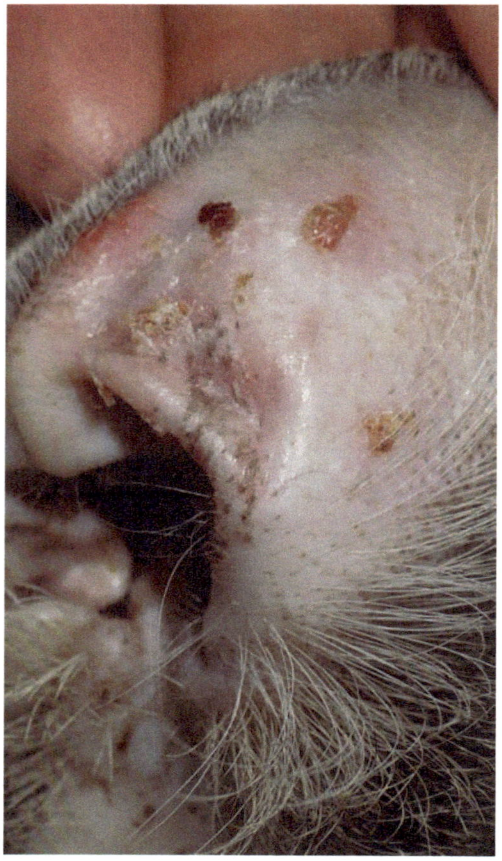

Figure 11.2K Pinnal crusts and erosions due to pemphigus foliaceus.

Algorithm 11.1 Treatment of canine pemphigus foliaceus.

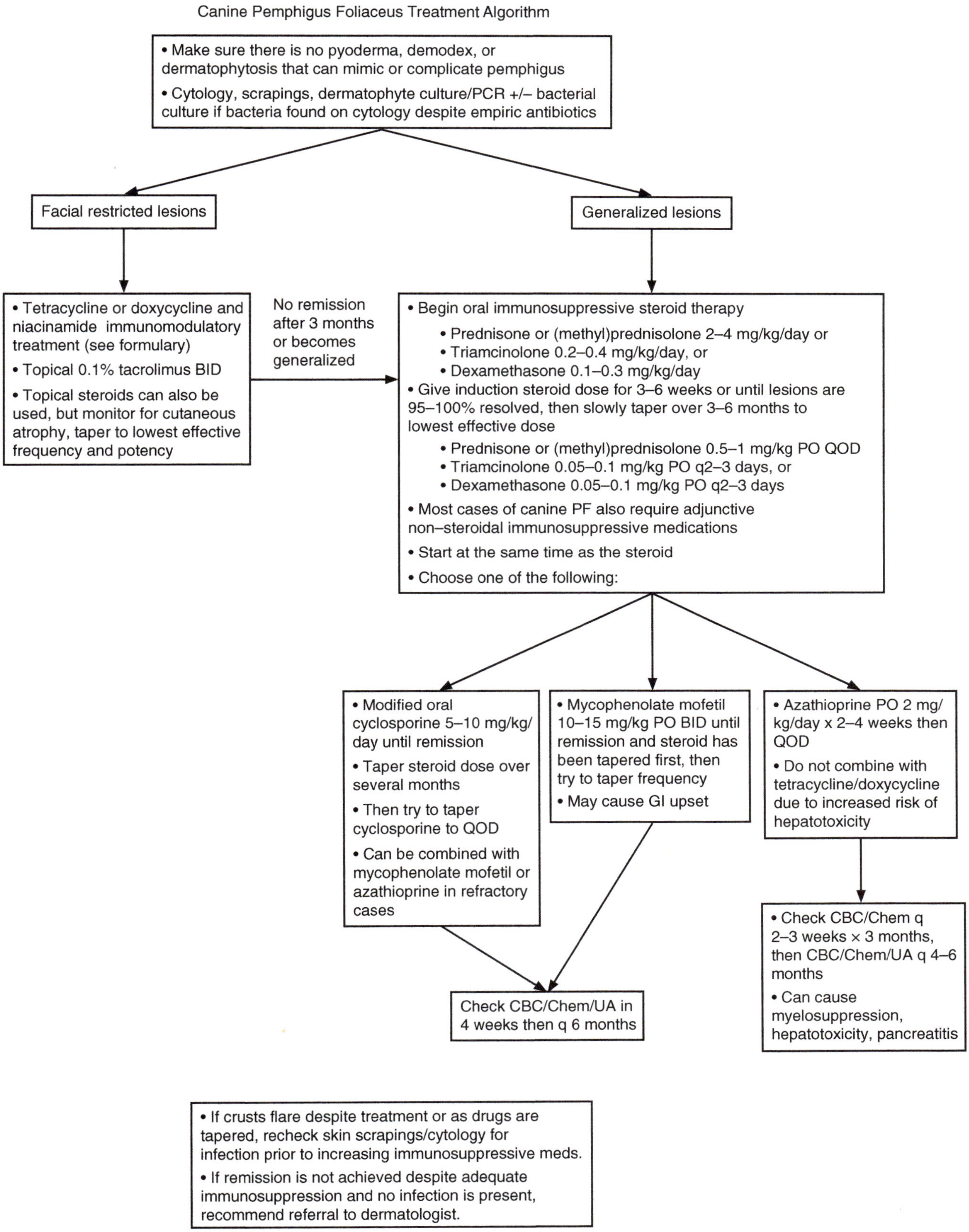

Algorithm 11.2 Treatment of feline pemphigus foliaceus.

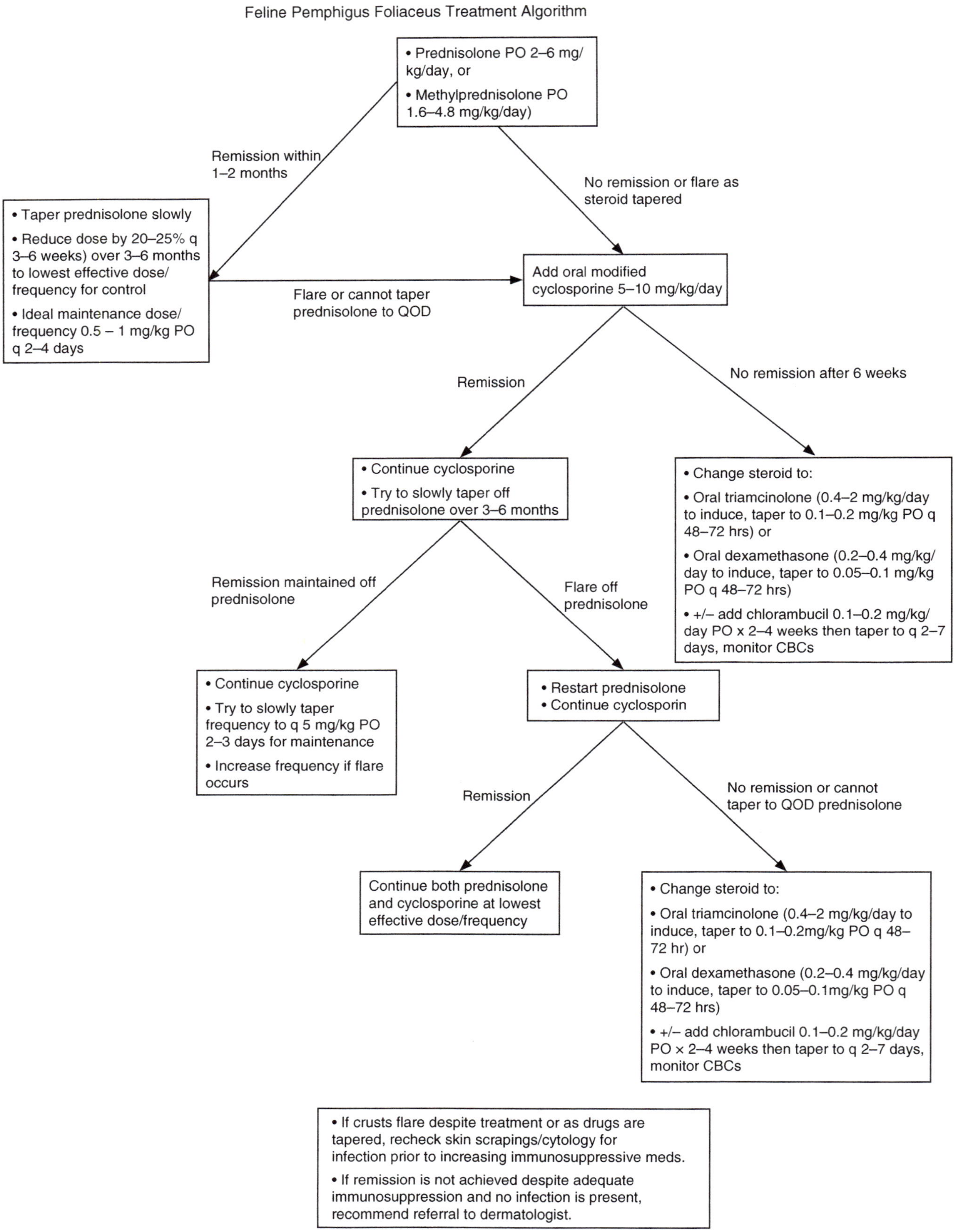

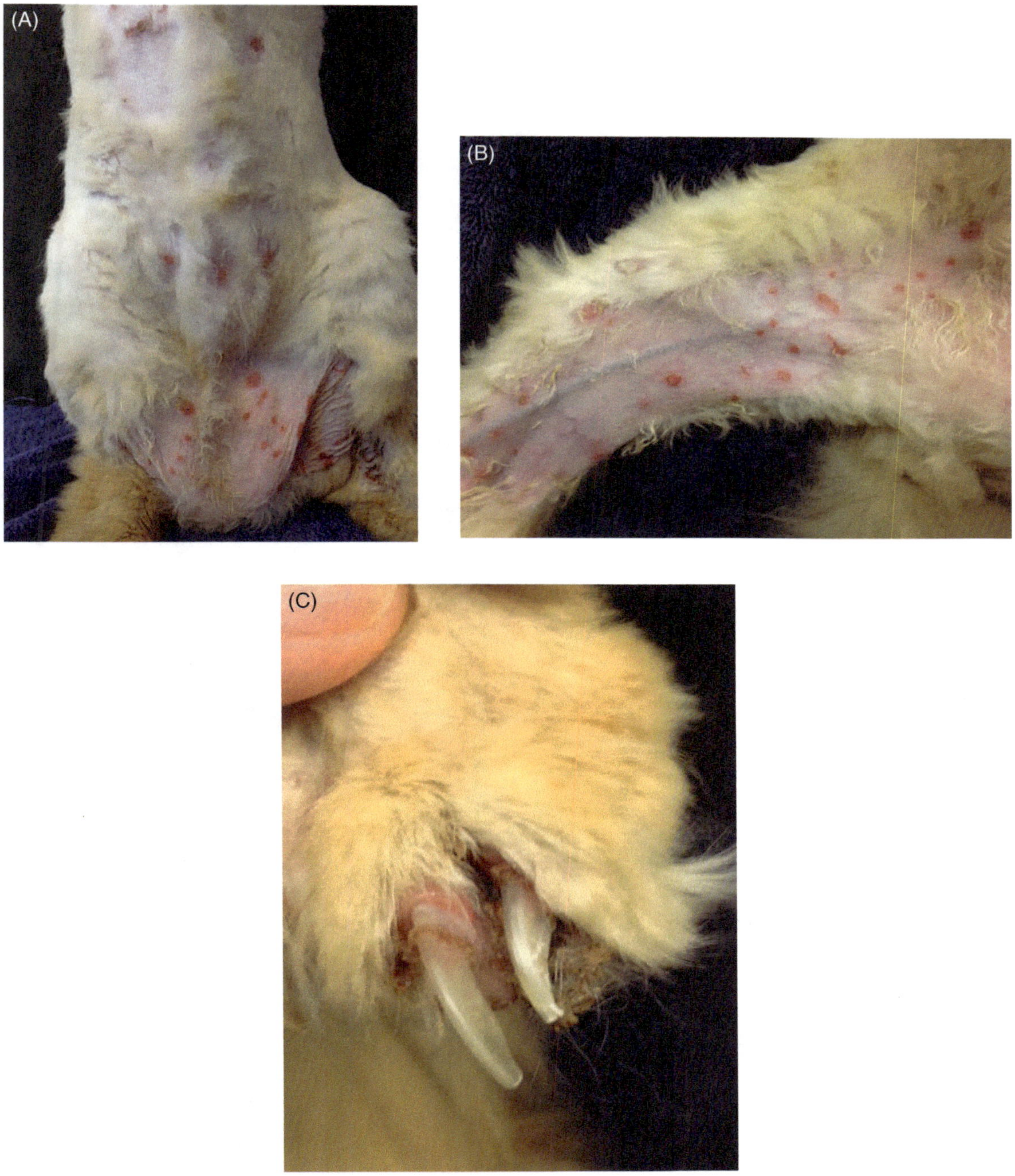

Figures 11.3A–C Numerous oval skin ulcerations and nailbed ulcers in a cat with pemphigus vulgaris. *Source:* Images courtesy of Dr. Trish Ashley, DACVD.

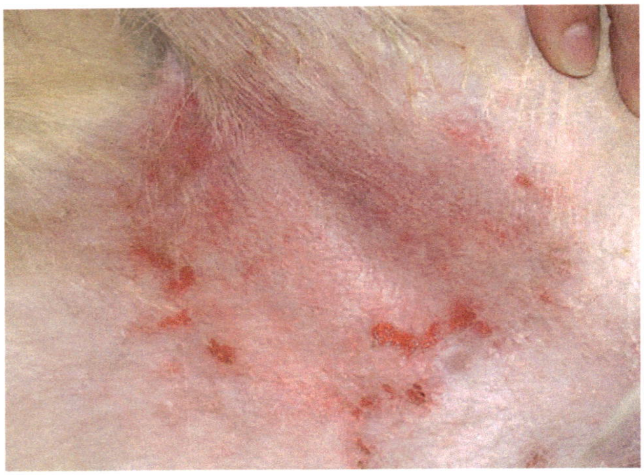

Figure 11.4 Oval to serpiginous inguinal ulcerations in a Sheltie with vesicular cutaneous lupus erythematosus.

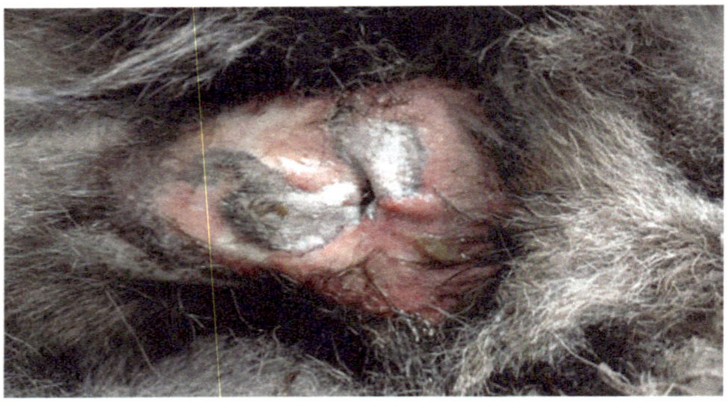

Figure 11.5A A dog with mucocutaneous lupus erythematosus (MCLE) causing painful anal mucosal ulcerations.

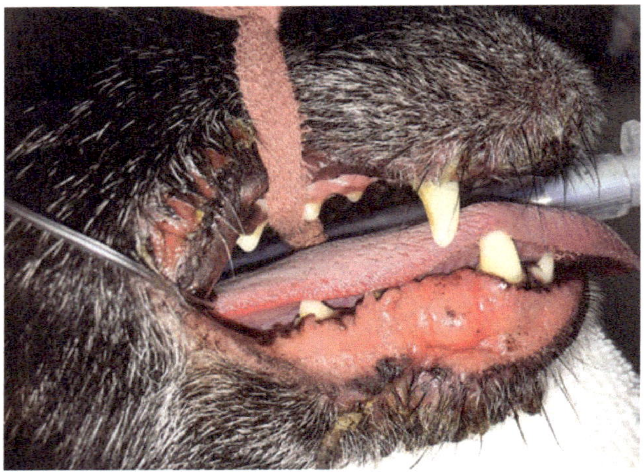

Figure 11.5B Mucocutaneous lip ulceration and crusting due to MCLE.

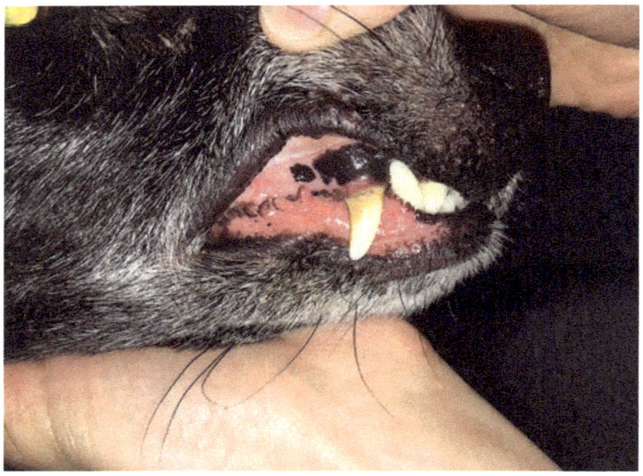

Figure 11.5C The same dog as in Figure 11.2B two months after treatment with doxycycline/niacinamide.

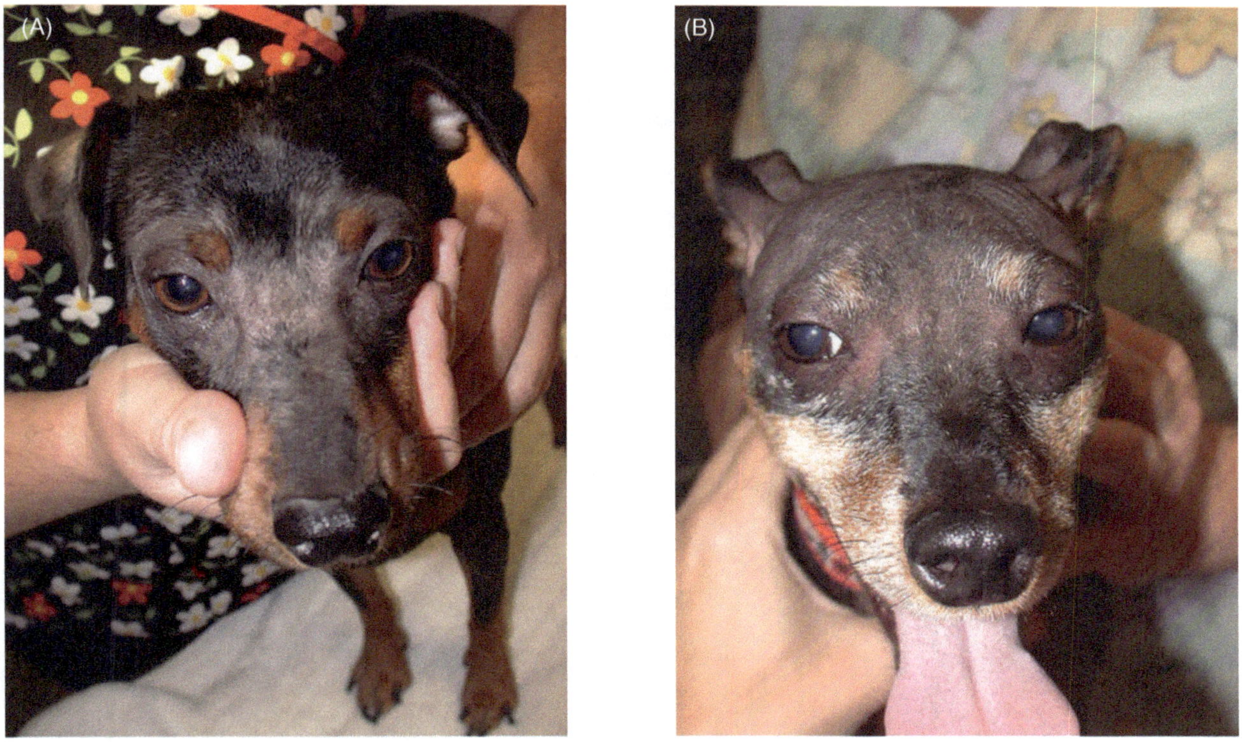

Figures 11.6A and B A dog with patchy alopecia due to alopecia areata.

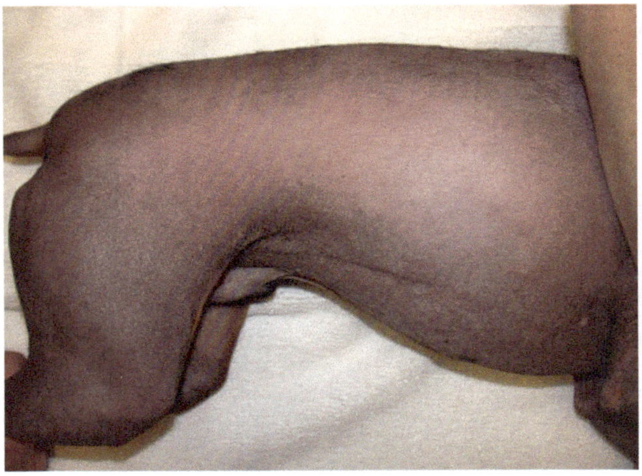

Figure 11.6C Alopecia universalis in a Miniature Pinscher.

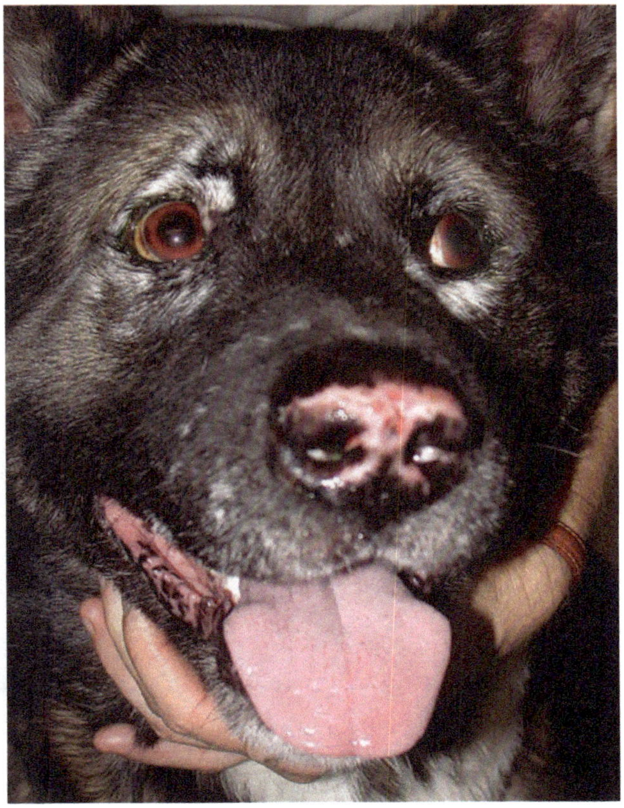

Figure 11.7 Patchy facial leukotrichia, nasal planum depigmentation, and uveitis in an Akita with uveodermatologic syndrome.

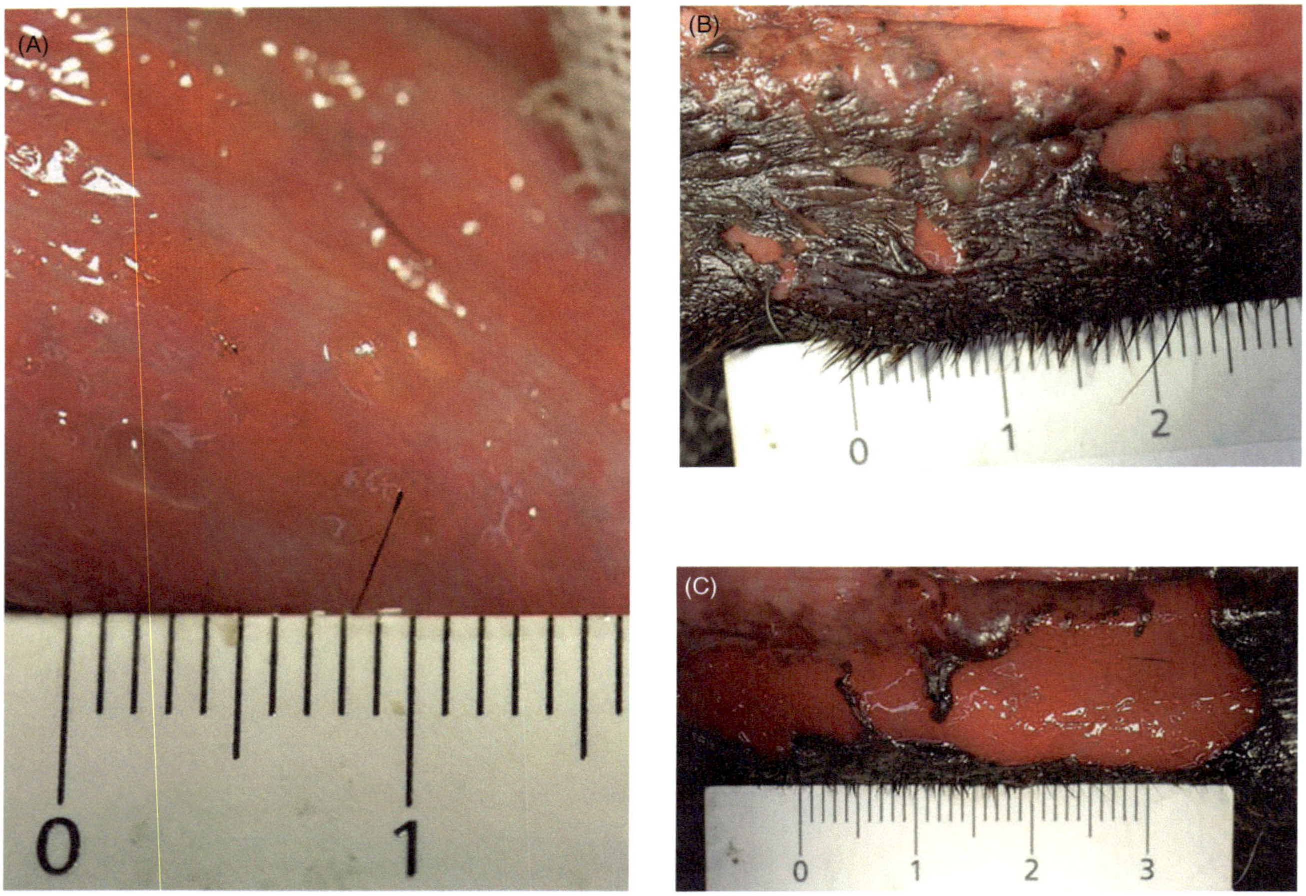

Figures 11.8A–C A Great Dane with epidermolysis bullosa acquisita, demonstrating lesions progressing from fluid-filled vesicles to punctate to confluent, full thickness ulceration of lip mucosa. *Source:* Images courtesy of Dr. Charlie Walker, BVetMed CertSAD MRCVS.

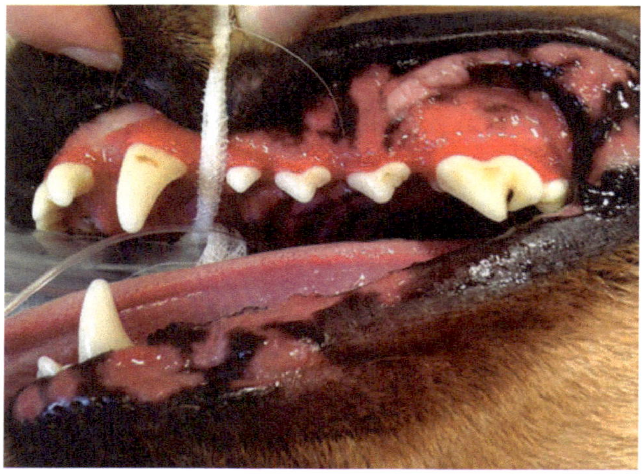

Figure 11.8D Mucosal and gingival ulcerations in a dog with mucous membrane pemphigoid. *Source:* Image courtesy of Dr. Trish Ashley, DACVD.

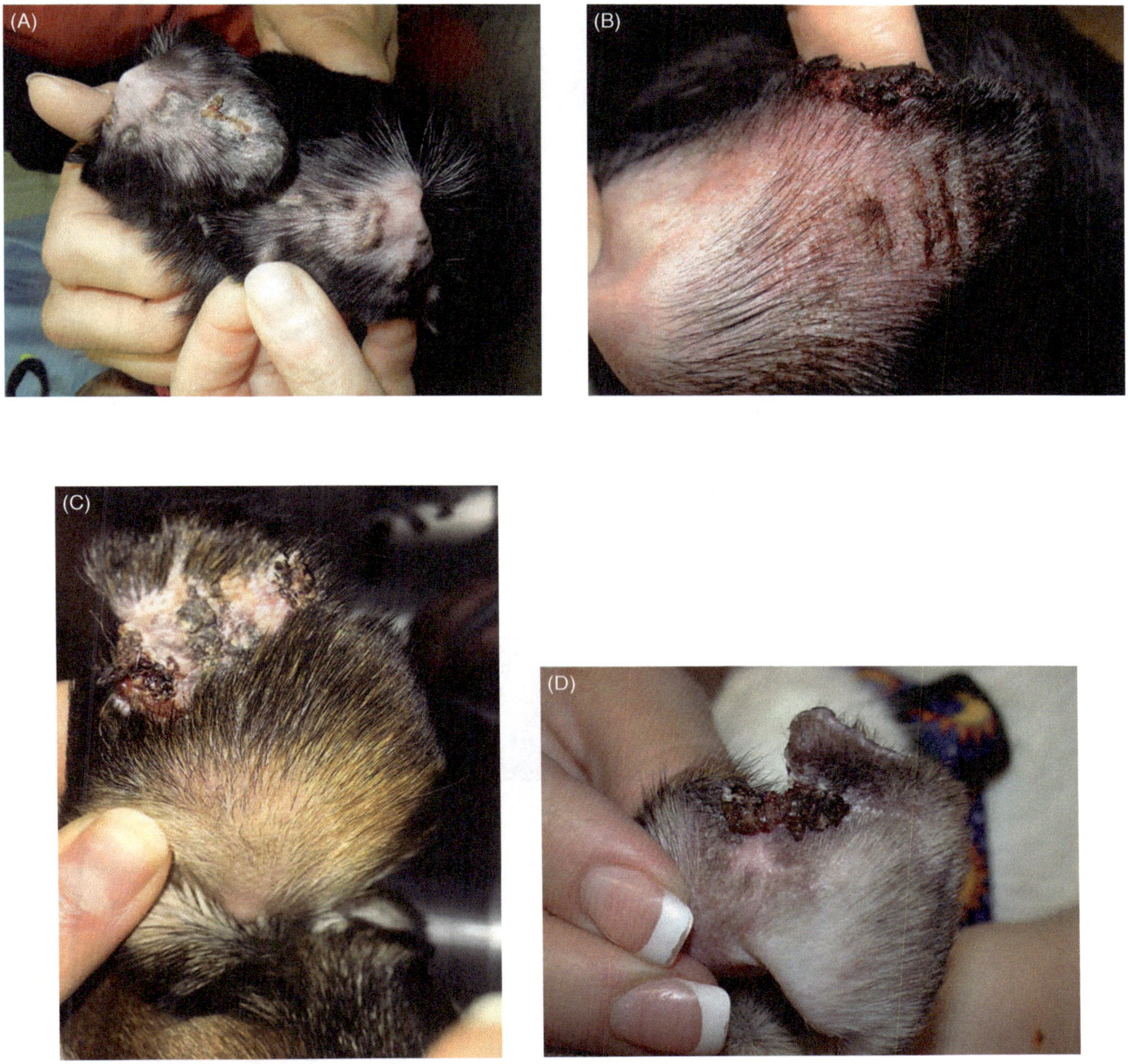

Figures 11.9A–D Pinnal vasculitis causing pinnal crusting, ulceration, and deformation.

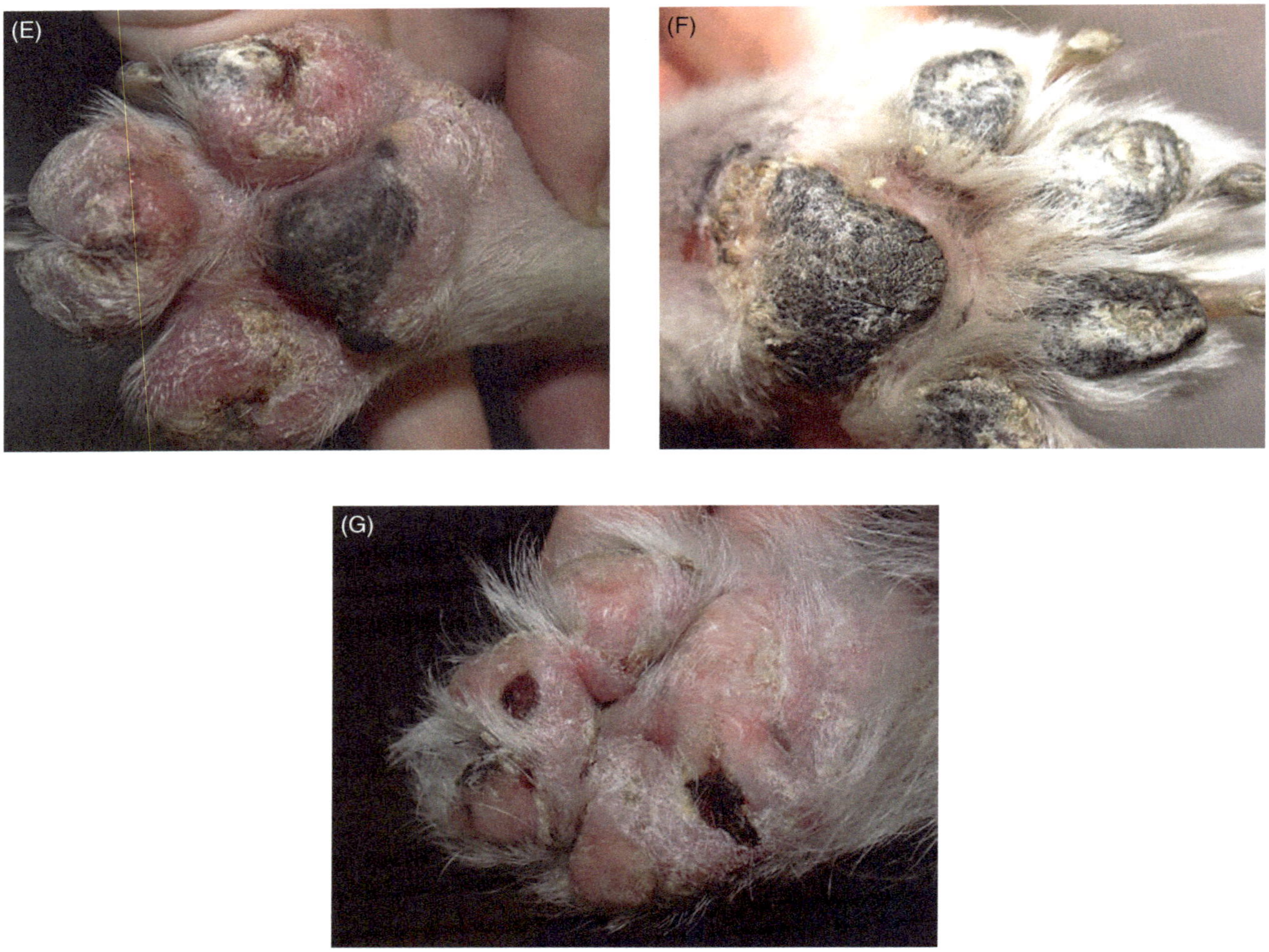

Figures 11.9E–G Paw pad crusting and erosion due to vasculitis.

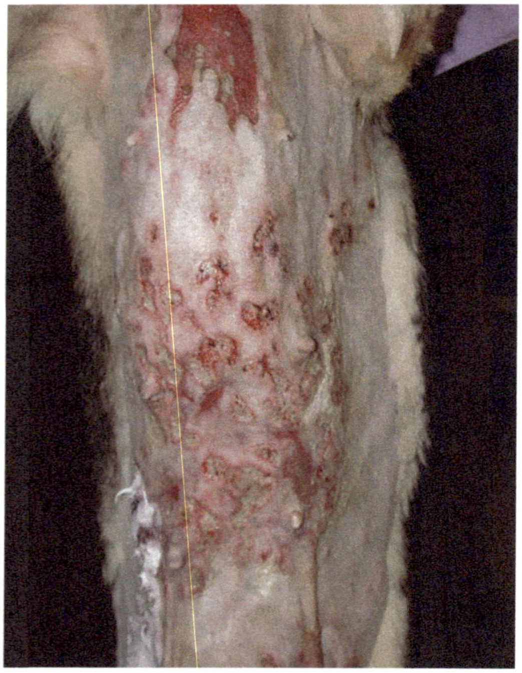

Figure 11.9H Vasculitis on the thorax of a septic German Shepherd.

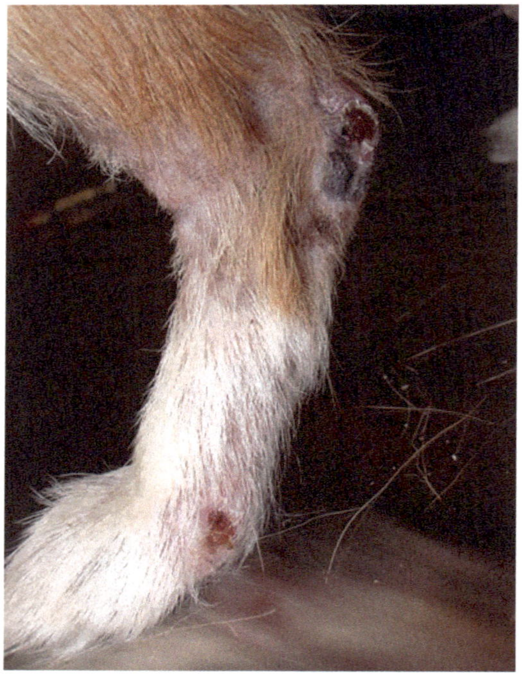

Figure 11.9I Crusts and ulcerations on the hocks due to vasculitis.

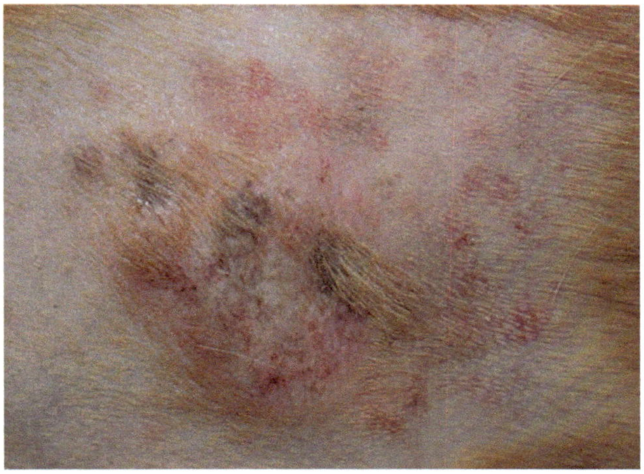

Figure 11.9J Truncal vasculitis triggered by tick borne disease.

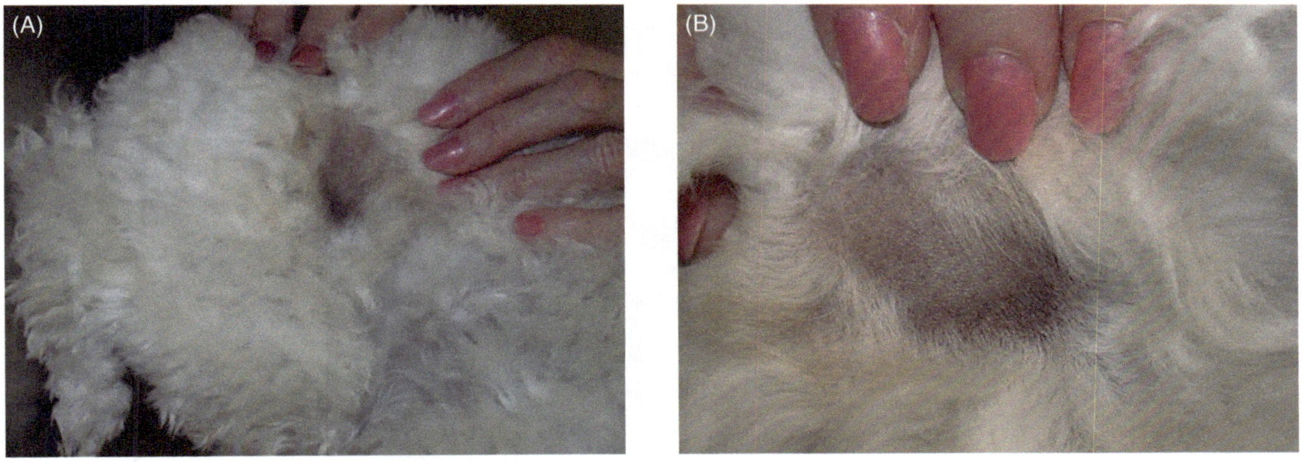

Figures 11.10A and B Rabies vaccine-induced vasculitis on the right lateral thigh of a Bichon.

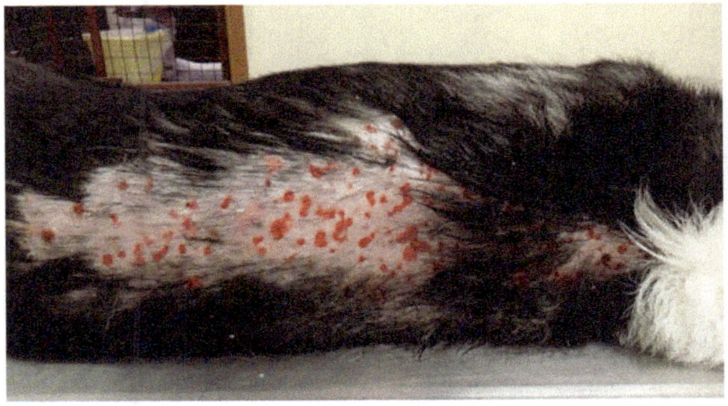

Figure 11.11A Numerous erythematous erosions in a Collie due to an adverse drug reaction to trimethoprim sulfa.

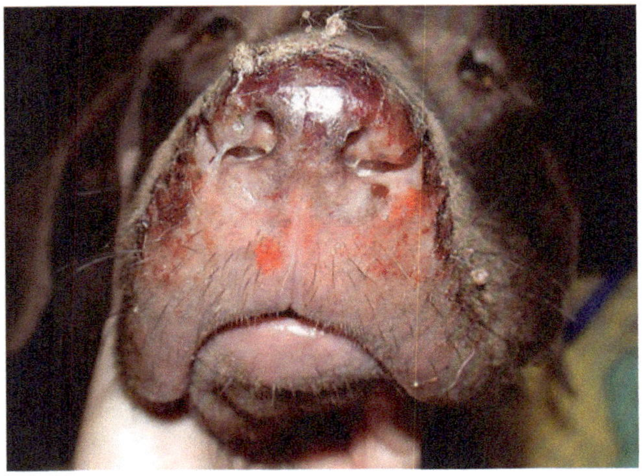

Figure 11.11B Muzzle and nasal planum ulceration caused by a drug eruption to cephalexin.

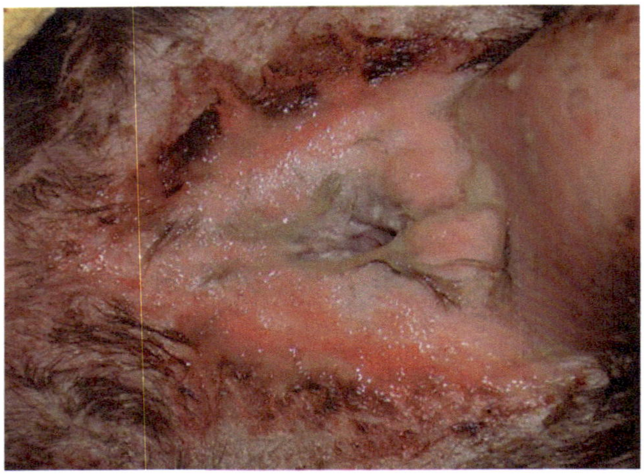

Figure 11.11C Ulcerated anal mucosa in the same dog as 11.11B.

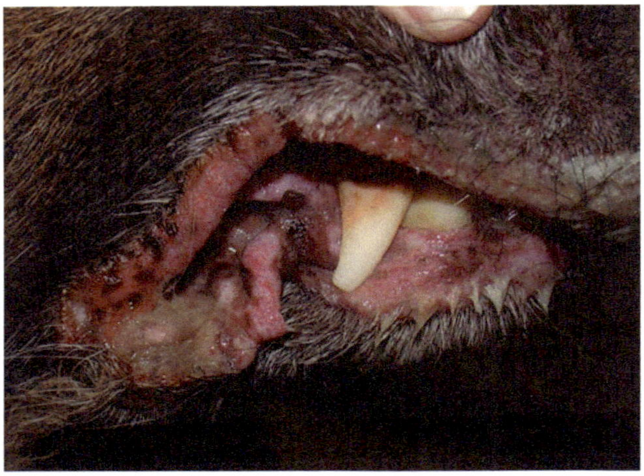

Figure 11.11D Lip mucocutaneous ulcerations in a dog which had an adverse drug reaction to carprofen.

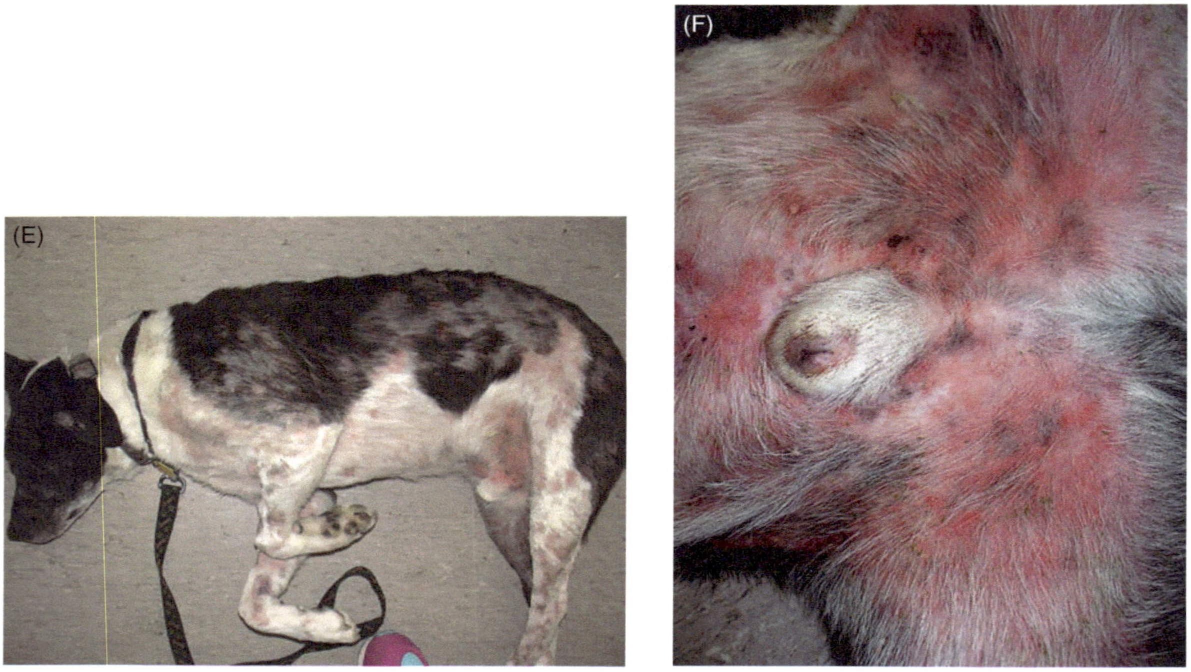

Figures 11.11E and F Patchy alopecia, crusts, and inflamed papules/macules in a dog with a drug reaction to cephalexin; biopsy demonstrated drug-induced pemphigus foliaceus.

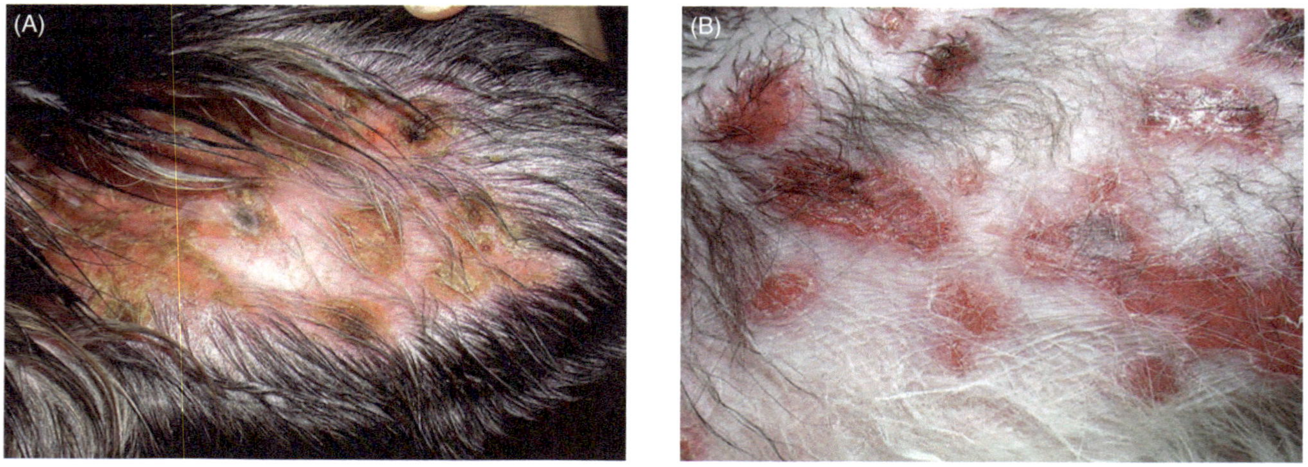

Figures 11.12A–B Erythematous crusted erosions on the inner pinna and inguinal area of a dog due to erythema multiforme.

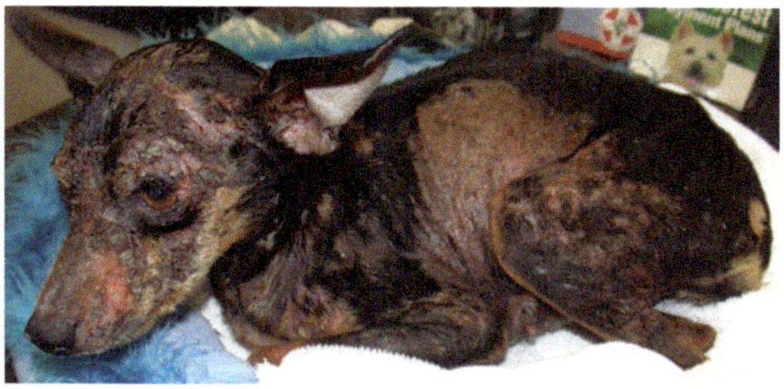

Figure 11.12C Severe erythema multiforme with secondary MRSA infection; the dog had been treated for several weeks at a primary clinic prior to specialty referral and unfortunately died of sepsis and renal failure shortly after presentation.

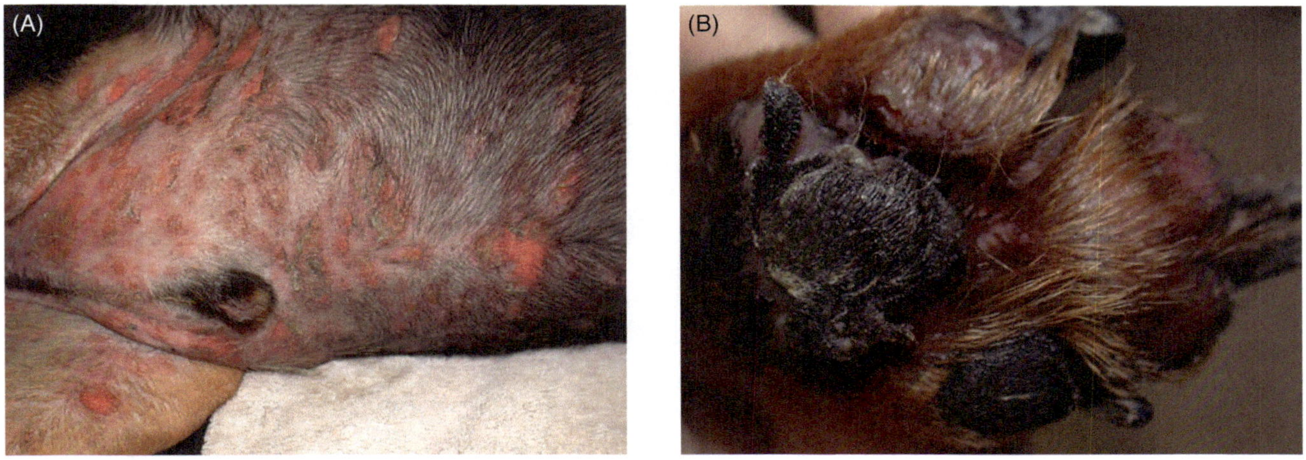

Figures 11.13A and B Toxic epidermal necrolysis in a Miniature Pinscher; full thickness ulcerations were present on the groin, paw pads and oral cavity; the dog died. Disease onset occurred within a few days of multiple vaccinations.

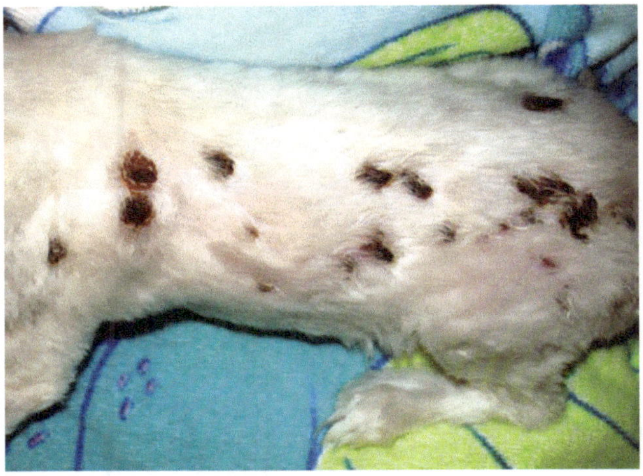

Figure 11.14A Crusting, draining, truncal lesions due to sterile panniculitis.

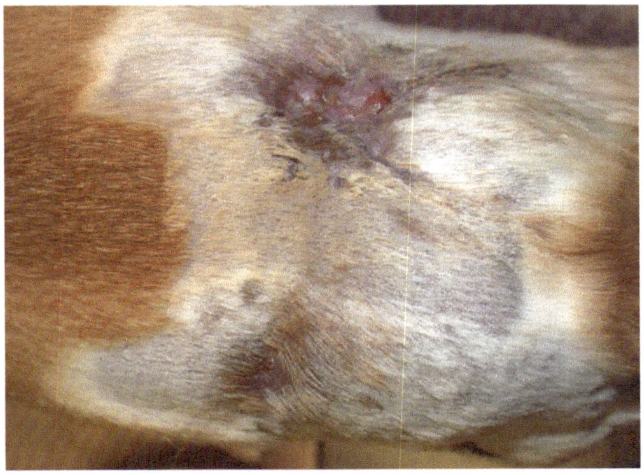

Figure 11.14B In this Chihuahua with sterile panniculitis, severe, atrophic scarring occurred.

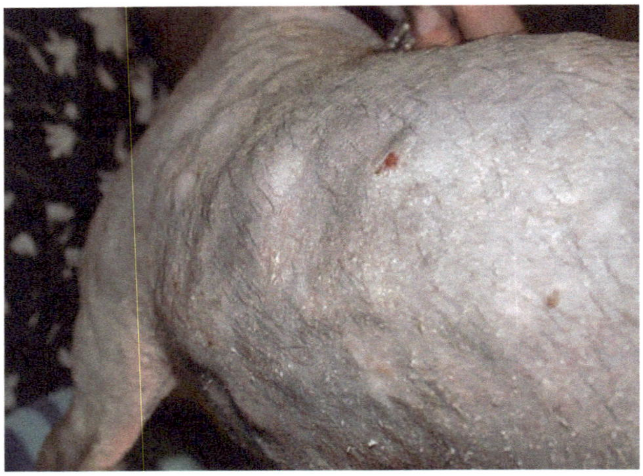

Figure 11.14C A Chihuahua with sterile panniculitis, note the irregular swelling of the truncal fat.

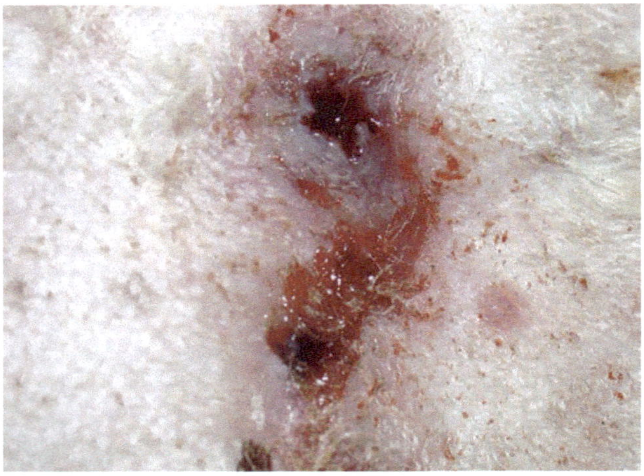

Figure 11.14D Hemorrhagic oily exudate from a draining tract caused by sterile panniculitis.

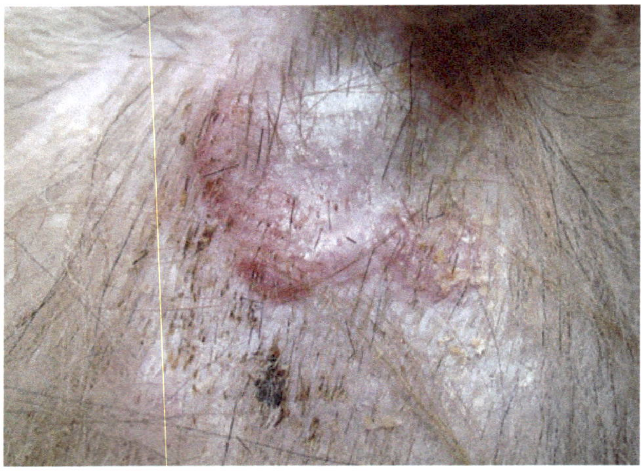

Figure 11.15A A pink, raised, flat topped plaque in a Collie due to sterile granuloma.

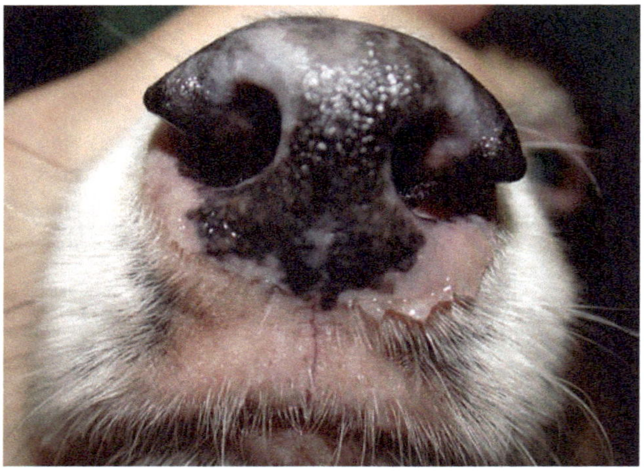

Figure 11.15B Patchy depigmentation of the nasal planum and frontal muzzle; biopsy showed sterile granulomatous inflammation.

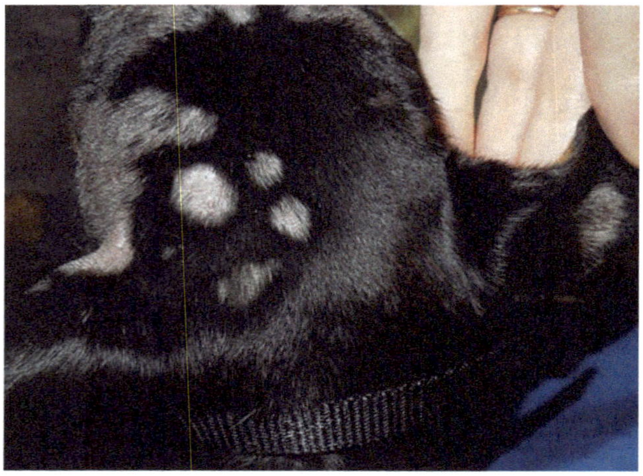

Figure 11.15C Patchy alopecia on the dorsal head of a Miniature Pinscher with histopathology consistent with sterile granuloma.

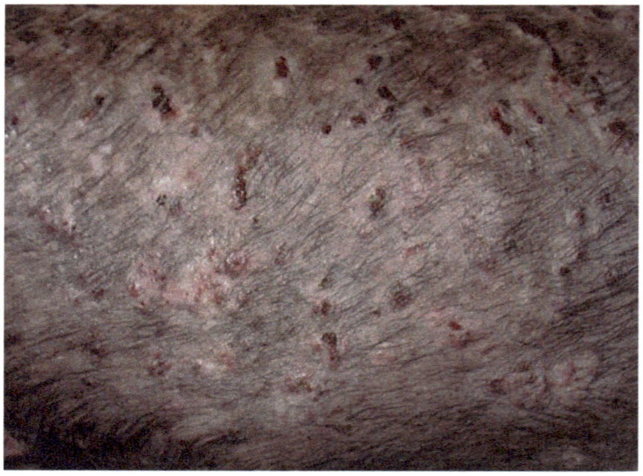

Figure 11.15D This Labrador mix had generalized chronic alopecia and crusting due to sterile granulomatous dermatitis.

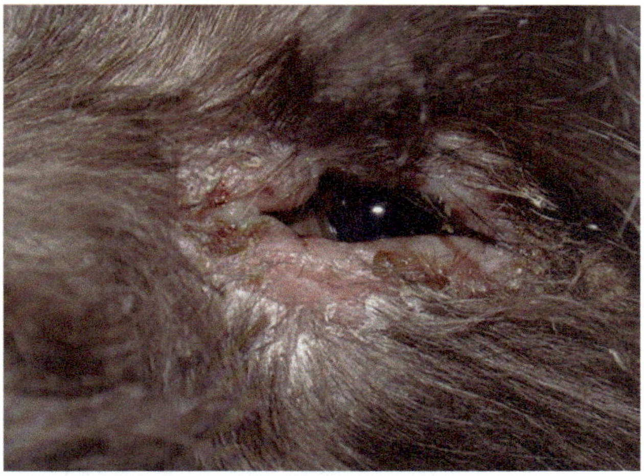

Figure 11.15E Inflamed, swollen/eroded, and crusted eyelids due to sterile granuloma/pyogranulomas.

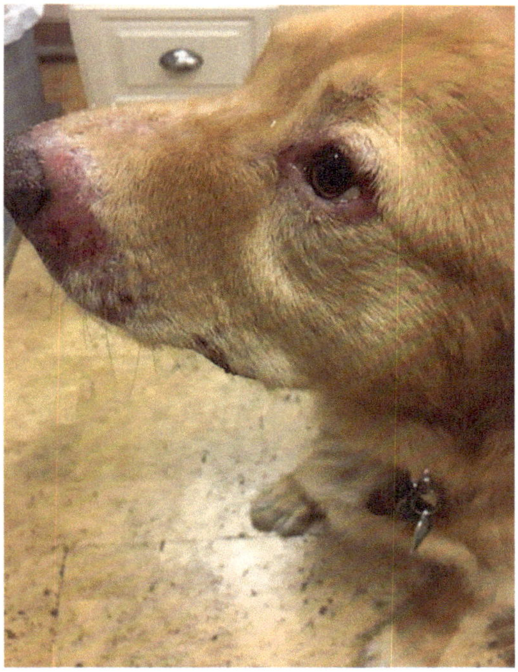

Figure 11.16A Juvenile cellulitis in a Golden Retriever mix; scarring alopecia is present on the distal muzzle and eyelids but the non-haired nasal planum is spared. *Source:* Image courtesy of Dr. Carine Laporte, DACVD.

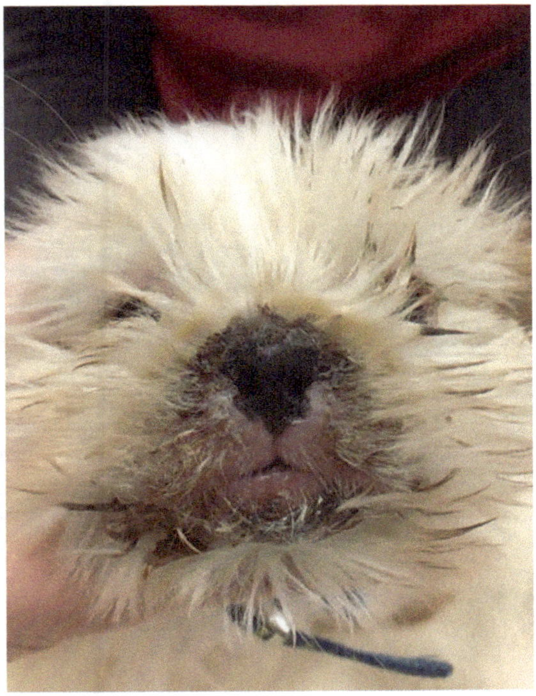

Figure 11.16B A Poodle mix puppy with marked crusting and thickened inflamed skin on the distal muzzle due to juvenile cellulitis. *Source:* Image courtesy of Dr. Carine Laporte, DACVD.

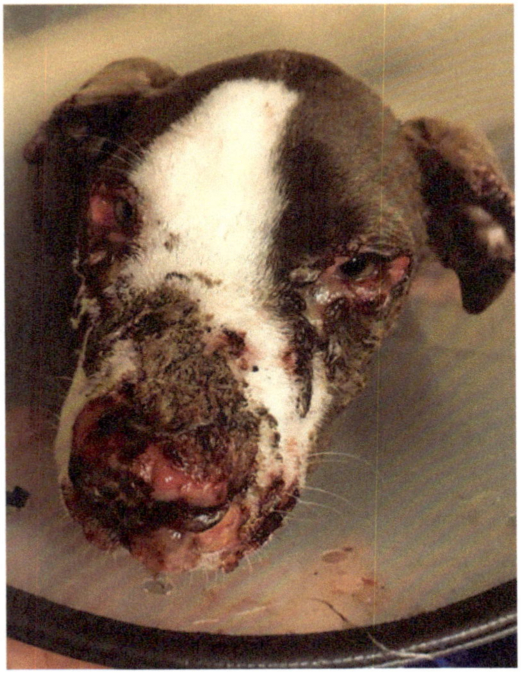

Figure 11.16C In this Pitbull puppy with juvenile cellulitis, a severe secondary bacterial infection is contributing to inflammation and nasal planum dermatitis. *Source:* Image courtesy of Sara Morar, DVM.

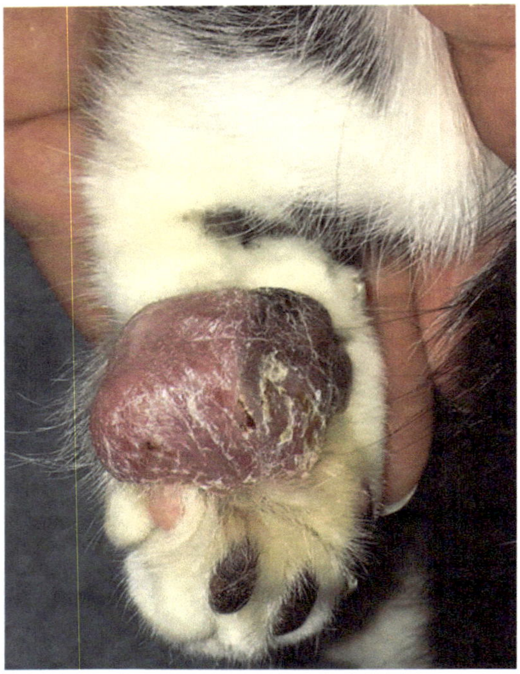

Figure 11.17A Plasma cell pododermatitis causing extensive ballooning paw pad swelling.

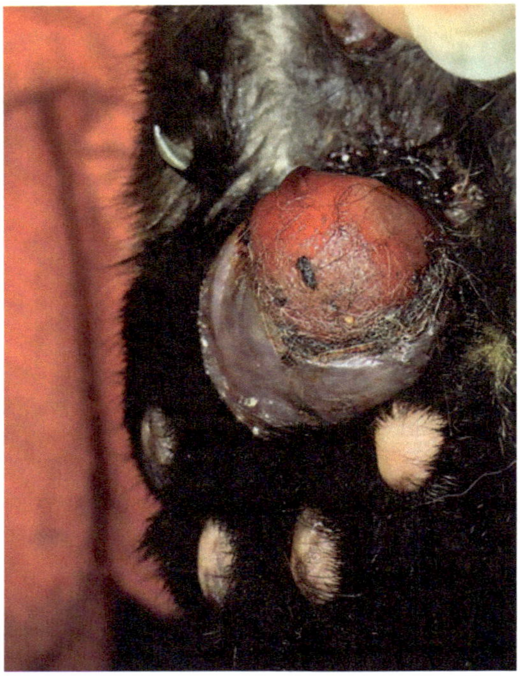

Figure 11.17B Severe plasma cell pododermatitis resulting in paw pad ulceration.

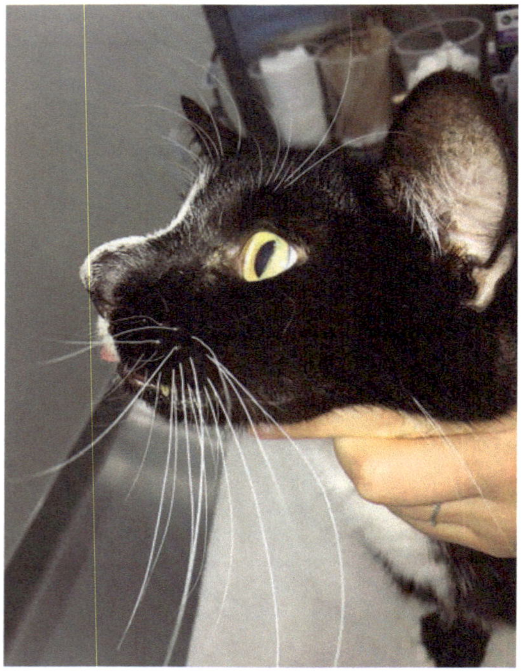

Figure 11.17C Nasal swelling also caused by plasmacytic inflammation in a cat with concurrent plasma cell pododermatitis.

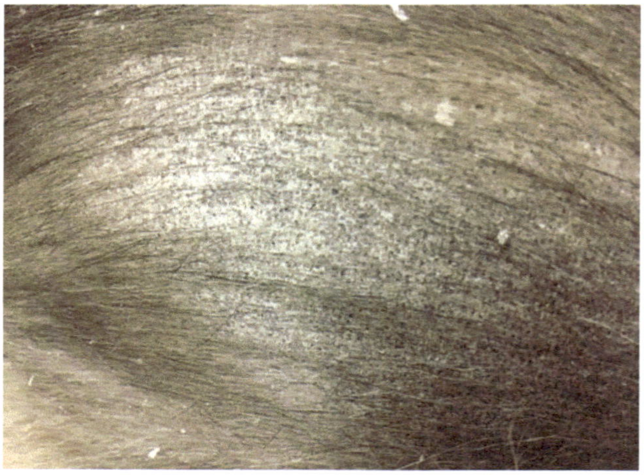

Figure 11.18A Extensive scaling and hypotrichosis which was found on biopsy to be due to pseudopelade. *Source:* Image courtesy of VIN and Becky Arthur, DVM.

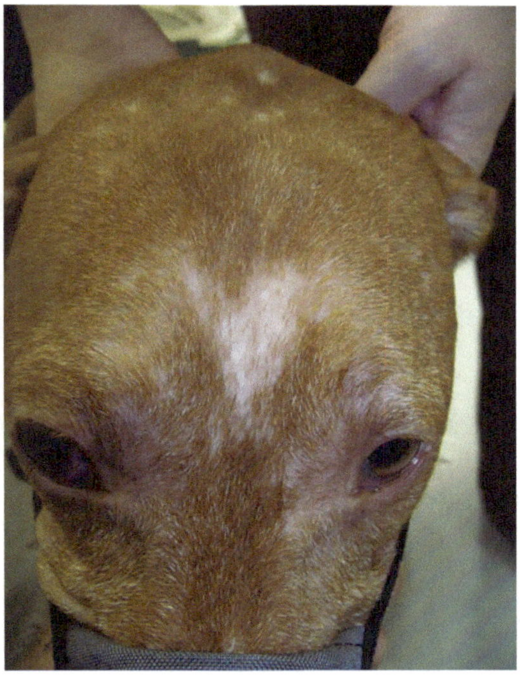

Figure 11.18B Patchy alopecia due to pseudopelade on the head of a Vizsla. *Source:* Image courtesy of VIN and Jennifer Prior, DVM.

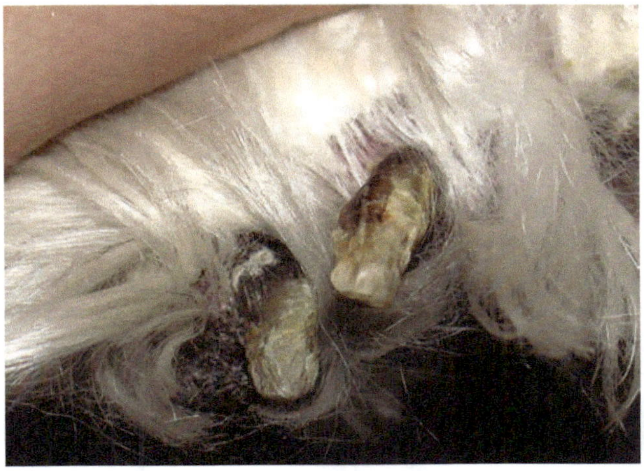

Figure 11.19A Lupoid onychitis in a West Highland White Terrier; nails normalized with pentoxifylline and a hypoallergenic diet; after three months pentoxifylline was discontinued and the toenails continued to be normal.

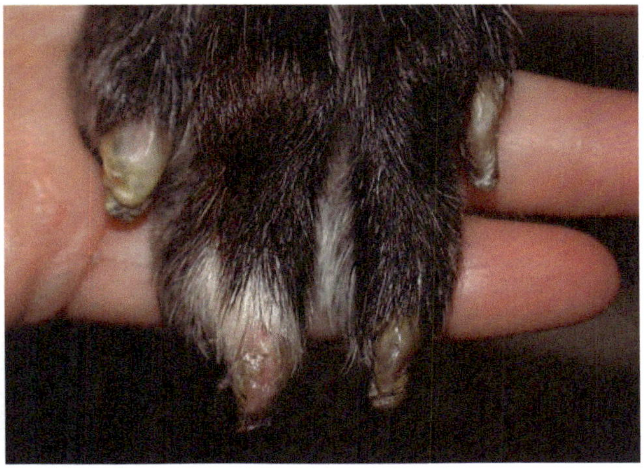

Figure 11.19B A Greyhound with lupoid onychitis; he responded well to doxycycline and niacinamide.

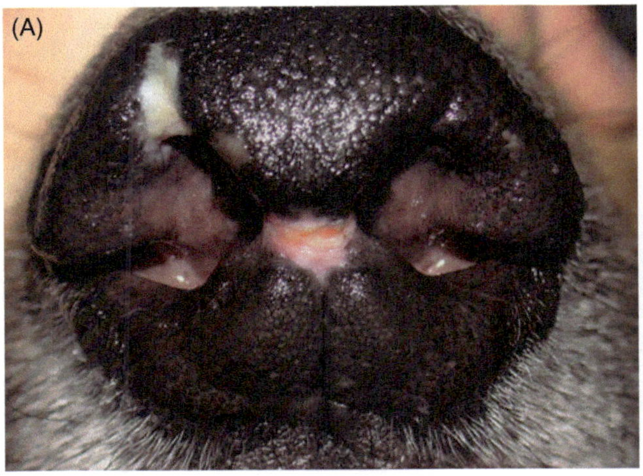

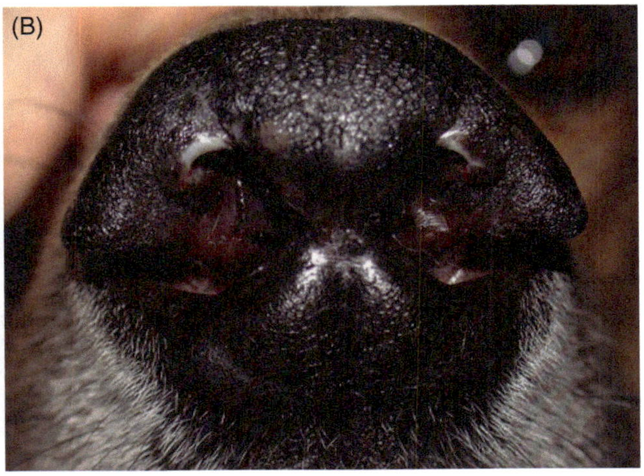

Figures 11.20A and B A Hound mix with nasal arteritis pre- and post-treatment with cyclosporine.

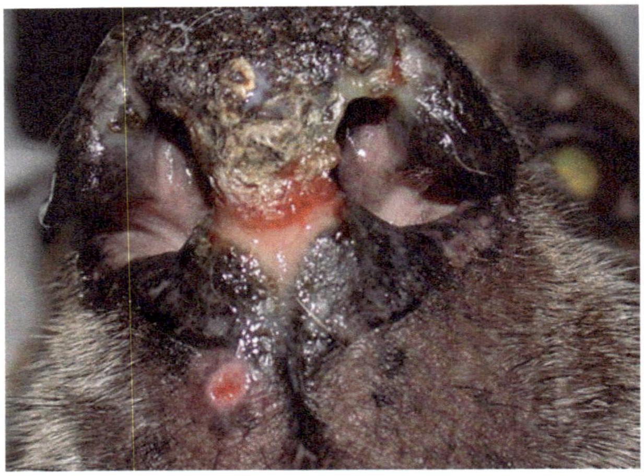

Figure 11.20C A Bloodhound with nasal arteritis and a severe secondary nasal bacterial pyoderma causing marked crusting.

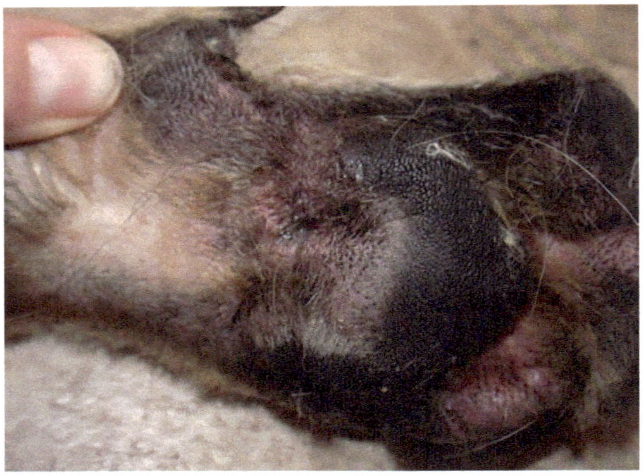

Figure 11.21A A German Shepherd dog with metacarpal fistulas; irregular, firm scarring and small draining tracts with seropurulent exudate are present just proximal to the metacarpal pad.

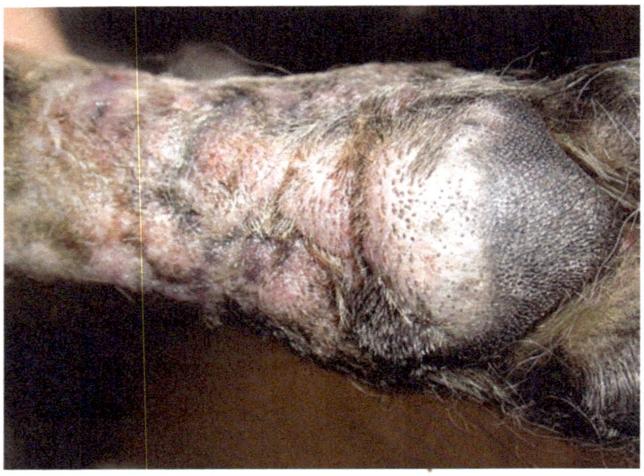

Figure 11.21B In this German Shepherd with metacarpal/metatarsal fistulas, more extensive scarring and fistulation are progressing proximally.

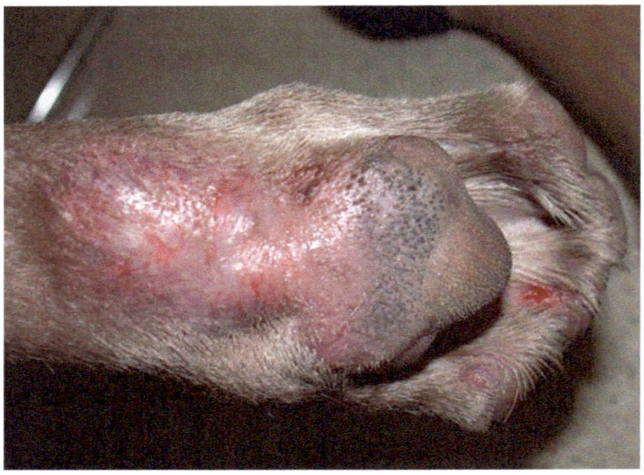

Figure 11.21C A Weimaraner dog with swelling and draining tracts caused by metatarsal fistulas; small areas of similar swelling were present on the toes as well. He responded well to doxycycline and topical tacrolimus.

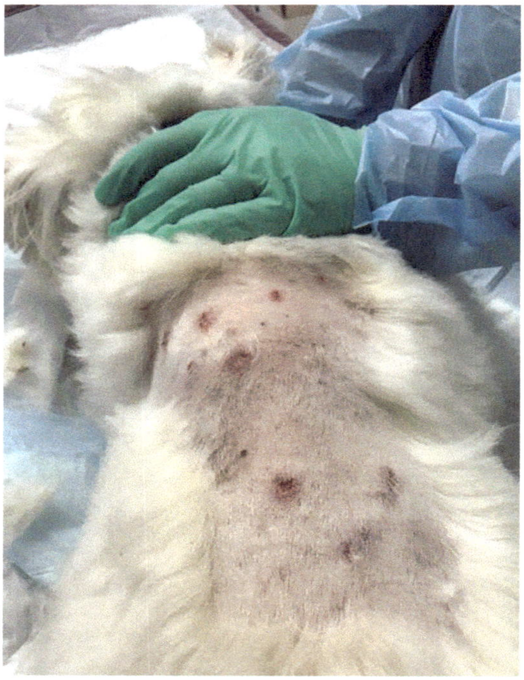

Figure 11.22 Acute dorsal truncal, draining tracts and nodules in a dog with Sweet's syndrome; he was also febrile, lethargic, and had diarrhea; biopsies and cultures demonstrated sterile neutrophilic inflammation.

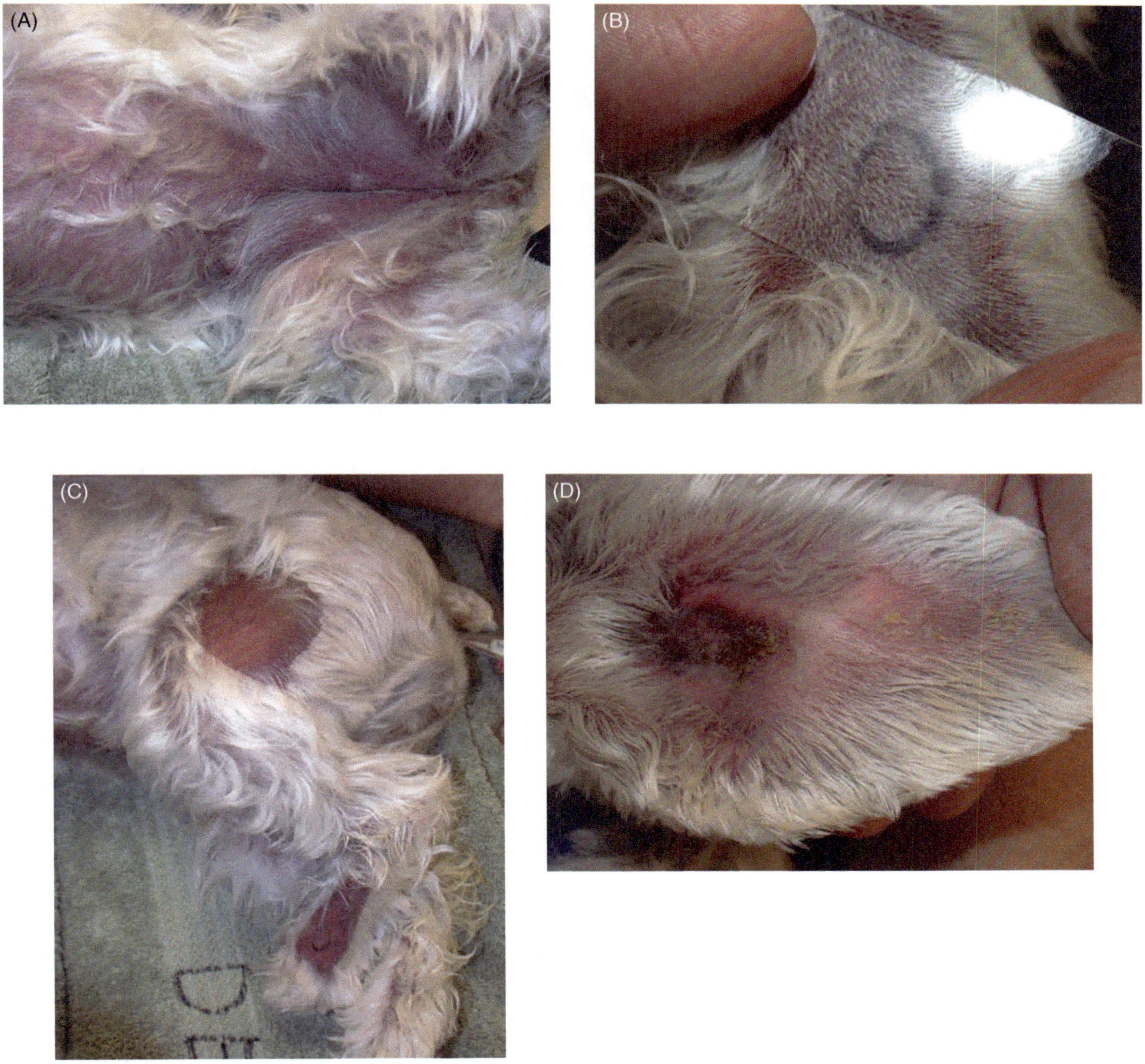

Figures 11.23A–D Acute purplish skin discoloration and pinnal crusting in a critically ill Miniature Schnauzer with superficial suppurative necrolytic dermatitis; the discoloration did not blanche on diascopy (B), indicating vascular leakage of red blood cells was the cause for the skin discoloration.

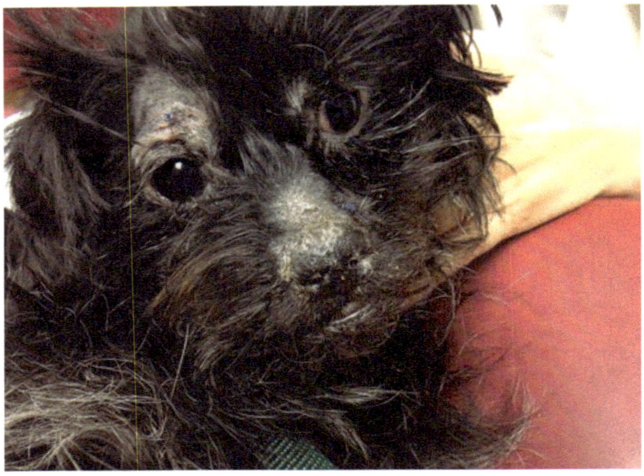

Figure 11.24A Crusting on the periocular areas, dorsal muzzle, and nasal planum in a dog; biopsy results and labwork including ANA (antinuclear antibody) were consistent with SLE. *Source:* Image courtesy of Dr. Andrew Simpson, DACVD.

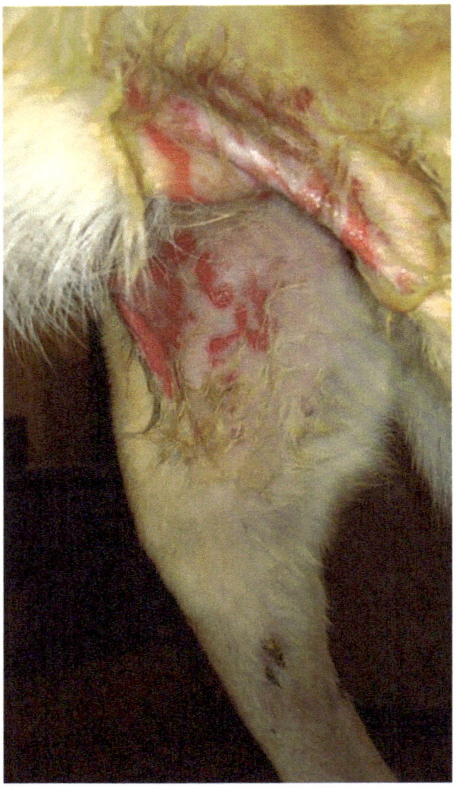

Figure 11.24B Serpiginous inguinal ulcerations in a dog with systemic lupus erythematosus. *Source:* Image courtesy of Dr. Andrew Simpson, DACVD.

Table 11.2 Typical glucocorticoid doses for treatment of autoimmune and immune-mediated disorders (use low end of dose range for dogs and high end of dose range for cats).

Steroid	Induction dose	Maintenance dose
Prednisone/Prednisolone	2–4 mg/kg/day	0.5–1 mg/kg q 48 hours
Methylprednisolone	1.6–4 mg/kg/day	0.5–1 mg/kg q 48 hours
Dexamethasone	0.2–0.4 mg/kg/day	0.05–0.1 mg/kg q 48–72 hours
Triamcinolone	0.4–2 mg/kg/day	0.1–0.2 mg/kg q 48–72 hours

Common side effects of steroids include increased thirst, urination, appetite, weight gain, hepatopathy, increased risk of diabetes, hypertension, increased risk of infections (urinary tract and cutaneous), calcinosis cutis.
Monitoring: CBC, Chemistry panel, UA every six months to evaluate for liver enzymes elevations, blood and urine glucose for evidence of diabetes and evidence of urinary tract infections.

Table 11.3 Non-steroidal immunosuppressant or immunomodulatory drugs as adjunctive or primary treatments of autoimmune/immune-mediated diseases.

Drug	Dose	Indications	Side effects	Monitoring
Azathioprine	2 mg/kg/day for 2–4 wk, tapering to q48h.	Adjunctive therapy for treatment for many AI diseases, including pemphigus, vasculitis.	Vomiting, diarrhea, hepatotoxicity, myelosuppression, pancreatitis, opportunistic infections. DO NOT USE IN CATS	CBC, platelet count, Chemistry q2–3 wk for the first 3 mo then q6 mo.
Cyclosporine modified	5–10 mg/kg/day with attempts to taper to 5 mg/kg q48h.	Adjunctive treatment for many AI diseases (pemphigus [especially in cats], vasculitis, VCLE). Primary treatment in sebaceous adenitis, alopecia areata, pseudopelade, erythema multiforme, TEN, panniculitis, and perianal fistulas.	Vomiting, diarrhea, gingival hyperplasia, urinary tract infection, hirsutism, papillomatosis.	CBC, Chemistry panel, UA q6–12 mo.
Chlorambucil	Dogs: 0.1–0.2 mg/kg/day for 2–4 wk then q2–7d. Cats: 0.1–0.2 mg/kg PO q24h; usually ½ of a 2 mg tablet once daily for larger cats. Alternate dosing schedule: 2 mg PO q48h for cats >4 kg and 2 mg PO q72h for cats <4 kg.	Used as adjunctive therapy in refractory AI diseases (primarily pemphigus, vasculitis).	Myelosuppression, vomiting, diarrhea, anorexia.	CBC, platelet count, Chemistry panel q2–3 wk for 2–3 mo then q6 mo.
Dapsone	Dogs: 1 mg/kg q8h.	Used as adjunctive therapy in refractory pemphigus. Effective in treatment of neutrophilic vasculitis.	Myelosuppression, vomiting, diarrhea, neuropathies, cutaneous drug eruptions. DO NOT USE IN CATS	CBC, platelet count, Chemistry panel, UA every 2–3 wk for first 3 mo then q3–4 mo.
Doxycycline	5 mg/kg q12h or 10 mg/kg q24h.	Used as principle treatment combined with niacinamide in treatment for discoid lupus erythematosus, certain forms of vasculitis (vaccine-induced), symmetric onychitis, or pemphigus erythematosus (facially localized pemphigus). Can be used as adjunctive therapy for many AI/immune-mediated diseases. Cats: Sole treatment for plasma cell pododermatitis.	Vomiting, diarrhea, hepatopathy. Esophagitis can occur in cats, follow each dose with 15–30 ml water.	Periodic CBC, Chemistry panel; possible increase in risk of hepatotoxicity if combined with other potentially hepatotoxic drugs such as azathioprine.
Hydroxychloroquine	5–10 mg/kg/day.	Has been used in treatment of refractory canine discoid lupus erythematosus, systemic lupus erythematosus, and exfoliative cutaneous lupus erythematosus (as sole therapy or combined with CSA).	None reported in dogs; GI symptoms reported in people.	There is little information regarding safety in dogs; consider periodic CBC, Chemistry panel monitoring. In patients with cardiac abnormalities, consider ECG monitoring and routine eye exams.

(*Continued*)

Table 11.3 Non-steroidal immunosuppressant or immunomodulatory drugs (Continued)

Drug	Dose	Indications	Side effects	Monitoring
Leflunomide	Dogs: 2–4 mg/kg/day. Cats: 10 mg/cat/day then taper to q2–3 days when in remission.	Adjunctive treatment for pemphigus. Treatment in histiocytic diseases (systemic histiocytosis, reactive histiocytosis).	Lethargy, GI disturbance, myelosuppression.	CBC, platelet count, Chemistry panel q2 wk for 2–3 mo then q4–6 weeks.
Mycophenolate mofetil	Dogs: 10–15 mg/kg q12h; can attempt taper once disease is in remission.	Adjunctive therapy for AI diseases, especially pemphigus in dogs.	Primarily GI (vomiting, diarrhea, hematochezia), occasionally myelosuppression.	CBC, platelet count, Chemistry panel at 2–4 weeks then q4–6 mo.
Niacinamide	250 mg q12h for dogs <10 kg; 500 mg q12h for dogs >10 kg.	Used as principle treatment combined with doxycycline in treatment for discoid lupus erythematosus, certain forms of vasculitis (vaccine-induced), symmetric onychitis, or pemphigus erythematosus (facially localized pemphigus). Can be used as adjunctive therapy for many AI/immune-mediated diseases.	Lethargy, vomiting, diarrhea, anorexia; caution for use in patients with seizure disorders.	No monitoring required.
Pentoxifylline	15–25 mg/kg q8–12h/day; once in remission can be tapered.	Used primarily in vasculitis cases and for treatment of symmetric onychitis.	Gastrointestinal (vomiting, diarrhea).	None
Sulfasalazine	10–40 mg/kg q8h.	Used primarily as adjunctive therapy in refractory pemphigus cases and other neutrophilic disorders.	Keratoconjunctivitis sicca, anemia, hepatotoxicity.	CBC, Chemistry panel q2 weeks for 6 weeks then q2–4 mo; tear production checked q2–4 weeks.
Tacrolimus 0.1% ointment	Applied topically to affected area twice daily for 2 wk then tapered to every 1–2d.	Often used as adjunctive treatment for discoid lupus erythematosus, localized problem areas of pemphigus and perianal fistulas.	Occasional local irritation, hair loss.	No monitoring required.

Further reading

Ackerman, A.L., May, E.R., and Frank, L.A. (2017). Use of mycophenolate mofetil to treat immune-mediated skin disease in 14 dogs – a retrospective study. *Vet. Dermatol.* 28 (2): 195–e44.

Banovic, F., Olivry, T., and Linder, K.E. (2014). Ciclosporin therapy for canine generalized discoid lupus erythematosus refractory to doxycycline and niacinamide. *Vet. Dermatol.* 25 (5): 483–e79.

Banovic, F., Robson, D., Linek, M. et al. (2017). Therapeutic effectiveness of calcineurin inhibitors in canine vesicular cutaneous lupus erythematosus. *Vet. Dermatol.* 28 (5): 493–e115.

Kim, H.J., Kang, M.H., Kim, J.H. et al. (2011). Sterile panniculitis in dogs: new diagnostic findings and alternative treatments. *Vet. Dermatol.* 22 (4): 352–359.

Mauldin, E.A., Morris, D.O., Brown, D.C., and Casal, M.L. (2010). Exfoliative cutaneous lupus erythematosus in German shorthaired pointer dogs: disease development, progression and evaluation of three immunomodulatory drugs (ciclosporin, hydroxychloroquine, and adalimumab) in a controlled environment. *Vet. Dermatol.* 21 (4): 373–382.

Mueller, R.S., Rosychuk, R.A., Jonas, L.D. et al. (2003). A retrospective study regarding the treatment of lupoid onychodystrophy in 30 dogs and literature review. *J. Am. Anim. Hosp. Assoc.* 39 (2): 139–150.

Olivry, T. and Linder, K.E. (2009). Dermatoses affecting desmosomes in animals: a mechanistic review of acantholytic blistering skin diseases. *Vet. Dermatol.* 20 (5–6): 313–326.

Olivry, T., Rossi, M.A., Banovic, F. et al. (2015). Mucocutaneous lupus erythematosus in dogs (21 cases). *Vet. Dermatol.* 26: 256–e55.

Plumb, D.C. (2018). *Plumb's Veterinary Drug Handbook*, 9e. Stockholm, Chichester: Wiley.

Rosenkrantz, W. (2004). Pemphigus: current therapy. *Vet. Dermatol.* 15 (2): 90–98.

Schulz, B.S., Hupfauer, S., Ammer, H. et al. (2011). Suspected side effects of doxycycline use in dogs – a retrospective study of 386 cases. *Vet. Rec.* 169 (9): 229.

Yager, J. (2014). Erythema multiforme, Stevens–Johnson syndrome and toxic epidermal necrolysis: a comparative review. *Vet. Dermatol.* 25 (5): 406–e64.

12

Endocrine skin diseases

Patricia Ashley, DVM, DACVD

Veterinary Allergy and Dermatology Services, Springfield, OR, USA

Clinical Atlas of Canine and Feline Dermatology, First Edition. Edited by Kimberly S. Coyner.

Companion website: www.wiley.com/go/coyner/dermatology

Table 12.1 Canine endocrine skin diseases.

Condition	Cutaneous symptoms	Systemic symptoms	Diagnosis	Treatment, expected response, monitoring, comments
Hypothyroidism (Figures 12.1A–12.1F; Chapter 2, Figures. 2.31 2.55; Chapter 3, Figures 3.28, 3.79, 3.91A) Seen in multiple breeds; Retrievers and Doberman Pinschers may be predisposed.	Variable; include alopecia from poor hair growth in areas of wear, bridge of nose, trunk, tail; thickened skin/mucinosis of face ("tragic expression"); dry brittle hair coat, seborrhea; recurrent bacterial or yeast infections; ceruminous otitis. Boxers, Irish Setters may have thickened hair coats.	Variable but include lethargy, weight gain, low exercise tolerance. Stunted growth in congenital cases.	↓TT4, ↓fT4 by equilibrium dialysis; ↑cTSH (however TSH can be normal in 25% of hypothyroid dogs). Sensitivity and specificity of testing improves when all 3 values assessed rather than individual tests. Response to supplement acceptable if testing inconclusive. Common clinical path changes: ↑cholesterol, +/– mild, non-regenerative anemia.	Oral levothyroxine; 0.02 mg/kg BID (best given on an empty stomach; may be able to reduce to once daily after response; monitor for recurrence of symptoms). Dogs with concurrent cardiac disease: Start with lower levothyroxine dose of 0.005 mg/kg BID and increase dose by 0.005 mg every 2 weeks to 0.02 mg/kg BID. Systemic signs respond within 2 weeks; Cutaneous signs may take 8–12 weeks to resolve and hair loss/scaling may temporarily worsen due to increased epidermal and follicular turnover. Desired 4–6 hr post pill TT4 levels at or just above upper end of normal range.
Spontaneous hyperadrenocorticism (HAC, Cushing's disease): Pituitary dependent hyperadrenocorticism (PDH)/or adrenal tumor (AT) (Figures 12.2A–12.2D; Chapter 3, Figure 3.91B) Dachshunds, Boston Terriers, Boxers, and Poodles may be predisposed.	Variable; include dull hair coat; alopecia (mostly truncal) from poor hair growth; thin skin; comedones; seborrhea; milia; recurrent pyoderma; phlebectasia; calcinosis cutis.	Polyuria/polydipsia, polyphagia, weight gain, muscle atrophy, and weakness; panting, pendulous abdomen, hepatic enlargement, hypertension, clitoral enlargement, testicular atrophy.	Definitive tests: 1) Low dose (0.01 mg/kg) dexamethasone suppression test (LDDST): Lack of cortisol suppression at 4 and/or 8 hours; cortisol suppression at 4 hours and escape at 8 hours consistent with PDH. False positive results can occur with stress/ illness. 2) ACTH stimulation (cosyntropin 1ug/kg IV or 5ug/kg IM or IV, max dose 250ug): Exaggerated cortisol level one hour post cosyntropin. False negative and false positive results can occur. Adrenal tumors: Lack of cortisol suppression at 4 and 8 hours after high dose (0.1 mg/kg) dexamethasone suppression test. Adrenal imaging (ultrasound, CT, MRI), especially to differentiate pituitary vs adrenal etiology. Screening/supportive tests: ↑urine cortisol/creatinine ratio (UCCR), however, UCCR can be increased with stress and other systemic diseases. Common clinical path changes: ↑ALP, "stress" leukogram, ↑ cholesterol, triglycerides, ↓ urine concentration, proteinuria.	Pituitary-dependent options:[a] 1) Trilostane: Most common dosing is 1–2 mg/kg PO BID, but published doses vary from 2.2–6.7 mg/kg PO q24h to off-label low dose of 0.21–1.1 mg/kg PO BID. Dosing adjustments should be made on a case by case basis. Evidence suggests larger dogs respond to a lower mg/kg dose. See Table 12.2 for more monitoring details. 2) Mitotane (o,p'-DDD, Lysodren): 25–50 mg/kg/day for induction phase; 35–50 mg/kg divided twice a week for maintenance. 3) Ketoconazole: 5–15 mg/kg PO BID. 4) L-Deprenyl: 1–2 mg/kg/day (less effective; not a first choice). [a] See Chapter 20 for important details regarding monitoring. Adrenal tumor: Adrenalectomy. If surgery refused or inappropriate, mitotane can be used palliatively at 50–75 (up to 150) mg/kg/day divided; longer time to remission than PDH. When post-ACTH cortisol in normal range, maintenance therapy of 75–200 mg/kg/week, divided, is started. Relapse is common. Monitor ACTH stim every 1–2 months or based on patient's clinical symptoms. (This is extralabel use of mitotane.) Ketoconazole and trilostane may be effective (at doses above for PDH). These medications are not adrenolytic and will not slow tumor growth. Skin changes regress in 3–4 months. Some lesions of calcinosis cutis may be permanent.

Iatrogenic hypercortisolemia (Figures 12.3A–12.3E)	Same as spontaneous condition.	Same as spontaneous condition.	ACTH stim: ↓ post-ACTH cortisol. History of corticosteroid use or application. Supportive tests: ↑ALP; ↑UCCR	Wean/taper off exogenous cortisone over 2 weeks. May take 3–4 months for cutaneous symptoms to resolve.
Atypical Cushing's disease (ACD) Debated whether a separate condition from HAC. May be a congenital adrenal hyperplasia-like syndrome.	Same as HAC.	Same as HAC.	Same as HAC except adrenal function tests are normal. High post ACTH 17-hydroxyprogesterone.	Treat as for Cushing's disease; treatment of preference is debated. Scottish Terriers with ACD may have very high 17-OHP and trilostane should not be used in these patients (trilostane may increase 17-OHP). Lignans plus melatonin can be tried: For details, see University of Tennessee Clinical Endocrinology Service website, treatment option considerations for hyperadrenocorticism in dogs. Most reported cases of ACD are adrenal tumors, which may secrete cortisol intermittently or in normal amounts but secrete excessive sex hormones. Another theory is this is not a separate condition and that reference ranges for HAC may be too high in some labs.
Food-induced Cushing's disease (Possibly a subset of Atypical Cushing's disease.)	Same as for HAC.	Same as for HAC.	Normal ACTH response and LDDST tests, suppressed endogenous ACTH levels; bilaterally enlarged adrenal glands; >100% increase in UCCR 3 hr after a meal.	Administer trilostane or mitotane 2 hr prior to meal; monitor as recommended for spontaneous HAC.
Topical corticosteroid application (Figures 12.4A–12.4C; Chapter 3, Figures 3.134A and 3.134B)	Alopecia, thin skin/dermal atrophy, milia, pyoderma; pinnae most often affected; ventral skin more susceptible.	Uncommon but can see hypothalamic–pituitary–adrenal axis suppression with chronic and excessive use.	Hx of cortisone application; biopsy; may have suppressed ACTH stim.	Identify and stop topical steroid-product. Can take several weeks to months to return to normal. Can progress to calcinosis cutis.
Alopecia X/Hair Cycle Arrest: See Chapter 13				
Pituitary dwarfism Reported in several breeds; most commonly in German Shepherd and Carnelian Bear dogs.	Short hair coat of mostly primary hairs (head and extremities are spared); progresses to alopecia and hyperpigmentation, thin skin, comedones.	Stunted growth apparent after 2 mo of age. May also have adrenal, thyroid, and gonadal insufficiency. May express fear or aggressiveness; shortened life span.	Hx, clinical exam findings; insulin-induced prolonged hypoglycemia; growth hormone (GH) stimulation tests, which need to be interpreted in light of thyroid and adrenal function tests.	1) Growth hormone (GH) injections (bovine, 10 IU SQ EOD × 30 days; porcine, 2 IU SQ EOD for 4–6 weeks); may be of limited availability. 2) Medroxyprogesterone acetate, 5–10 mg/kg SQ every 3 weeks until response, then every 6 weeks. Side effects of progestin treatment include risk of immune suppression, mammary neoplasia, pyometra. Poor long-term prognosis.

(*Continued*)

Table 12.1 Canine endocrine skin diseases (Continued)

Condition	Cutaneous symptoms	Systemic symptoms	Diagnosis	Treatment, expected response, monitoring, comments
Calcinosis cutis (Figures 12.5A and 12.5B; Chapter 3, Figures 3.112 and 3.128)	Firm, small, white to pink plaques with surrounding erythema; progress to large, hard, ulcerated plaques; can progress to dermal ossification. More common on head and trunk. Secondary bacterial infection common.	Most often a sequela of iatrogenic or spontaneous hypercortisolemia; less often associated with hypercalcemia of infection.	Biopsy; confirmation of underlying cause.	Identify and treat underlying cause. Topical DMSO gel applied once daily (wear gloves to apply, apply a quarter sized amount and massage in to affected skin, rotate sites treated each day). Monitor serum Ca^{2+} if using DMSO on large areas. Minocycline (anecdotal info.): 5 mg/kg/day PO; aluminum hydroxide antacid; anecdotal info.): 1, 2, or 3 tabs PO BID for small, medium, or large dogs, respectively. Therapies can be done in combination. "Gets worse before it gets better;" takes weeks to months to resolve. Dermal ossification will not resolve.
Exogenous estrogen-related alopecia (Figures 12.6A–12.6D)	Alopecia of, most often, ventral neck, ventrolateral chest, abdomen, lateral thighs.	None reported.	Hx of owner use of transdermal estradiol (hormone replacement therapy) or chronic administration of oral estriol for treatment of incontinence. Biopsy, +/− high serum estrogen concentrations.	Prevent exposure to transdermal or oral hormone; owner should consult physician about altering or stopping therapy. Improves within 3–5 mo of removing exogenous estradiol.
Spontaneous hyperestrogenism (Figures 12.7A–12.7C; Chapter 3, Figure 3.131) Most common in intact female and male dogs; associated with ovarian cysts or neoplasia and testicular Sertoli cell tumors.	Alopecia, often symmetrical starting in perineal area progressing cranially; comedones on ventrum and vulvar skin. Female dogs: Enlarged vulva, +/− gynecomastia. Male dogs: Alopecia, gynecomastia, comedones, +/− linear preputial erythema (pathognomonic), +/− macular to diffuse hyperpigmentation ventrum, perineal area.	Female dogs: Increased risk for pyometra, vulvar edema or overt estrus; can develop aplastic anemia. Male dogs: Attractive to other male dogs, +/− palpable testicular tumor; prostate enlargement, infection.	R/o other endocrinopathies; palpable testicular tumor; abdominal ultrasound; measurement of baseline estrogen may be problematic but supportive if high. Skin biopsy supportive of endocrine alopecia but changes not specific for hyperestrogenism.	Thoracic radiographs to r/o metastasis. Intact dogs: Castration or ovariohysterectomy. Spayed female dogs: R/o exogenous estrogen administration; retained ovarian tissue.

Spontaneous hyperandrogenism (Figure 12.8) Usually from testicular neoplasia (interstitial cell tumor).	Seborrhea oleosa, secondary pyoderma; +/− symmetrical truncal alopecia; hypertrophy of circumanal and tail gland tissue; hyperpigmented macules on scrotum, perineal area, ventrum.	+/− palpable testicular mass. May shows signs of aggression, hypersexual behavior.	Clinical symptoms, high testosterone levels, response to castration.	Castration. Will take 2–4 months for hair coat to return to normal. Antiseborrheic shampoo pending improvement; treat secondary pyoderma. Some glandular thickening may not revert to normal.
Tail gland hyperplasia (Figure 12.9; Chapter 3, Figure 3.83) Predisposition: Intact male dogs/cats.	Dogs: Hyperplasia of sebaceous and circumanal glands resulting in large patch of alopecia, scaling, greasy seborrhea, and often hyperpigmentation about 2.5–5 cm from base of tail on dorsal surface. With progression, glandular hypertrophy can become cystic and secondarily infected. Cats: Most commonly present with increased oily secretions on tail. Can become hypotrichotic to alopecic, scaly and crusted in some cases.	None	Clinical signs, biopsy.	Neutering intact animals (stops progression, but may not reverse; antiseborrheic topical agents may help control follicular plugging and secondary infection. In cats, topical 0.1% retinoic acid gels can be effective but can be irritating. If occurring in neutered animal, evaluation for a functional adrenal tumor may be needed.

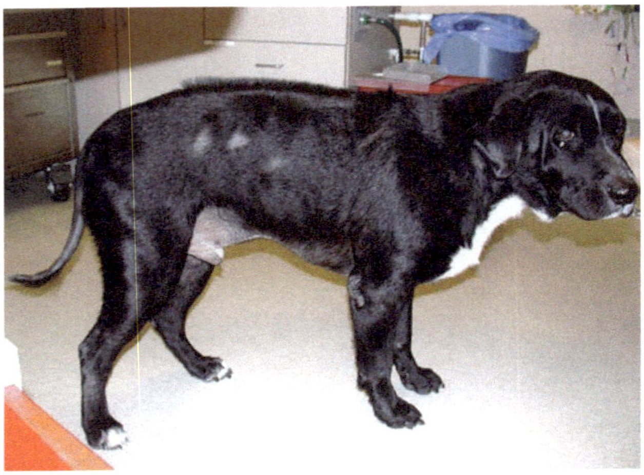

Figure 12.1A A hypothyroid Labrador demonstrating almost complete alopecia of the tail, a tragic facial expression, and patchy truncal alopecia due to secondary bacterial pyoderma.

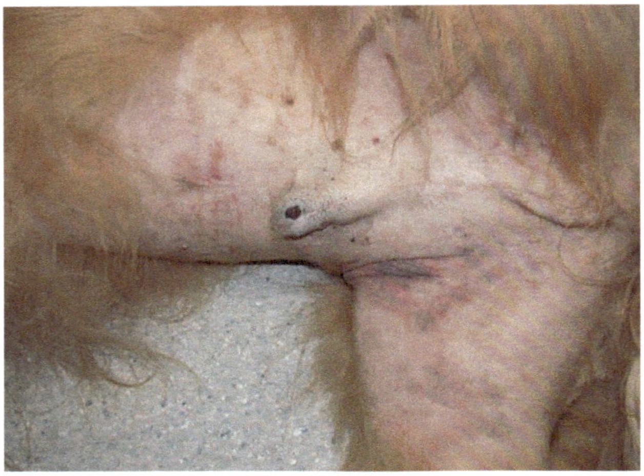

Figure 12.1B A Golden Retriever with hypothyroidism caused inguinal alopecia, comedones, and pyoderma.

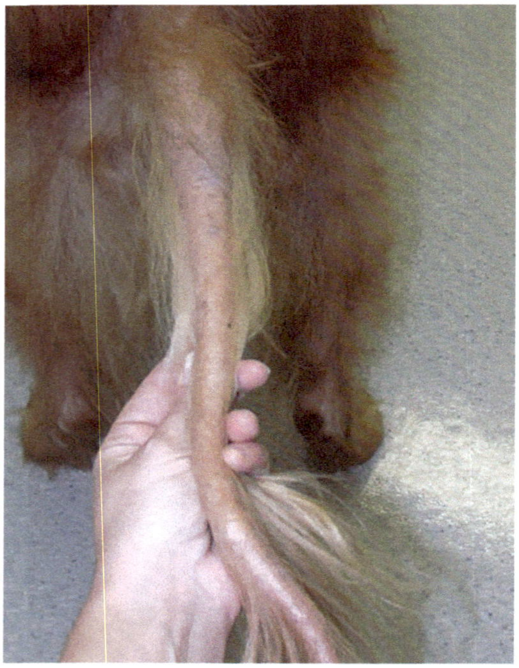

Figure 12.1C Tail alopecia in a Golden Retriever caused by hypothyroidism.

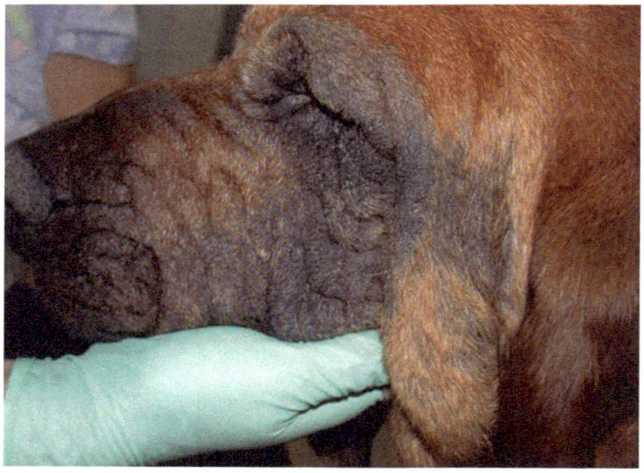

Figure 12.1D Hypothyroidism in this Bloodhound caused severe secondary bacterial and yeast skin infections.

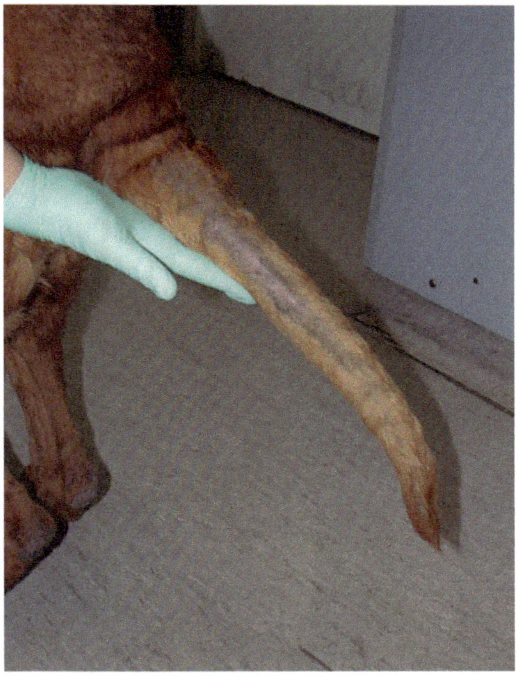

Figure 12.1E The same patient as in 12.1D; note the alopecia on the tail.

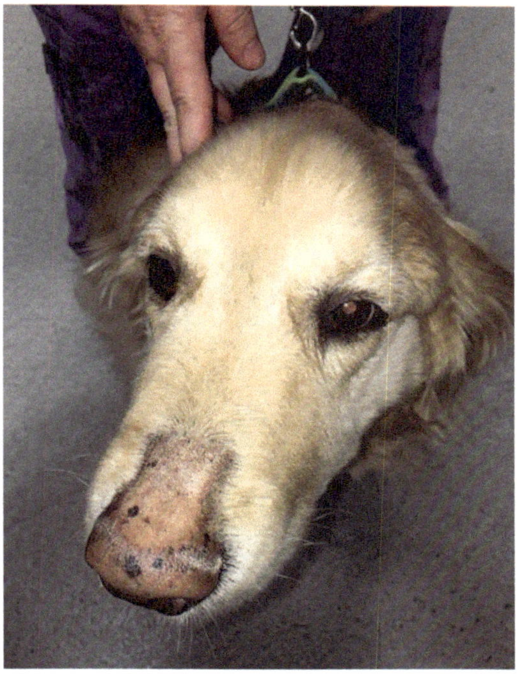

Figure 12.1F Alopecia on the dorsal nose caused by hypothyroidism.

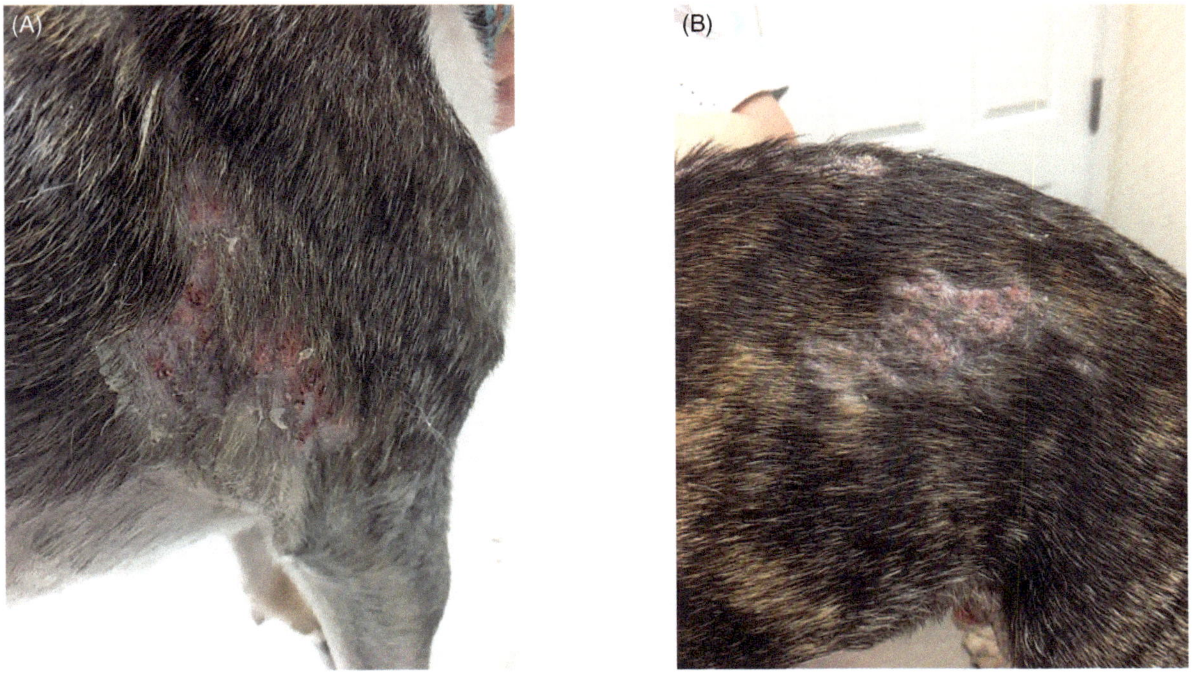

Figures 12.2A–C Cushing's disease in a Boston Terrier which caused calcinosis cutis and secondary bacterial pyoderma.

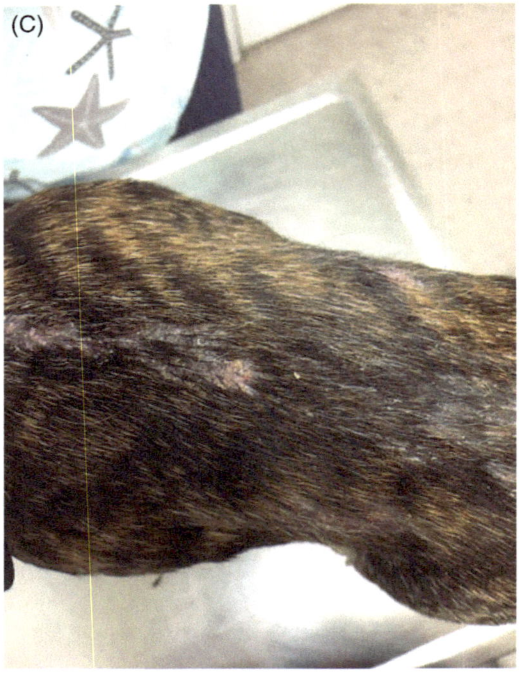

Figures 12.2A–C (Continued)

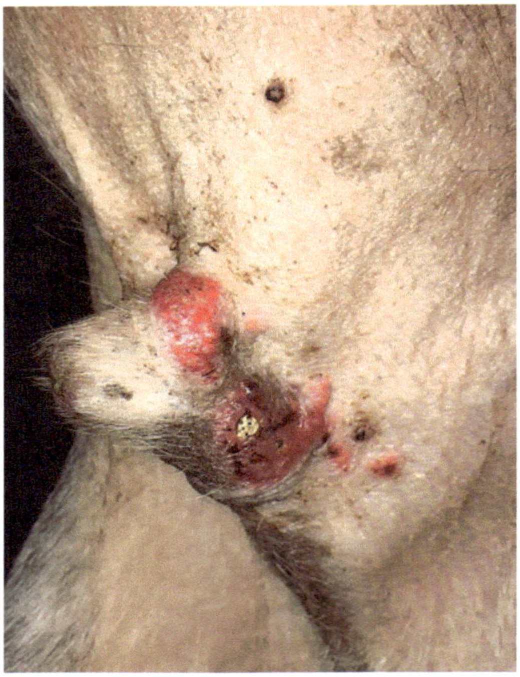

Figure 12.2D Red, raised, gritty plaques on the groin of this dog due to calcinosis cutis.

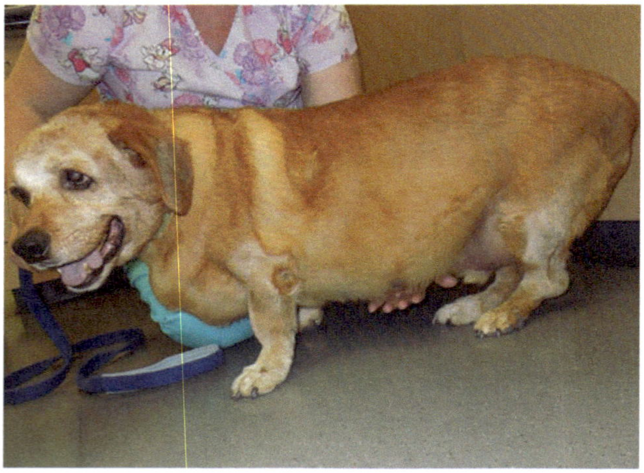

Figure 12.3A Iatrogenic Cushing's disease in a dog on prolonged daily steroids; there is abdominal distention and limb muscle atrophy.

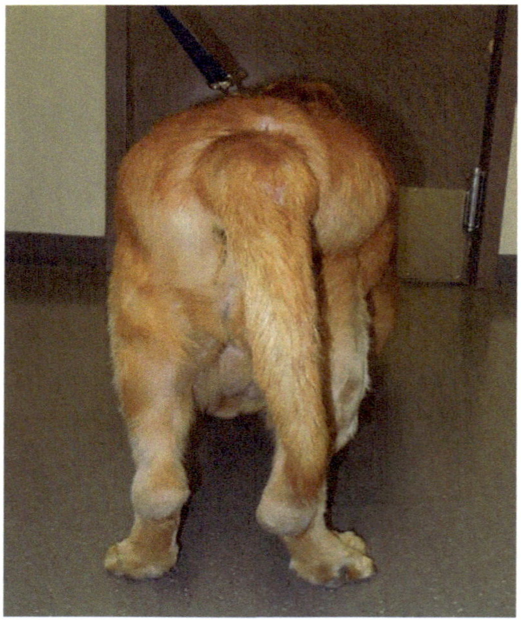

Figure 12.3B Prominent fat redistribution on the dorsal lumbar area caused by chronic steroid administration.

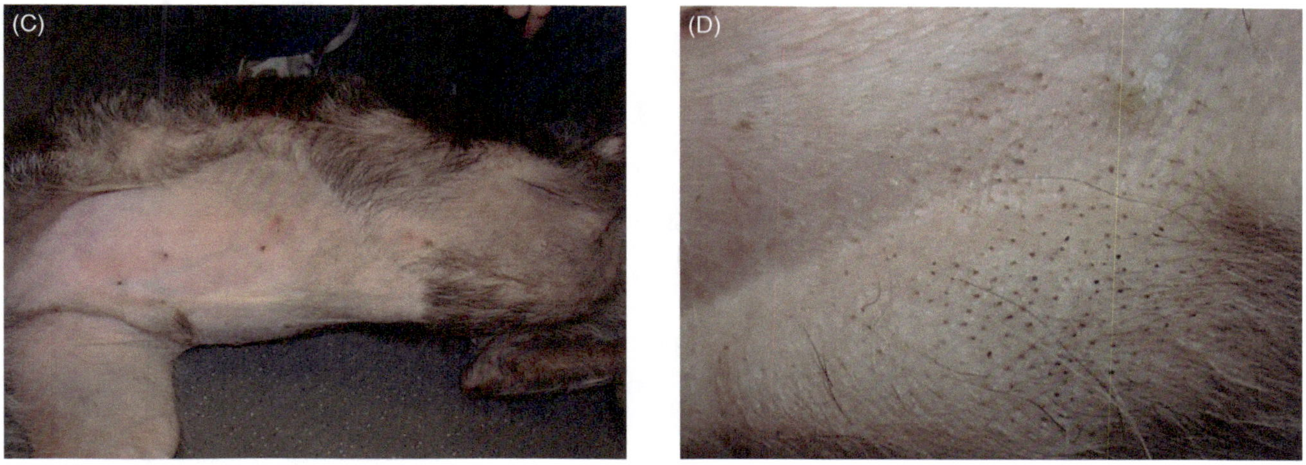

Figures 12.3C and D Extensive ventral truncal alopecia, cutaneous atrophy, and comedones in an Addisonian dog treated with an excessive dose of steroids.

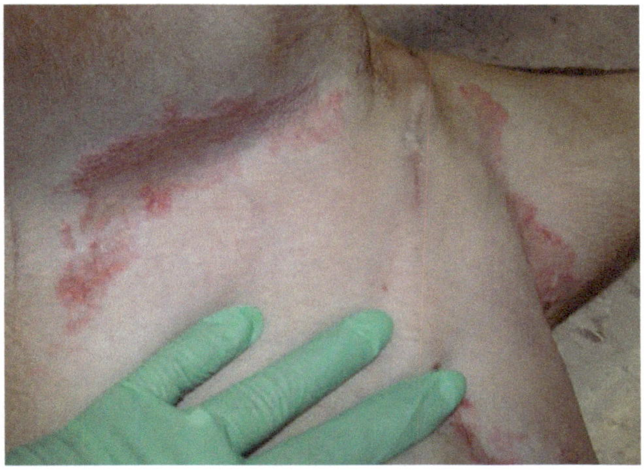

Figure 12.3E Iatrogenic Cushing's in a Pitbull, which caused ventral truncal alopecia as well as calcinosis cutis.

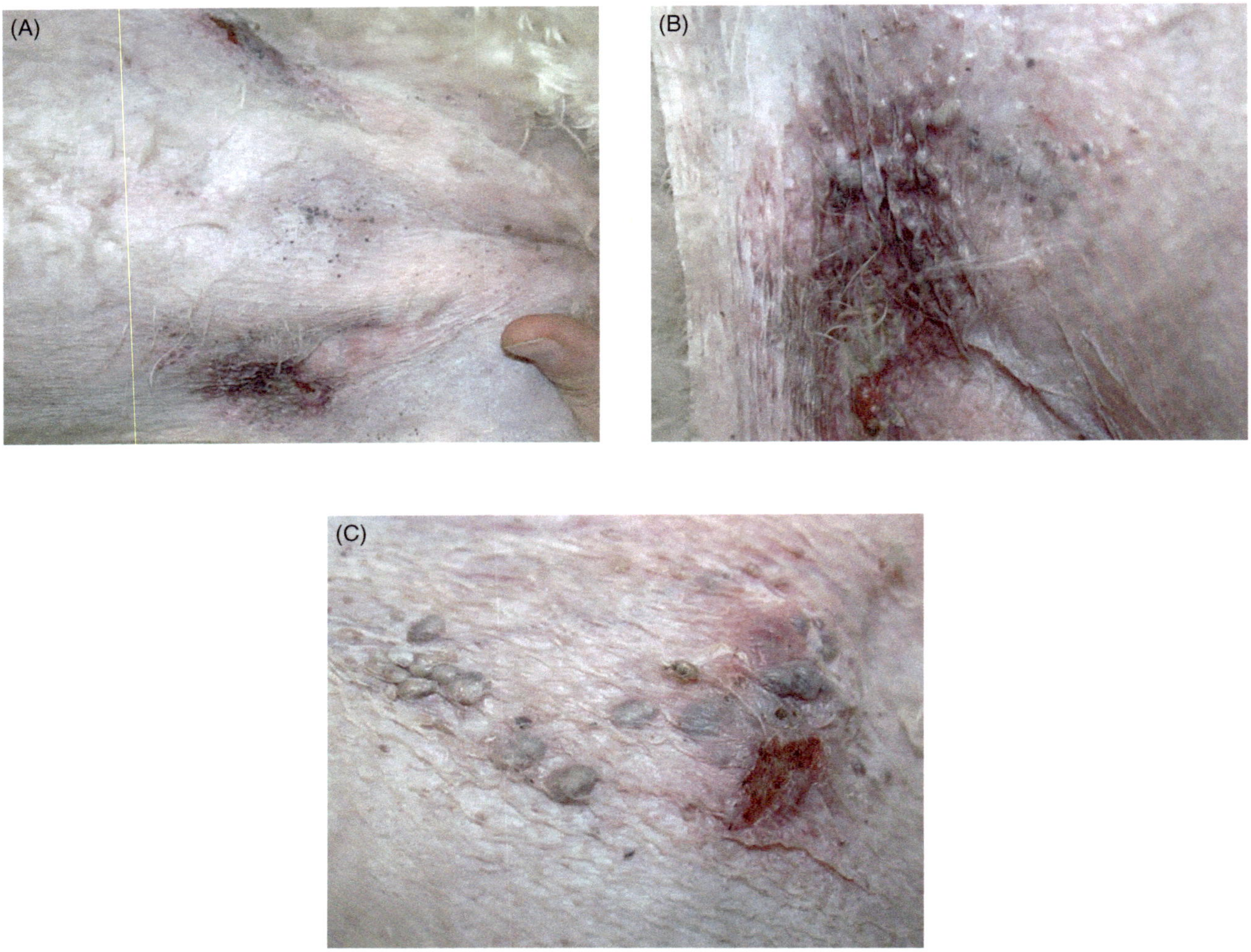

Figures 12.4A–C Prolonged use of a potent topical steroid ointment caused cutaneous atrophy, tearing, and milia (cystic plugged follicles).

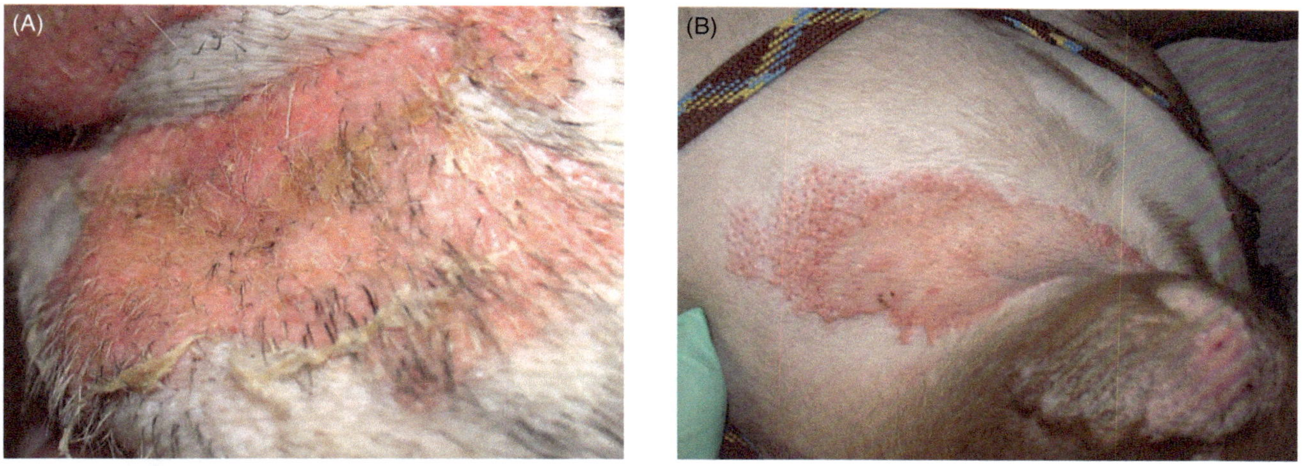

Figures 12.5A and B Calcinosis cutis causing red, raised, slightly crusted plaques on the axilla and groin of a dog treated with chronic high dose of prednisone.

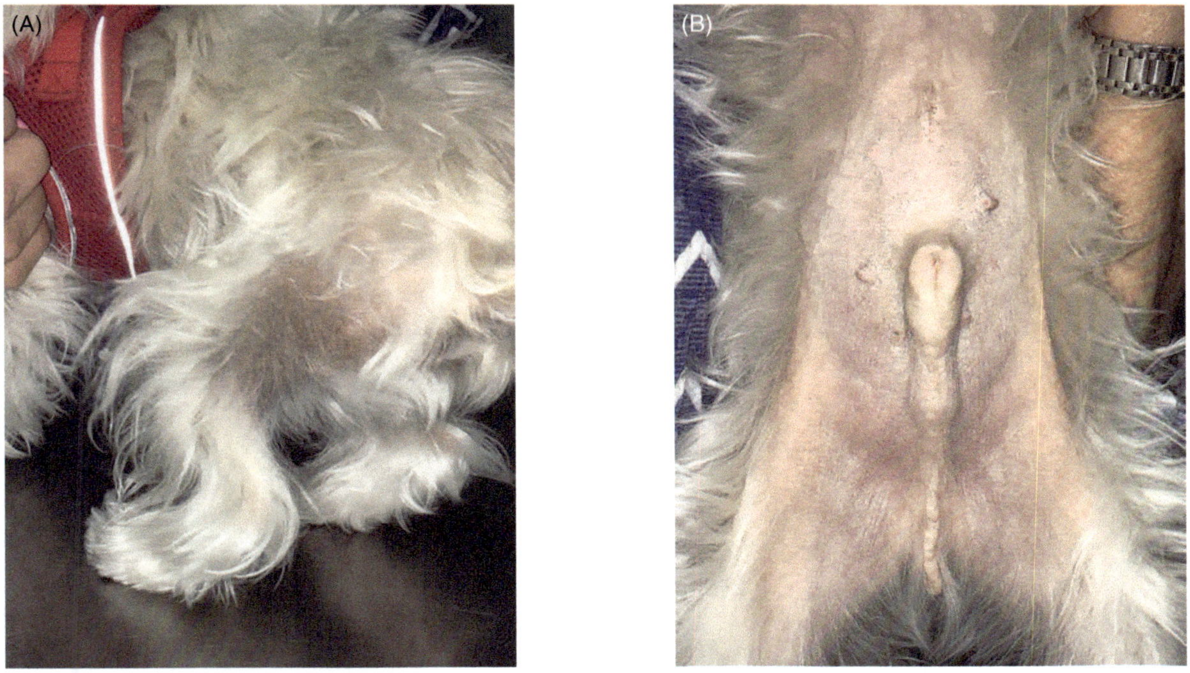

Figures 12.6A and B Alopecia on the thigh and ventral trunk of a dog due to chronic exposure to the owner's transdermal hormone replacement gel (estrogen); note the comedones and prominent nipples in this young, neutered, male dog. The dog's thigh contacted the owner's forearm where the gel was placed each day.

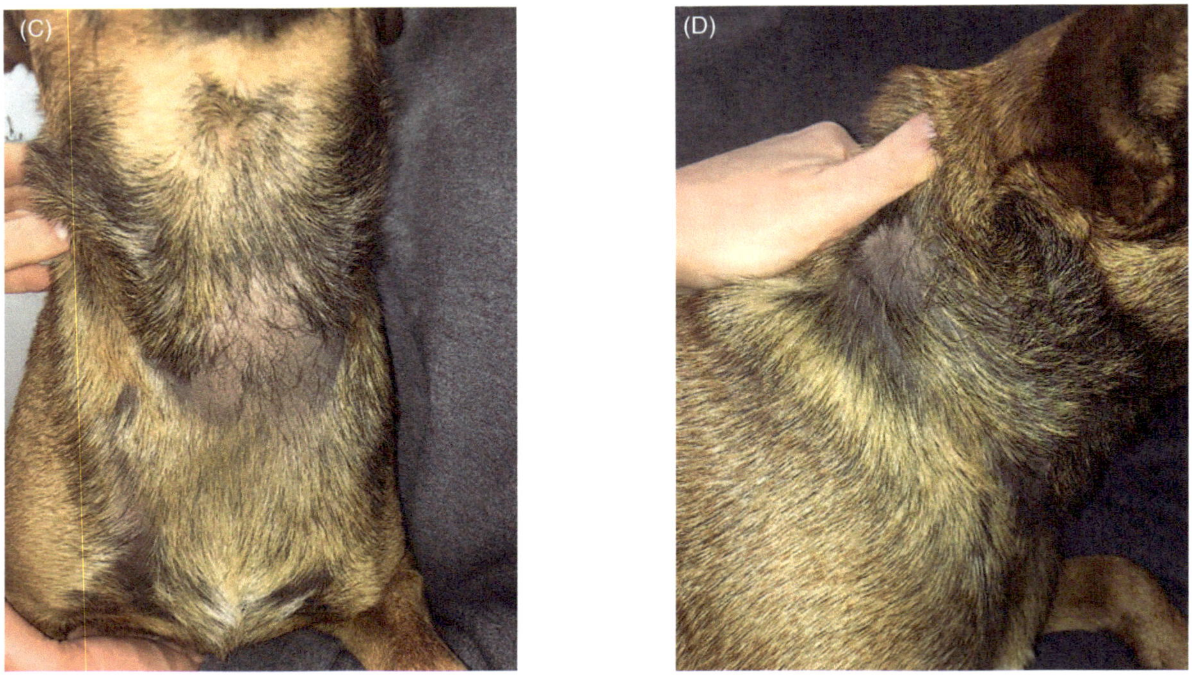

Figures 12.6C and D Circumferential hypotrichosis and hyperpigmentation on the neck of a dog treated with chronic daily estriol as treatment for incontinence.

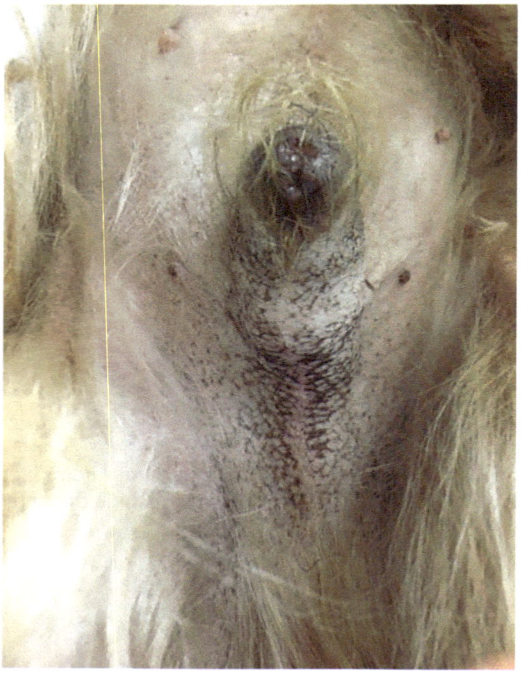

Figure 12.7A Linear preputial dermatosis caused by a testicular tumor in an older, intact, male dog.

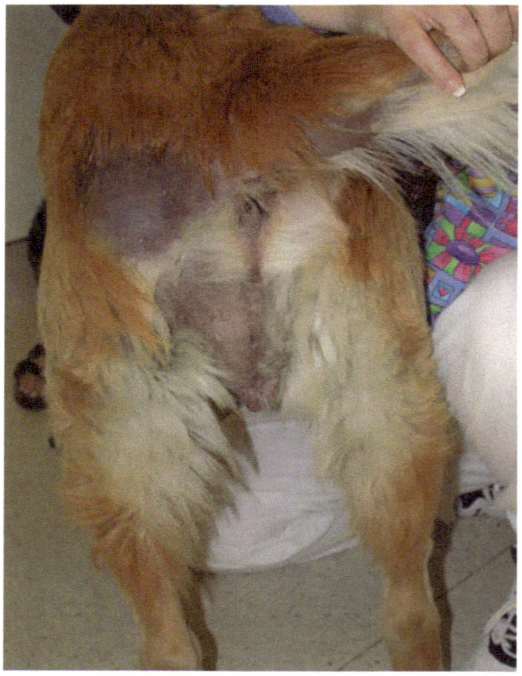

Figure 12.7B A dog with a Sertoli cell tumor causing alopecia and hyperpigmentation on the perineal area and ventral tail.

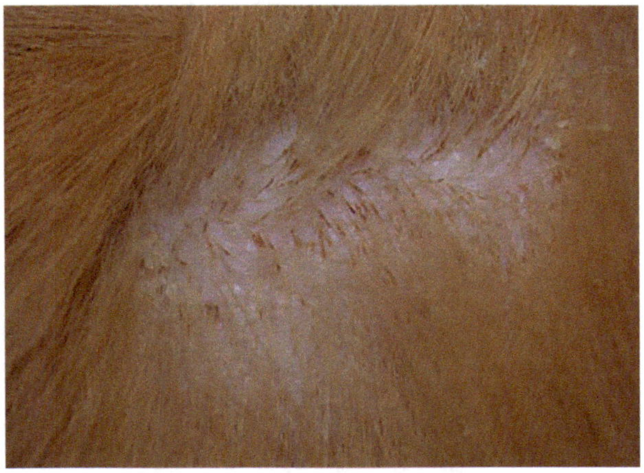

Figure 12.7C The same dog as in Figure 12.7B also had hormone-induced follicular casting.

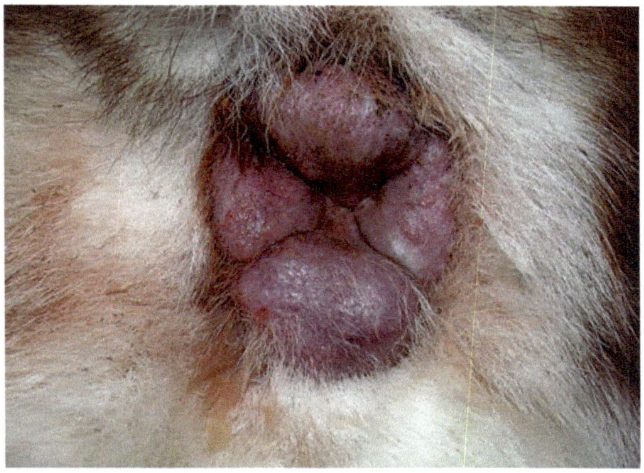

Figure 12.8 Perianal gland hyperplasia due to elevated testosterone levels in a dog.

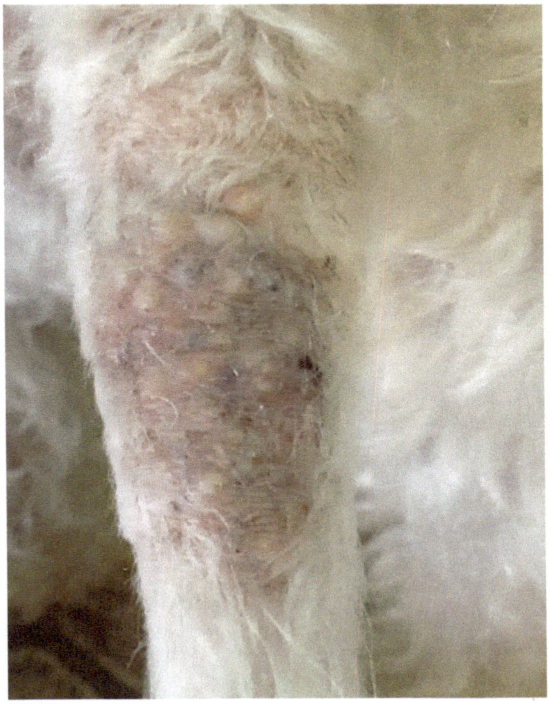

Figure 12.9 Tail gland hyperplasia causing alopecia and small follicular cysts on the dorsal proximal tail. *Source:* Image courtesy of VIN and Robin Rainford, DVM.

Table 12.2 Trilostane treatment and monitoring (from Vetoryl® package insert). Ten to fourteen days after starting treatment, do 4–6 hour post-dosing ACTH stimulation test as well as serum chemistry including electrolytes. If physical exam is acceptable, take action according to Table 12.2:

Post-ACTH cortisol levels		**Action**
μg/dl	**nMol/L**	
<1.45	<40	Stop treatment. Restart at a decreased dose
1.45–5.4	40–150	Continue on the same dose
>5.4–9.1	>150–250	EITHER: Continue on current dose if clinical signs are well controlled OR: Increase dose if clinical signs of hyperadrenocorticism are still evident
>9.1	>250	Increase dose

Alternatively, pre- and 3-hour post-trilostane cortisol concentrations, in one study to date (Macfarlane, Parkin, and Ramsey, 2016), have been shown to be as accurate in assessing control as cortisol measured after ACTH stimulation testing. (Use values listed in Table 12.2.) This information should be assessed in light of exam findings, electrolytes/serum chemistry values, and owner assessment.
When acceptable control is achieved, the patient should be monitored via exams and blood work in four weeks and every three months thereafter. This information is not all-inclusive regarding management of the Cushing's patient. The reader is encouraged to review other appropriate texts and resources for more in-depth information on management of hyperadrenocorticism.

Table 12.3 Endocrine skin diseases of cats.

Condition	Cutaneous symptoms	Systemic symptoms/clinical pathology changes	Diagnosis	Treatment, expected response, monitoring, comments
Hyperthyroidism Common endocrinopathy in cats; usually from thyroid adenoma.	In 30% of cats: Excessive shedding, matting/unkempt haircoat, seborrhea, overgrown claws, traumatic alopecia, arteriovenous fistulae, thin skin, and truncal alopecia in chronic cases.	Polyphagia, polydipsia, polyuria, weight loss, hyperactivity, tachycardia, arrhythmias, vomiting, diarrhea. 10% of cats are lethargic. High liver enzymes, polycythemia.	High TT4, high fT4 10% of hyperthyroid cats have a normal T4 T3 suppression test.	Thyroidectomy Radioactive iodine (I131). Antithyroid drugs (methimazole, carbimazole). Please refer to appropriate endocrinology text for treatment and monitoring details. Low Iodine diet (<0.32 ppm).
Hypothyroidism Forms: Congenital (rare), spontaneous (adult cats, rare), and iatrogenic (secondary to hyperthyroid treatment).	Congenital: Full but dry, dull haircoat of secondary hairs. Spontaneous: Dull coat, puffy face. Iatrogenic: Seborrhea, decreased grooming, alopecia of pinnae, pressure points, tail base, symmetric alopecia of neck, trunk.	Congenital form: Stunted growth, lethargy, poor appetite, death. Spontaneous: Lethargy, poor appetite, obesity. Iatrogenic: Transient lethargy. High cholesterol, mild anemia.	TT4 but poor specificity; fT4. Too few cases to establish testing protocol.	Not well established. 0.05–0.2 mg l-thyroxine PO every 12–24 hr. Systemic symptoms improve in 1 week; cutaneous symptoms improve in 2–3 months.
Hyper adrenocorticism (HAC) (Figures 12.10A and 12.10B) Spontaneous and iatrogenic forms (both rare); pituitary-dependent more common than adrenal tumor.	Thin, fragile skin (spontaneous tearing); alopecia of trunk/ventrum; easy bruising. Seborrheic skin and dull hair coat. Curling of ear tips seen in iatrogenic form only.	Polyuria, polydipsia; muscle atrophy; +/− lethargy, weight loss. Secondary diabetes mellitus (DM) common and often hard to regulate until HAC addressed.	Protocols for adrenal function testing not well established but are reported; reader is referred to Boland and Barrs (2017) and Feldman, Nelson, and Reusch (2015) for more detailed references. Dexamethasone suppression testing more sensitive than ACTH stim test. Use 0.1 ml/kg dexamethasone IV. Use imaging to differential between pituitary and adrenal-dependent HAC.	Iatrogenic: Discontinue steroid administration. Spontaneous HAC (pituitary or adrenal-dependent): Poor prognosis. Reports of treatment success with trilostane: 0.5–12 mg/kg or 15–30 mg cat PO q12–24h. Mitotane also tried; less successful. Adrenalectomy. Close monitoring of blood glucose necessary as hypoglycemia/reduction in insulin needs likely when HAC controlled. Reader is referred to more detailed endocrinology texts (Feldman, Nelson, and Reusch, 2015) for further discussion.

Feline acquired skin fragility (Figures 12.11A and 12.11B) Usually middle-aged and older cats.	Severely fragile and thin skin that tears due to minor trauma such as scratching or restraint. Skin is NOT hyperextensible.	In cases associated with underlying illness, cats display with accompanying systemic symptoms.	R/o Cushing's disease, diabetes mellitus. If not associated with Cushing's, has been seen with liver disease, nephrosis, phenytoin administration, histoplasmosis, and FIP (feline infectious peritonitis). Some cases idiopathic. Biopsy very difficult; histopathology shows atrophic dermis with disorganized collagen fibers, thin to no panniculus.	Grave prognosis regardless of cause. Surgical repair not possible. Non-advanced cases from spontaneous or iatrogenic Cushing's will resolve with treatment/removal of causative agent.
Diabetes mellitus (DM) (Figure 12.12)	Not common but can see bacterial pyoderma, yeast dermatitis (*Candida*), seborrhea, thin skin, and xanthomas.	Reader is referred to endocrinology texts (e.g. Feldman, Nelson, and Reusch, 2015) for more detailed information.	Reader is referred to endocrinology texts (e.g. Feldman, Nelson, and Reusch, 2015) for more detailed information.	Reader is referred to endocrinology texts (e.g. Feldman, Nelson, and Reusch, 2015) for more detailed information.
Acromegaly (Figure 12.13) Male cats; associated with pituitary tumor.	Mild to moderately thickened skin, enlarged claws.	Enlarged paws, skull; prognathism, increased interdental spaces, cardiac failure, PU/PD, +/− insulin-resistant DM.	The diagnosis is made by consideration of history, and suggestive physical examination and labwork findings. Serum insulin-like growth factor – 1 (IGF-1) is usually elevated. Radiographs may reveal cardiomegaly/organomegaly, hyperostosis of the skull, mandibular protrusion, spondylosis of the spine, and periosteal joint tissue reaction. Computed tomography or MRI are useful for identifying pituitary masses.	Irradiation of pituitary tumor is the preferred treatment. Transsphenoidal hypophysectomy may be an option at specialized veterinary centers; post-surgical treatment with cortisone, thyroid supplementation +/- desmopressin is necessary. Medical treatments with a somatostatin analogue (octreotide), or dopamine agonist (l-deprenyl) have not been successful in cats.

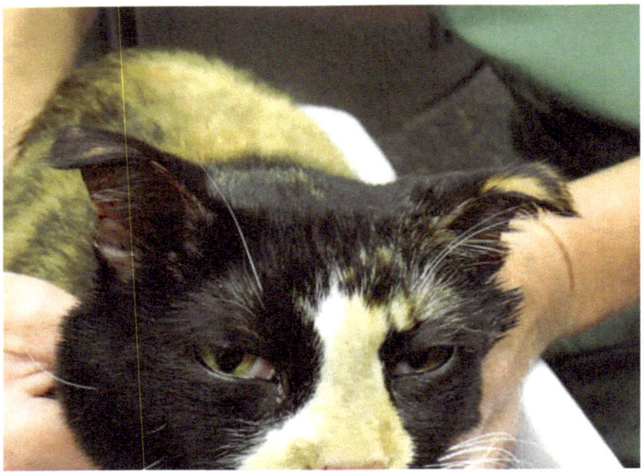

Figure 12.10A Iatrogenic Cushing's in a cat due to prolonged exogenous steroids caused bilateral drooping of the pinnal tips. *Source:* Image courtesy of VIN and Sue Fluhr, DVM.

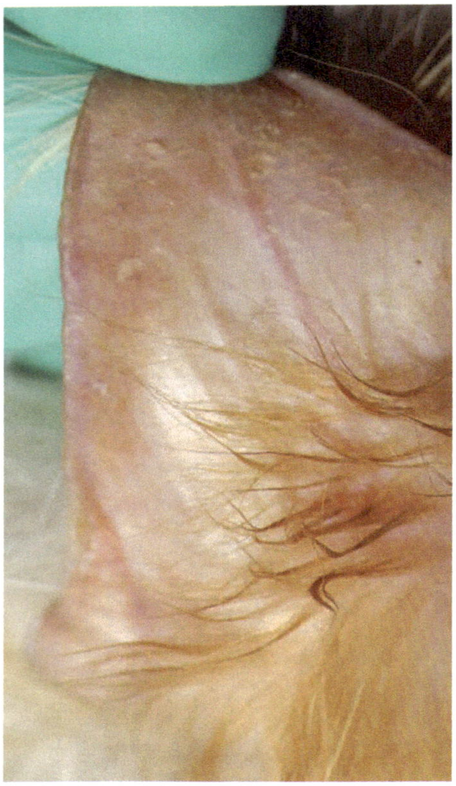

Figure 12.10B In this atopic cat prolonged administration of a topical steroid-containing solution on the ear caused complete alopecia and cutaneous atrophy with scaling.

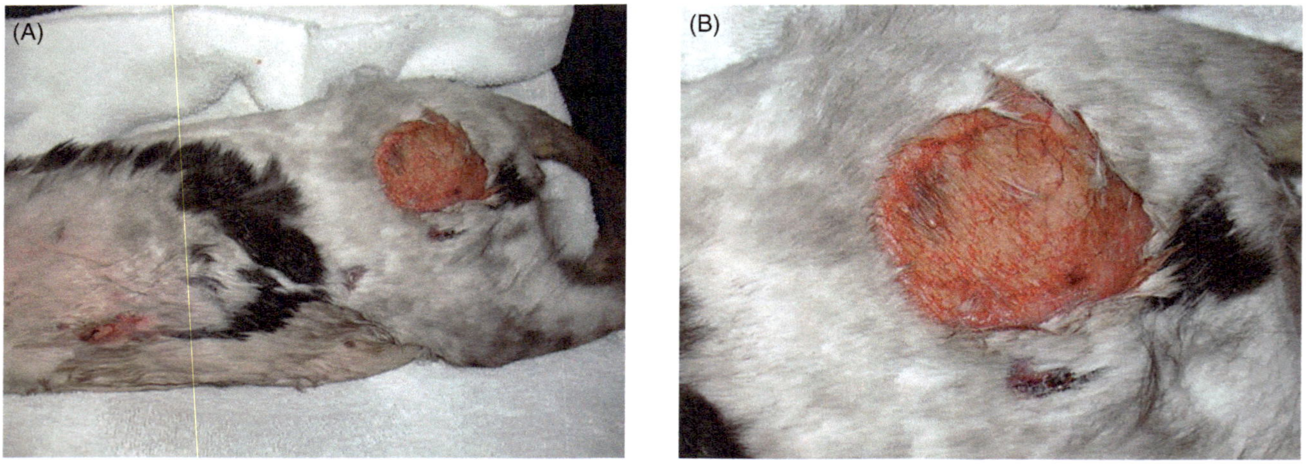

Figures 12.11A and B Feline acquired skin fragility in a diabetic and Cushingoid cat.

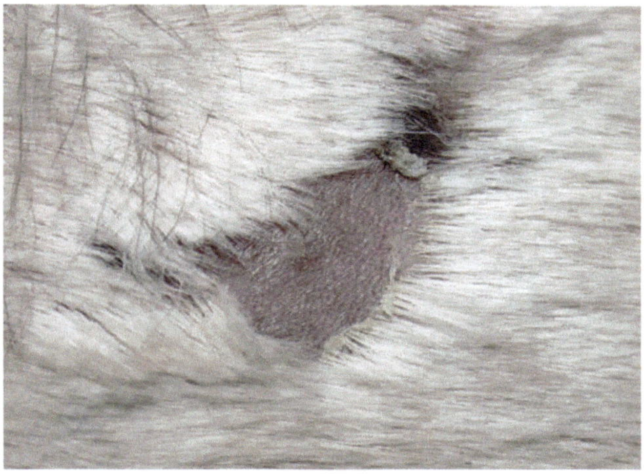

Figure 12.12 The same cat as in Figures 12.11A and 12.11B also had multifocal epidermal collarettes due to a secondary bacterial pyoderma.

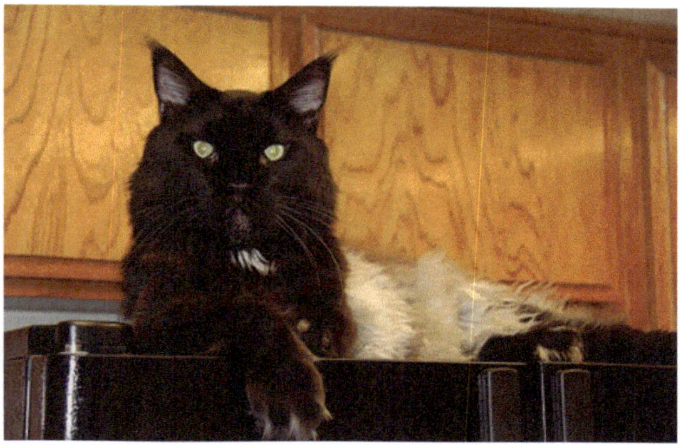

Figure 12.13 Acromegaly in a cat; note the enlarged skull and prognathism. *Source:* Image courtesy of VIN.

References/Further reading

Berger, D.J., Lewis, T.P., Schick, A.E. et al. (2015). Canine alopecia secondary to human topical hormone replacement therapy in six dogs. *J. Am. Anim. Hosp. Assoc.* 51 (2): 136–142.

Boland, L.A. and Barrs, V.R. (2017). Peculiarities of feline hyperadrenocorticism: update on diagnosis and treatment. *J. Feline Med. Surg.* 19 (9): 933–947.

Feldman, E., Nelson, R., Reusch, C. et al. (2015). *Canine and Feline Endocrinology*, 4e. Philadelphia, PA: Saunders.

Galac, S., Kars, V.J., Voorhout, G. et al. (2008). ACTH-independent hyperadrenocorticism due to food-dependent hypercortisolemia in a dog: a case report. *Vet. J.* 177 (1): 141–143.

Macfarlane, L., Parkin, T., and Ramsey, I. (2016). Pre-trilostane and three-hour post-trilostane cortisol to monitor trilostane therapy in dogs. *Vet. Rec.* 179: 597.

McKnight, C.N., Lew, L.J., and Gamble, D.A. (2018). Management and closure of multiple large cutaneous lesions in a juvenile cat with severe acquired skin fragility syndrome secondary to iatrogenic hyperadrenocorticism. *J. Am. Vet. Med. Assoc.* 252 (2): 210–214.

Mecklenburg, L., Linek, M., and Tobin, D.J. (2009). *Hair Loss Disorders in Domestic Animals*. Ames, Iowa: Wiley-Blackwell.

Miller, W., Griffin, C., and Campbell, K. (2014). *Mueller and Kirk's Small Animal Dermatology*, 7e. Philadephia, PA: Saunders.

Valentin, S., Cortright, C., Nelson, R. et al. (2014). Clinical findings, diagnostic test results, and treatment outcome in cats with spontaneous hyperadrenocorticism: 30 cases. *J. Vet. Intern. Med.* 28: 481–487.

13

Non-endocrine alopecia

Patricia Ashley, DVM, DACVD

Veterinary Allergy and Dermatology Services, Springfield, OR, USA

Clinical Atlas of Canine and Feline Dermatology, First Edition. Edited by Kimberly S. Coyner.

Companion website: www.wiley.com/go/coyner/dermatology

Table 13.1 Non-endocrine alopecia of dogs.

	Clinical features	Diagnostic test(s)[a]	Treatment(s)	Prognosis/expected response/ monitoring/comments
Localized Alopecia				
Post-clipping alopecia (hair cycle arrest) (Figure 13.1)	Lack of hair growth >3 months after clipping.	Hx, elimination of other causes of hair cycle arrest (endocrine disorders), +/−biopsy.	No treatment recommended.	May take 1–2 years to resolve.
Traction alopecia	Focal hair loss where hair retaining device placed.	History, biopsy.	Pentoxifylline may help in early lesions; owner education; surgical removal of scar.	Scarring may be permanent.
Congenital follicular/ ectodermal dysplasia	Hypotrichosis to alopecia noted at <8 weeks of age.	Consider signalment (age), biopsy.	No treatment available.	May or may not be hereditary.
Regional to Multifocal Alopecia				
Color dilution alopecia (Figures 13.2A–13.2H; Chapter 6, Figures 6.11A and 6.11B and 6.40)	Broken hairs, hypotrichosis, eventual alopecia of dilute colored hairs. Secondary pyoderma can occur.	Signalment: Color dilute breed. Trichogram: Melanin clumping in hairs. Biopsy.	Minimize trauma to hair coat. Anecdotal reports of melatonin stimulating hair growth (see doses listed for Cyclic Flank Alopecia).	No systemic signs; life-long condition. Reported in many breeds.
Black hair follicular dysplasia (Figures 13.3A and 13.3B, Chapter 3, Figure 3.93)	Broken hairs, hypotrichosis, eventual alopecia of black/pigmented hairs. Secondary pyoderma can occur.	PE: Only dark hairs affected Trichogram: Melanin clumping in hairs. Biopsy.	Minimize trauma to hair coat. Anecdotal information to try melatonin (see doses listed for Cyclic Flank Alopecia).	No systemic signs; life-long condition.
Non-color, breed-related follicular dysplasia (Figure 13.4; Chapter 6, Figure 6.21)	Regional alopecia recognized in several breeds, including Irish Water Spaniels, Portuguese Water Dogs, Curly-coated Retrievers, and Doberman Pinschers. Alopecia of caudal dorsum, ventral neck progressing to most of trunk usually starting 2–4 years of age. Weimaraner: Diffuse truncal alopecia starting at 1–3 years of age; secondary pyoderma can occur. Husky and Malamute: Loss of truncal guard hairs and change of hair color to red-orange starting 3 mo to 3–4 years of age.	Signalment, trichogram, biopsy, and elimination of endocrine disorders.		No systemic signs; life-long condition. In the author's opinion, some cases of "cyclic follicular dysplasia" described in Airedales, Boxers, and other breeds are cases that could be called canine recurrent flank alopecia. Therefore treatment with oral melatonin can be justified (see doses for Cyclic Flank Alopecia).

Cyclic flank alopecia (canine recurrent flank alopecia, seasonal flank alopecia) (Figures 13.5A–13.5C; Chapter 2, Figure 2.32A; Chapter 6, Figures 6.5 and 6.23) Predisposed breeds: English Bulldogs, Airedale Terriers, Boxers, Schnauzers.	Geographic alopecia of flanks +/− dorsum; hyperpigmented skin. Onset: Fall or spring but varies with latitude.	PE, elimination of other causes of hair cycle arrest, biopsy.	Many self-resolve in 3–8 mo. Melatonin Oral: 3–6 mg BID – TID; some use 0.5 mg/kg BID. Give for 4–6 weeks. *Ensure melatonin supplement does not contain xylitol.* SQ constant release implants, 24 mg, available from http://melatoninimplants.com. Caution: Implants occasionally associated with SQ abscessation and efficacy compared to oral form not evaluated.	No systemic symptoms. May or may not recur in subsequent years. Permanent alopecia in some cases.
Pattern alopecia (Figures 13.6A–13.6D; Chapter 2, Figure 2.32B, Chapter 3, Figure 3.47; Chapter 6, Figure 6.10)	Miniaturized hairs, symmetrical hypotrichosis, pinnae, base of pinnae, ventral neck, caudal thighs. Young adult, short-coated breeds (Dachshund, Boston Terrier, Boxer, etc.).	PE, signalment, +/−biopsy.	No treatment necessary; melatonin may trigger hair growth.	No systemic symptoms.
Follicular lipidosis Rottweilers, Dachshund (1 case); young dogs.	Alopecia of mahogany hairs of face and paws.	PE, biopsy.	No treatment.	No systemic symptoms.
Generalized Alopecia				
"Alopecia X"/Hair cycle arrest (Figures 13.7A–13.7D; Chapter 3, Figure 3.92; Chapter 6, Figures 6.41 and 6.49) Most common in young adult Nordic and plush-coated breeds (e.g. Husky, Malamute, Chow, Pomeranian, Samoyed) and Poodles.	Progressively dull coat, alopecia, hyperpigmentation, +/− scaling on trunk, caudal thighs, neck, perineal area, tail. Spares head and distal extremities. Hair regrows after trauma (e.g. biopsy, infection). Usually no systemic symptoms.	Signalment, rule out other causes of non-inflammatory alopecia (e.g. hypothyroidism, sex hormone abnormalities, Cushing's disease, follicular dysplasia).	Various treatment options; response to treatment is often temporary: 1) Neuter/spay intact dogs. 2) Oral melatonin: 3–12 mg BID–TID based on size. Allow 4–6 weeks for response; helps about 40% of dogs. Avoid in diabetic patients, and make sure the supplement does not contain xylitol. 3) Some recommend concurrent use of phytoestrogens (lignans) in cases of high estrogen and cortisol levels (see https://vetmed.tennessee.edu/vmc/dls/Endocrinology/Pages/News-and-Articles.aspx for more information. [b] 4) Mitotane: Induction of 15–25 mg/kg daily, then same dose twice weekly. (Editor's note: The use of aggressive and potentially toxic therapies for this cosmetic condition is not recommended).	Cosmetic disorder which does not warrant aggressive treatment; consider risk vs. benefit if considering treatment. Condition not well understood. Relapse of alopecia after all treatments is common; recommended to discontinue treatment when a response is seen to restart therapy when alopecia recurs.

(*Continued*)

Table 13.1 Non-endocrine alopecia of dogs (Continued)

	Clinical features	Diagnostic test(s)[a]	Treatment(s)	Prognosis/expected response/ monitoring/comments
Alopecia X (cont.)			[b] 5) Trilostane: (0.5 - 1 mg/kg) BID. Note: Published doses for treatment of Alopecia X with trilostane are high and vary greatly (3–30 mg/kg q12h). Yet hyperadrenocorticism can be managed with trilostane doses as low as 0.5–1 mg/kg q12h. In light of this, and that Alopecia X is considered a cosmetic condition, the authors encourage starting a lower twice daily dose (0.5–1 mg/kg), adjusting dose if needed based on response and monitoring. See more discussion on hyperadrenocorticism in Table 12.1. [b] Adrenal function tests must be monitored as for Cushing's disease. 6) Microneedling (using a Dermaroller) has reports of success; requires heavy sedation or general anesthesia. 7) Medroxyprogesterone injections; 5–10 mg/kg SQ once a month. Should not be used in intact female dogs; possible side effects include behavior changes, mammary enlargement, diabetes mellitus, alopecia of injection site. 8) Deslorelin, a synthetic GnRH agonist, implants (4.7 mg/dog) have reported success in intact male dogs.	
Color dilution alopecia	See comments under "Multifocal/regional alopecia"			
Anagen/telogen effluvium (defluxion)	Patchy to diffuse alopecia; "shedding to bald;" trunk most often affected. Follows significant stress, illness, postpartum, or after chemotherapy (especially doxorubicin) in some dogs, especially dogs with continuously growing haircoats. Anagen effluvium occurs within days and telogen effluvium within 1–3 months of the insult.	History, trichogram; +/− biopsy.	No treatment necessary.	Hair will regrow within 1–3 months.
Non-color breed-related follicular dysplasia	See comments under "Multifocal/regional alopecia"			

[a] It is beyond the scope of this text to discuss histopathology findings. The reader is referred to more detailed texts (e.g. Miller, Griffin, and Campbell, 2014; Gross et al. 2008) for dermatohistopathology descriptions if needed.
PE, physical exam; Hx, history.

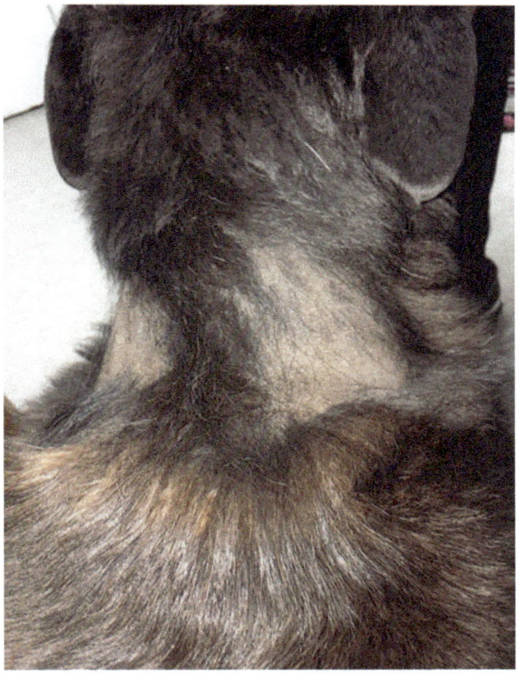

Figure 13.1 Post-clipping alopecia on the neck of a dog; the area was shaved for skin mass removal three months prior.

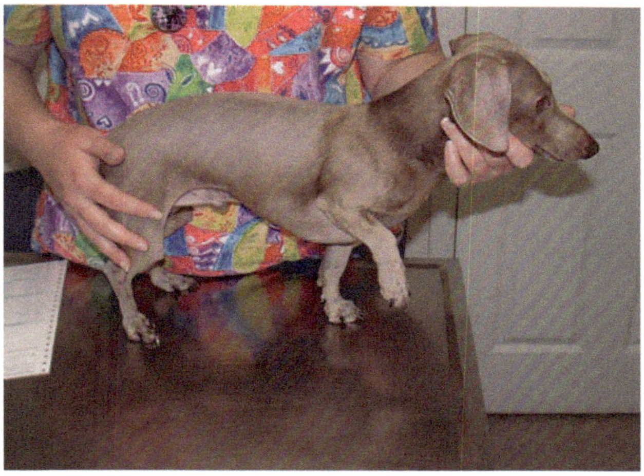

Figure 13.2A Color dilution alopecia in a blue Miniature Dachshund.

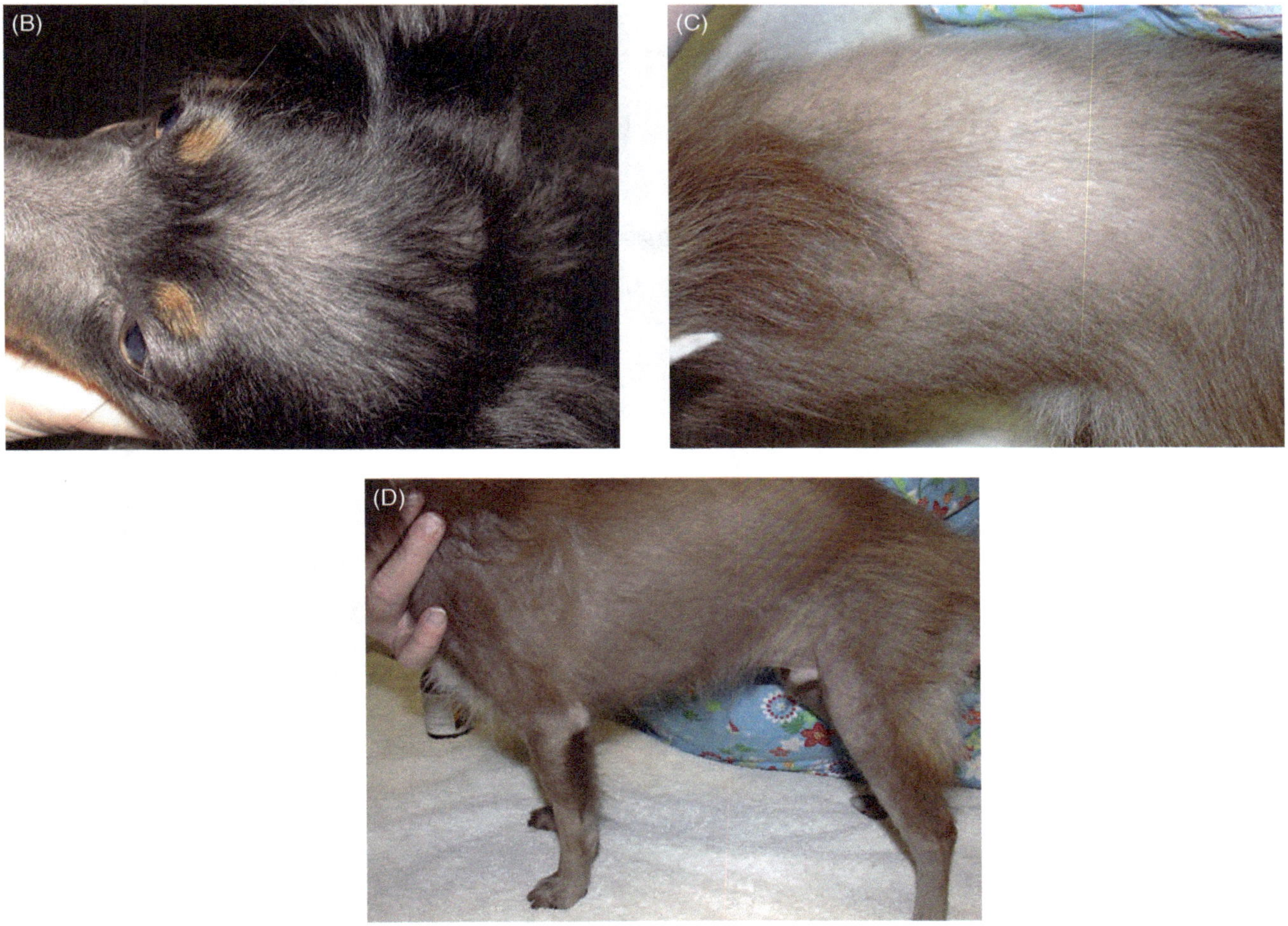

Figures 13.2B–D Color dilution alopecia in two Pomeranian dogs.

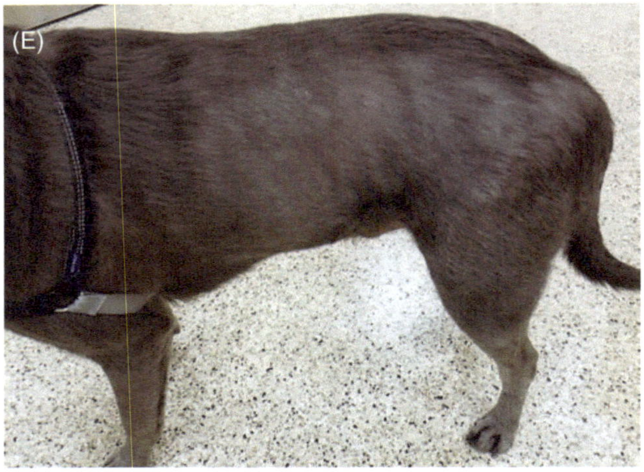

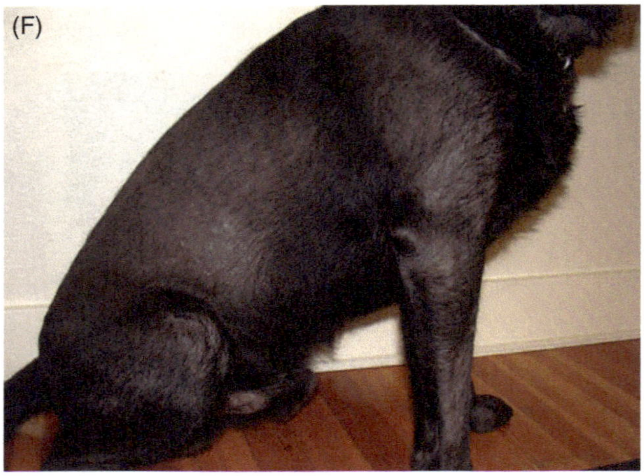

Figures 13.2E and F Color dilution alopecia in two silver Labrador dogs. *Source:* Image 13E courtesy of Dr. Amy Shumaker, DACVD; Image 13.3F courtesy of Dr. Trish Ashley, DACVD.

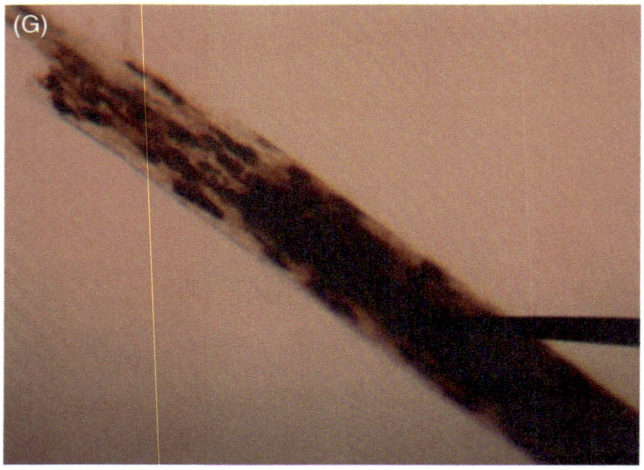

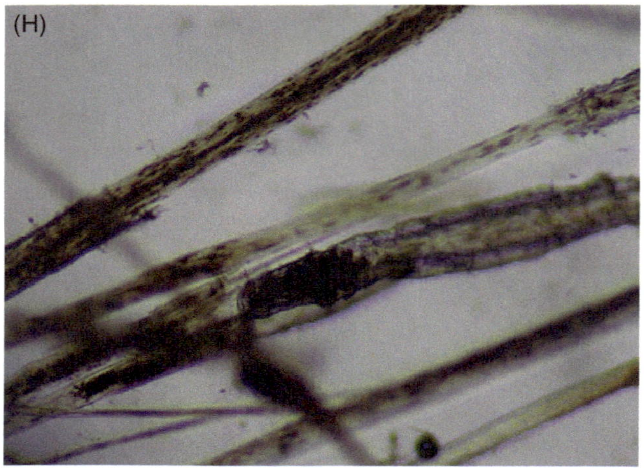

Figures 13.2G and H Trichograms of a color dilute dog demonstrating pigment clumping in the hair cortex (Fig. 13.2G is 10×, Fig. 13.2H is 4×).

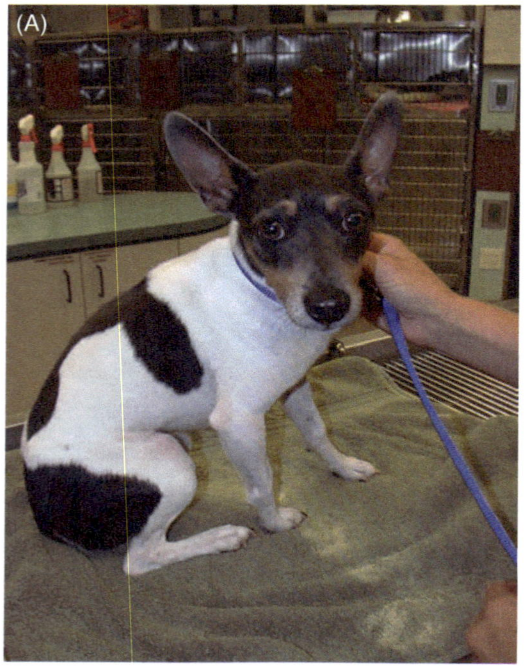

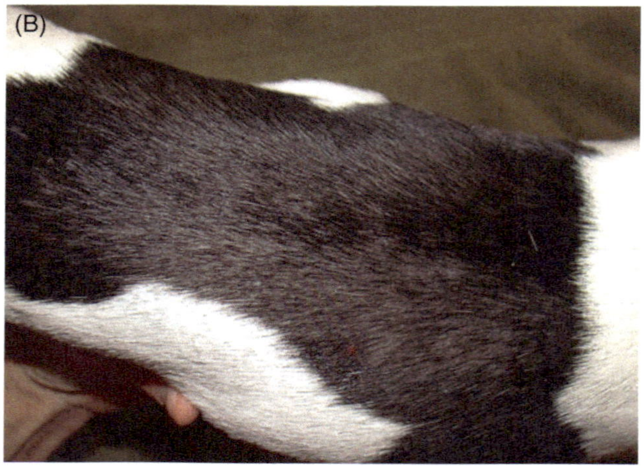

Figures 13.3A and B Black hair follicular dysplasia in a Terrier.

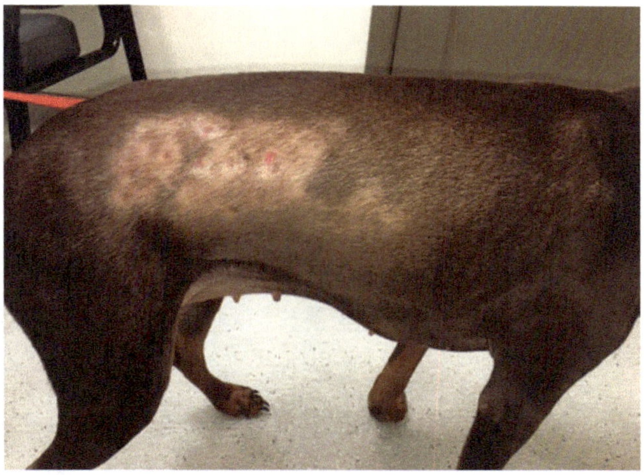

Figure 13.4 A young Doberman with follicular dysplasia.

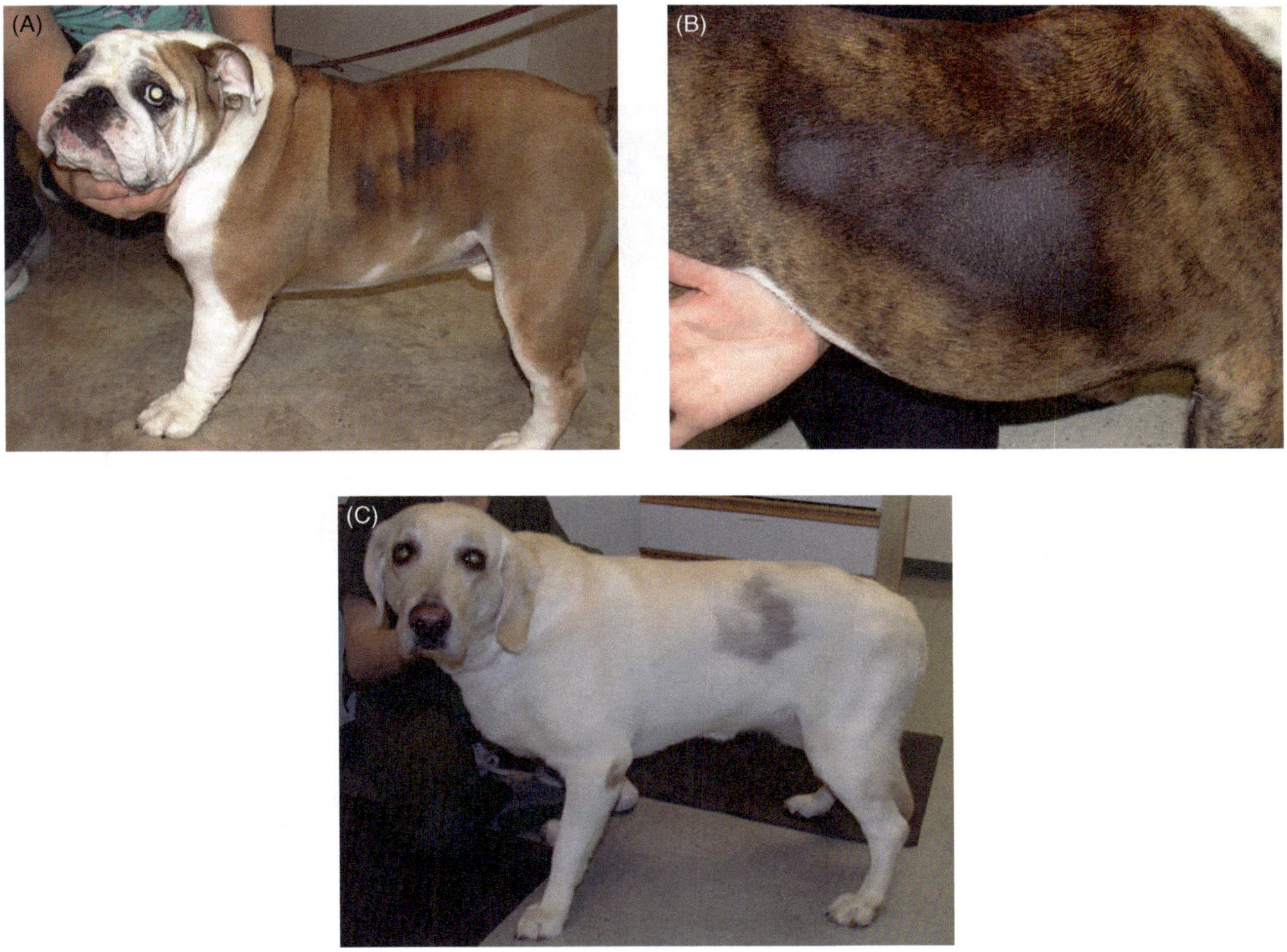

Figures 13.5A–C Canine recurrent flank alopecia.

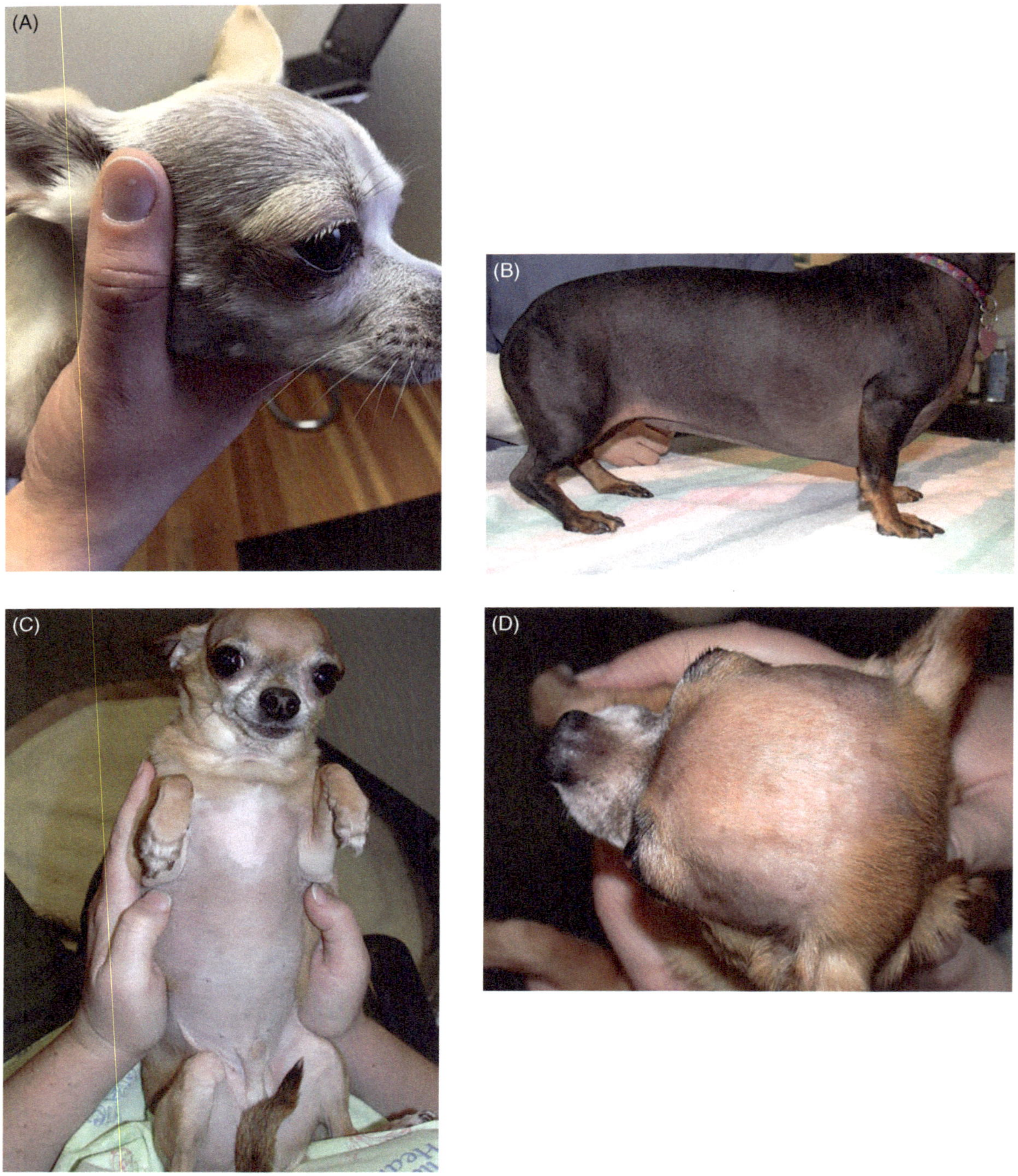

Figures 13.6A–D Canine pattern alopecia. *Source:* Images 13.6A and B courtesy of Dr. Trish Ashley, DACVD.

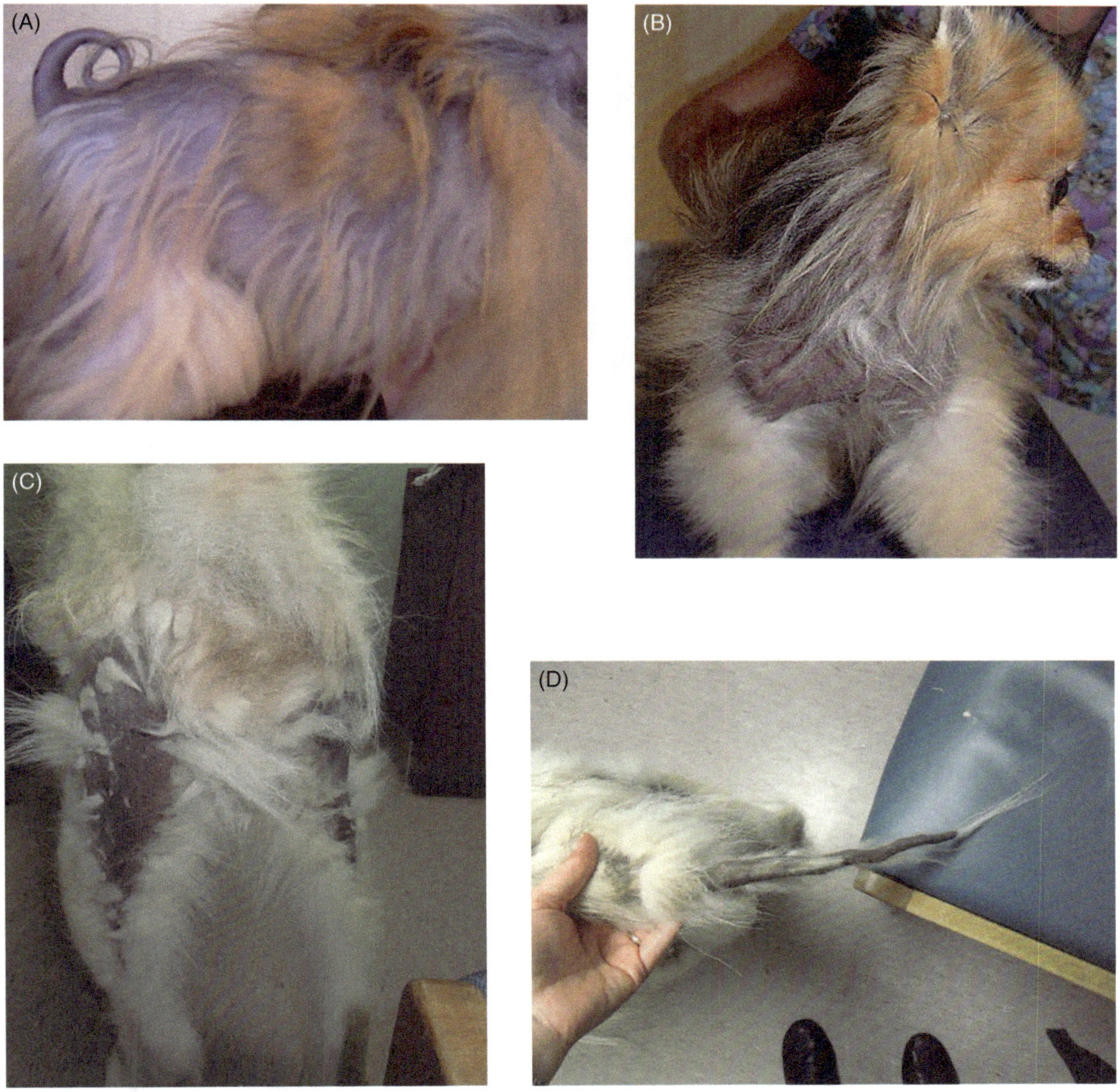

Figures 13.7A–D Canine Alopecia X. *Source:* Images 13.8A and B courtesy of Dr. Trish Ashley, DACVD.

Table 13.2 Non-endocrine alopecia of cats.

Condition	Cutaneous symptoms	Systemic symptoms/Clinical pathology changes	Diagnosis	Treatment/expected response/ monitoring/comments
Congenital hypotrichosis Autosomal recessive condition; reported in Birman, Burmese, Siamese, and Devon Rex cats	Non-color associated hair loss starting in first few weeks of life. Birman cats may also have abnormal or no whiskers, claws, or lingual papillae.	Affected Birman cats lack a thymus. Otherwise healthy.	Clinical appearance. Biopsy: Only small, fine secondary hairs; decreased number of, or absent, hair follicles, sebaceous and apocrine glands.	No specific treatment. Appropriate antiseborrheic topical therapy when indicated.
Hair shaft disorder of Abyssinian cats	Primary hairs, whiskers are rough, dull and have a visible onion-shaped bulge usually at tip of hair; hair susceptible to fracture.	No systemic symptoms.	Clinical history and exam; trichogram. Biopsy: No follicular abnormalities.	No specific treatment; minimize trauma to the hair shafts.
Pili torti Unusual congenital condition.	Flattening and twisting of secondary hair shafts. Fragile hairs susceptible to breakage. Seborrheic dermatitis and otitis; paronychia; accentuated skin folds.	May have ocular abnormalities (blepharitis, cataracts, corneal opacities).	Trichogram, biopsy.	Some kittens die at a young age; others report to do well past 1 year of age.
Feline preauricular "alopecia"	Symmetrical, non-inflammatory, thin hair coat between the pinnae and the eyes of cat.	None	Clinical appearance and no diagnostics indicated.	This is a normal hair pattern of cats that is more noticeable in short- than long-haired cats.
Feline pinnal alopecia (Figure 13.8) Siamese cats predisposed.	Periodic, patchy to complete pinnal non-inflammatory alopecia.	None	Breed, clinical appearance, and otherwise healthy. Helpful to rule out demodicosis and dermatophytosis.	Self-resolving. Once infectious causes eliminated, no further diagnostics/treatment indicated.
Feline psychogenic alopecia Indoor and Asian breed cats appear predisposed.	Barbered alopecia of ventrum +/− medial thighs, medial forelegs. Pulling or over-grooming of hair. Can create focal erythemic plaques or streaks. Nail chewing reported. Uncommon disorder and most cases suspected to be behavioral over-grooming are actually allergic dermatitis.	No systemic symptoms but may show stress response to noises, strangers, other animals. May display ptyalism, tachycardia, tachypnea, increase or decrease in food intake.	Elimination of other causes of pruritus: Skin scrapes/parasite treatment trial, dermatophyte culture or PCR. Elimination diet: 8 or more weeks. Behavioral evaluation/thorough history of home environment and changes. Lack of response to anti-inflammatory doses of corticosteroids + positive response to anti-anxiety therapy.	Clomipramine: 0.5 mg/kg PO q24h; can increase to 1 mg/kg if no response. Fluoxetine: 1 mg/kg PO q24h. Amitriptyline: 0.5 mg/kg PO BID. Buspirone: 5 mg tablets: 2.5–7.5 mg per cat PO 2–3 times per day. Endorphin blocker: Naloxone 1 mg/kg SC (may be effective for several weeks). See Chapter 20, Table 20.7. Address suspected cause(s) of stress; pheromone therapy. Environmental enrichment.

Mural folliculitis (Figures 13.9A and 13.9B)	Multifocal to generalized alopecia that is clinically non-inflammatory.	Variable.	Histopathologic evaluation shows inflammation suggestive of auto-immune disorder targeting the hair follicle.	If this is seen on biopsy, rule out infectious causes such as dermatophyte and *Demodex* and question history for signs of underlying allergies, consider food trial. If no etiology found, consider repeating biopsies; can progress to more apparent cutaneous lymphoma. Idiopathic cases reported but rare.
Mucinotic mural folliculitis Very rare condition.	Generalized alopecia most pronounced on the head; skin of face, including eyelids, thickened.	Often lethargic. Reports of some cats living with the condition long-term. 3/7 cats in one case series were FIV positive (Gross, Olivry, Vitale, and Power, 2001).	Biopsy; labwork to assess metabolic health and test retroviral status.	Poorly responsive to medications (corticosteroids and cyclosporine tried).
Pseudopelade (Chapter 11, Figure 11.18A) Very rare.	Variably-sized, often symmetrical non-inflamed areas of alopecia. May have abnormal or sloughing claws.	No other symptoms reported.	Biopsy: Though clinically non-inflammatory, histology shows inflammation suggestive of auto-immune dermatosis.	Generally poorly responsive to treatment but anecdotal reports of improvement with cyclosporine or cyclosporine combined with triamcinolone. See also Chapter 11, Table 11.1.
Trichorrhexis nodosa Very rare condition.	Symmetric diffuse alopecia. May be associated with overgrooming or topical insecticide application plus underlying (subclinical) hair keratin defect.	None	Trichogram: Nodes or swellings of hair shafts in affected area. Hair shaft often fractures at a node leaving "frayed" ends abutting each other.	Stop any topical treatments; address any cause of trauma to the hairs (such as pruritus, overgrooming).
Feline paraneoplastic alopecia (Figures 13.10A–13.10D) Usually in cats 10 years and older. Always associated with neoplasia, usually pancreatic or bile duct carcinoma.	Dramatic hair loss of ventrum, then legs, face. Foot pads, nasal planum may be involved. Alopecic skin appears shiny (not fragile); pads appear smooth. Large sheets of scale and crusting may be present. Acute and rapidly progressive signs. Secondary *Malassezia* infections common.	Cats are usually systemically ill when cutaneous symptoms develop.	Skin biopsy: Histopathologic findings are unique to this condition. Ultrasound, exploratory laparotomy to locate malignancy.	Grave prognosis. Complete tumor resection leads to resolution of cutaneous signs, but neoplasia has usually metastasized by time of diagnosis. Most cats euthanized within 8 weeks of onset of alopecia.

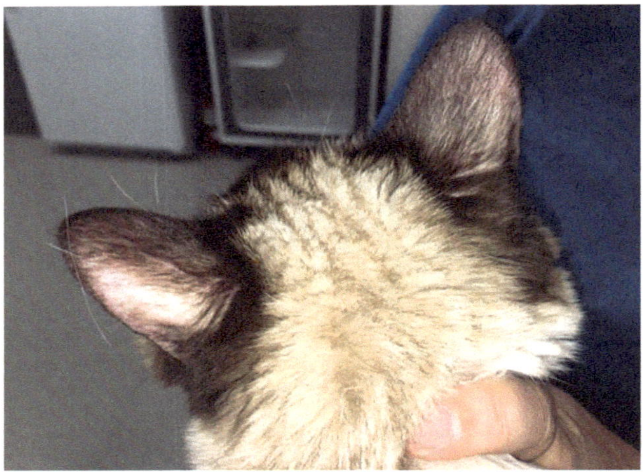

Figure 13.8 Non-inflammatory, bilaterally symmetric, outer pinnal hypotrichosis in a Siamese cat.

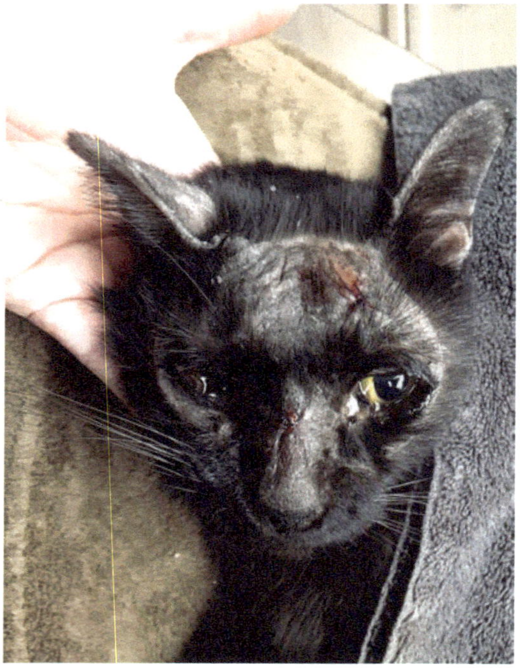

Figures 13.9A Feline mural folliculitis causing patchy facial and pinnal alopecia *Source:* Image courtesy of VIN and Emily Black, DVM.

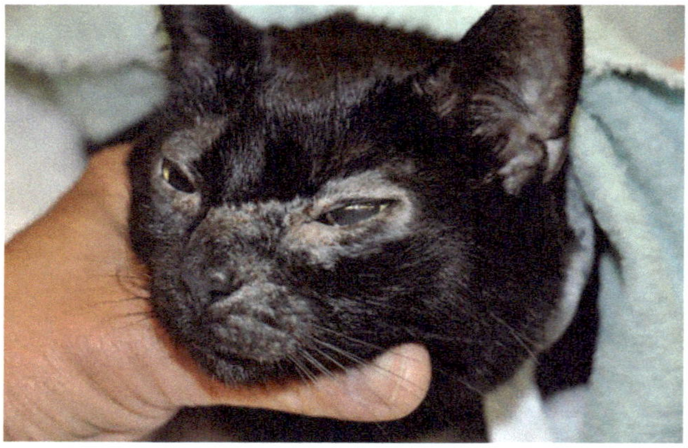

Figures 13.9B Patchy alopecia and slight crusting of the eyelids and muzzle due to feline mural folliculitis *Source:* Image courtesy of Dr. William Miller, DACVD.

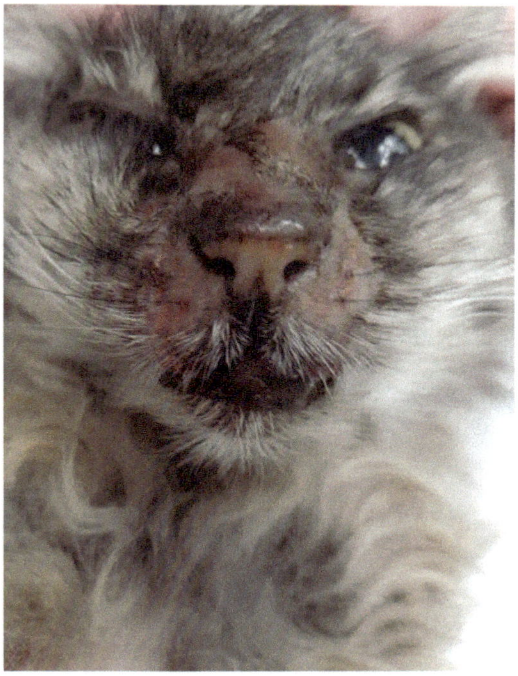

Figure 13.10A Facial hair loss with easily epilated fur caused by paraneoplastic alopecia due to a liver tumor *Source:* Image courtesy of VIN and Eric Clough, DVM.

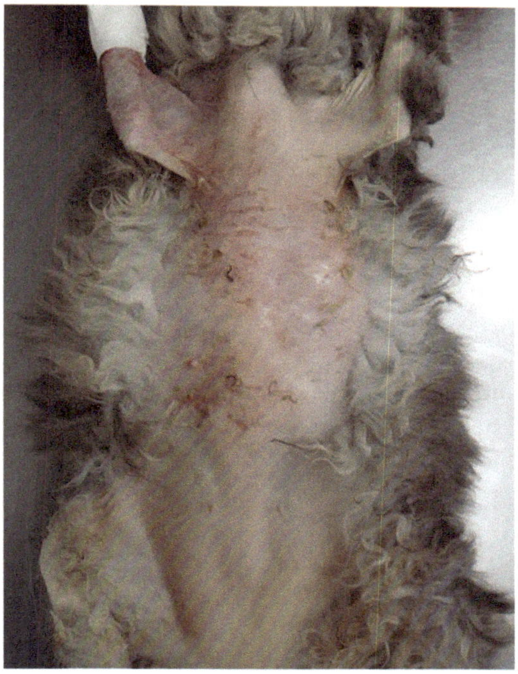

Figure 13.10B The same cat as Figure 12.12A; note marked ventral truncal alopecia with a shiny appearance to the skin. *Source:* Image courtesy of VIN and Eric Clough, DVM.

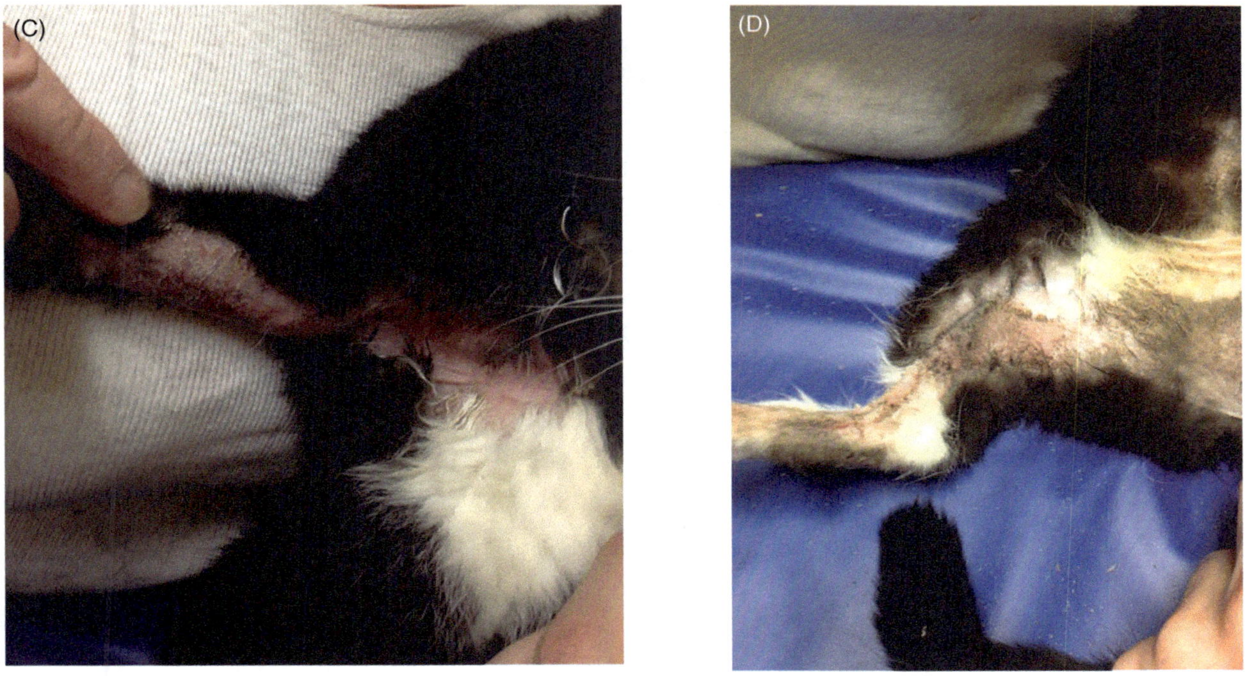

Figures 13.10C–D Paraneoplastic alopecia in a cat causing easily epilated fur on the medial limbs. *Source:* Images courtesy of VIN and John Ley, DVM.

References/Further reading

Frank, LA. (2014) Non-inflammatory Alopecia, It's not always Hormonal. Proceedings of the North American Veterinary Dermatology Forum, Phoenix, AZ, USA (12–14 Apr 2014). Ames, Iowa: Wiley.

Frank, L.A. (2017). Alopecia X in a Pomeranian. *Clinician's Brief* https://www.cliniciansbrief.com/article/alopecia-x-pomeranian.

Gross, T.L., Ihrke, P.J., Walder, E.J. et al. (eds.) (2008). *Skin Diseases of the Dog and Cat, Clinical and Histopathologic Diagnosis*, 2e. Ames, Iowa: Blackwell Science.

Gross, T.L., Olivry, T., Vitale, C.B., and Power, H.T. (2001). Degenerative mucinotic mural folliculitis in cats. *Vet. Dermatol. Oct* 12 (5): 279–283.

Guaguere, E. and Prelaud, P. (1999). *A Practical Guide to Feline Dermatology*. Merial.

Mecklenburg, L., Linek, M., and Tobin, D.J. (2009). *Hair Loss Disorders in Domestic Animals*. Ames, Iowa: Wiley Blackwell.

Miller, W., Griffin, C., and Campbell, K. (2014). *Mueller and Kirk's Small Animal Dermatology*, 7e. Philadephia, PA: Saunders.

Stoll, S., Dietlin, C., and Nett-Mettler, C.S. (2015). Microneedling as a successful treatment for alopecia X in Pomeranian siblings. *Vet. Dermatol.* 26 (5): 387–390.

14

Diagnosis and treatment of acute and chronic otitis

Kimberly S. Coyner, DVM, DACVD

Dermatology Clinic for Animals, Lacey, WA, USA

14.1 Approach to otitis

- Otitis externa is a common medical problem in dogs and less common in cats.
- When presented with a case of acute otitis (see Algorithm 14.1), always obtain otic cytology and swabs for mites in order to accurately identify and treat infection, and perform otoscopic examination to screen for ear canal foreign bodies or masses.
- If the ear canal is too painful or swollen for otoscopic examination, treatment of infection and a tapering two to three weeks course of oral anti-inflammatory steroids may be needed prior to recheck and otoscopic examination.
- If cerumen/debris in ear canals prevent full otoscopic examination (Figures 14.1A–14.1E), then gently cleaning the ear canal with a ceruminolytic flush may be needed +/− in severe cases sedation or anesthesia for deep flush using a 5–8F red rubber catheter and a 12–20 cc syringe through the otoscope head to guide safe flushing and avoid iatrogenic ear canal or tympanum trauma (Figure 14.2); video otoscopic guided ear flushing has the benefit of increased magnification to visualize deep ear canal structures (Figure 14.3).
- Use cuffed ET tube for anesthetic procedures to prevent aspiration of ear flush fluid if the tympanum is not intact; for sedated procedures if any coughing is observed then immediately stop the procedure.
- Instill ceruminolytic agent for five minutes to loosen debris.
- Dogs: Flush ears with mild cleaner or 0.9% NaCl.
- Cats: Use warmed saline only!
- If tympanum ruptured, flush out cleaners with saline.
- Use separate flushing materials/solution for each ear.
- Repeat ear flush q7–10 days until infection controlled.
- Continue at-home preventative cleaning q3–7 days.
- Treat infection topically and recheck otic cytology and examination in two to three weeks to ensure infection has resolved.
- If otitis persists or recurs more often than two to three times/year, or in cases with chronic otitis, then further workup is indicated (see Algorithm 14.2) to identify a potentially resistant bacterial infection +/− otitis media, as well as to identify and address the underlying primary cause(s) for otitis, including:
  - Hypersensitivity (atopy, food allergy, contact hypersensitivity)
  - Parasite
  - Ear canal foreign body
  - Ear canal tumor or polyp
  - Endocrinopathy
  - Immune-mediated disease
  - Keratinization disorder

14.2 Otoscopic examination

- Otoscopic examination is a skill which requires practice to master; it is helpful to first practice otoscopy on sedated or anesthetized animals to develop correct technique.
- Grasp the pinna and gently pull the ear canal up and outward to help straighten it and facilitate insertion of the otoscopic cone.
- It is important to be able to recognize normal ear canal and tympanum anatomy (Figures 14.4A–14.4D) in order to be able to recognize abnormalities (Figures 14.5A–14.5H).
- Using an otoscope head with magnification is often helpful, as is video otoscopy if available.

14.3 Choice of otic medications

- Bacterial otitis
  - Antiseptic flushes containing silver or chlorhexidine commercial otic solution.

Clinical Atlas of Canine and Feline Dermatology, First Edition. Edited by Kimberly S. Coyner.

Companion website: www.wiley.com/go/coyner/dermatology

Algorithm 14.1 Diagnostic and treatment steps for acute otitis externa.

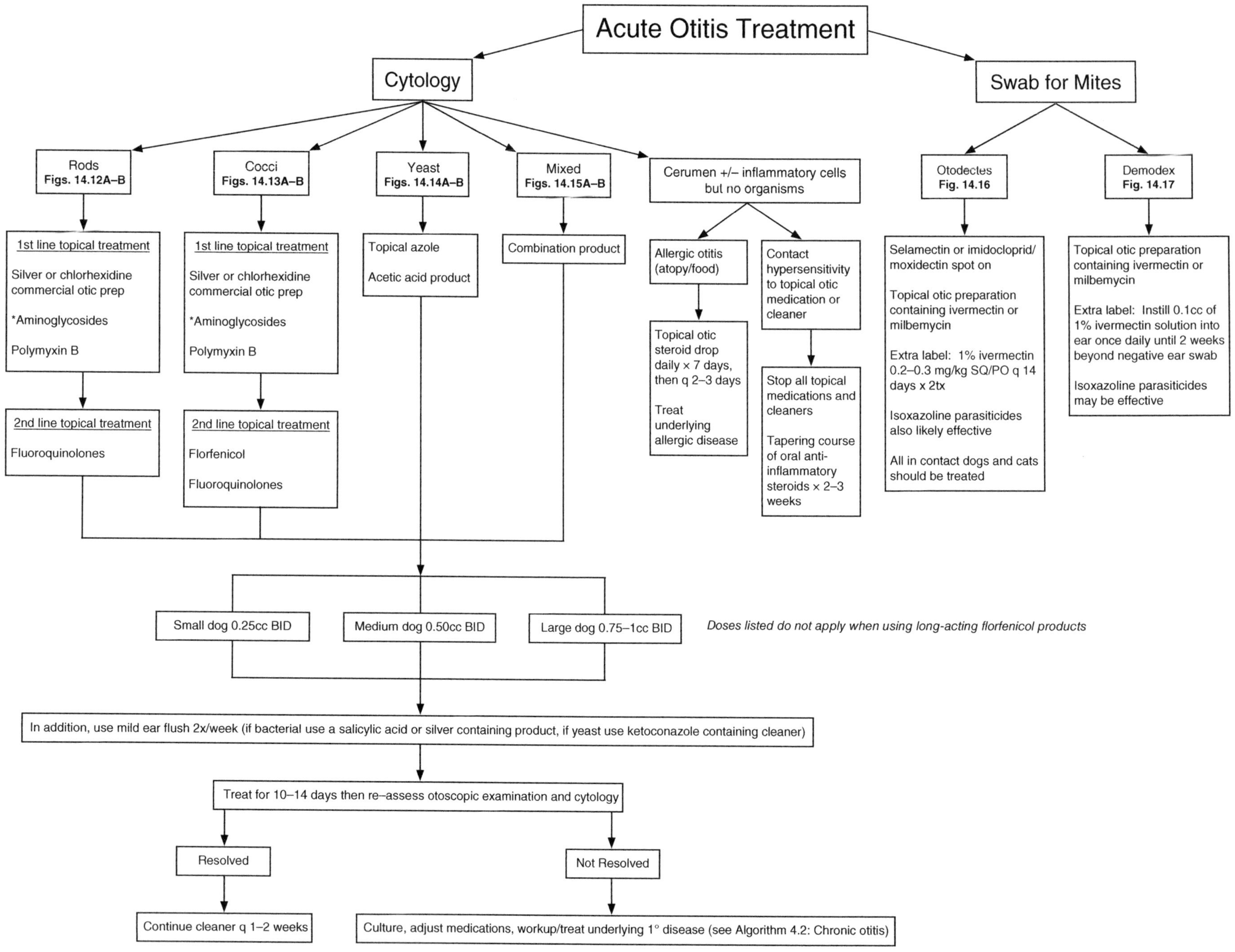

**Aminoglycoside antibiotics should not be used if tympanum is ruptured.*

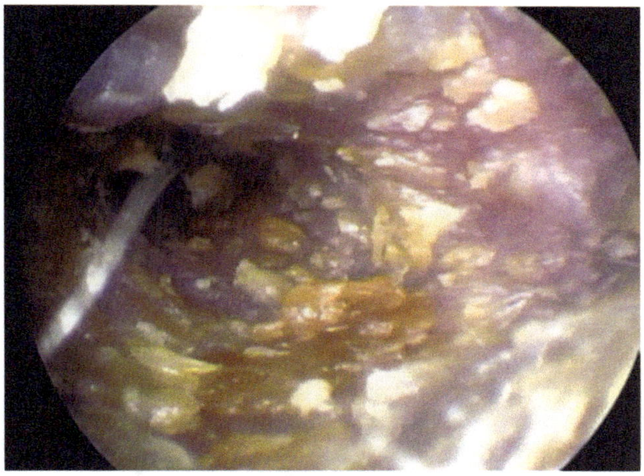

Figure 14.1A Accumulated exudate and cerumen on the canal walls and obstructing the horizontal canal in this allergic dog will prevent adequate penetration of topical antimicrobial otic medications.

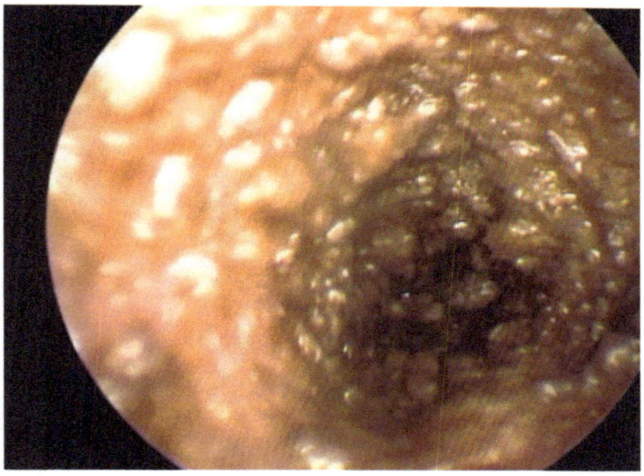

Figure 14.1B This atopic dog had chronic *Malassezia* otitis which did not resolve with prior ear medications due to severe accumulation of cerumen and exudate which sequesters the yeast organisms away from antifungal medications.

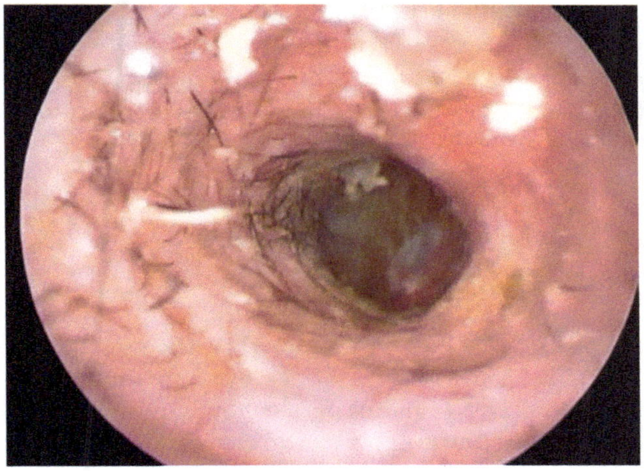

Figure 14.1C After the exudate was flushed out, the tympanum was revealed to be thickened and abnormal, suggesting otitis media also contributed to chronic infection; the dog's otitis resolved with topical antifungal drops combined with a four-week course of oral antifungal medication and allergy hyposensitization therapy to treat the underlying atopy.

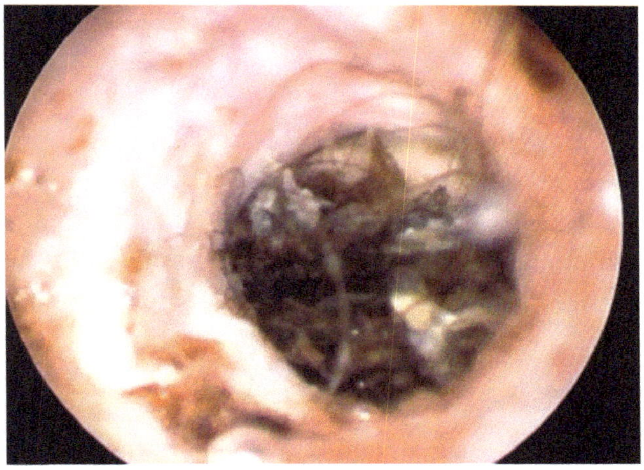

Figure 14.1D This Miniature Poodle also had chronic otitis unresponsive to treatment; otoscopic examination revealed a plug of fur and cerumen obstructing the horizontal canal which was causing inflammation as well as sequestering infection.

  - Antibiotic drops or ointments (i.e. neomycin, gentamycin).
  - Reserve fluoroquinolones for resistant *Pseudomonas* and for cases with questionable tympanum.
- Yeast otitis
  - Acetic acid/boric acid flushes may be effective but can be irritating in some dogs.
  - Antifungal products (i.e. clotrimazole, miconazole, ketoconazole, thiabendazole, nystatin).
- Use steroid containing products to reduce inflammation.
- Do not tell owners to count drops, it is more accurate and effective to deliver a measured dose of ear medication into the ear canal.
  - The average ear canal volume is 2.7 ml
  - 1 ml = 15–20 drops
- Repackage ointments and solutions into dropper bottles or Yorkers and provide syringes to owners to facilitate dosing:
  - Small dog: 0.25 cc BID
  - Medium dog: 0.50 cc BID
  - Large dog: 0.75–1.0 cc BID
  - Doses above do not apply when using long-acting florfenicol products
- Long acting veterinary labeled florfenicol/terbinafine otic preparations may be appropriate for otitis in which cocci bacteria and yeast are found on otic cytology, however florfenicol is ineffective for *Pseudomonas* and should not be empirically used for otitis in which rods are present cytologically unless culture and sensitivity data indicate bacterial susceptibility.

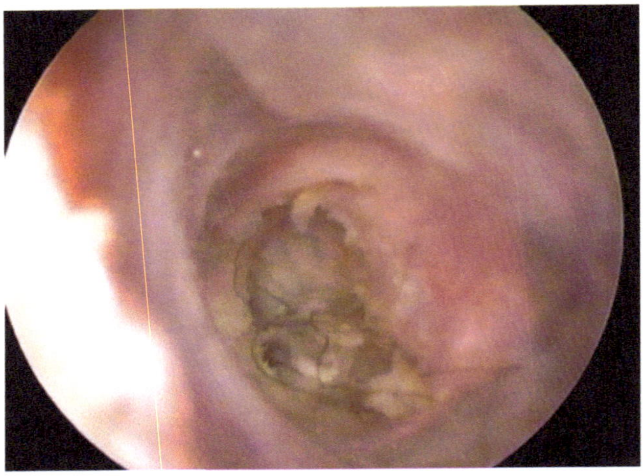

Figure 14.1E Same dog as Fig. 14.1D; When the plug of fur/cerumen was removed, the underlying tympanum was thickened/abnormal, consistent with otitis media; otitis resolved with antibiotics based on culture and did not recur.

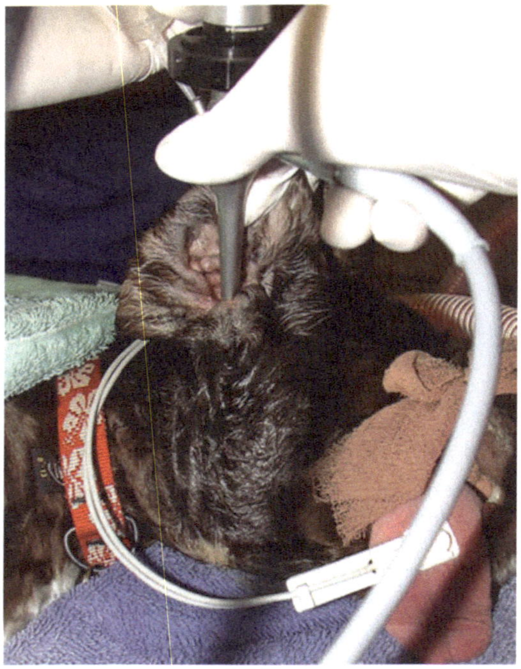

Figure 14.3 A Cocker Spaniel with chronic otitis due to atopy undergoing video otoscopy under anesthesia to flush out deep ear debris and evaluate the tympanum.

- Use of a long-acting veterinary labeled ketoconazole/hydrocortisone preparation may be considered in difficult to treat dogs with *Malassezia* otitis externa.
- Avoid compounded long-acting otic preparations except as a last resort in dogs which will not tolerate application of appropriate labeled otic medications; the carrier used in compounded otic medications can cause ototoxicity and deafness and is very difficult to remove from the middle ear (Fig 14.5I).

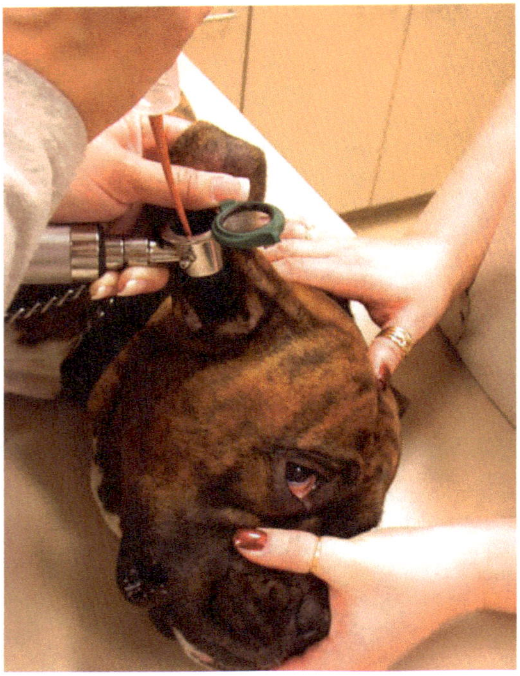

Figure 14.2 Deep ear flush using a handheld otoscope to guide a catheter through the otoscope cone and into the deep canal to flush out accumulated debris; the dog is lightly sedated.

14.4 Indications for systemic steroid/antibiotic therapy in otitis treatment

- Proliferative otitis which prevents effective topical therapy (Figure 14.6).
- Severe ulcerative and/or purulent otitis.
- Owner inability to apply topical medications.
- Adverse reaction to topical medications.
- Topical therapy is not effective.
- Otitis media (controversial, Figures 14.1E, 14.5H).

14.5 Choice of otic cleanser/flushes

- Ear cleaning solutions can have several properties:
  - Ceruminolytic – help cleaning by emulsifying waxes/lipids.
  - Drying – reduce moisture accumulation in the ear canal.
  - Antimicrobial – antibacterial and/or antifungal.
  - Combination products.
- Ceruminolytics
  - Use for ears that form large amounts of waxy exudate which needs to be dissolved.
  - Potent ceruminolytic agents include surfactants (DSS) and detergents to emulsify waxes and lipids.
  - Milder ceruminolytic agents in commercial ear cleaners include propylene glycol, glycerin, and mineral oil.

Algorithm 14.2 Diagnostic and treatment steps for chronic otitis.

How to address chronic/recurrent otitis

Identify and treat 1° cause

- Atopy — **Figs. 14.18A–C**
  - 6 mo–5 yr, usually bilateral
  - Seasonal or non–seasonal
  - Often steroid responsive
  - Can occur in any breed, but some breeds more commonly atopic
- Food allergy — **Figs. 14.19A–C**
  - Any age, usually bilateral
  - Non–seasonal
  - Not usually very steroid responsive
  - Can occur in any breed, but some breeds more commonly food allergic
- Contact allergy — **Fig. 14.20**
  - Suspect if inflammation or pain worsens with topical medications.
- Parasite — **Figs. 14.21A–D**
  - Otodectes
    - Most common cause of feline otitis
  - Demodex
    - May or may not have concurrent skin disease
    - More common in young or immunosuppressed
  - Usually bilateral
- Tumor/polyp — **Figs. 14.22A–D**
  - Usually unilateral
  - Polyps more common in young cats
  - Tumors more common in older pets
- Foreign body — **Figs. 14.23A–D**
  - Usually unilateral
- Endocrinopathy — **Figs. 14.24A–B**
  - Hypothyroidism, hyperadrenocorticism
  - Usually bilateral, older dogs
  - Usually other skin or systemic signs
- Keratinization disorder — **Figs. 14.25A–B**
  - Sebaceous adenitis
    - More common in Standard Poodles, Akitas
  - Primary seborrhea
    - Very rare, Cocker Spaniels
- Immune-mediated — **Figs. 14.26A–E**
  - Usually bilateral
  - Often other skin lesions present
  - Pemphigus, juvenile cellulitis, erythema multiforme, vasculitis, drug eruption

Flush out accumulated exudate

- Take samples for cytology +/– culture
- If the canal is swollen, pretreat with tapering oral anti-inflammatory steroids x 2–3 weeks and start topical otic antibiotics — **Figs. 14.27A–B**
- Sedate (medetomidine +/– opioid), +/– anesthetize with cuffed ET tube
- Instill squalene based ear flush to soften cerumen × 5 min.
- Use 5–8 F red rubber catheter and 12–20cc syringe, guided through otoscope, or video-otoscope — **Figs. 14.2–14.3**
- Syringe flush with mild ceruminolytic ear cleaner or saline
- If tympanum is not intact, flush with saline
- After flushing all exudate out, aspirate canal dry, instill antibiotic +/– steroid drops
- Continue topical ear medications based on cytology +/– culture 4 weeks
- Send home mild ear flush to begin at home ear cleaning in 4–5 days, clean twice a week, NOT daily; separate cleaner and medicated drops by 8–12 hrs
- Continue tapering oral anti–inflammatory steroids 2–4 weeks beyond deep ear flush

Treat infection

- Obtain in clinic cytology at every visit to enable interpretation of culture results, guide empiric treatment decision pending culture results, and assess response to therapy and when to adjust or discontinue therapy — **Figs. 14.28A–B**
- In cases of bacterial otitis unresponsive to prior empiric therapies, obtain culture to guide topical +/– systemic antibiotic choice

Topical Treatment

- Use syringes to measure topical otic medications (not applicable for long-acting otic preps)
  - Small animals < 10#: 0.25cc per dose
  - Medium animals 11–50#: 0.50cc per dose
  - Large dogs > 50#: 0.75–1.0cc per dose
- Tell owners to **not** clean ears prior to instilling antibiotic drops
- Use long acting florfenicol otic preps based on cytology +/– culture results
  - Cocci +/– yeast
  - Not ideal empiric choice if rods present on cytology; not effective for *Pseudomonas*
- Do not use long-acting compounded otic medications except as last resort if dog will not allow owners to safely apply topical otic medications

Systemic Treatment

- Use oral antibiotics based on culture x 4 weeks in addition to topical medications if canals are severely inflamed/ulcerated/proliferative
- Use oral antiyeast medication x 4–6 weeks if yeast otitis media suspected
- Use of a 4–6 week course of oral antibiotics for otitis media is controversial and only recommended if based on culture of middle ear exudate sample

When to refer for surgery

- End–stage otitis (**Figs. 14.29A–B, Fig. 14.5D**)
- Recurrent otitis media despite appropriate medical treatment
- Recurrent benign ear canal mass or polyp after initial removal or benign mass which cannot be removed
- Malignant ear canal neoplasia
- Multi-drug resistant bacterial otitis media with no available antibiotic options

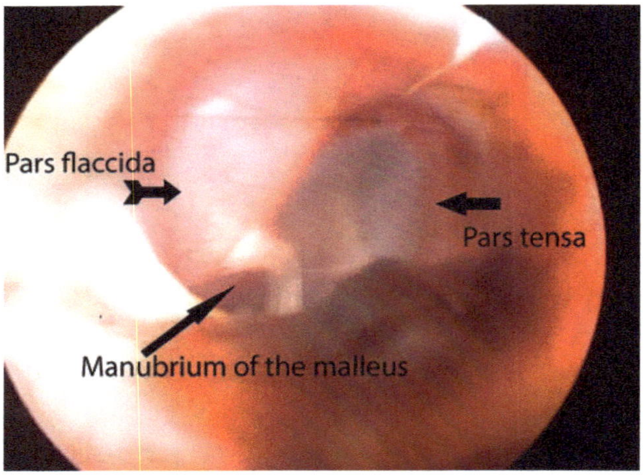

Figure 14.4A A normal canine tympanum with anatomic locations labeled.

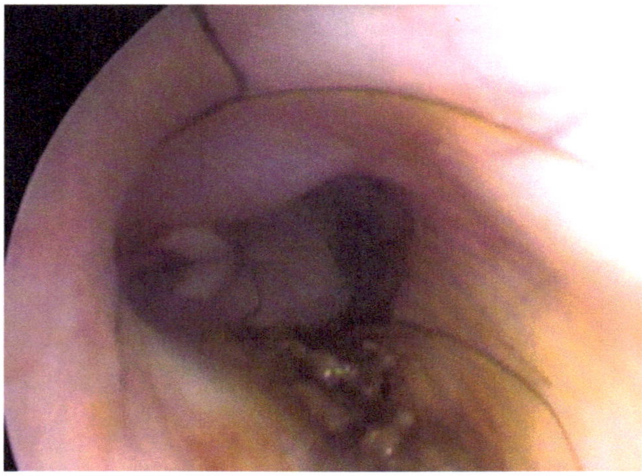

Figure 14.4B A normal feline tympanum; the whitish structure which can be seen behind the pars tensa is the boney septum of the bulla, a normal structure. There is normal cerumen present on the ventral aspect of the proximal horizontal canal.

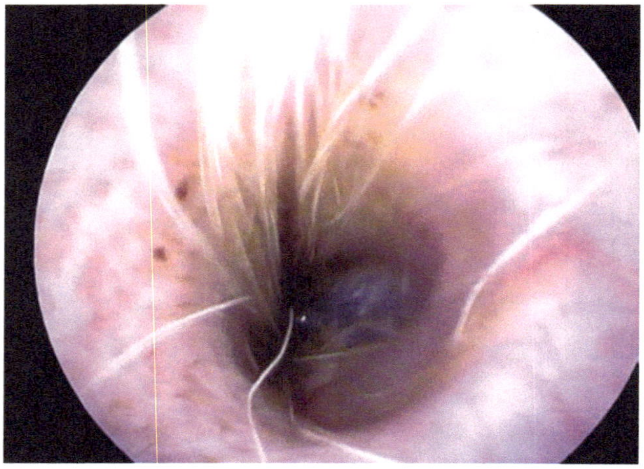

Figure 14.4C Some dogs have hair which grows from the epitympanic recess; this can be a normal variation which can complicate otitis due to tendency to accumulate cerumen which is difficult to dislodge.

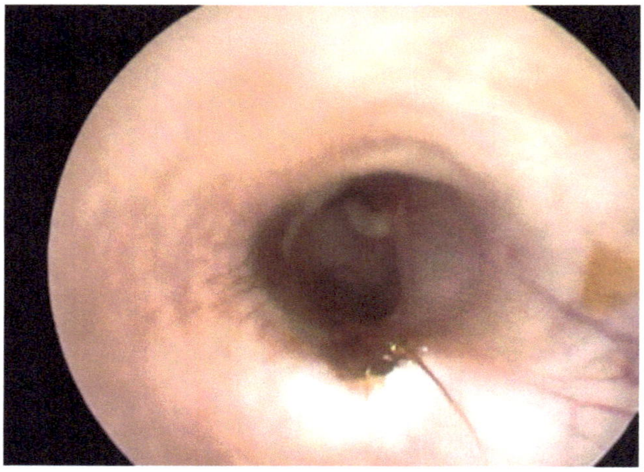

Figure 14.4D This dog's tympanum was normal, however increased middle ear pressure due to anesthesia caused the pars flaccida to bow outward, mimicking a mass.

  - Most ceruminolytics and detergents are contraindicated with ruptured tympanum.
  - Squalene is a milder surfactant cleanser, may be safer if tympanum ruptured.
- Drying agents can be used for prevention of "swimmer's ear."
  - Examples of drying agents in commercial ear cleaners include: alcohol, boric acid, benzoic acid, salicylic acid, acetic acid, aluminum acetate, sulfur, silicone dioxide.
- Antimicrobial ingredients
  - Ingredients in commercial ear cleaners which have antimicrobial properties include propylene glycol, acetic acid, salicylic acid, sulfur, silver, aloe vera, chlorhexidene, alcohol, miconazole, ketoconazole.
  - Often incorporated into a combination ear cleaner.
- Use a mild ceruminolytic/mild drying formulation for routine cleaning, for prevention of cerumen accumulation, and for ears which tend to be moist.
- Products with antimicrobial properties can also be helpful in preventing recurrent otitis.

14.6 Educate owners on how to correctly use ear flushes

- Instill product until canal is full, don't touch cleaner bottle tip to ear canal.
- Massage ear canal gently for 20–30 seconds.
- Allow the pet to shake their head, then wipe out excess with dry cotton balls, never Q tips.
- Cleanse one to two times weekly for most ears, two to three times weekly for infected ears.

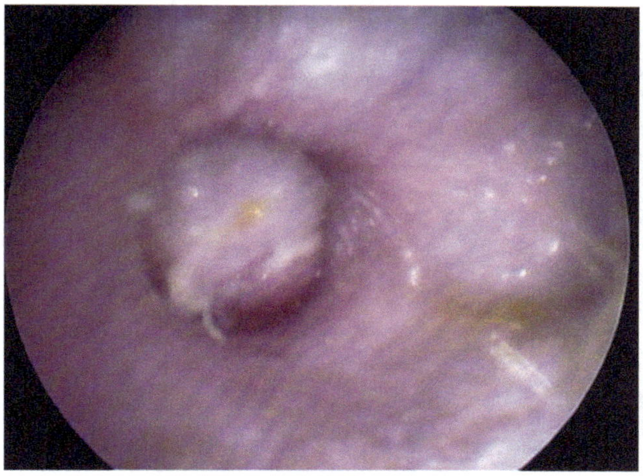

Figure 14.5A An ear canal mass in a dog; histopathology revealed an inflammatory polyp secondary to chronic allergic and bacterial otitis.

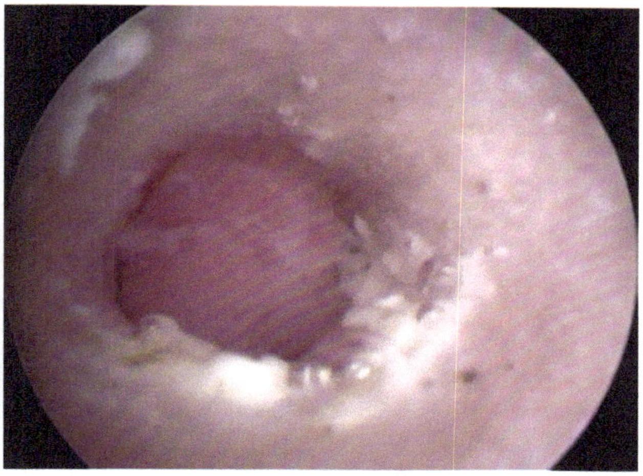

Figure 14.5B An inflammatory polyp in a cat.

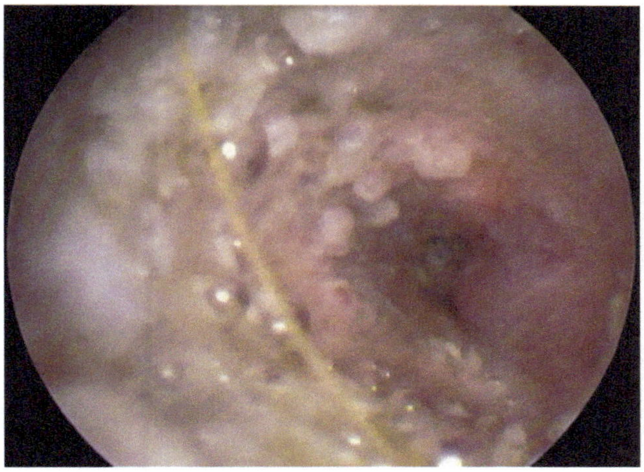

Figure 14.5C Early polypoid otitis in a Cocker Spaniel with chronic allergic and bacterial otitis; the entire canal is lined with small masses of ceruminous gland hyperplasia; this ear can still be salvaged by aggressive treatment with oral and topical steroids for four to six weeks, treatment of infection, and treatment of underlying allergic disease.

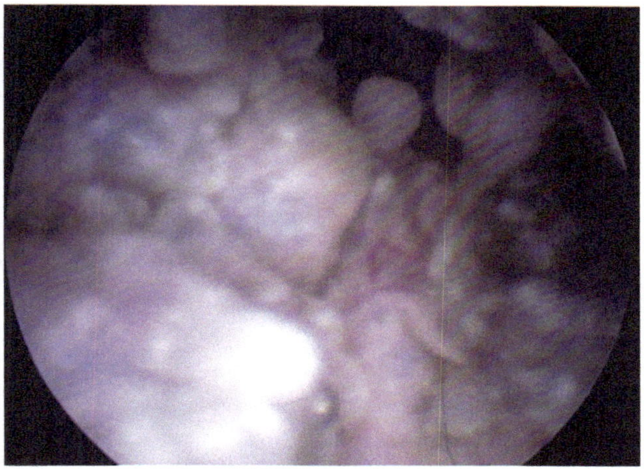

Figure 14.5D End stage hyperplastic otitis in a different Cocker Spaniel; the changes in this ear canal cannot be reversed and total ear canal ablation will likely be needed.

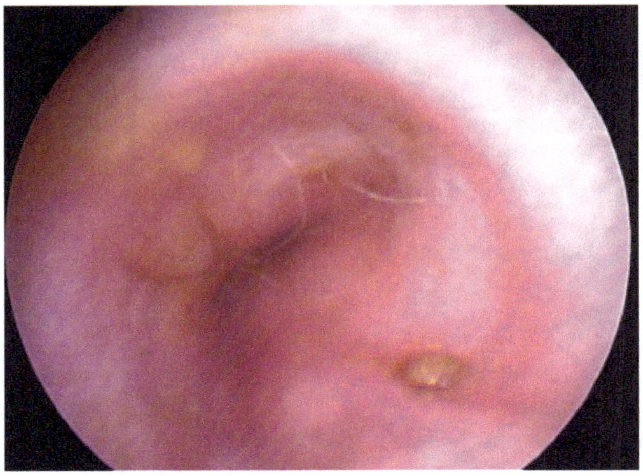

Figure 14.5E French Bulldogs often have anatomically very stenotic canals which contribute to treatment difficulty in this breed.

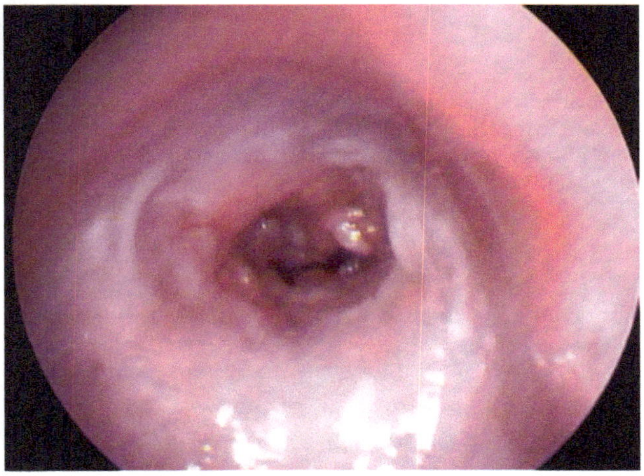

Figure 14.5F In this dog, an infiltrative horizontal canal mass has caused partial canal stricture.

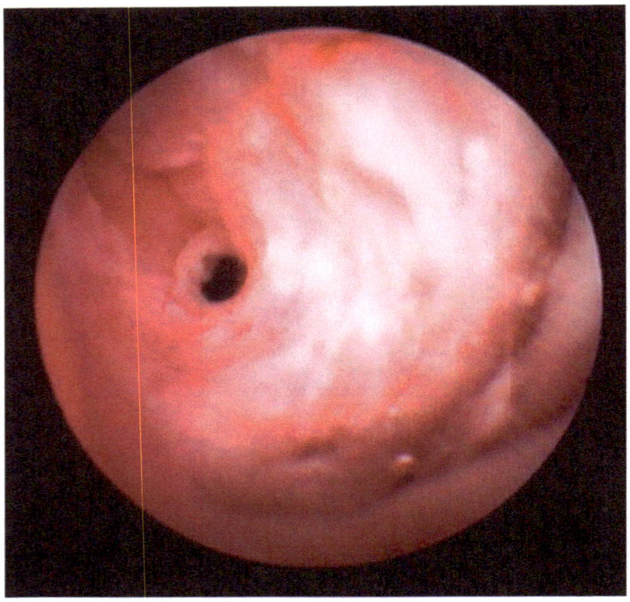

Figure 14.5G This dog's chronic otitis was due to a stricture which narrowed the canal by 90%, it was unknown if the stricture was congenital or acquired due to prior ear canal trauma. Total ear canal ablation is indicated.

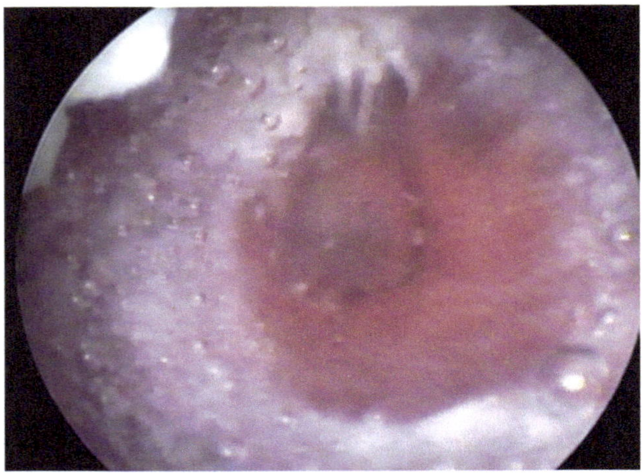

Figure 14.5H This thickened and abnormal tympanum which is bowing outward indicates otitis media is present.

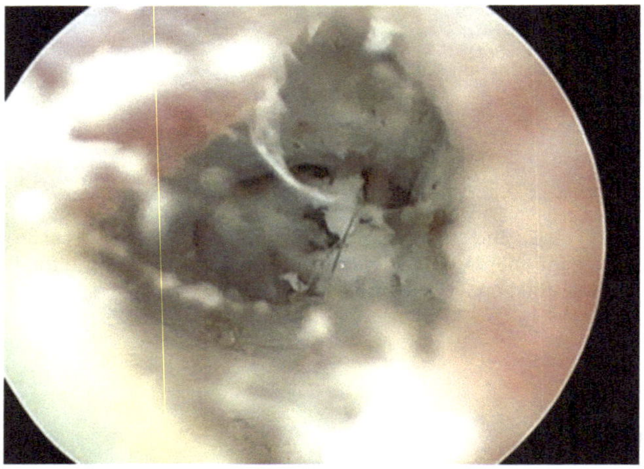

Figure 14.5I This atopic dog had chronic otitis and deafness with ear canal pain after multiple administration of compounded antibiotic "ear packs" which had ruptured the tympanum and filled the middle ear; removal of the gooey substance was extremely difficult and time consuming.

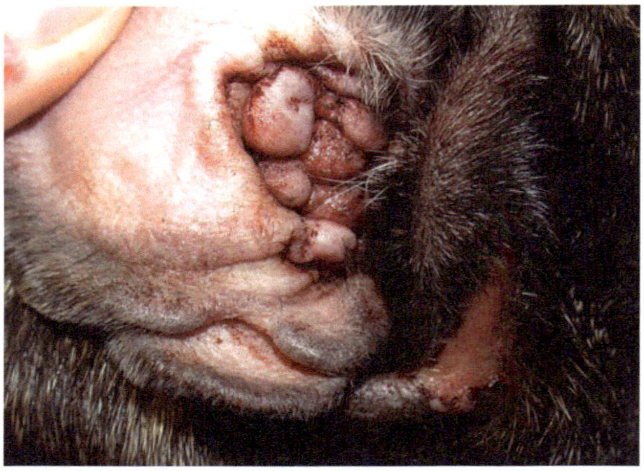

Figure 14.6 This atopic dog with chronic bacterial and yeast otitis has developed severe external canal hyperplasia and stenosis which prevents penetration of topical otic medications, and oral steroids are indicated to reduce canal swelling and facilitate medication administration.

- In general, do not clean before instilling antibiotic ear drops as it will dilute the drops.
  - In cases of *Pseudomonas* otitis, instillation of a Triz-EDTA containing product 15 minutes prior to antibiotic drops can facilitate antibiotic penetration through bacterial cell walls.
- If the pet ever seems painful/irritated by a cleanser or ear medication, consider contact hypersensitivity.
- Do not use out of date ear cleaners as they can be contaminated by bacteria.
  - A study cultured the tips of the bottles as well as bottle contents of client-used ear flush bottles (Bartlett, Rosenkrantz, and Sanchez, 2011).
  - Contamination rates increased for out of date products, larger bottles, and products containing Triz-EDTA.

14.7 Diagnosis and treatment of otitis media

- Common in chronic otitis externa.
- Clinical signs:
  - Recurrent otitis is the most common symptom.
  - +/– Horner's, mild head tilt, facial palsy (Figure 14.7).

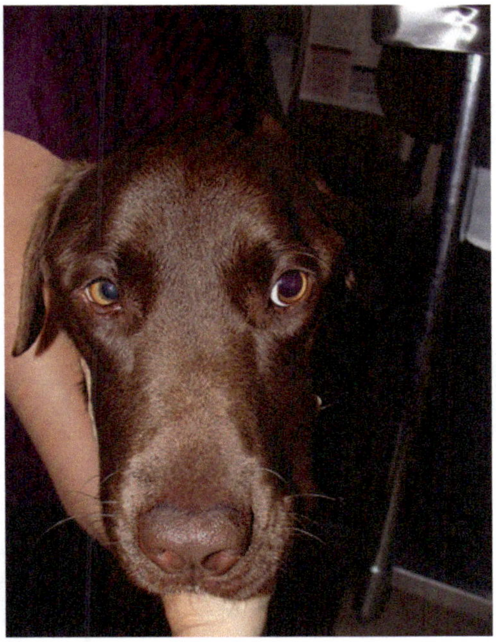

Figure 14.7 A Labrador with Horner's syndrome caused by chronic bacterial otitis media and middle ear neoplasia.

- Diagnosis:
  - Otoscopic exam: Tympanum thickened, bowing outward, opaque, +/− torn (Figures 14.8A and 14.8B, 14.9A and 14.9B).
  - An intact tympanum does not rule out otitis media.
  - In chronic infections >6 mo, 50–90% have otitis media, and 70% have intact but abnormal tympanum.
  - Bulla radiographs: May be normal or show opacified bulla and/or thickened bullae walls.
  - CT scan: More sensitive; not as available.
- Treatment
  - Treat bacterial otitis media with systemic antibiotics based on culture for one to two months.
  - Treat yeast otitis media with systemic antifungal medication for one to two months.
  - Myringotomy to sample middle ear for culture may be needed to guide antibiotic therapy, as external ear pathogens may not be the same as middle ear.

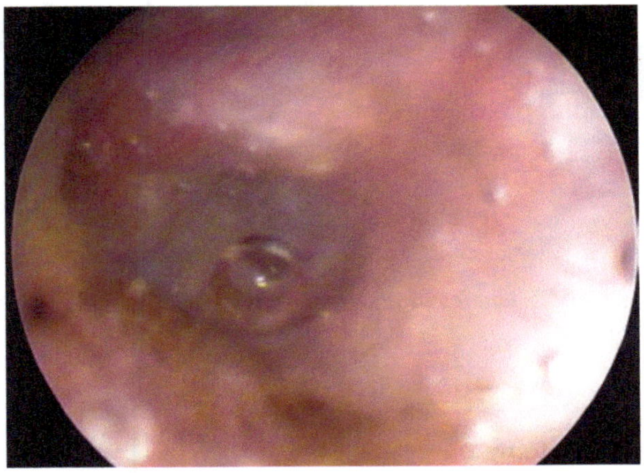

Figure 14.8A An air bubble escaping from a small tear in the tympanum.

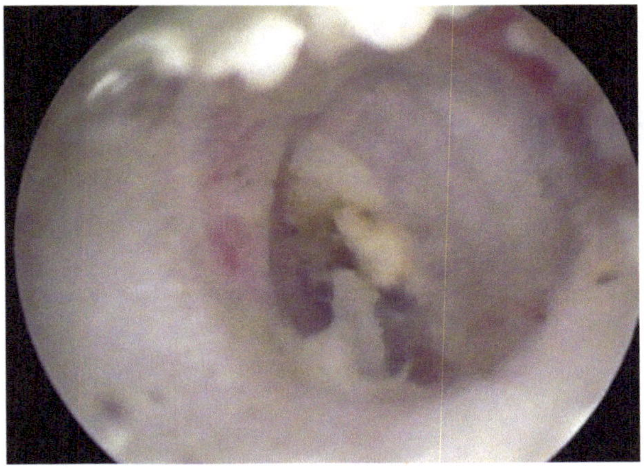

Figure 14.8B This dog's tympanum was intact but very thickened and abnormal due to otitis media.

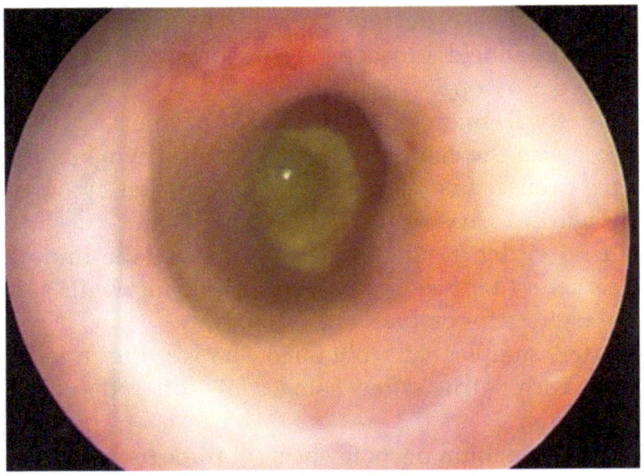

Figure 14.9A On initial view of the proximal horizontal canal of this dog with otitis media, only a pool of purulent exudate can be seen.

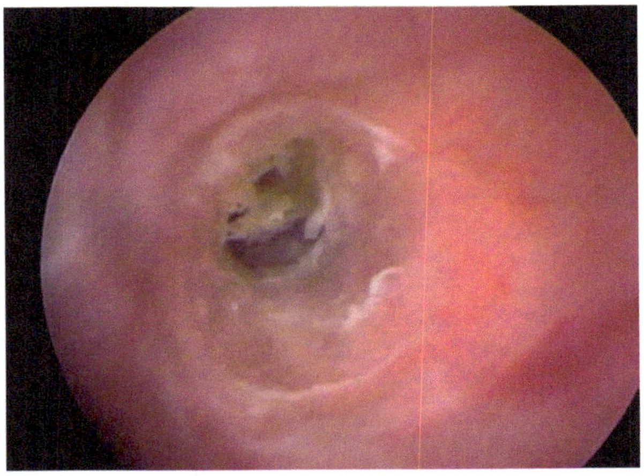

Figure 14.9B When the exudate was flushed out, there is no recognizable tympanum, just residual shreds on the canal wall, and the underlying bulla is visible.

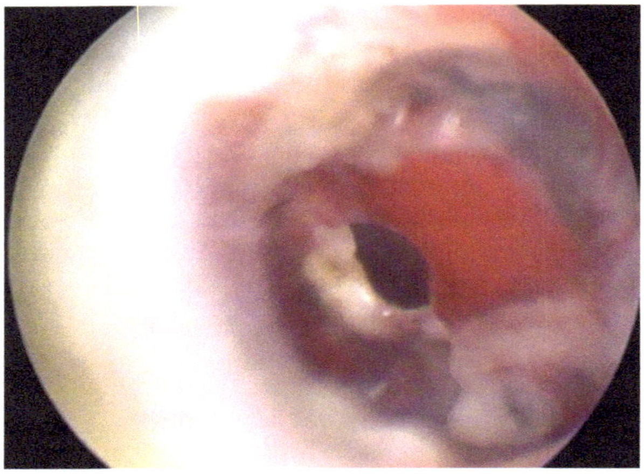

Figure 14.10A A myringotomy incision in the tympanum of a cat with a head tilt.

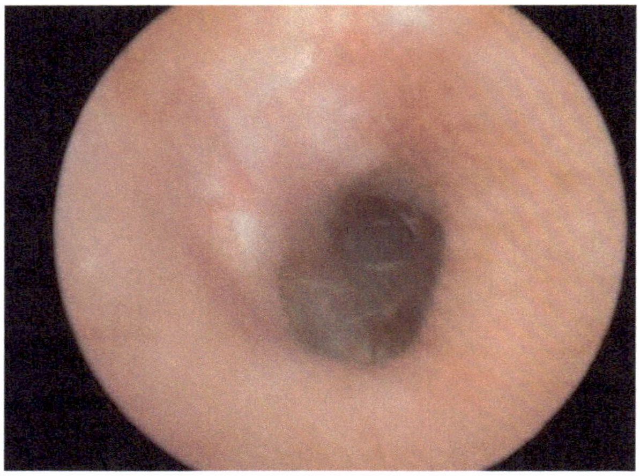

Figure 14.10B The tympanum of a Cavalier King Charles Spaniel with deafness due to primary secretory otitis media (PSOM).

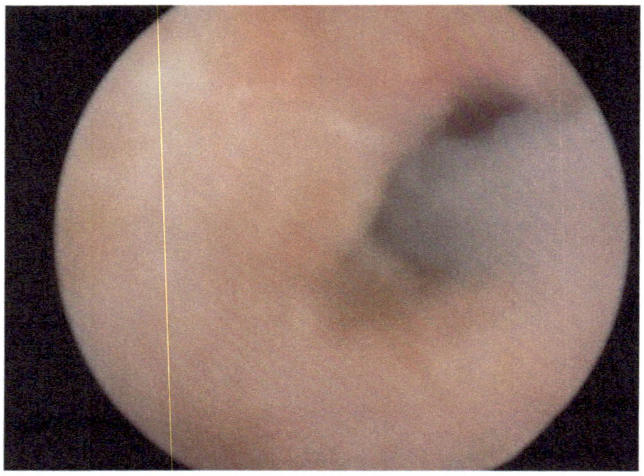

Figure 14.10C Image taken after myringotomy and during saline middle ear flush to remove middle ear mucous.

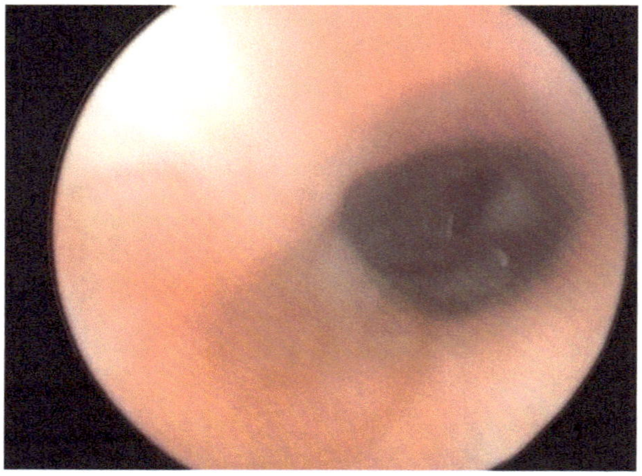

Figure 14.10D Post myringotomy; the incision in the pars tensa is visible.

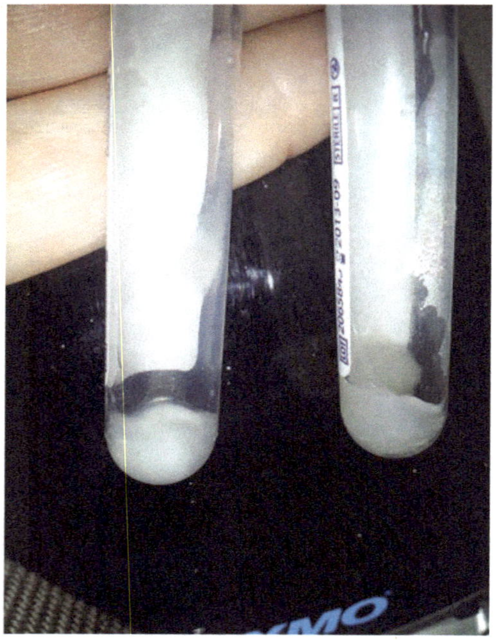

Figure 14.10E PSOM mucous collected from the patient.

- Myringotomy
  - Performed if tympanum is intact but abnormal to obtain samples for cytology and culture.
  - Informed owner release for potential complications (i.e. temporary Horner's, facial nerve paralysis, vestibular disease, deafness).
  - Use handheld otoscope/sterile otoscope cone or video otoscope.
  - Use sterile micro culturette swab or tomcat catheter to incise the caudoventral quadrant of tympanum/pars tensa, first sample for culture, then cytology (Figures 14.10A–14.10E).
  - If no visible exudate on swab, the use the tomcat catheter to infuse 1–2 cc sterile saline into bulla and reaspirate for culture and cytology.
  - After samples are obtained, lavage the middle ear with warm saline using a 5F soft red rubber catheter.
  - The tympanum normally heals in three to five weeks if infection is controlled.

- Pending culture results, start empiric topical and oral antibiotics based on cytology and continue medications based on culture for one to two months;
  - Avoid aminoglycosides.
  - Don't use ear flushes (or use only saline flushes) for two to three weeks post myringotomy.
- Tapering anti-inflammatory steroids for two to three weeks and pain medications are indicated.
- Advise owner to monitor for any signs of ototoxicity from topical medications and discontinue otic medications if adverse symptoms occur.

- If otitis continues to recur then consider bulla osteotomy.
- Cholesteatoma
  - Middle ear cholesteatoma can occur as a complication of chronic otitis media.
  - An epidermoid cyst lined by a keratinizing epithelium containing keratin debris (Figures 14.11A and B).
  - The cyst expands, and destroys adjacent tissue, including the bone of the tympanic bulla.
  - Two theories:
    - Migration of the stratified squamous epithelium from the external auditory meatus into the infected middle ear cavity through a perforated ear drum.
    - Pars flaccida retracts into the middle ear due to inflammation and/or negative pressure then the pocket fills with keratin.
  - History of chronic otitis, pain on opening of the mouth and on temporomandibular joint palpation.
  - Neurological abnormalities, including head tilt, facial palsy, and ataxia can occur.
  - Treatment is surgery to remove all keratin debris and stratified squamous epithelium (bulla osteotomy).
  - High (50%) risk of recurrence.

14.8 When to refer for surgery

- End-stage otitis (Figures 14.5D, 14.29A–14.29B).
- Recurrent otitis media despite appropriate medical treatment.
- Recurrent benign ear canal mass or polyp after initial removal or benign mass which cannot be removed.
- Malignant ear canal neoplasia.
- Multi-drug resistant bacterial otitis media with no available antibiotic options.

14.9 Ototoxicity

- Topical otic medications and flushes can sometimes cause ototoxicity, with potential symptoms including decreased hearing, deafness, and vestibular disease.
- Medication volume/vehicle, treatment duration, and pre-existing otic inflammation can influence risk of ototoxicity.
- Cats and younger animals are especially predisposed to ototoxicity.
- There is conflicting information in the literature about ototoxicity of topical medications in the canine ear; most information about topical medication ototoxicity is derived from studies on guinea pigs and chinchillas.
- There have been a few studies in dogs with ruptured eardrums using brainstem auditory evoked response (BAER) results after application of topical medications, and these studies found that topical medications which had *no* significant effect on BAER (i.e. were not ototoxic) included marbofloxacin, clotrimazole, gentamycin (diluted to 0.14% in Triz-EDTA), 0.2% chlorhexidene, and squalene (Mansfield et al. 1997; Merchant et al. 1995; Paterson, 2011).

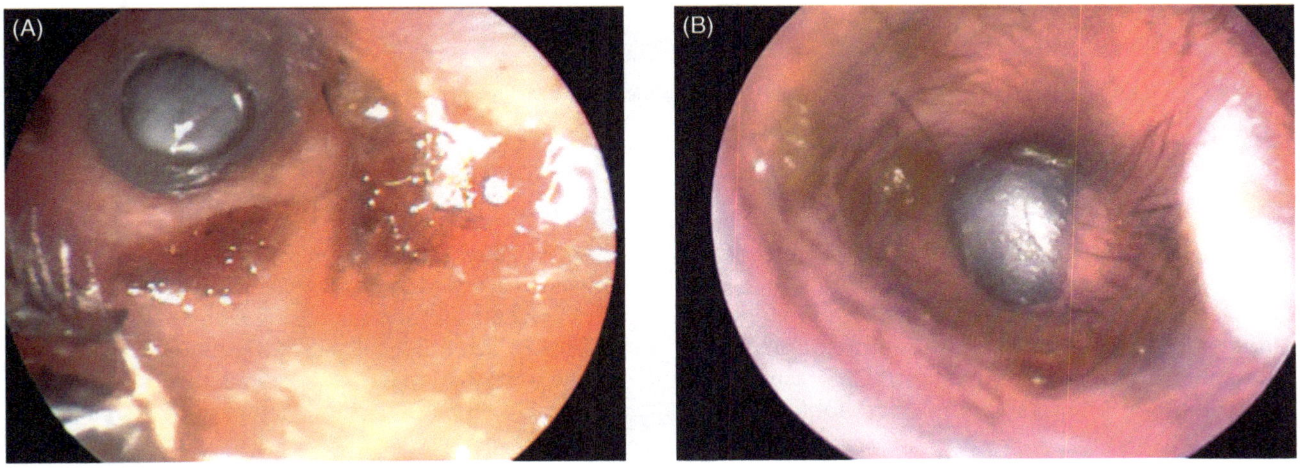

Figures 14.11A and B Middle ear cholesteatomas in two dogs with chronic otitis media.

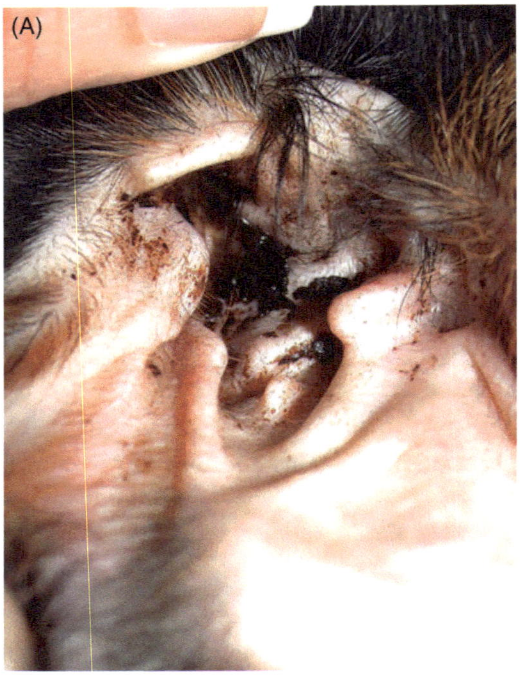

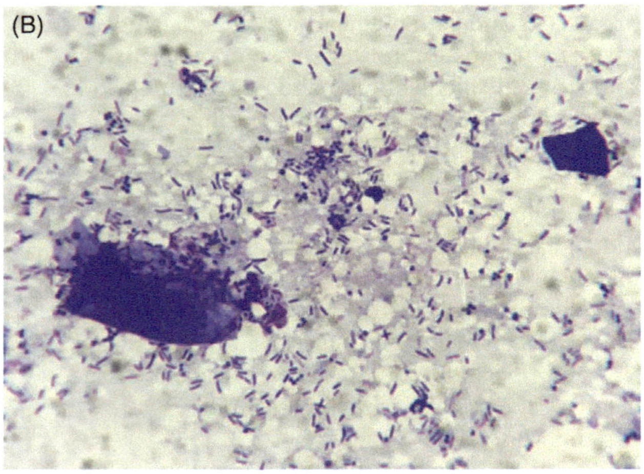

Figures 14.12A and B Clinical and cytological pictures of bacterial otitis externa due to rod bacteria with fewer cocci; atopy was the primary underlying cause. 100×

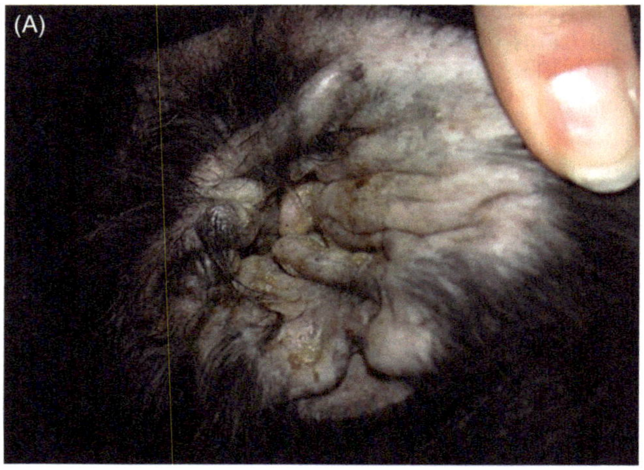

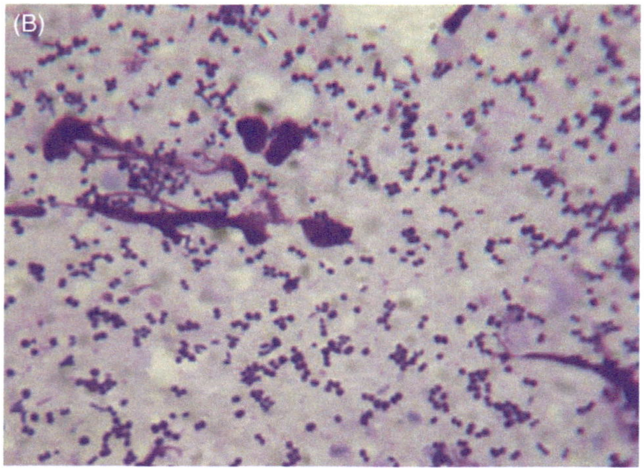

Figures 14.13A and B Clinical and cytological pictures of bacterial otitis externa due to cocci bacteria, likely *Staphylococcus*; atopy was the primary underlying cause. 100×

- Silver sulfadiazine cream diluted 50 : 50 in sterile water had variable effect on BAER.
- Conversely, topical medications which were found to *suppress* BAER in dogs (i.e. were ototoxic) included 1% tobramycin, 2.5% ticarcillin, DSS, carbamide peroxide, and triethanolamine. See Table 14.1 for more information.
- The literature in cats is even more sparse. Topical gentamycin was found to be ototoxic when applied into the bulla at concentrations ranging from 3–10% (Copner Webster, Carroll, Benitez, and McGee, 1971), 2% chlorhexidene was found to be both vestibulotoxic and ototoxic, and 0.05% chlorhexidene was found to be vestibulotoxic (Igarishi and Suzuki, 1985; Igarishi and Oka, 1988a,b).

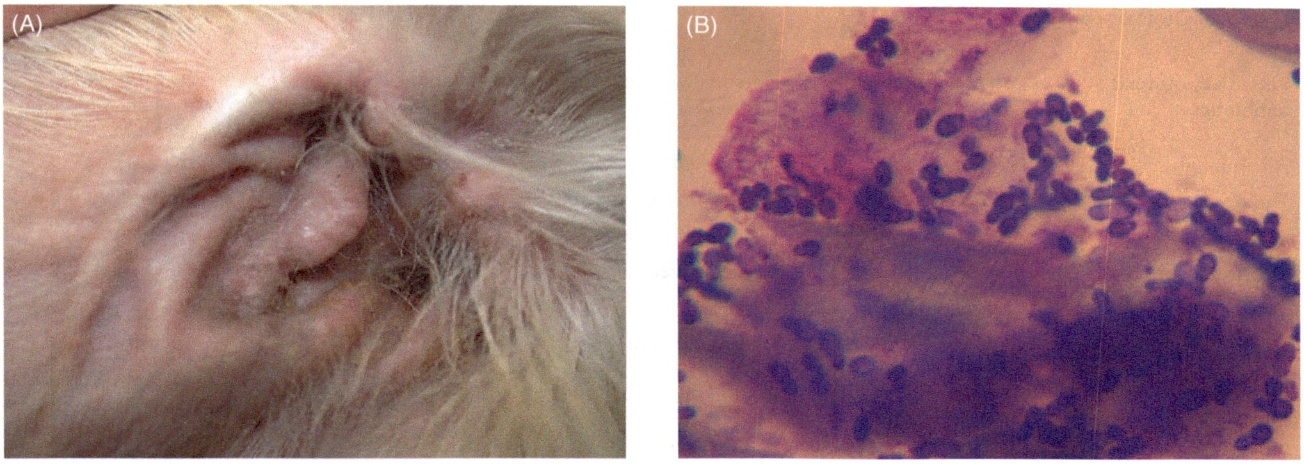

Figures 14.14A and B Clinical and cytological pictures of bacterial otitis externa due to *Malassezia* yeast; atopy was the primary underlying cause. 100×

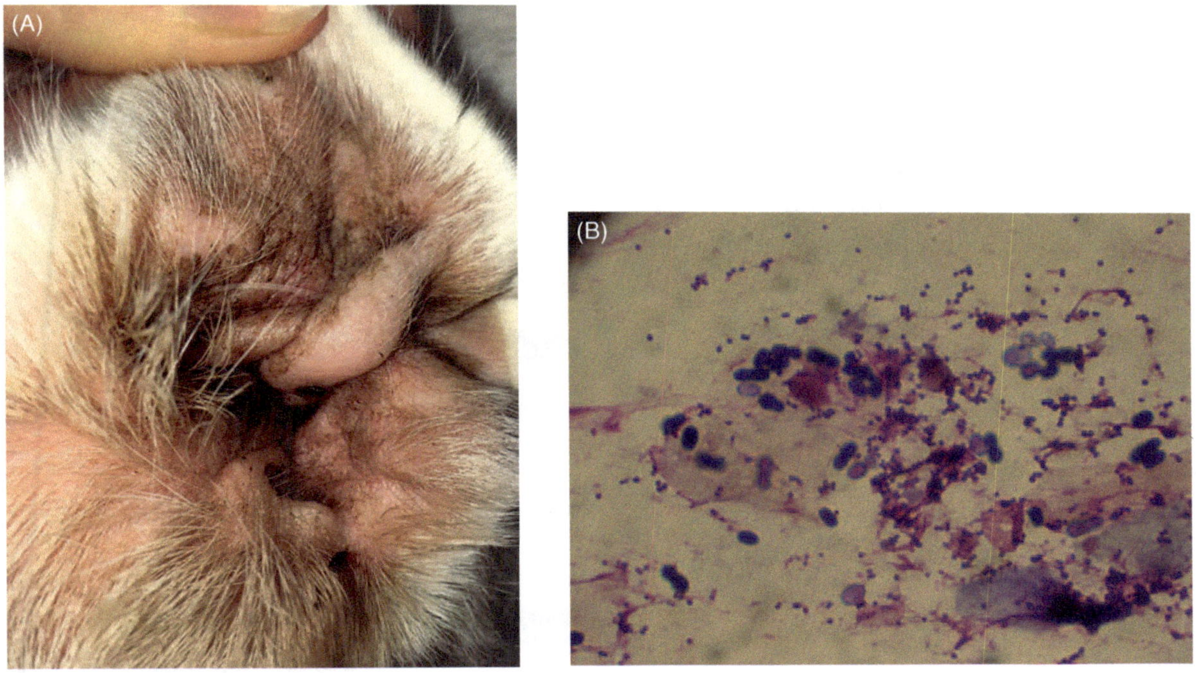

Figures 14.15A and B Clinical and cytological pictures of mixed bacterial and yeast otitis externa; atopy was the primary underlying cause. 100×

- In humans, topical antifungal products which have been found *not* to be ototoxic include clotrimazole, fluconazole, ketoconazole, econazole, and miconazole. Conversely, topical antifungal products which have been found to be *ototoxic* include acetic acid, boric acid, cresylate, and Gentian violet.
- If a patient is presented with symptoms suggestive of ototoxicity, flushing prior otic medications out of the ear canal with warmed sterile 0.9% saline is needed.
- Discontinue all topical otic medications and flushes. There are no published studies on the use of medications to treat ototoxicity, and any information on treatments is anecdotal.
  - In rodent studies, coadministration of steroids or antioxidants such as N-acetylcysteine or glutathione were helpful to reduce ototoxicity of topical or systemic ototoxic medications, but no studies have evaluated utility or efficacy of these medications after ototoxicity has already occurred.

Table 14.1 Ototoxic agents.

Potentially ototoxic antibiotics	Potentially ototoxic antifungals	Potentially ototoxic antiseptics	Potentially ototoxic ceruminolytic agents	Miscellaneous agents
All aminoglycosides	Amphotericin B	Acetic acid	Carbamide peroxide	Cytoxan
Bacitracin	Griseofulvin	Benzalkonium chloride	DSS	Dapsone
Chloramphenicol	Acetic acid	Cetrimide	Propylene glycol	Detergents
Erythromycin	Boric acid	Chlorhexidene	Polyethylene glycol	DMSO
Gramicidin	Cresylate	Ethanol	Triethanolamine	Diphenylhydrazine
Oxytetracycline	Gentian violet	Iodine and iodophors	Toluene	Cisplatin
Minocycline				Potassium bromide
Polymyxin B				Salicylates
Tetracycline				
Ticarcillin				
Vancomycin				

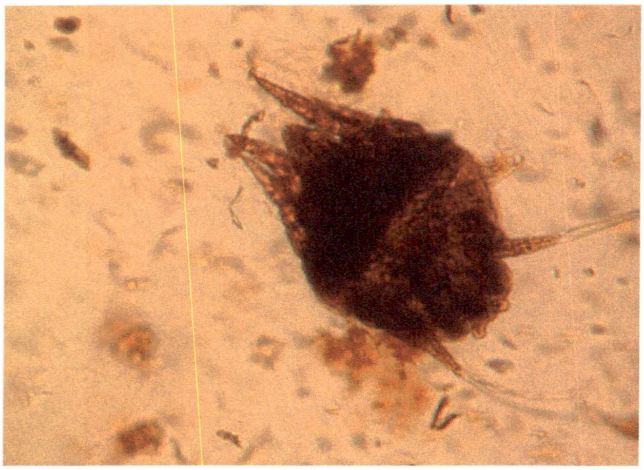

Figure 14.16 *Otodectes cynotis* found in a dog with chronic recurrent otitis externa. 4×

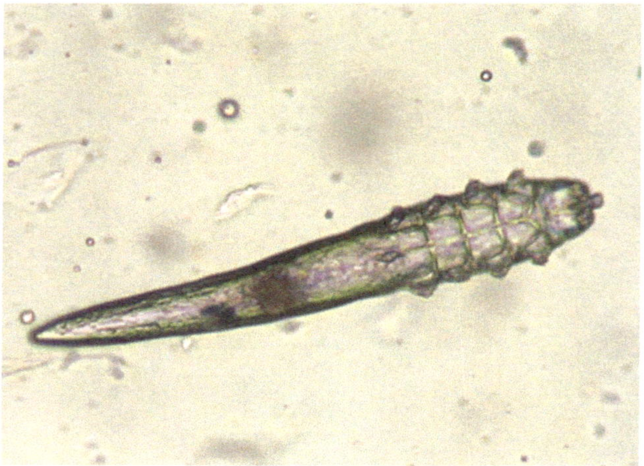

Figure 14.17 A *Demodex canis* mite. 10× with digital zoom.

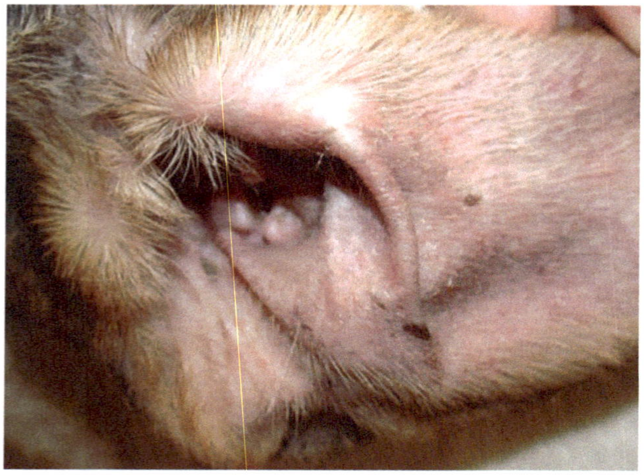

Figure 14.18A Allergic otitis due to atopy in a dog.

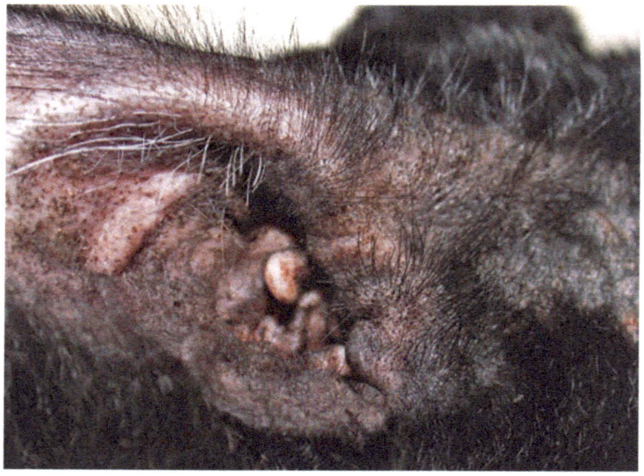

Figure 14.18B Allergic otitis due to atopy in a cat.

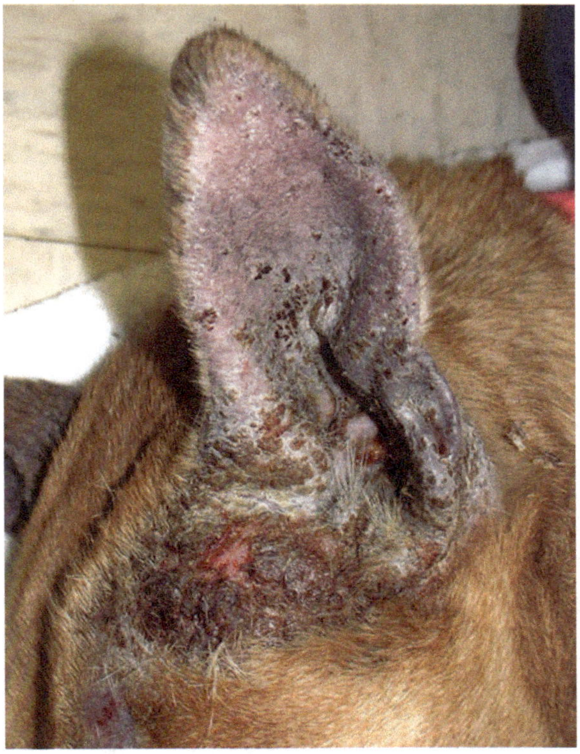

Figure 14.18C Severe inflammation and excoriations in an atopic dog with secondary bacterial otitis externa.

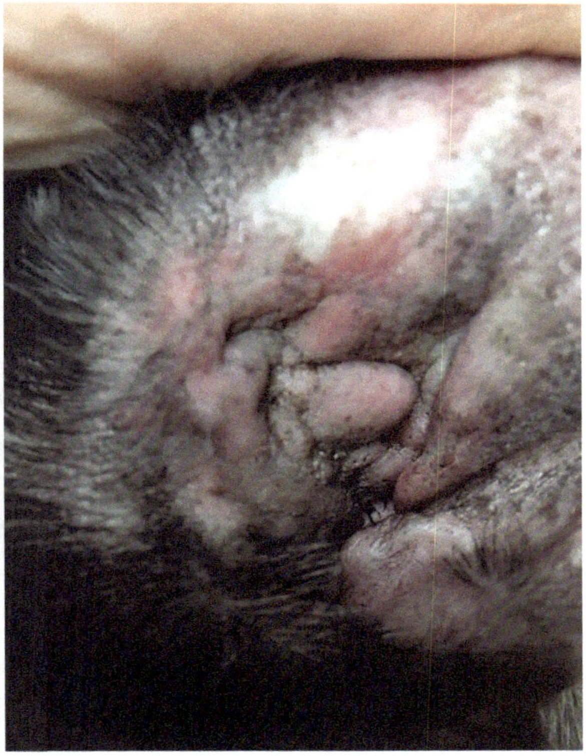

Figure 14.19A A food allergic dog with otitis externa.

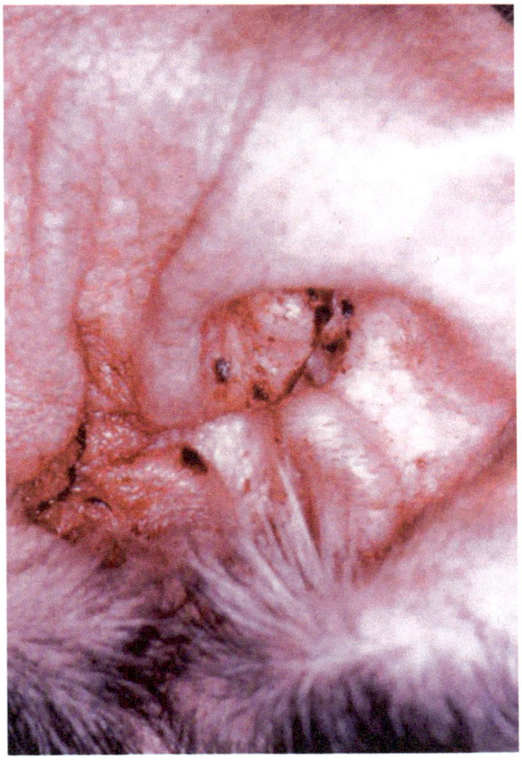

Figure 14.19B A food allergic dog with severe ear canal swelling; the dog was referred for total ear canal ablation.

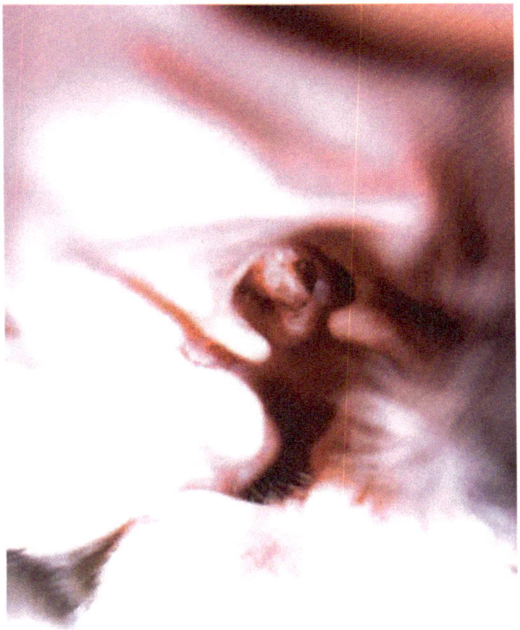

Figure 14.19C The same dog as in Figure 14.19B after a tapering course of steroids, treatment of yeast otitis, and a hypoallergenic diet trial.

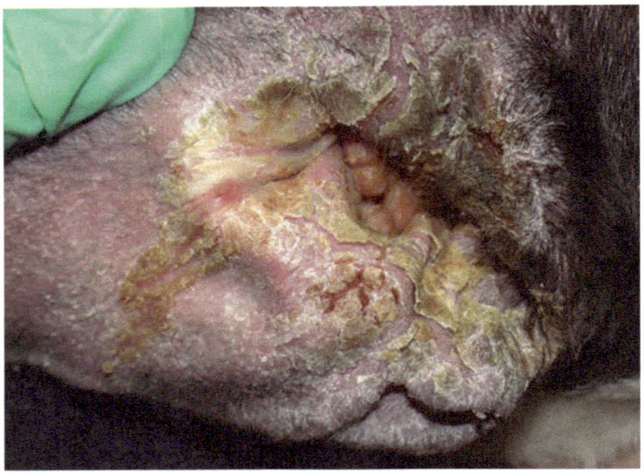

Figure 14.20 This atopic dog had severe bacterial otitis which was complicated by a contact reaction to xenodine ear drops.

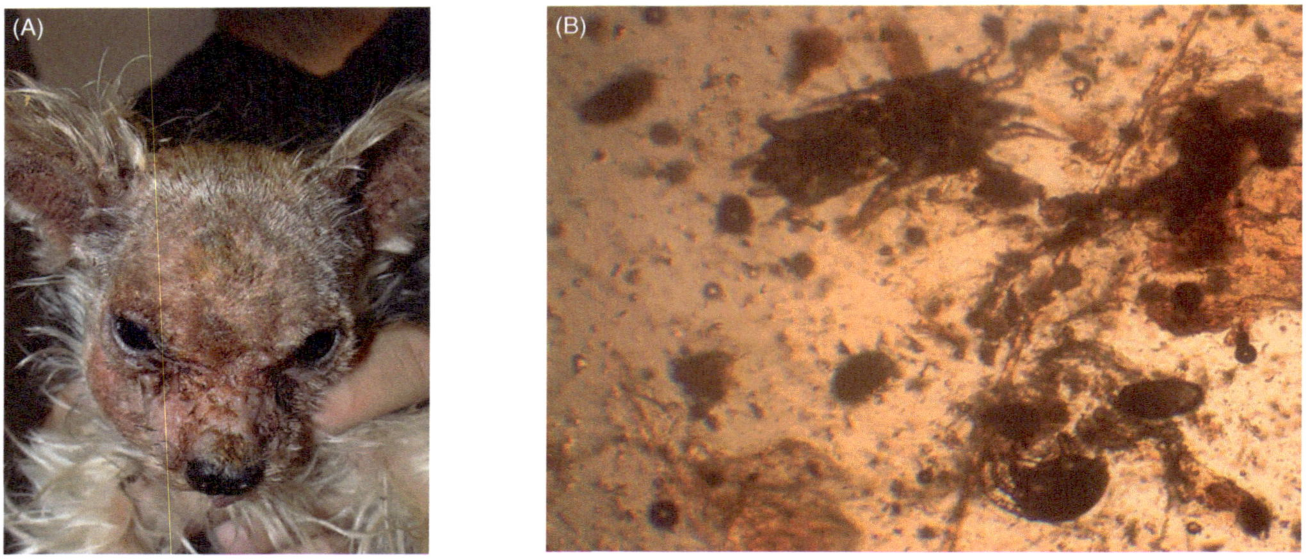

Figure 14.21A and B A dog with severe *Malassezia* otitis and dermatitis triggered by *Otodectes* infestation. (14.21B 4× magnification)

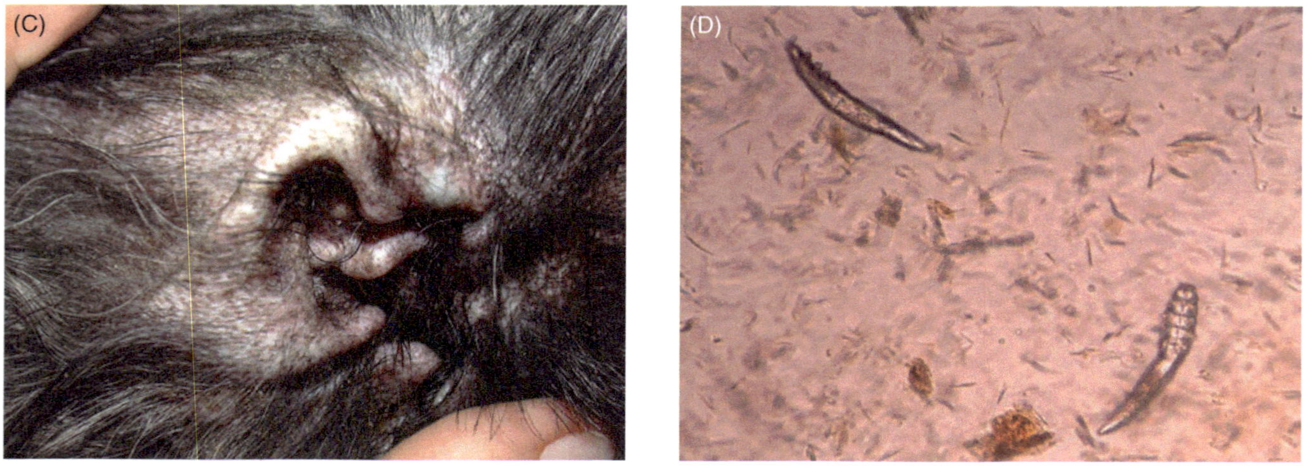

Figures 14.21C and D An elderly dog with otitis externa due to otic demodicosis. (Fig. 14.21D 10× magnification)

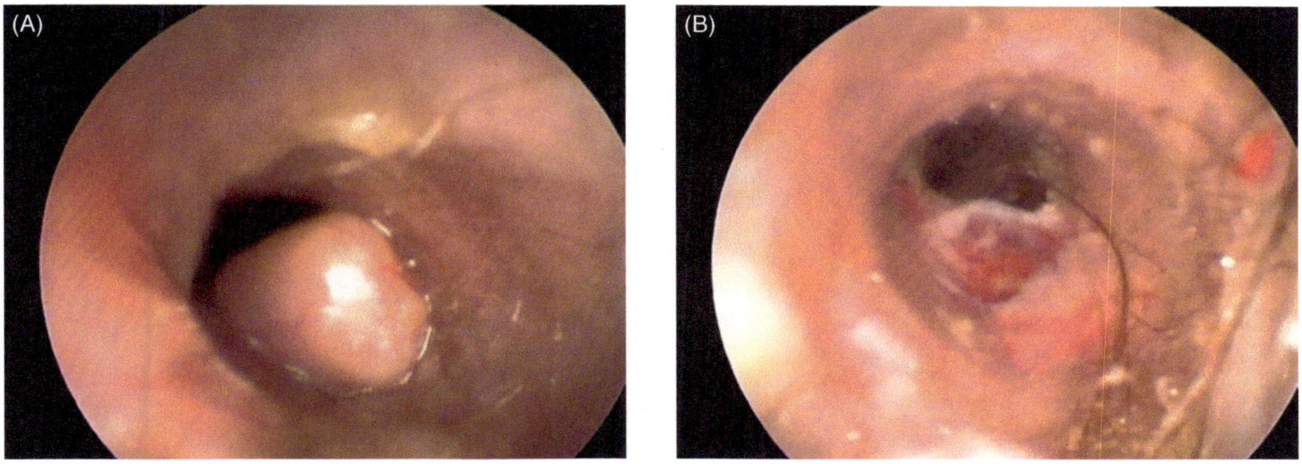

Figures 14.22A and B Chronic allergic and bacterial otitis in a Shih Tzu triggered this benign ear canal tumor which was successfully removed.

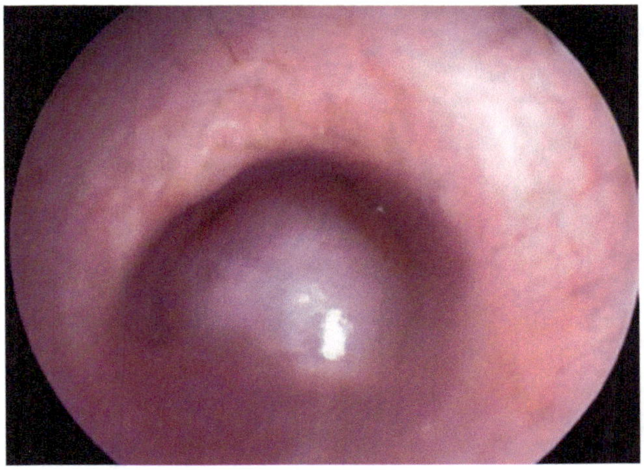

Figure 14.22C An inflammatory otic polyp in a cat.

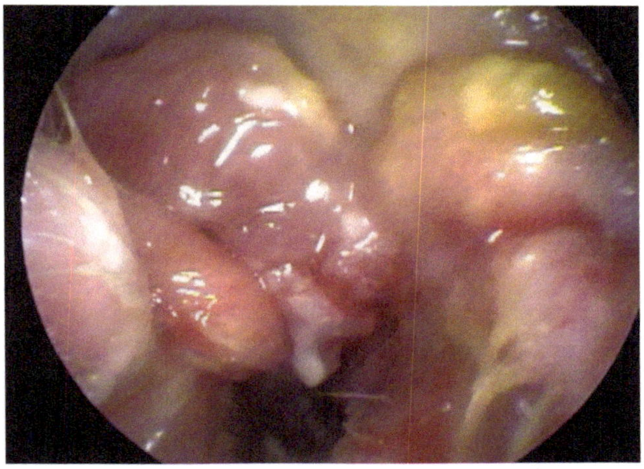

Figure 14.22D Squamous cell carcinoma in the ear of a dog was the trigger for its chronic bacterial otitis.

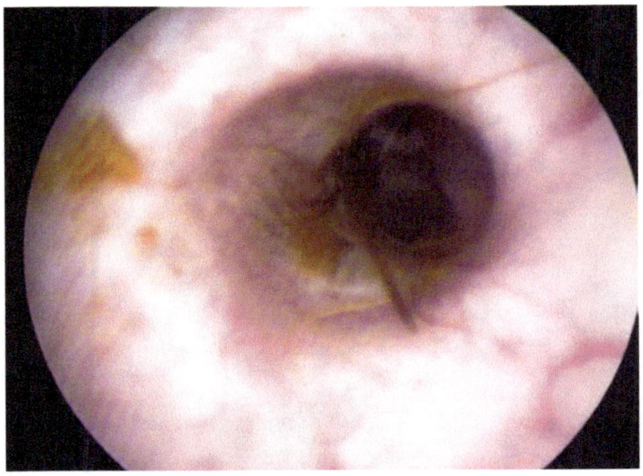

Figure 14.23A This dog had acute head and ear shaking due to a foxtail (grass awn) which can be seen just in front of the tympanum.

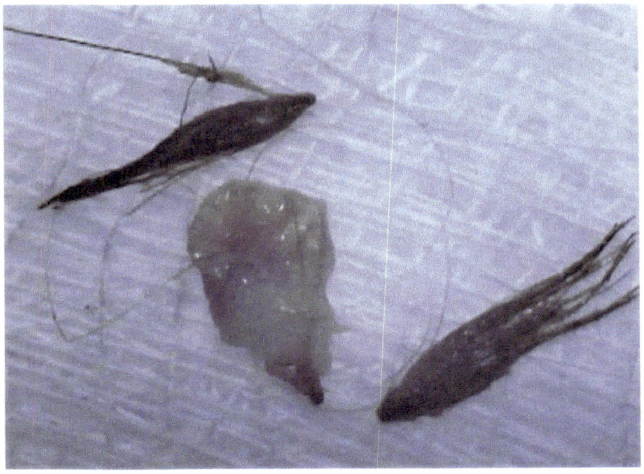

Figure 14.23B In a different case, chronic otitis triggered by foxtails had led to growth of an inflammatory polyp.

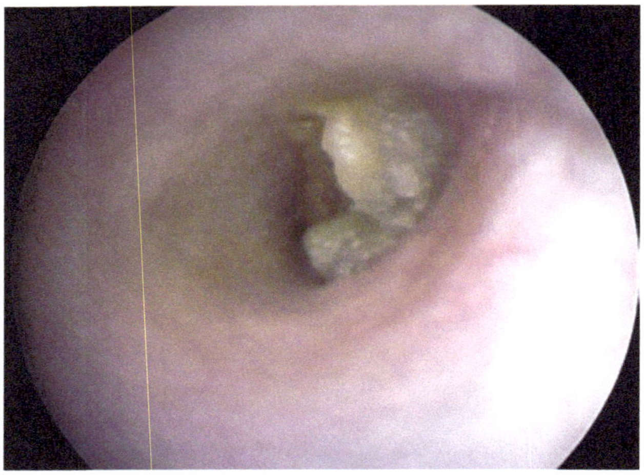

Figure 14.23C This cat was shaking its head/ears due to a ceruminolith which obstructed the horizontal canal.

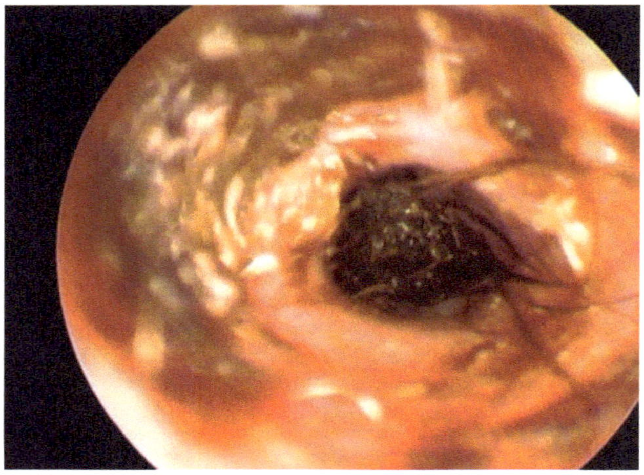

Figure 14.23D A large concretion of fur and cerumen in the ear canal of a dog with chronic *Malassezia* otitis due to underlying atopy.

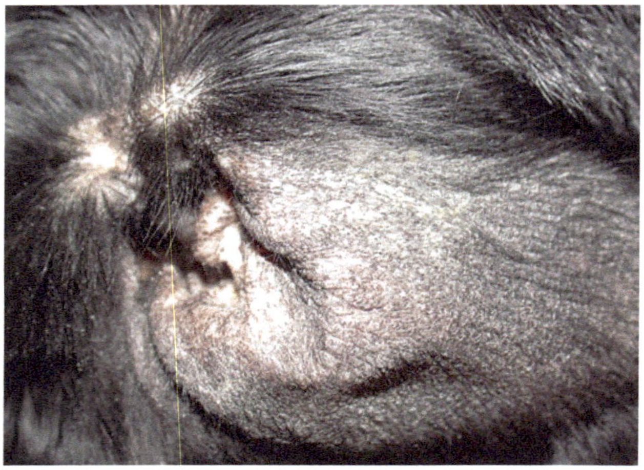

Figure 14.24A Ceruminous otitis externa due to underlying hypothyroidism.

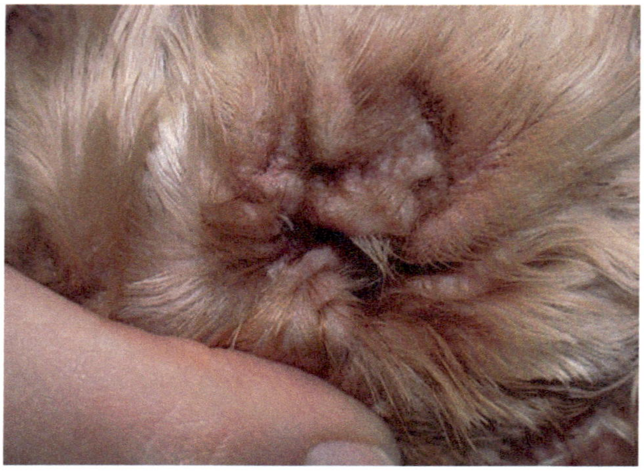

Figure 14.24B Chronic yeast otitis externa triggered by hypothyroidism.

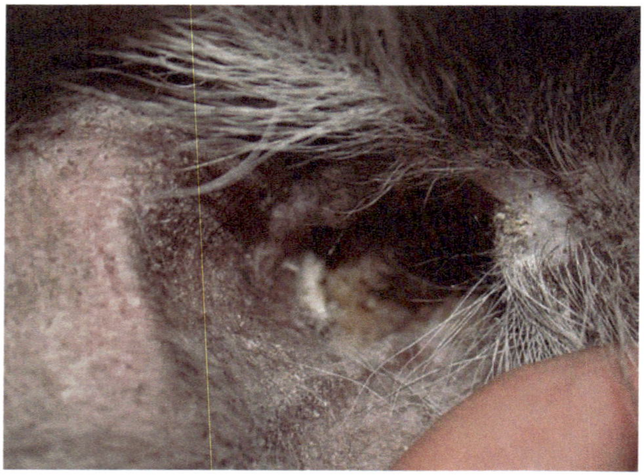

Figure 14.25A Scaling and adherent, brown, epithelial debris on the canal walls of a dog with sebaceous adenitis.

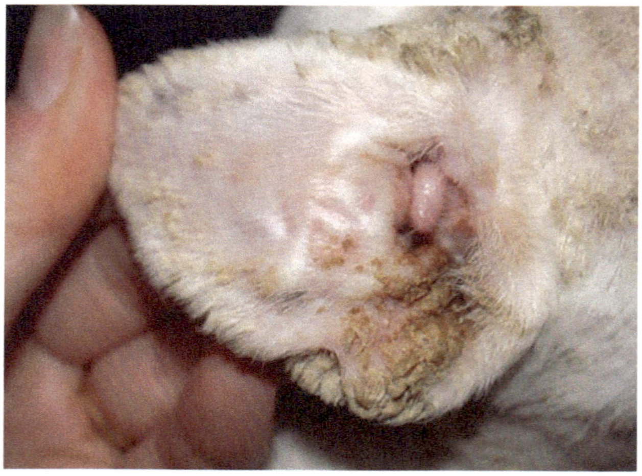

Figure 14.25B Otitis externa due to underlying ichthyosis in a young American Bulldog.

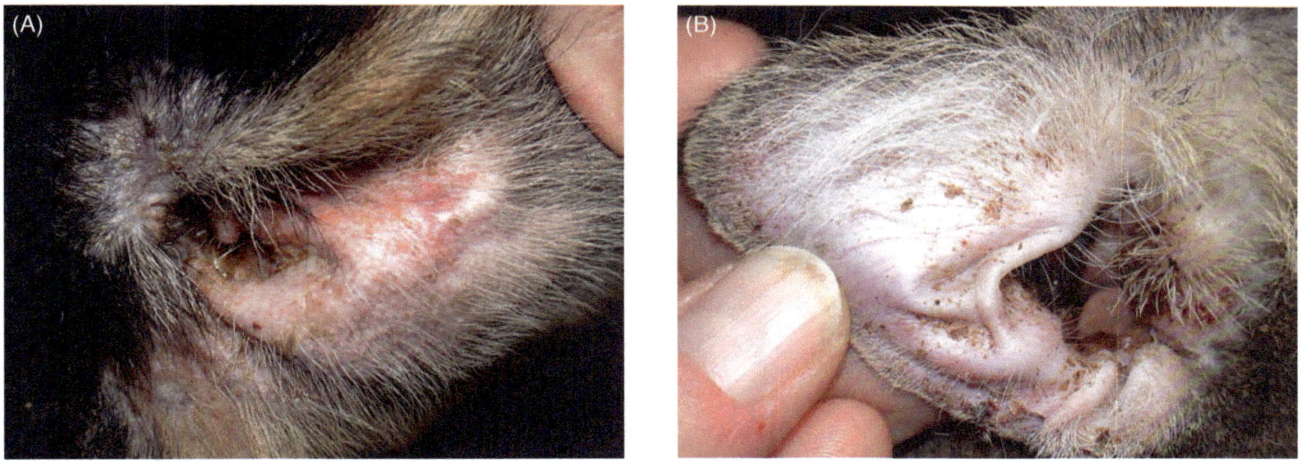

Figure 14.26A and B Otitis externa in a dog (14.26A) and cat (14.26B) with pemphigus foliaceus; typical pustular and crusting lesions were present on the face and trunk as well.

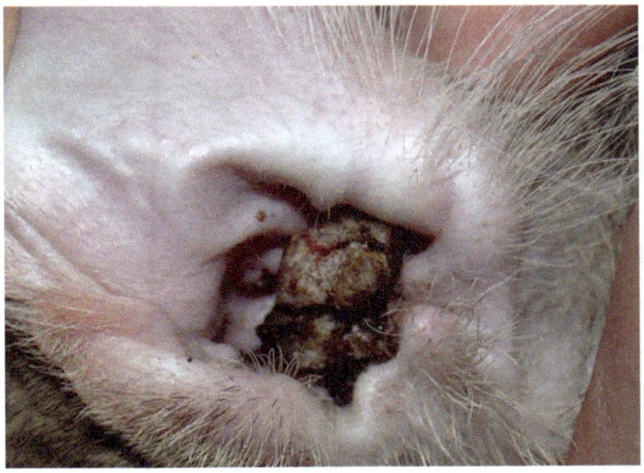

Figure 14.26C Otitis externa in a cat due to proliferative necrotizing otitis externa.

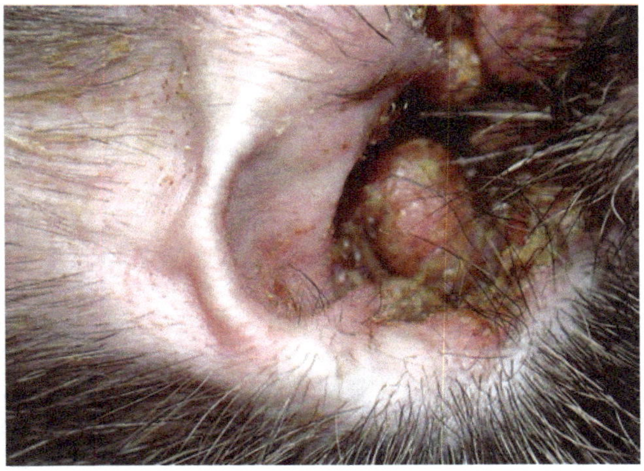

Figure 14.26D Otitis externa due to erythema multiforme.

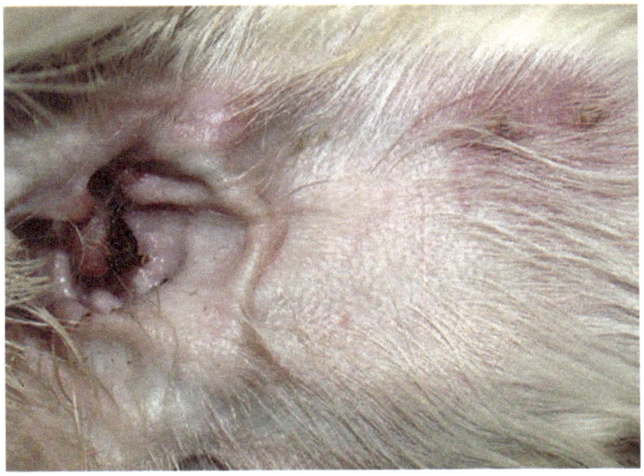

Figure 14.26E Otitis externa and pinnal crusts in a puppy with juvenile cellulitis.

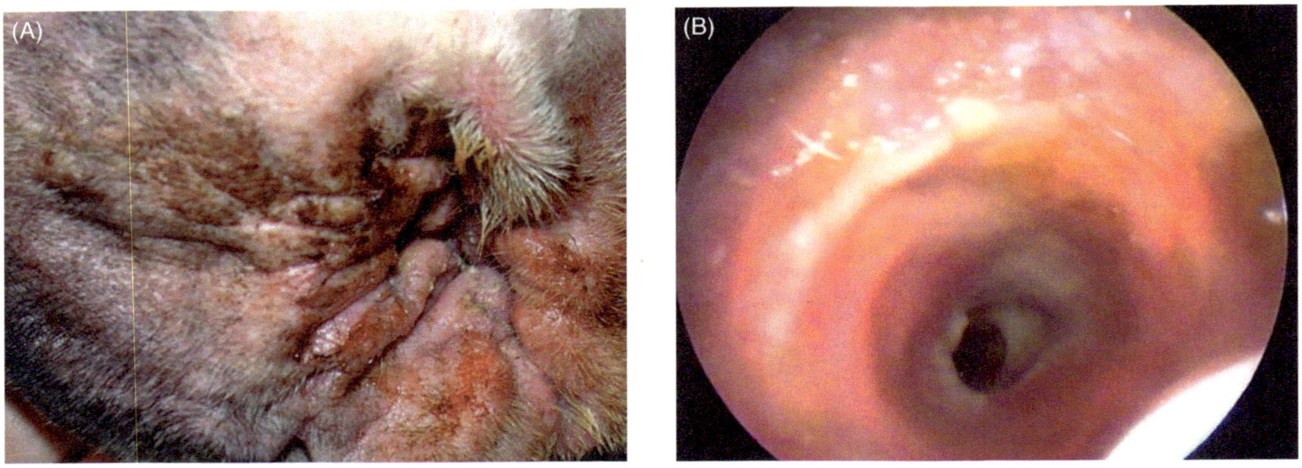

Figure 14.27A and B Severe *Pseudomonas* otitis externa due to underlying atopy; oral and topical steroids in addition to antibiotics are indicated to reduce canal swelling and exudate.

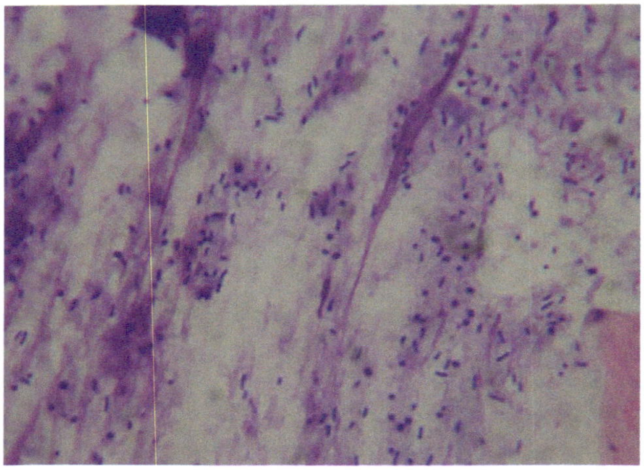

Figure 14.28A Cytology of bacterial otitis. 100×

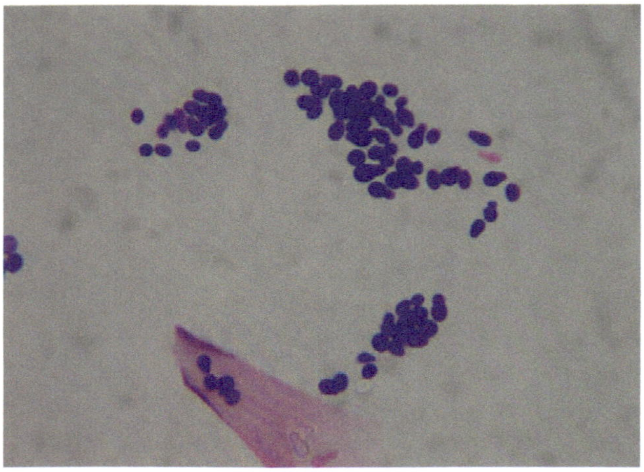

Figure 14.28B Cytology of *Malassezia* otitis. 100×

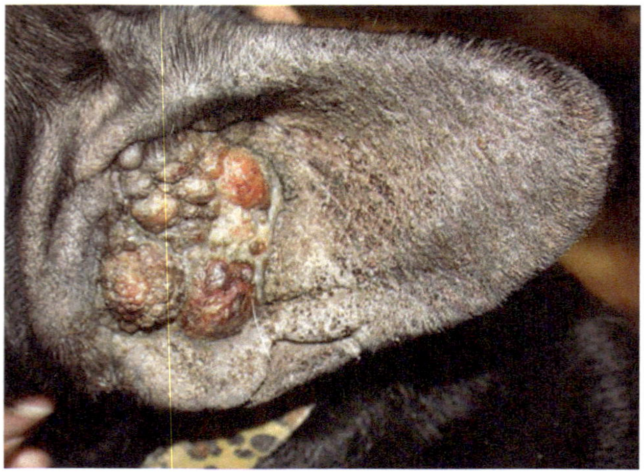

Figure 14.29A End stage proliferative otitis in a young French Bulldog; total ear canal ablation is indicated.

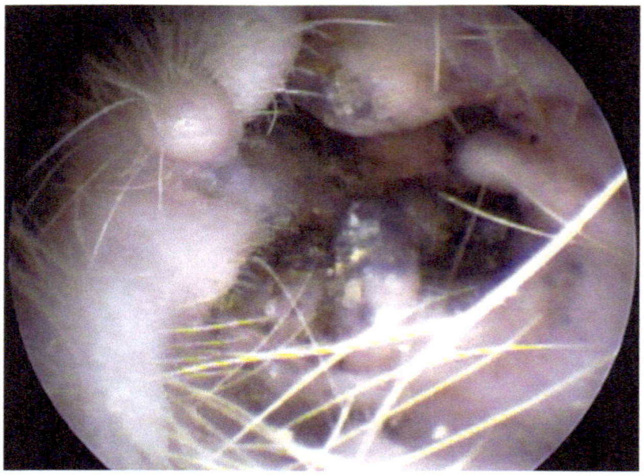

Figure 14.29B This cat has complete ear canal occlusion due to apocrine cystomatosis, total ear canal ablation is indicated.

References/Further reading

Angus, J.C. (2004). Otic cytology in health and disease. *Vet. Clin. North Am. Small Anim. Pract.* 34 (2): 411–424.

Bartlett, S.J., Rosenkrantz, W.S., and Sanchez, S. (2011). Bacterial contamination of commercial ear cleaners following routine home use. *Vet. Dermatol.* 22 (6): 546–553.

Bloom, P. (2009). A practical approach to diagnosing and managing ear disease in dogs. *Compend. Contin. Educ. Vet.* 31 (5): E1–E5.

Cole, L.K. (2004). Otoscopic evaluation of the ear canal. *Vet. Clin. North Am. Small Anim. Pract.* 34 (2): 397–410.

Cole, L.K. (2010). Anatomy and physiology of the canine ear. *Vet. Dermatol.* 21 (2): 221–231.

Cole, L.K., Kwochka, K.W., Kowalski, J.J., and Hillier, A. (1998). Microbial flora and antimicrobial susceptibility patterns of isolated pathogens from the horizontal ear canal and middle ear in dogs with otitis media. *J. Am. Vet. Med. Assoc.* 212 (4): 534–538.

Copner Webster, J., Carroll, R., Benitez, J., and McGee, T. (1971). Ototoxicity of topical gentamicin in the cat. *J. Infect. Dis.*, Supplement: Second International Symposium on Gentamicin: An Aminoglycoside Antibiotic 124: S138–S144.

Gortel, K. (2004). Otic flushing. *Vet. Clin. North Am. Small Anim. Pract.* 34 (2): 557–565.

Gotthelf, L. (2005). *Small Animal Ear Diseases*, 2e. St. Louis: Elsevier.

Gotthelf, L.N. (2004). Diagnosis and treatment of otitis media in dogs and cats. *Vet. Clin. North Am. Small Anim. Pract.* 34 (2): 469–487.

Greci, V., Travetti, O., Di Giancamillo, M. et al. (2011). Middle ear cholesteatoma in 11 dogs. *Can. Vet. J.* 52 (6): 631–636.

Griffin, C. (2009). Otitis: anatomy every practitioner should know. *Compend Contin. Educ. Vet.* 31 (11): 504–512.

Griffin, C.E. (2006). Otitis techniques to improve practice. *Clin. Tech. Small Anim. Pract.* 21 (3): 96–105.

Haynes, D., Rutka, J., Hawke, M., and Roland, P. (2007). Ototoxicity of ototopical drops: an update. *Otolaryngol. Clin. North Am.* 669–683.

Igarashi, Y. and Oka, Y. (1988a). Mucosal injuries following intratympanic application of chlorhexidine gluconate in cats. *Arch. Otorhinolaryngol.* 245 (5): 273–278.

Igarashi, Y. and Oka, Y. (1988b). Vestibular ototoxicity following intratympanic application of chlorhexidine gluconate in the cat. *Arch. Otorhinolaryngol.* 245 (4): 210–217.

Igarashi, Y. and Suzuki, J. (1985). Cochlear ototoxicity of chlorhexidine gluconate in cats. *Arch. Otorhinolaryngol.* 242 (2): 167–176.

Kennis, R.A. (2013). Feline otitis: diagnosis and treatment. *Vet. Clin. North Am. Small Anim. Pract.* 43 (1): 51–56.

Mansfield, P. and Miller, S. (2000). Ototoxicity of topical preparations. In: *Small Animal Ear Diseases*, 2e (ed. L.N. Gotthelf), 149. Elsevier.

Merchant, S., Neer, T., Tedford, B. et al. (1995). Ototoxicity assessment of a topical chlorhexidene otic preparation in dogs. *Prog. Vet. Neurol.* 4: 72–75.

Mansfield, P.D. et al. (1997). The effects of four commercial ceruminolytics on the middle ear. *J. Am. Anim. Hosp. Assoc.* 33: 479–486.

Munguia, R. and Daniel, S.J. (2008). Ototopical antifungals and otomycosis: a review. *Int. J. Pediatr. Otorhinolaryngol.* 72: 453–459.

Murphy, K.M. (2001). A review of techniques for the investigation of otitis externa and otitis media. *Clin. Tech. Small Anim. Pract.* 16 (4): 236–241.

Nuttall, T. and Cole, L.K. (2007). Evidence-based veterinary dermatology: a systematic review of interventions for treatment of *Pseudomonas* otitis in dogs. *Vet. Dermatol.* 18 (2): 69–77.

Paterson S. Safety of otic treatment and cleaners as supported by BAER testing. In: Proceedings of the NAVC Conference 2011.

Paterson, S. (2016). Topical ear treatment - options, indications and limitations of current therapy. *J. Small Anim. Pract.* 57 (12): 668–678.

Paterson, S. and Tobias, K. (2013). *Atlas of Ear Diseases of the Dog and Cat.* Oxford UK: Wiley Blackwell.

Risselada, M. (2016). Diagnosis and management of cholesteatomas in dogs. *Vet. Clin. North Am. Small Anim. Pract.* 46 (4): 623–634.

15

Metabolic/nutritional/keratinization dermatologic disorders

Amy Shumaker, DVM, DACVD

VCA Southshore (Weymouth) Animal Hospital, South Weymouth, MA, USA

Clinical Atlas of Canine and Feline Dermatology, First Edition. Edited by Kimberly S. Coyner.

Companion website: www.wiley.com/go/coyner/dermatology

Table 15.1 Keratinization, metabolic, and nutritional disorders.

Disease	Clinical signs	Additional tests	Diagnosis	Treatment
Seborrhea (secondary) (Figures 15.1–15.14) Most commonly secondary to bacterial or yeast skin infections and other inflammatory skin diseases including demodicosis/ other external parasitism, dermatophytosis, cutaneous lymphoma, atopy; also endocrinopathies, nutritional or keratinization disorders (i.e. sebaceous adenitis, ichthyosis), environmental factors (low humidity).	Seborrhea sicca: Focal, multifocal to diffuse, white to gray nonadherent scales. Coat is generally dry, dull, and flaky. Seborrhea oleosa: Associated with greasy skin and coat, and patients are often malodorous.	Skin scrapings for mites. Cytology: Often associated with bacterial and *Malassezia* infections. In older dogs, lab work should be performed to evaluate for endocrinopathy. Biopsy in cases occurring in very young or very old dogs if screening skin diagnostics/labs are not explanatory.	Clinical signs, results of appropriate diagnostic tests.	Correct underlying cause (e.g. endocrinopathy) and treat secondary infections. Animals with long coats should be clipped for best response to topical therapy. Benzoyl peroxide shampoos can be used for seborrhea oleosa but can be drying with long-term use; change to milder shampoo as condition improves. For seborrhea sicca, hypoallergenic and moisturizing shampoos or sulfur/salicylic acid-based shampoos are helpful, followed by a cream rinse. Antiseborrheic spot on applications also helpful adjunctive therapies.
Vitamin A responsive dermatosis (Figure 15.15) Breed predisposition: Cocker Spaniel.	Most prominent lesions are hyperkeratotic plaques with superficial fronds and follicular plugging. Additional lesions include scaling, crusting, alopecia, and papules.	Pyoderma and *Malassezia* can appear similar; cytology and treatment of any secondary infection should be performed before consideration of this disease and biopsy.	Clinical signs, ruling out and treating secondary infections. Biopsy: Marked follicular hyperkeratosis.	1000 IU/kg vitamin A daily with fatty meal until resolution; can often decrease to every other day for maintenance.
Sebaceous adenitis (Figure 15.12, Figures 15.16A–D; Chapter 2, Figure 2.41A and 2.41B; Chapter 3, Figures 3.45, 3.51, 3.84, 3.110; Chapter 6, Figures 6.33A and 6.33B and 6.56A and 6.56B)	Various presentations and can vary based on breed and type of coat (short coat vs. long coat). Symptoms can wax and wane. Long-coated breeds (Poodles, Akitas, German Shepherd Dogs, Samoyed) may initially just have coat color changes or straightening of coat.		Biopsy: Granulomatous inflammation targeted at sebaceous glands, secondary follicular and epidermal hyperkeratosis; complete loss of sebaceous glands in chronic cases.	Topical moisturizing antiseborrheic/ keratolytic shampoos (avoid benzoyl peroxide and tar), humectants, or oil treatments are recommended for all cases, are synergistic with cyclosporine, and reduce scaling more effectively than cyclosporine alone. Spot on lipid treatments may be helpful between baths.

Breed predisposition: Akita, Standard Poodles, Vizslas, German Shepherds, Samoyeds, Springer Spaniels, Havanese. Male predilection in some breeds.	Progression to dull, dry, brittle coat with scaling, follicular casting and hypotrichosis to alopecia. Secondary infection often present. Pruritus is variable. Short-coated breeds (Vizslas), lesions often present as annular areas of scaling and alopecia, often coalescing. Nonadherent, fine scaling present and follicular casting varies. Lesions generally affect head, base of pinnae, dorsum, but generally spares the limbs. Cats: Multifocal patches of scales, crusts, follicular casts, and alopecia. Lesions generally start on the head and neck and progress to body.			Oral omega-6 and Omega-3 supplementation. Oral vitamin A daily 1000 IU/kg +/− isotretinoin. Cyclosporine 5 mg/kg/day PO is the only treatment documented to cause regeneration of sebaceous glands histologically. Combo of vitamin A with tetracycline or doxycycline and niacinamide may be helpful in some cases.
Schnauzer comedo syndrome (Chapter 2, Figure 2.47; Chapter 3, Figure 3.108; Chapter 6, Figure 6.44)	Comedones along dorsum.	Skin scrapings for mites, cytology for infection.	Clinical signs, biopsy. Cytology to rule out secondary infections. Senior labwork in older dogs to rule out endocrinopathy.	Topical treatment of affected dorsum with cleansing and antiseborrheic products especially benzoyl peroxide or sulfur. Bathe twice weekly × 1 month then once weekly for maintenance. Use benzoyl peroxide only on affected areas to prevent excessive drying. Use human acne pads daily between baths. Control secondary bacterial infections with topical chlorhexidine spray/mousse/wipes or alternating chlorhexidine shampoo with antiseborrheic shampoo.

(*Continued*)

Table 15.1 Keratinization, metabolic, and nutritional disorders (Continued)

Disease	Clinical signs	Additional tests	Diagnosis	Treatment
Nasodigital hyperkeratosis (Figure 15.17; Chapter 3, Figure 3.2; Chapter 6, Figures 6.14A and 6.14B) Older dogs, Cocker Spaniels, Boxers, and English Bulldogs predisposed.	This condition can result as an inherited disorder, concurrent with other disorders, due to breed anatomic abnormalities (brachycephalic breeds), or due to senile changes. The nasal planum becomes dry, hard, and hyperkeratotic (thick crusts). Fissures, erosions, and ulcers may develop. The digital pads can develop hyperkeratotic changes involving the entire pad, however, more frequently involves the margins of weight bearing pads, and accessory carpal and tarsal pads. Pads can develop fissures and erosions and result in lameness.		Clinical signs, cytology to rule out nasal mucocutaneous pyoderma. Senior labwork with thyroid profile in older animals. Biopsy: Need to rule out possible other diseases that can cause crusting/ hyperkeratosis including pemphigus, zinc-responsive dermatitis, drug eruptions, infections, cutaneous lymphoma.	Severe cases may need trimming with scissors or scalpel blade; presoaking with propylene glycol can be helpful. Frequent use of hydration followed by antiseborrheic topicals; soak paws/nose in water or apply wet compress to hydrate then apply a keratolytic agent (50% propylene glycol, salicylic acid), or a balm containing vegetable and essential oils), +/− tretinoin gel. Apply daily until adequate hydration then as needed for maintenance.
Callus (Figure 15.18; Chapter 3, Figure 3.87)	Round to oval, hyperkeratotic, lichenified plaque generally overlying bony prominences, primarily the elbows and hocks. Deep-chested dogs (e.g. Great Danes) may be subject to callus formation on the sternum. Laying on harder and/or rough surfaces is a predisposing factor. Callus formation is a normal protective response of the skin to damage and inflammation induced from pressure. Can become secondarily infected. Hygromas, fluid-filled sacs/bursas, may also be a sequela to repeated trauma over pressure points.	May need to consider skin scrapes to rule out demodicosis or DTM to rule out dermatophytosis if lesion is at an unusual location (can occur if patient sits or lays in an unusual position).	Often diagnosed based on clinical signs and location.	Encourage the patient to lay on padded surfaces. Can use special wraps that are padded for that site (e.g. elbow pad). Surgical correction should be done with caution as these are mobile sites and generally sites that would create tension on sutures.

Xeromycteria (a.k.a. parasympathetic nose, neurogenic KCS (keratoconjunctivitis sicca)) (Figure 15.19; Chapter 3, Figure 3.5)	Unilateral drying, crusting, and hyperkeratosis of the nasal planum due to impaired innervation of the lacrimal gland secondary to an inflammatory, traumatic, or neoplastic process or can be secondary to otitis media.	Schirmer's tear test may be low on the ipsilateral side.	Clinical signs, cytology to rule out nasal mucocutaneous pyoderma.	Topical hydrating therapies as for idiopathic nasodigital hyperkeratosis. Pilocarpine 2% ophthalmic 1–2 drops PO in food daily. Lubrication of the affected eye with ophthalmic emollients.
Ear margin dermatosis (Chapter 3, Figure 3.36) Predisposed breeds: Dachshunds, dogs with pendulous ears.	Seborrhea/follicular casting +/− patchy alopecia occurs on pinnal margins. Can progress to thickened adherent debris/fissuring and discomfort, head shaking/ear tip trauma.	Skin scrapings for mites, cytology for secondary infection.	Consider signalment, clinical signs. Biopsy: Marked surface and follicular ortho- or parakeratotic hyperkeratosis. If pinnal marginal ulceration is present then this is consistent with a pinnal vasculitis and not seborrhea.	Soften hardened debris with water then gently wash with keratolytic shampoo (benzoyl peroxide or sulfur/salicylic acid) followed by a hydrating conditioner (+/− application of a steroid cream or ointment if pinnal inflammation results from the shampoo) QOD until debris is removed, then prn for control. 1–2 times weekly application of spot on antiseborrheic treatments may be helpful.
Canine acne (Figures 15.20A–15.20D) Predisposed breeds (short-coated breeds): Bulldogs, Boxers, Doberman Pinschers, Great Danes, etc.	Chin and lip papules that can enlarge (progress to furuncles) that can drain and ulcerate. Local trauma/rubbing of the chin (during play, chewing toys, etc.) pushes the short muzzle hairs under the skin, creating furunculosis.	Skin scrapings/hair plucks to rule out demodicosis. Cytology to evaluate for secondary infection.	Clinical appearance, appropriate skin diagnostics.	With mild lesions (early onset) may respond to behavior modification to prevent self-trauma. Benzoyl peroxide shampoos, gels, or wipes can be used daily initially until resolution then as needed. Secondary infections should be treated with topical therapies (mupirocin ointment, benzoyl peroxide) +/− a 4–6 week course of oral antibiotics in severe cases. Topical steroids (fluocinolone with DMSO or betamethasone) can be used daily until remission then tapered. A 2 week course of tapering oral corticosteroids can be helpful in more severe cases.

(*Continued*)

Table 15.1 Keratinization, metabolic, and nutritional disorders (Continued)

Disease	Clinical signs	Additional tests	Diagnosis	Treatment
Feline acne (Figures 15.21A–15.21C; Chapter 3, Figure 3.34) Affects cats of any age or gender status.	Clinical signs vary from presence of comedones on chin and occasionally upper lips to progression of papules, pustules, folliculitis/furunculosis, and cellulitis. Lesions can be associated with secondary bacterial or *Malassezia* infections or dermatophytes. Follicular cysts may develop. Scarring may occur in severe cases. Pruritus is variable and often present in more severely affected animals.	Cytology +/− cultures to evaluate presence of bacteria and *Malassezia*. Dermatophyte culture, skin scrapings for feline *Demodex*.	Clinical signs, appropriate diagnostic tests to rule out infection.	Treatment is based on severity of presentation: Comedone phase: Can use antiseborrheic wipes or human acne wipes; caution with benzoyl peroxide products which can cause irritation. Papular/cystic phase: May need topical medicated cream/ointment (clindamycin, erythromycin, metronidazole, or mupirocin). Topical retinoic acids can be helpful applied daily for 4 weeks then every other day to twice weekly for maintenance. Steroids can be used in cases with severe inflammation: Prednisolone/ methylprednisolone 1 mg/kg/day tapering q5 days or dexamethasone SP injection at 0.2 mg/kg IM or SC. Oral isotretinoin (2 mg/kg/d) in refractory cases.
Zinc responsive dermatosis (Figures 15.22A–15.22C; Chapter 2, Figure 2.40; Chapter 3, Figures 3.20, 3.39, 3.44, 3.62; Chapter 6, Figures 6.4, 6.34) Breed predisposition: Alaskan Malamutes and Siberian Huskies (Syndrome I).	Focal to multifocal areas, erythema, alopecia, crusts, and scaling. Most commonly affected areas are mucocutaneous junctions, distal extremities, footpads (hyperkeratosis), and frictional areas. Secondary infections are common. Pruritus is often present. Two syndromes: Syndrome I: Zinc malabsorption. Syndrome II: In rapidly growing dogs/young adults fed zinc-deficient diet, a diet high in phytates or minerals that interfere with zinc absorption.	Screen dietary history to ensure that a balanced AAFCO (American Association of Feed Control Officers) diet is being fed without unnecessary supplements; avoid diets high in phytates/grains and boutique diets without AAFCO certification. Skin scrapings/plucks to rule out *Demodex* and skin cytology for secondary infections.	Consider breed, diet history, appropriate diagnostics for infection. Biopsy: Marked epidermal and follicular parakeratosis.	Syndrome II: Dietary modification. Syndrome I: Oral zinc methionine or zinc sulfate dose based on elemental zinc content 2–3 mg/kg/day with food • Zinc methionine is 21% zinc, so 238 mg zinc methionine contains 50 mg elemental zinc. • Zinc sulfate is 23% zinc, so 110 mg zinc sulfate contains 25 mg elemental zinc. • Zinc gluconate is 14.3% zinc, so 100 mg zinc gluconate contains 14 mg elemental zinc. if poor response can add in low dose corticosteroids to increase absorption. Daily essential fatty acids can be helpful. Intact female dogs may benefit from neutering.

Necrolytic migratory erythema (Figure 15.23; Chapter 2, Figure 2.71; Chapter 3, Figures 3.4, 3.21, 3.63, 3.90C) a.k.a. superficial necrolytic dermatitis, metabolic epidermal necrosis, or hepatocutaneous syndrome.	Erythema, crusting, and ulceration often involving the muzzle, distal limbs, elbows, hocks, and ventrum. Crusting and erosion of mucocutaneous junctions (oral, genital, anal). Footpads are often crusted and hyperkeratotic and may be very pruritic. Occurs due to end stage liver disease or pancreatic glucagonoma; may have concurrent signs of systemic illness, or polyuria and polydipsia subsequent to concurrent diabetes mellitus.	CBC may reveal anemia; chemistry panel may reveal elevated liver enzymes, hyperglycemia, elevated bile acids, hypoalbuminemia. Cytology of crusted skin lesions and paws often showed secondary pyoderma and/or *Malassezia* infections.	Skin biopsy: Marked parakeratotic hyperkeratosis overlying inter/intracellular epidermal edema and basal epidermal cell hyperplasia. Abdominal ultrasound may reveal a "swiss cheese" or "honey-comb" vacuolar pattern to the liver or may reveal a pancreatic tumor. Amino acid levels: Low (especially glutamine and arginine).	For glucagonoma: Surgical excision of an identifiable glucagonoma. If nonoperable, treatment with octreotide initially at 2 ug/kg SQ BID. For hepatic disease, supportive medications can include: S-adenosylmethionine (sAME) 18–22 mg/kg PO daily, vitamin E 400 IU PO q12 hr, ursodiol 10 mg/kg/day PO. Nutritional supplementation 1 whole egg/4.5 kg/day, oral zinc supplementation and fatty acids can be helpful. Parenteral amino acid supplementation may be beneficial (Aminosyn® or procalamine at 25 ml/kg IV over 6–8 hours); repeat 1–2 times weekly until clinical improvement then give q2–6 weeks for control. Glucocorticoids can temporarily reduce skin inflammation but are not recommended as they can precipitate or worsen diabetes mellitus. Oral amino acid supplementation anecdotally helpful; specific products include Promod® (hydrolyzed collagen), at a dose of 1 scoop per 10 pounds of dog per day; or Procel (whey protein) 1 tsp. per 20–25 lb of dog per day.
Exfoliative dermatitis associated with thymoma (Figures 15.24A–15.24D) Usually middle to older aged cats.	Non-pruritic to mildly pruritic scaling/crusting that starts on head/ neck and becomes generalized. Can develop brown sebaceous debris on claw folds, interdigital skin, periocular, and perioral areas. Secondary yeast overgrowth can cause pruritus.	Skin changes precede signs of tumor; can see dyspnea, coughing, decrease in appetite and weight. Rare reports of concurrent myasthenia gravis and megaesophagus.	Skin scrapings, cytology, dermatophyte culture to rule out infections. Biopsy: Interface dermatitis with apoptosis which can mimic erythema multiforme and graft vs. host disease but less apoptosis noted in exfoliative dermatitis. Radiographs or ultrasound evaluation can reveal mediastinal thymoma.	Resection of thymoma leads to resolution of symptoms. There are some cases of exfoliative dermatitis that were NOT associated with underlying thymoma; thymoma may just be one cause of this reaction pattern.

(*Continued*)

Table 15.1 Keratinization, metabolic, and nutritional disorders (Continued)

Disease	Clinical signs	Additional tests	Diagnosis	Treatment
Xanthomas (Figure 15.25)	Small, white to yellow papules, nodules with surrounding erythema. Rarely diffuse dermal thickening. Most often on head, extremities, bony prominences. May be pruritic or painful.	Usually secondary to hyperlipidemia (as from diabetes mellitus, glucocorticoid use, progesterone administration or feeding a high fat diet); can be secondary to idiopathic hyperlipidemia. Rare cases in metabolically healthy cats.	Fine needle aspirates. Biopsy: Infiltration of foamy macrophages, presence of multinucleate giant cells.	Treat underlying condition (e.g. address diabetes, feed prescription low fat diet for idiopathic hypertriglyceridemia). Minimize trauma to the skin.
Split paw pad disease (Figure 15.26) Suspected to be related to an anatomical defect in paw pad cornification; exposure to moisture and friction can precipitate splitting event. Young adult dogs are affected.	Splitting of paw pad and loss of superficial layers of pad in an axis parallel to contact surface; pain or pruritus cause subsequent self-trauma which exacerbates paw pad trauma. Often starts with one pad then similar lesions develop on other pads. Repeated episodes can lead to irregular hyperkeratotic pads. Adjacent haired skin is normal and no lesions are present on other parts of the body. Lameness often occurs but resolves when pads heal and dogs are normal between events.		Biopsy (of leading edge/ margin of the split): Necrosis of superficial epidermis resembling a burn; separation of necrotic epidermis from underlying viable epidermis, ulceration and crusting occur.	Immunosuppressive medications are of no benefit since this is not an immune-mediated condition. Protective boots, walking on soft surfaces, and avoidance of moisture can be helpful. When lesions occur, treat symptoms with pain medications and an Elizabethan collar to prevent self-trauma until pad heals. Topical mupirocin antibiotic ointment and dilute chlorhexidine soaks can be used if secondary infection occurs; routine use of oral antibiotics is not recommended due to risk of promoting antibiotic resistance.

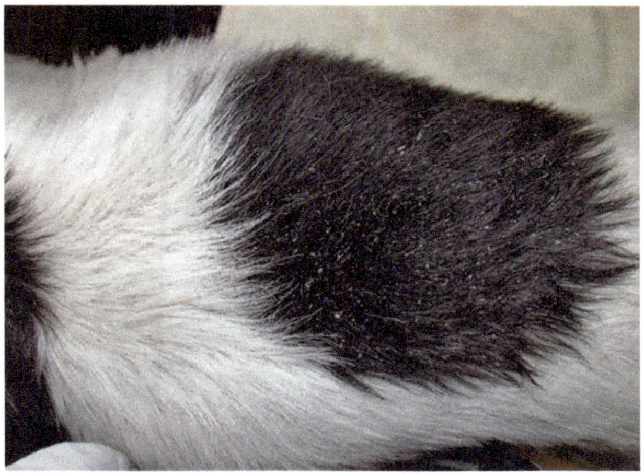

Figure 15.1 Fine, greasy, dorsal truncal seborrhea secondary to a bacterial skin infection.

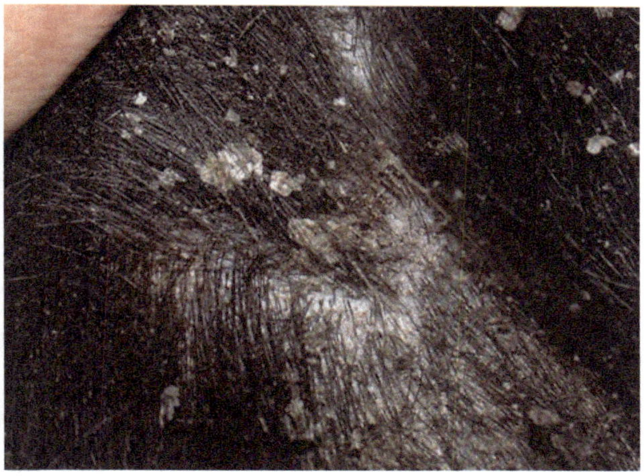

Figure 15.2 Larger, greasy, truncal scaling due to bacterial pyoderma secondary to atopic dermatitis.

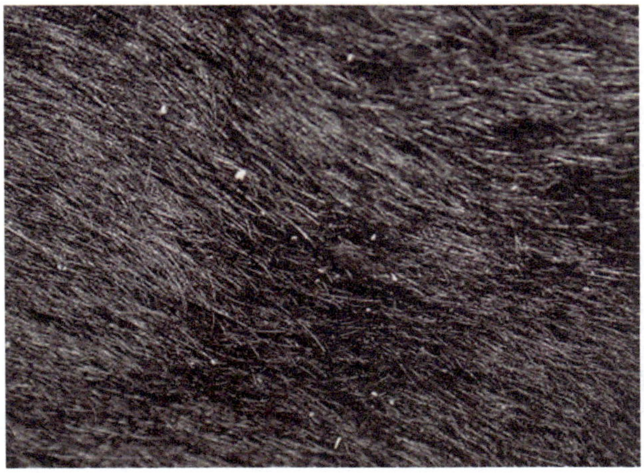

Figure 15.3A This atopic Cocker Spaniel had generalized, fine, dry, truncal scaling and was very pruritic despite oclacitinib.

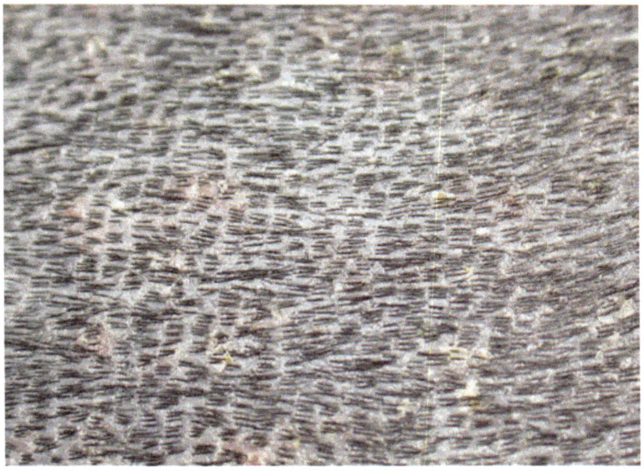

Figure 15.3B When the dog was shaved for intradermal allergy testing, a generalized bacterial truncal folliculitis was revealed as the cause for the scaling and itch.

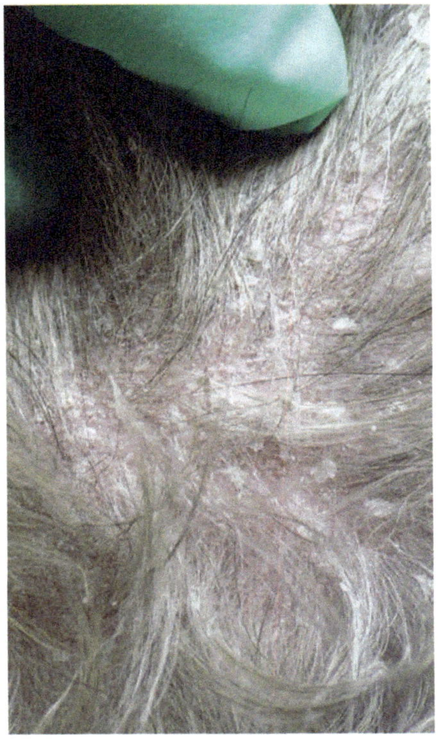

Figure 15.4 Greasy, adherent scaling due to bacterial pyoderma secondary to atopic dermatitis.

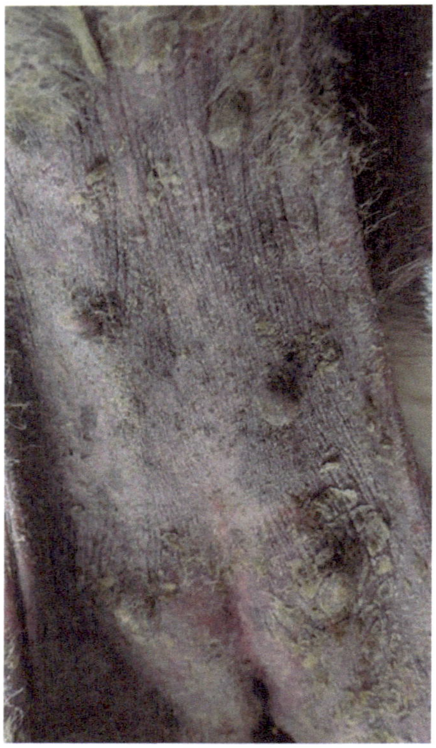

Figure 15.5 Oily seborrhea due to bacterial and yeast skin infections secondary to underlying hypothyroidism and atopy.

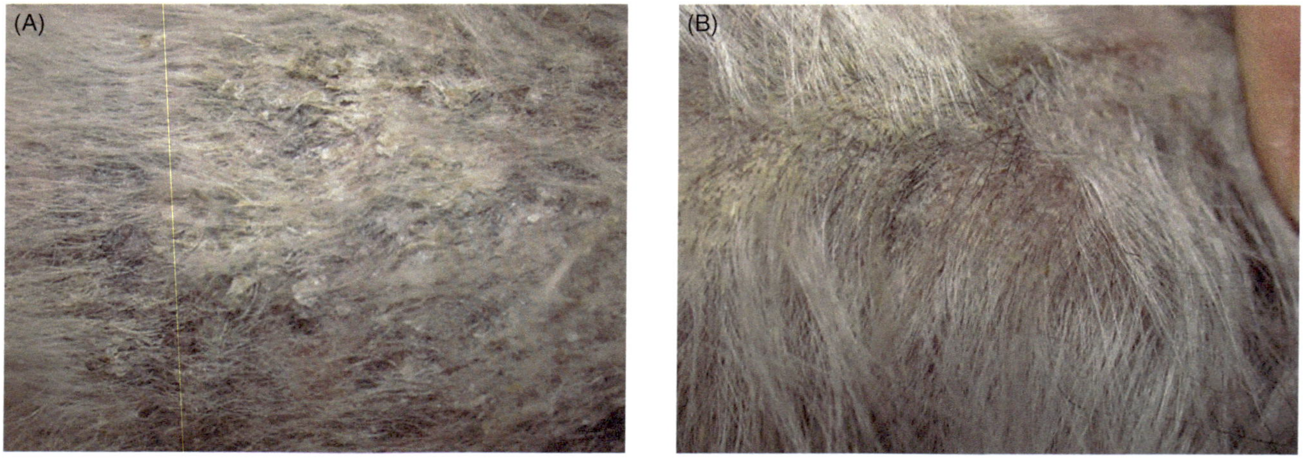

Figures 15.6A and B Adherent scaling and follicular casting due to generalized demodicosis.

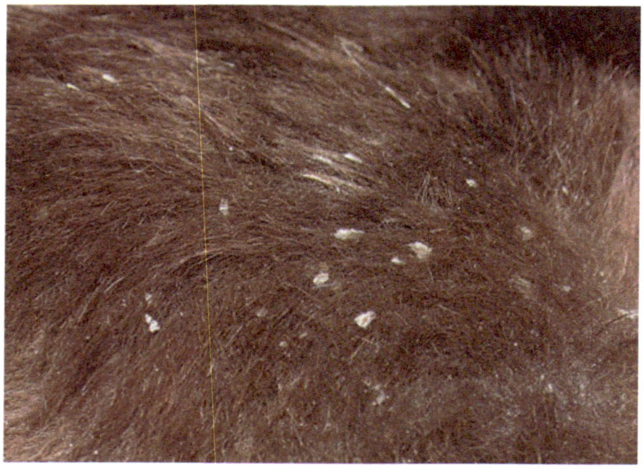

Figure 15.7 Exfoliative scaling in a Cocker Spaniel due to *Cheyletiella* infestation.

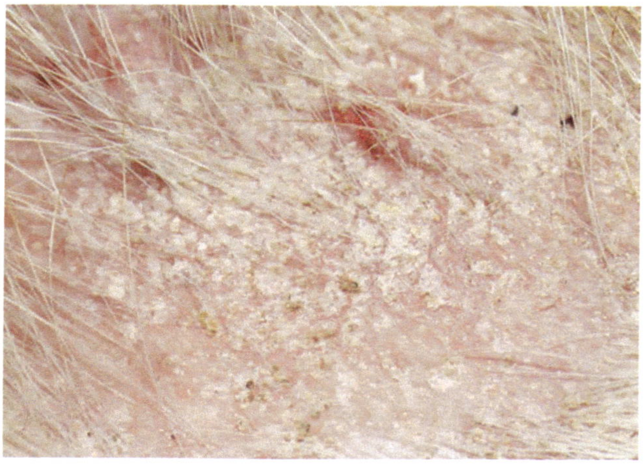

Figure 15.8 Adherent silver scaling and alopecia due to leishmania infection.

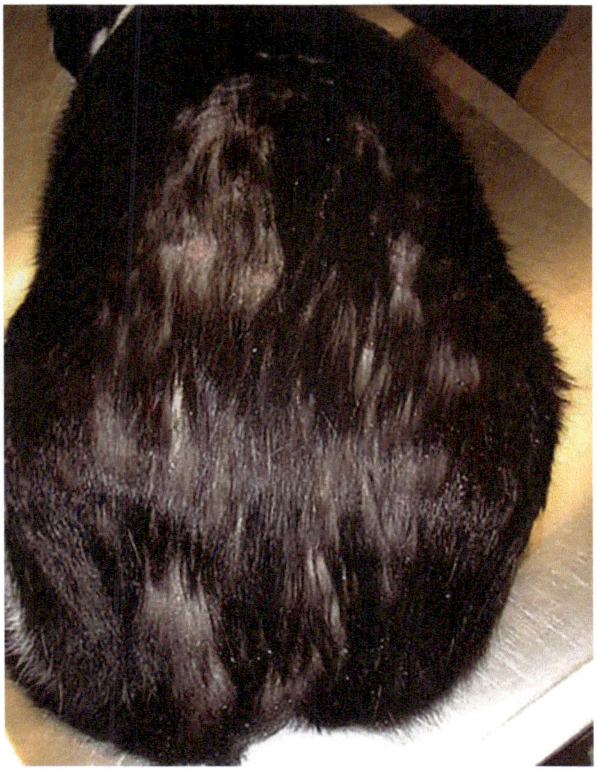

Figure 15.9 Dorsal lumbar scaling and patchy hypotrichosis due to dermatophytosis.

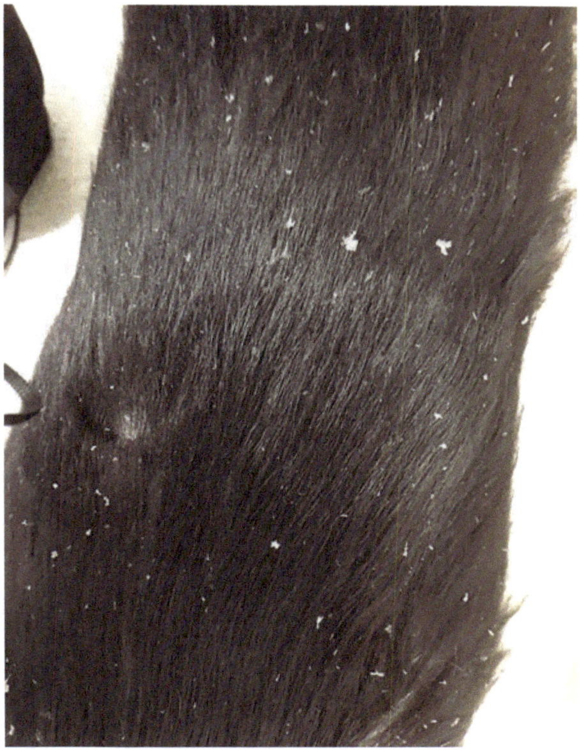

Figure 15.10 Exfoliative truncal scaling in a dog due to cutaneous epitheliotropic lymphoma.

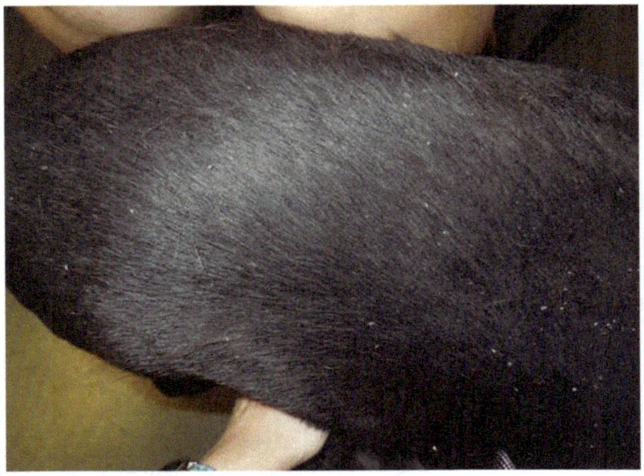

Figure 15.11 Truncal seborrhea in an older Labrador due to underlying hyperadrenocorticism and a secondary bacterial folliculitis.

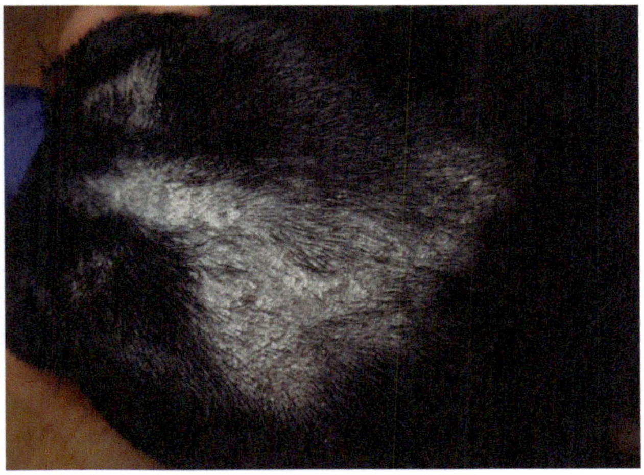

Figures 15.12 Adherent scaling and follicular casting due to sebaceous adenitis.

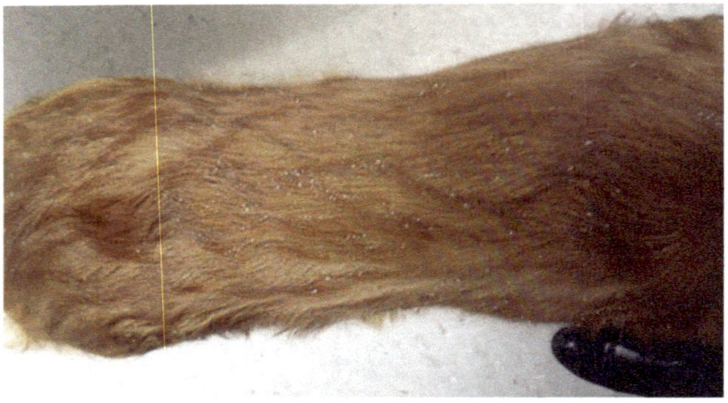

Figure 15.13 Truncal seborrhea in a Golden Retriever with ichthyosis.

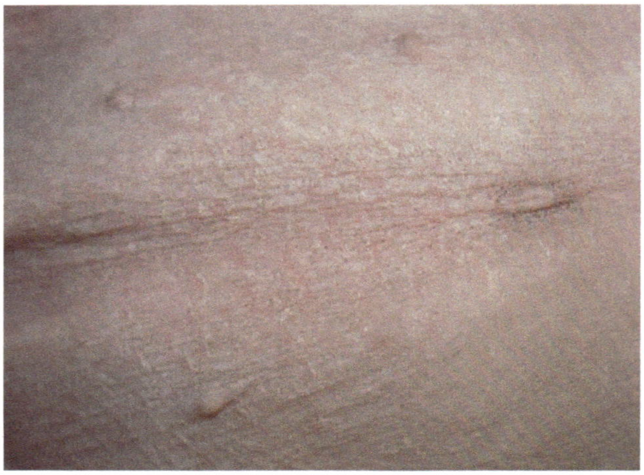

Figure 15.14 Inguinal, silvery, adherent, fish scale-like seborrhea in an American Bulldog puppy with ichthyosis.

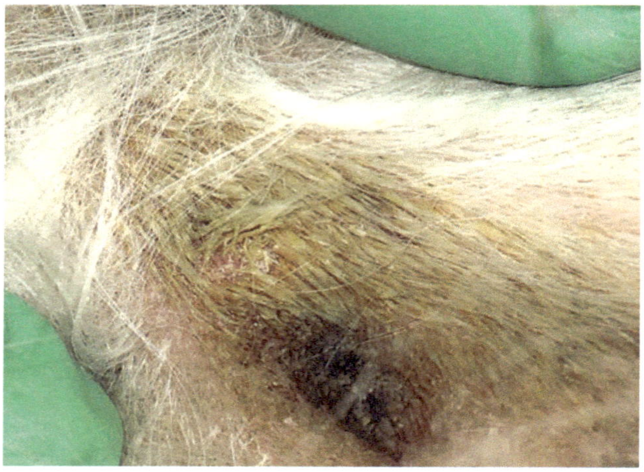

Figure 15.15 Hyperkeratotic fronds and follicular casting due to vitamin A responsive dermatosis on the inguinal area of a Cocker Spaniel.

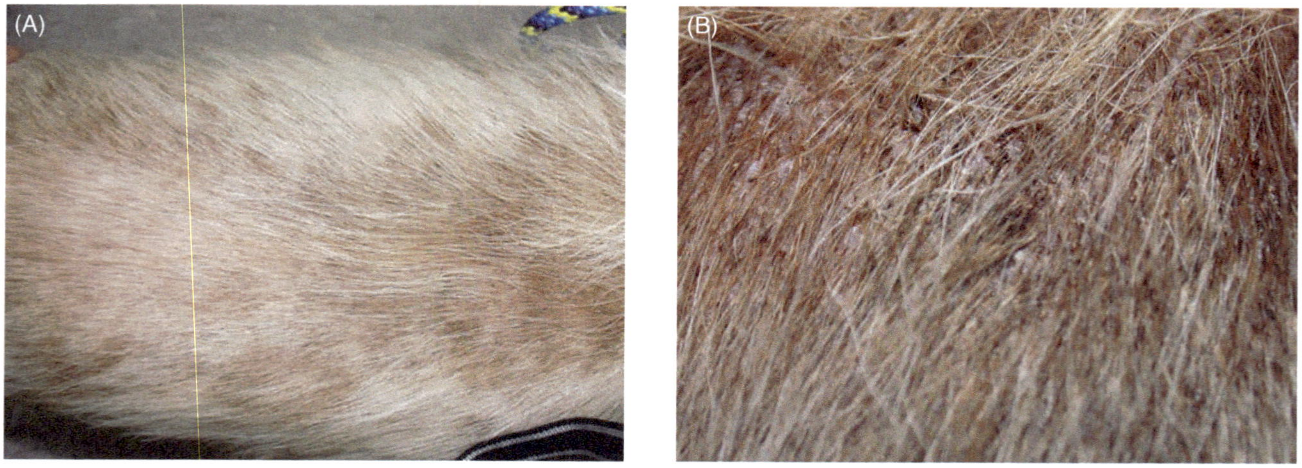

Figures 15.16A and B Truncal hypotrichosis with a coarse, rough coat in a mixed breed dog; on closer inspection there was moderate follicular casting typical for sebaceous adenitis.

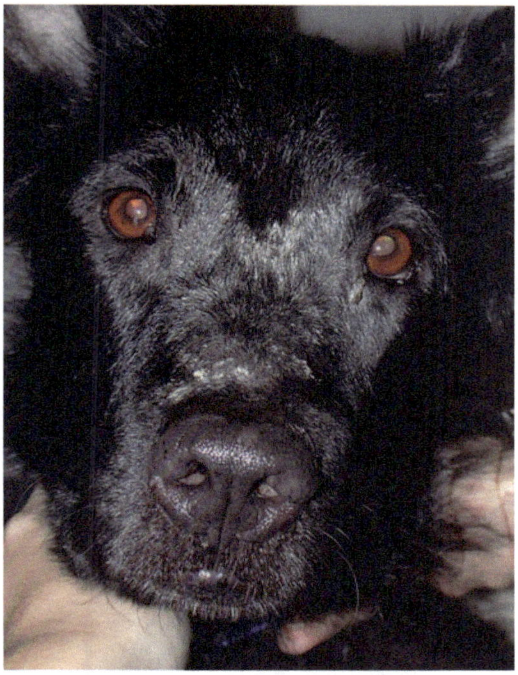

Figure 15.16C Facial hypotrichosis and follicular cast formation due to sebaceous adenitis.

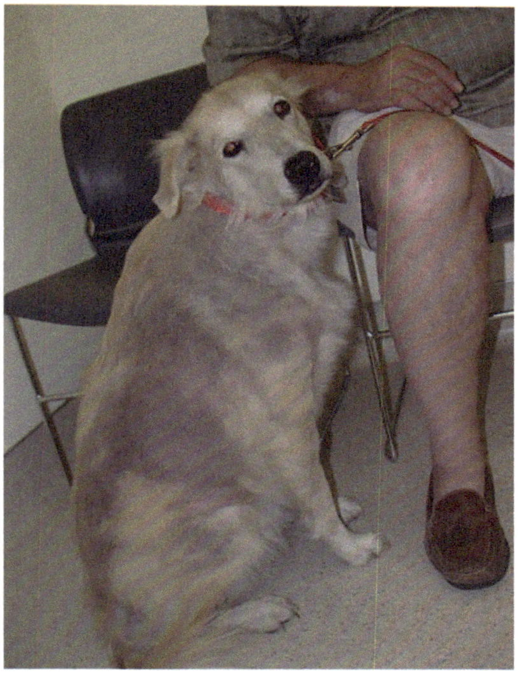

Figure 15.16D Truncal hypotrichosis and scaling caused by sebaceous adenitis.

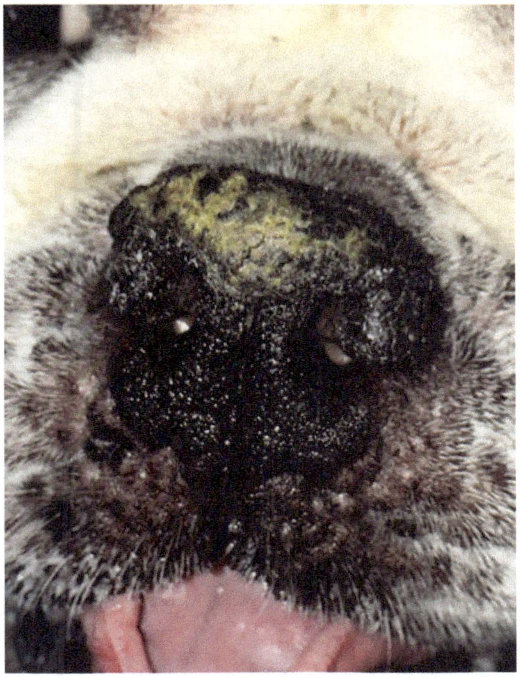

Figure 15.17 Idiopathic nasal hyperkeratosis in an English Bulldog.

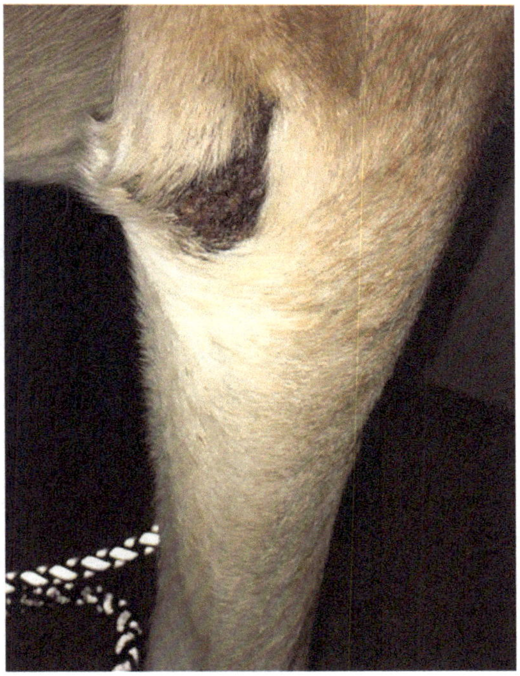

Figure 15.18 An elbow callus in a large breed dog; focal, alopecic, thickened lesion on the lateral elbow.

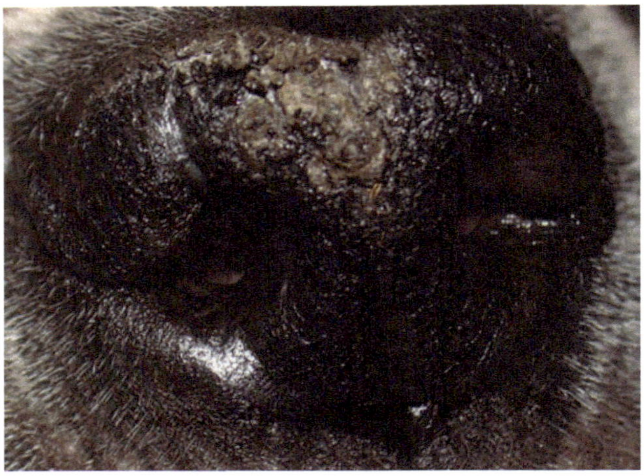

Figure 15.19 Chronic unilateral nasal hyperkeratosis in a dog due to parasympathetic nose.

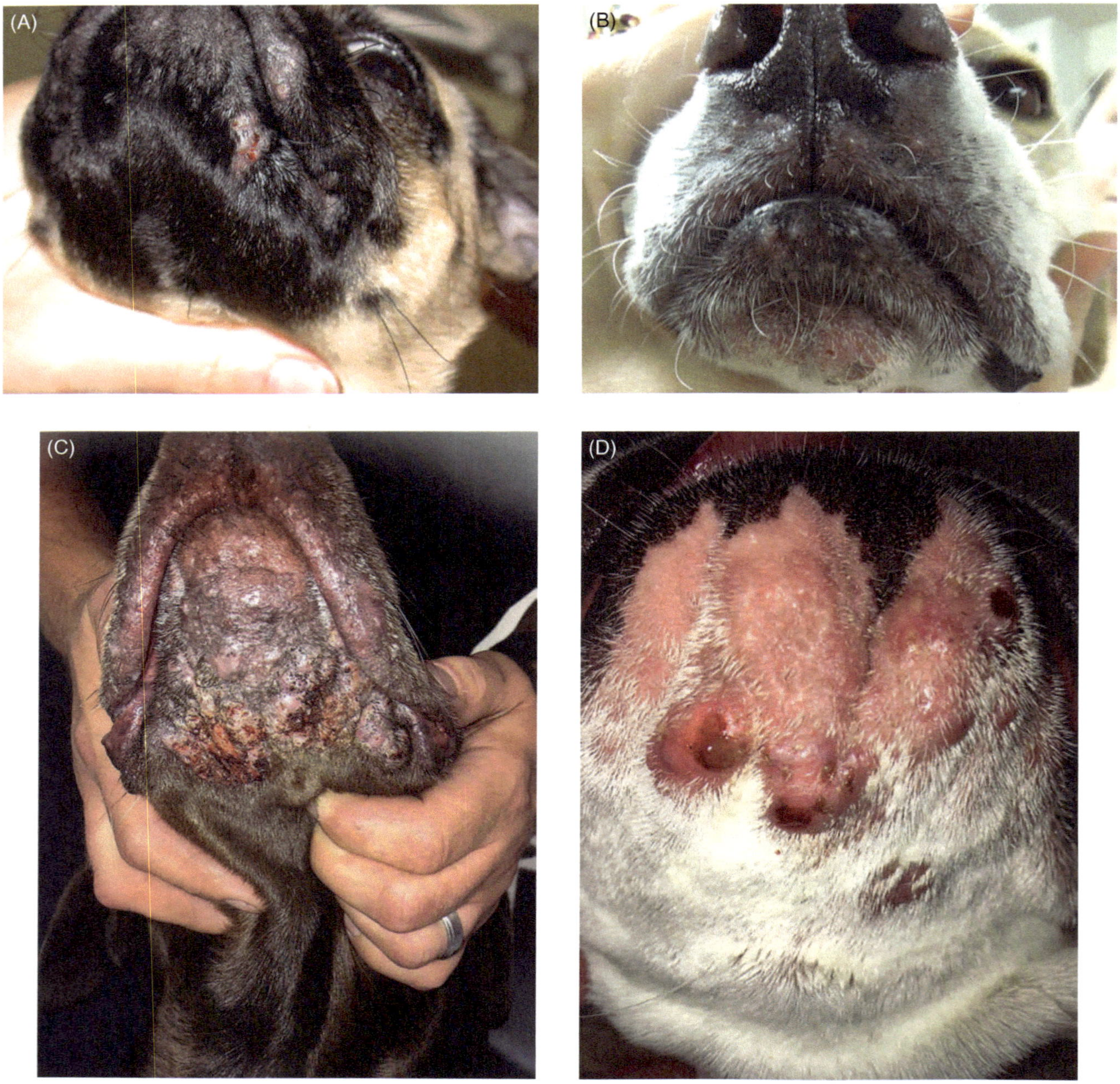

Figures 15.20A–D Canine acne.

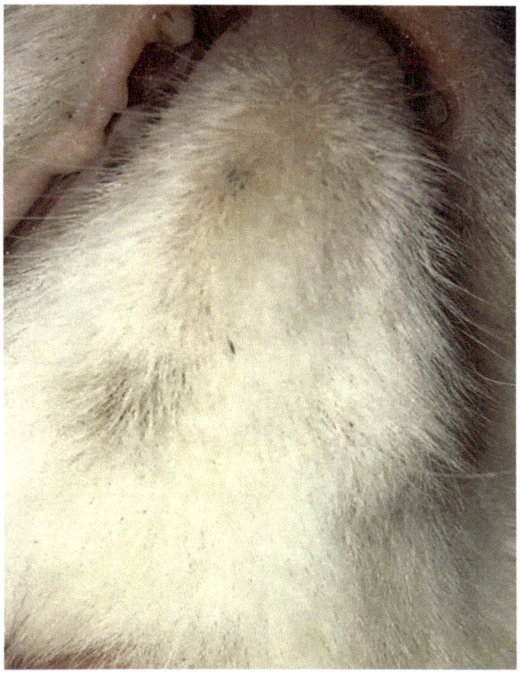

Figure 15.21A Mild, dark, chin debris and comedones due to feline acne.

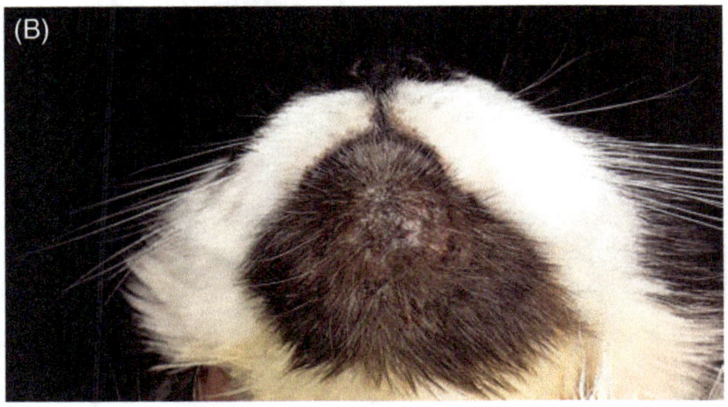

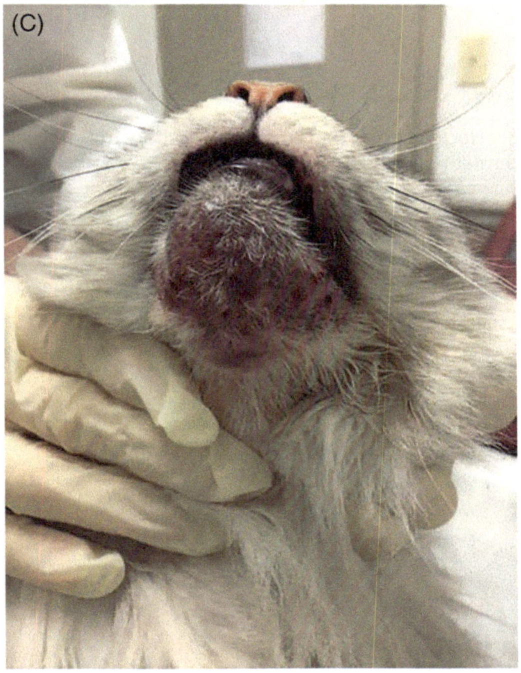

Figures 15.21B and C More severe cases of feline acne with painful cystic chin furunculosis. Source: Image 15.21B courtesy of VIN and Ray Snopek, DVM; Image 15.21C courtesy of VIN and Elizabeth Noyes, DVM.

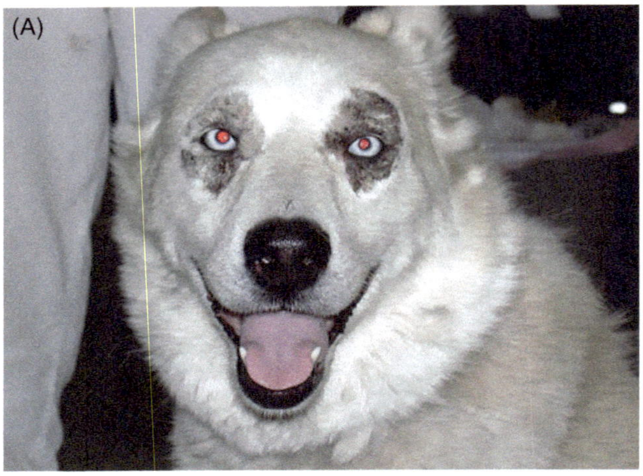

Figure 15.22A Periocular crusting in a Siberian Husky with zinc responsive dermatosis.

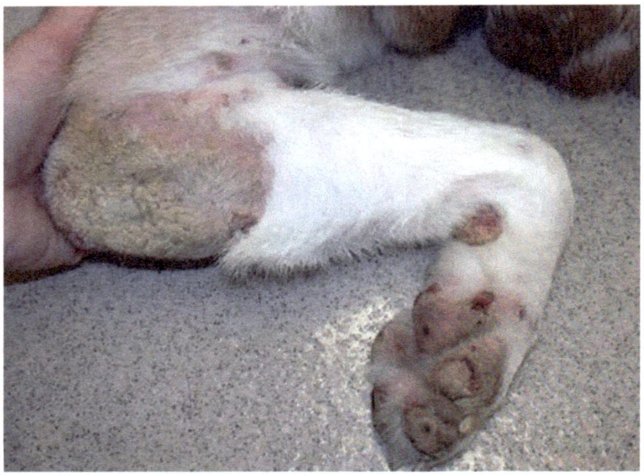

Figure 15.22B Paw pad and elbow hyperkeratosis secondary to zinc responsive dermatitis.

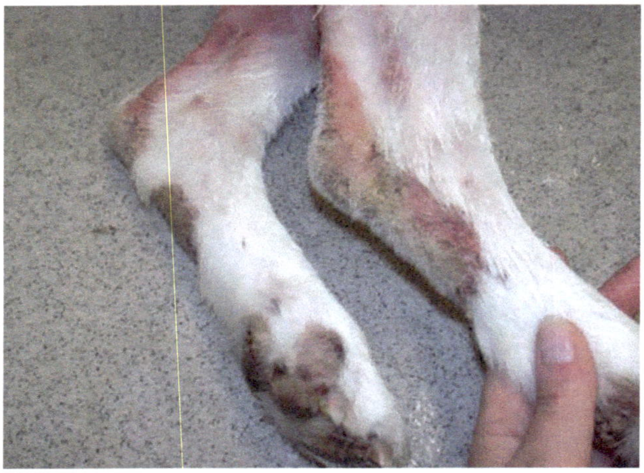

Figure 15.22C Hock and paw pad crusting secondary to zinc responsive dermatitis in husky.

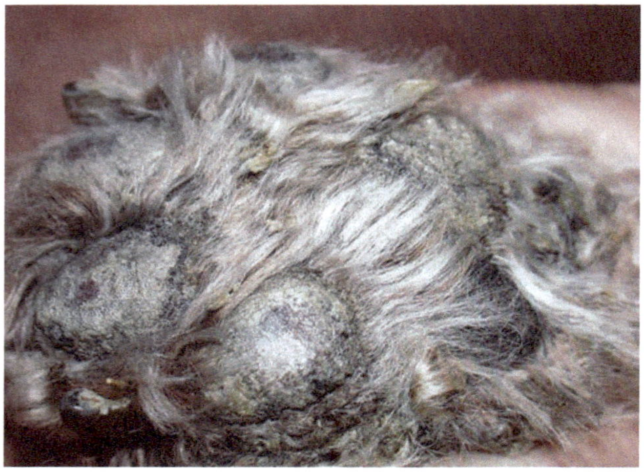

Figure 15.23 Marked paw pad hyperkeratosis and fissuring due to hepatocutaneous syndrome.

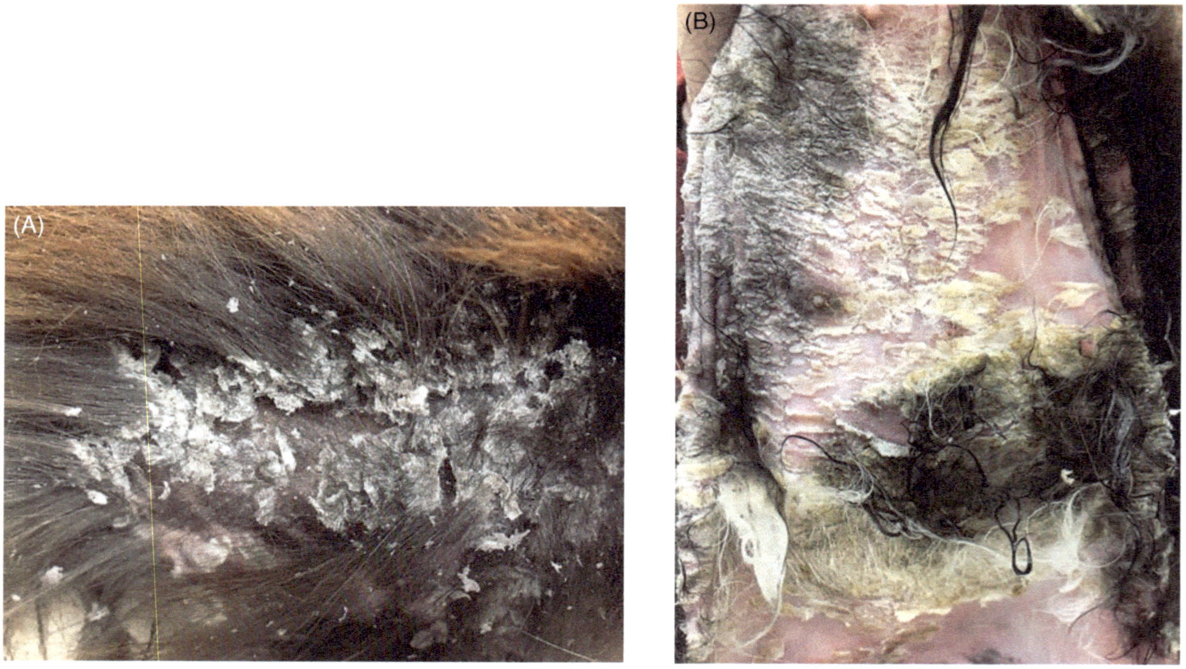

Figures 15.24A and B Generalized exfoliative dermatitis in a cat caused by a thymoma.

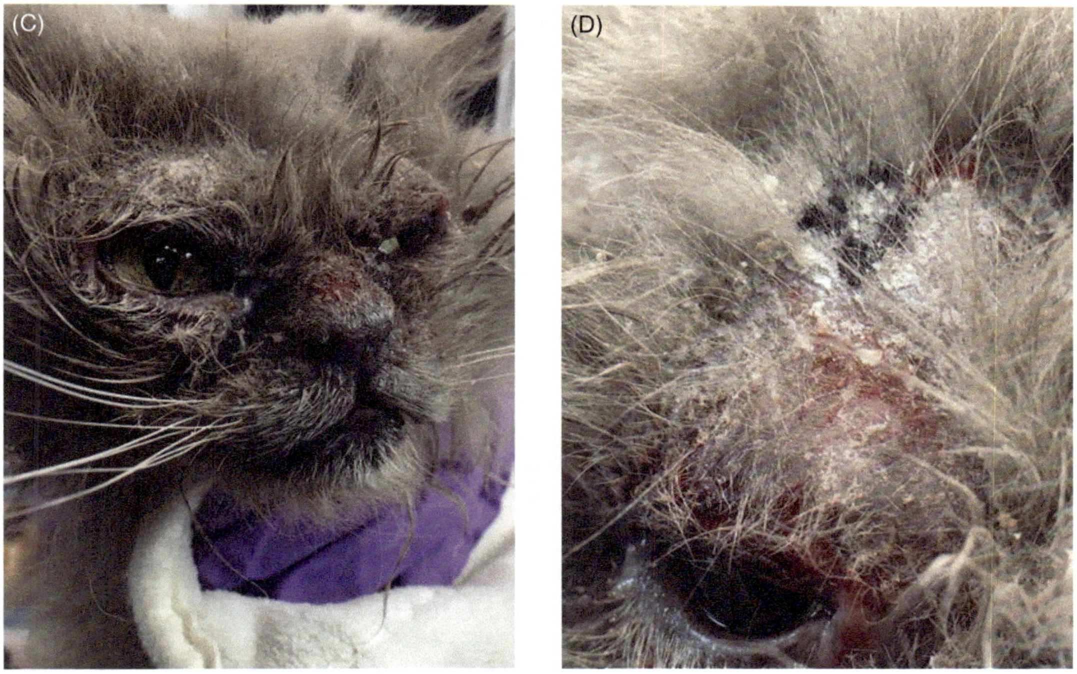

Figures 15.24C and D Exfoliative dermatitis in this cat was triggered by likely hepatic lymphoma and complicated by secondary bacterial and *Malassezia* infections causing marked pruritus; the dark circle in Figure 15.24D is a marker to denote the planned site of skin biopsy.

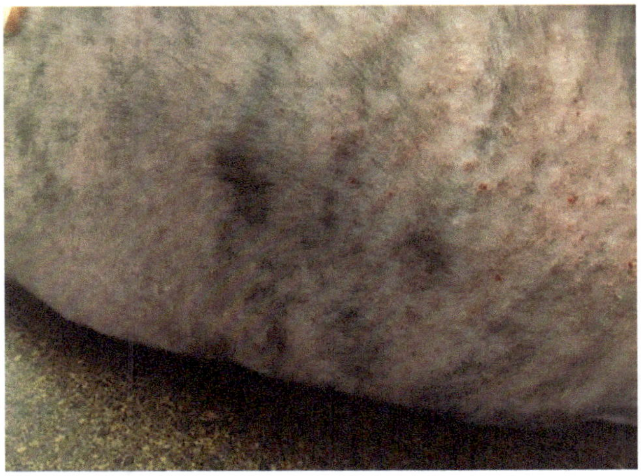

Figure 15.25 Generalized, raised, crusted, truncal papules in a pruritic cat; biopsy revealed xanthomas. Source: Image courtesy of Dr. Ann Trimmer, DACVD.

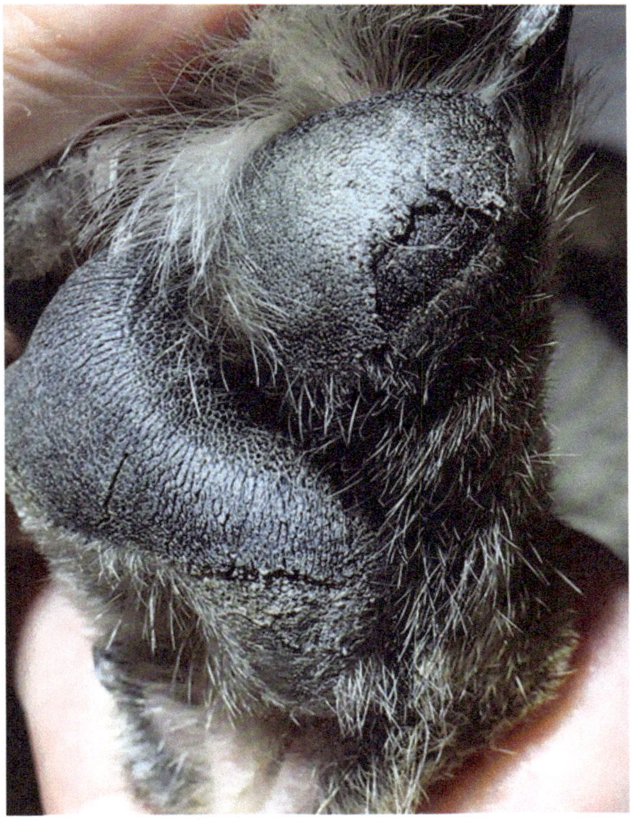

Figure 15.26 Split paw pad syndrome in a young German Shepherd; ulcerative peripheral pad lesions would wax and wane depending on activity and heal spontaneously regardless of therapy.

Further reading

Bach, J.F. (2013). A case of necrolytic migratory erythema managed for 24 months with intravenous amino acid and lipid infusions. *Can. Vet. J.* 54 (9): 873–875.

Catarino, M., Combarros-Garcia, D., Mimouni, P. et al. (2018). Control of canine idiopathic nasal hyperkeratosis with a natural skin restorative balm: a randomized double-blind placebo-controlled study. *Vet. Dermatol.* 29 (2): 134–e53.

Jazic, E., Coyner, K.S., Loeffler, D.G. et al. (2006). An evaluation of the clinical, cytological, infectious and histopathological features of feline acne. *Vet. Dermatol.* 17 (2): 134–140.

Lam, A.T., Affolter, V.K., Outerbridge, C.A. et al. (2011). Oral vitamin A as an adjunct treatment for canine sebaceous adenitis. *Vet. Dermatol.* 22 (4): 305–311.

Linek, M., Rüfenacht, S., Brachelente, C. et al. (2015). Nonthymoma-associated exfoliative dermatitis in 18 cats. *Vet. Dermatol.* 26 (1): 40–45. e12-3.

Lortz, J., Favrot, C., Mecklenburg, L. et al. (2010). A multicentre placebo-controlled clinical trial on the efficacy of oral ciclosporin A in the treatment of canine idiopathic sebaceous adenitis in comparison with conventional topical treatment. *Vet. Dermatol.* 21 (6): 593–601.

Oberkirchner, U., Linder, K.E., Zadrozny, L. et al. (2010). Successful treatment of canine necrolytic migratory erythema (superficial necrolytic dermatitis) due to metastatic glucagonoma with octreotide. *Vet. Dermatol.* 21 (5): 510–516.

Outerbridge, C.A., Marks, S.L., and Rogers, Q.R. (2002). Plasma amino acid concentrations in 36 dogs with histologically confirmed superficial necrolytic dermatitis. *Vet. Dermatol.* 13 (4): 177–186.

White, S.D., Bourdeau, P., Rosychuk, R.A.W. et al. (2001). Zinc-responsive dermatosis in dogs: 41 cases and literature review. *Vet. Dermatol.* 12 (2): 101–109.

16

Congenital/hereditary dermatologic disorders

Heide Newton, DVM, DACVD

Dermatology for Animals, Tucson, AZ, USA

Clinical Atlas of Canine and Feline Dermatology, First Edition. Edited by Kimberly S. Coyner.

Companion website: www.wiley.com/go/coyner/dermatology

Table 16.1 Congenital/hereditary dermatologic disorders.

Disease	Clinical signs	Diagnosis	Treatment
Primary seborrhea Rare disorder. Breeds: American Cocker Spaniel, English Springer Spaniel, West Highland White Terrier, Basset Hound, Persian and Himalayan cats. Onset of symptoms <1 year of age.	Variable including ceruminous hyperplastic otitis externa, dull coat with excessive scale, greasy malodorous skin, follicular casts, scaly or crusty pruritic patches, digital hyperkeratosis, dry brittle claws. Secondary bacterial and yeast infections commonly occur.	Rule out other more common causes of clinical signs with cytology/skin scrapings for bacterial/yeast/*Demodex* infections, labwork for endocrinopathy, hypoallergenic diet trial. Biopsy/dermatopathology: Marked keratinization defect with ortho to parakeratotic hyperkeratosis, follicular keratosis and variable keratinocyte apoptosis.	Topical treatments with moisturizing and antiseborrheic products (shampoo, spray, spot on, ear cleaners). For greasy seborrhea: Benzoyl peroxide, acetic/boric acid or tar-based shampoo twice weekly for 3 weeks then once weekly for maintenance. Control secondary bacterial or *Malassezia* infections by alternating antiseborrheic shampoo with miconazole/chlorhexidine shampoos or sprays/mousse/wipes every 1–2 days on affected areas. For recurrent *Malassezia*, oral ketoconazole daily × 14 days then pulse. Second-line/refractory: Vitamin A 1000 IU/kg/day PO. Retinoids (isotretinoin or acitretin) have been used in the past but are expensive and difficult for veterinarians to obtain, though compounded isotretinoin may be inconsistently available.
Idiopathic facial dermatitis of Persian and Himalayan cats (Chapter 6, Figure 6.63)	Dirty appearance to face (periocular, perioral, chin) with adherent black exudate, inflamed skin and variable severity of pruritus.	Clinical signs. Rule out infectious or allergic causes of clinical signs with skin scrapings, cytology, dermatophyte culture, hypoallergenic diet trial. Biopsy/dermatopathology is non-diagnostic, with non-specific inflammation including eosinophils and hyperkeratosis/hyperplasia.	Control secondary bacterial or *Malassezia* infections using miconazole/chlorhexidine containing wipes +/− oral itraconazole or fluconazole 5 mg/kg PO daily × 14 days then pulse. Topical treatment with acetic/boric acid containing wipes q24–48h. Second-line/refractory (concurrent allergy likely): Allergen specific immunotherapy +/− prednisolone 1 mg/kg PO daily tapered to lowest effective dose or cyclosporine 7 mg/kg PO daily tapered after 2 months to lowest effective dose.

Ichthyosis (Figures 16.1A and 16.1B, Chapter 2, Figure 2.37, Chapter 6, Figure 6.31) Breeds: Parson Russell Terrier, West Highland White Terrier, Golden Retriever, Norfolk Terrier, Cavalier King Charles Spaniel, Soft-coated Wheaten Terrier, American Bulldog, others.	Excessive scale of variable size, color, and adherence; thickened nasal planum and digital pads, ceruminous otitis externa.	Clinical signs in early puppyhood. Rule out infectious or allergic causes of clinical signs with skin scrapings, cytology, dermatophyte culture, hypoallergenic diet trial if presents as adult. Biopsy/dermatopathology: Marked epidermal and follicular orthokeratotic hyperkeratosis +/− marked hypergranulosis.	This is an incurable disorder but topical treatments with moisturizing products (shampoos, sprays, spot on) can be helpful to reduce clinical signs. Typical regimen: Ceramide containing shampoo followed by rinse or spray twice weekly for 3 weeks then once weekly. Ceramide-containing spray or spot on up to daily between baths. Ceramide or acetic/boric acid ear flush weekly. Control secondary bacterial or *Malassezia* infections by alternating moisturizing shampoo with miconazole/chlorhexidine shampoos, or similar sprays/mousse/wipes every 1–2 days on affected areas. For recurrent *Malassezia*, oral ketoconazole daily × 14 days then pulse.
Nasal parakeratosis of Labrador Retrievers (Chapter 6, Figure 6.39) Onset between 6 and 12 months of age.	Band of tightly adhered keratin on dorsal aspect of nasal planum of variable thickness. Can develop fissures, erosions and ulcers.	Clinical signs. Biopsy/dermatopathology: Parakeratotic hyperkeratosis with lymphocytic to neutrophilic exocytosis and multifocal serous epidermal lakes.	This is an incurable disorder but topical treatment daily with moisturizing products such as 50% propylene glycol BID-TID can be helpful. Refractory cases usually respond to a topical steroid ointment or 0.1% tacrolimus ointment.
Dermatomyositis (Figures 16.2A–16.2D; Chapter 2, Figure 2.33B; Chapter 6, Figure 6.15) Breeds: Collie, Shetland Sheepdog, Beauceron Shepherd, Belgian Tervuren, Portuguese Water dog, others. Lesions usually occur between 8 weeks–6 months of age.	Alopecia, erythema, scale, crust, sometimes ulcers in areas of mechanical trauma such as face, muzzle, pinna, carpus/tarsus, digits, tail tip. Myositis may occur months after skin lesions and correlates with skin lesion severity.	Rule out other differentials including demodicosis, bacterial folliculitis, dermatophytosis. Biopsy/dermatopathology: Hydropic basal cell degeneration +/− subepidermal clefting. Follicular atrophy/fibrosis common and vasculitis may be present. Muscle biopsy may show inflammation, necrosis, and atrophy.	First-line treatment: Minimize trauma and sun exposure. Begin pentoxifylline 20–30 mg/kg PO q8–12h, vitamin E and omega-3 fatty acid supplementation. Second-line/refractory cases: Add immunomodulating treatment with oral doxycycline and niacinamide, tacrolimus ointment to localized lesions q12–24h. In severe cases, oral prednisolone 1 mg/kg/d × 2–3 weeks, tapered to lowest effective dose, ideally 0.25–0.5 mg q48h or lower; for steroid-sparing effect, add cyclosporine 5 mg/kg PO q24h × 4–8 weeks then taper to q48h.

(*Continued*)

Table 16.1 Congenital/hereditary dermatologic disorders (Continued)

Disease	Clinical signs	Diagnosis	Treatment
Dermatomyositis (cont).			Lesions in mildly to moderately affected dogs may resolve as dogs mature, but scarring is common and relapse or disease flares may occur. Severely affected dogs with myositis have a poor prognosis due to difficulties in eating/drinking and risk of aspiration pneumonia; steroids improve skin lesions but increase muscle atrophy and compound pneumonia risk.
Congenital alopecia (Figures 16.3A and 16.3B; Chapter 6, Figures 6.12, 6.66–6.68) Alopecic breeds: Mexican Hairless dog, Chinese Crested dog, Sphynx, others. Congenital alopecia can also rarely occur in numerous other breeds.	Juvenile onset alopecia. Follicular structural abnormalities cause development of comedones and numerous small follicular cysts which can be mild to severe depending on the patient. Some patients also show abnormalities of claws, teeth, or glands.	Clinical signs. Biopsy/dermatopathology: In some cases there is a complete absence of follicles, other cases have hypoplastic follicles. Chinese Crested dogs commonly develop numerous comedones and plugged cystic hair follicles.	Protect from sun exposure and trauma. Topical +/− oral retinoids may be considered in patients with severe follicular cyst formation.
Cutaneous asthenia (Ehlers Danlos) (Figures 16.4A and 16.4B) Breeds: Beagle, Dachshund, Boxer, St Bernard, German Shepherd dog, Yorkshire Terrier, Alaskan Malamute, English Springer Spaniel, Greyhound, Manchester Terrier, Welsh Corgi, Persian, Burmese, others.	Skin is excessively folded, hyperextensible, easily torn and/or excessively scarred.	Skin extensibility index (EI) = (vertical height of skin fold/body length) x 100 Dogs: EI > 14.5% Cats: EI > 19% Biopsies with Masson trichrome stain: May show abnormal collagen fibers, but may be inconclusive. Electron microscopy of skin biopsy: Abnormal collagen structure/organization.	No definitive treatment. Minimize trauma (clothing, nail trims, possibly declaw in cats). Vitamin C supplementation (dogs 500 mg PO q12h, cats 50 mg PO q12h) anecdotally helpful.
Mucinosis Figures 16.5A and 16.5B, Chapter 2, Figure 2.17; Chapter 6, Figures 6.53A and 6.53B) Breeds: Chinese Shar-Pei.	Excessive skin folding and vesicles containing thick, clear sticky fluid.	Clinical signs. Biopsy/dermatopathology: Excessive dermal mucin. Labwork to rule out hypothyroidism.	None needed as this is cosmetic problem. Evaluate and manage any concurrent hypothyroidism. Short tapering course of anti-inflammatory prednisolone can be helpful to reduce swelling in severely affected dogs.

Urticaria pigmentosa (Chapter 6, Figure 6.68) Breeds: Sphynx, Himalayan, Devon Rex.	Variably pruritic, yellow-tan to reddish brown macules or papules on head, neck, ventrum, tail, and extremities.	Biopsy/dermatopathology: Moderate to severe perivascular to diffuse dermal and subcutaneous mast cell infiltrates. Rule out allergic hypersensitivity with parasite prevention and hypoallergenic diet trial.	Hydroxyzine or other antihistamines +/− methylprednisolone or prednisolone 0.5–1 mg/kg/d × 2 weeks then taper to lowest effective dose ideally 0.25–0.5 mg/kg q48h or lower. For steroid-sparing effect, if needed add cyclosporine 5 mg/kg PO q24h × 4–8 weeks then taper to q48h.
Ulcerative nasal dermatitis of Bengal cats (Chapter 6, Figure 6.61B) Age of onset: 4–12 months old.	Dry scale gradually progressing to hyperkeratosis, crusts and fissures +/− hypopigmentation of nasal planum.	Clinical signs and signalment. Biopsy/dermatopathology: Marked epidermal parakeratosis and crusting with mixed inflammation.	This is an incurable disorder but topical therapies can be helpful to control symptoms. First-line treatment: topical treatment q24–48h with moisturizing products (such as petroleum jelly or lanolin), salicylic acid containing ointment. If moisturizing treatments are not helpful then 0.1% tacrolimus ointment applied twice daily is usually helpful. Second-line/refractory: prednisolone or methylprednisolone 0.5–1 mg/kg/d × 2 weeks then taper to lowest effective dose (ideally 0.25–0.5 mg/kg q48h or lower) or stop and continue topicals only.
Dermoid sinus, a.k.a. dermoid cyst (embryonic neural tube developmental defect (Figures 16.6A and 16.6B) Breeds: Boxer, English Bulldog, Kerry Blue Terrier, Golden Retriever, Rhodesian Ridgeback, Siberian Husky, Shih-tzu, Yorkshire Terrier, cats.	Solitary or multiple cystic swellings and/or draining tracts along dorsal midline. Meningitis possible in severe cases with connection of sinus to spinal cord.	Clinical signs, neurologic examination. Myelography, fistulogram, and/or MRI may be needed for severe cases with spinal cord involvement.	Surgical excision: in cases in which lesion penetrates into deep tissues, perform MRI or fistulogram to determine depth of lesion and plan surgery.
Acrodermatitis Breeds: Bull Terrier, Miniature Bull Terrier.	From birth, light/white skin pigmentation, retarded growth, and difficulty swallowing and chewing due to high arched palate. By 6–8 weeks of age, tightly adherent scale, crust, and erythema at face, elbows, hocks, and paws. With progression, splayed paws, pawpad fissures, paronychia, onychodystrophy, pawpad hyperkeratosis, and secondary *Malassezia* or bacterial infections.	Clinical signs and signalment. Cytology to rule out secondary infections. Biopsy/dermatopathology: Diffuse parakeratotic hyperkeratosis with focal crusting and intraepidermal pustules.	This is an incurable and lethal disorder and most patients are euthanized due to humane considerations before 2 years of age. Control secondary *Malassezia* or bacterial infections. Genetic testing available to identify carriers prior to breeding and affected dogs.

(*Continued*)

Table 16.1 Congenital/hereditary dermatologic disorders (Continued)

Disease	Clinical signs	Diagnosis	Treatment
Acral mutilation syndrome (Figure 16.7) Breeds: Miniature Pinscher, German Short Haired Pointer, English Pointer, English Springer Spaniel, French Spaniel. Age of onset: 2–12 months.	Sudden intense licking, biting, and severe self-mutilation of one or more paws; auto-amputation of claws, digits, and footpads often results if not restrained; no evidence of lameness or pain when walking.	Clinical signs, signalment, no response to pain stimuli at affected distal limbs (sensory neuropathy), nerve biopsy.	This is an incurable disorder and most patients are euthanized. E-collars, bandages, and close supervision to prevent self-trauma. Control secondary bacterial or *Malassezia* infections. Genetic testing available to identify carriers prior to breeding and affected dogs.
Congenital keratoconjunctivitis sicca (KCS) and ichthyosiform dermatosis in the Cavalier King Charles Spaniel (CKCS)	Curly or crimped coarse coat from birth; progressive pawpad hyperkeratosis; variable onychodystrophy and onycholysis; variable pruritus and hypotrichosis. Bilateral progressive, severe KCS.	Clinical signs and signalment, Schirmer tear test confirms KCS. Biopsy/dermatopathology: Irregular epidermal hyperplasia, with marked surface hyperkeratosis.	This is an incurable disorder and many patients are euthanized. Topical treatments with moisturizing products (shampoos, sprays, spot on) can be helpful to reduce clinical signs. See details of treatment for ichthyosis above. Management of KCS. Genetic testing available to identify carriers prior to breeding.
Exfoliative cutaneous lupus erythematous (Figures 16.8A–16.8D) Breed predispositions: German Short-haired Pointer. Autosomal recessive condition; breeders should be alerted. Onset of disease generally occurs in young adults.	Disease is characterized by scaling and alopecia. Lesions generally first noted on the muzzle, pinnae, and dorsum, with progression to involve the limbs and ventrum. Ulcerations may develop. Lymphadenopathy and pyrexia may be present. Joint pain with lameness may be present but joint fluid analysis is unremarkable.	Clinical signs, breed, rule out infectious causes of scaling. Biopsy/dermatopathology: Interface dermatitis and mural folliculitis with frequent basal cell apoptosis and inflammation of apocrine and sebaceous glands. ANA testing is negative.	Guarded to poor prognosis with generally poor response to treatment; most affected dogs are euthanized within 2 years of onset of disease. Mycophenolate mofetil recently described as a successful treatment in one case. Cyclosporine combined with hydroxychloroquine may improve and slow progression of the disease. Topical antiseborrheic and moisturizing products may be somewhat beneficial for symptomatic therapy.
Epidermolysis bullosa (Figures 16.9A–16.9B) Lesions usually develop shortly after birth. Predisposed breeds include Beaucerons, German Shorthair Pointers, Siamese cats.	Erosions to ulcers over bony prominences of face, pinna, pressure points on limbs, pawpads and/or in oral cavity in juvenile patients.	Clinical signs. Biopsy/dermatopathology: Subepidermal separation with little to no inflammation.	Minimize trauma. Control secondary bacterial infections. Mildly affected animals may have reasonable quality of life with environmental management; prognosis for severely affected animals is poor.

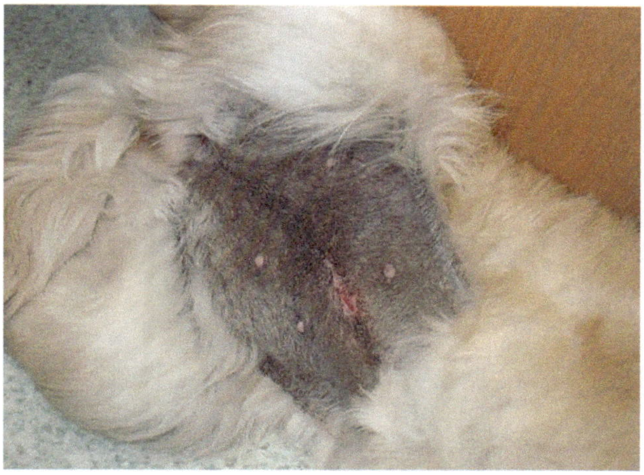

Figure 16.1A A young Golden Retriever with inguinal hyperpigmentation and adherent scaling due to ichthyosis.

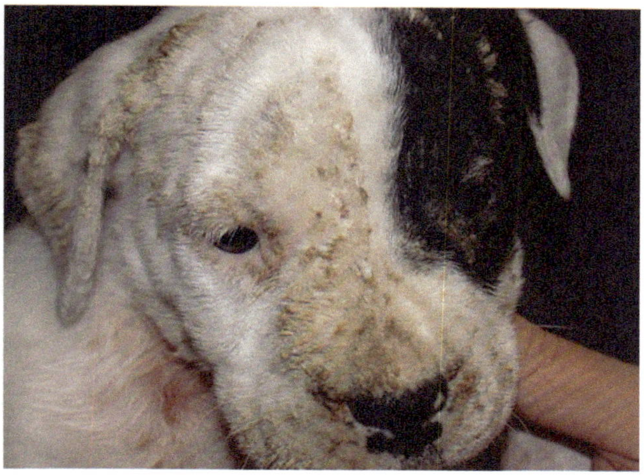

Figure 16.1B An American Bulldog puppy with adherent crusting on the face and pinna; a secondary *Malassezia* infection was also present.

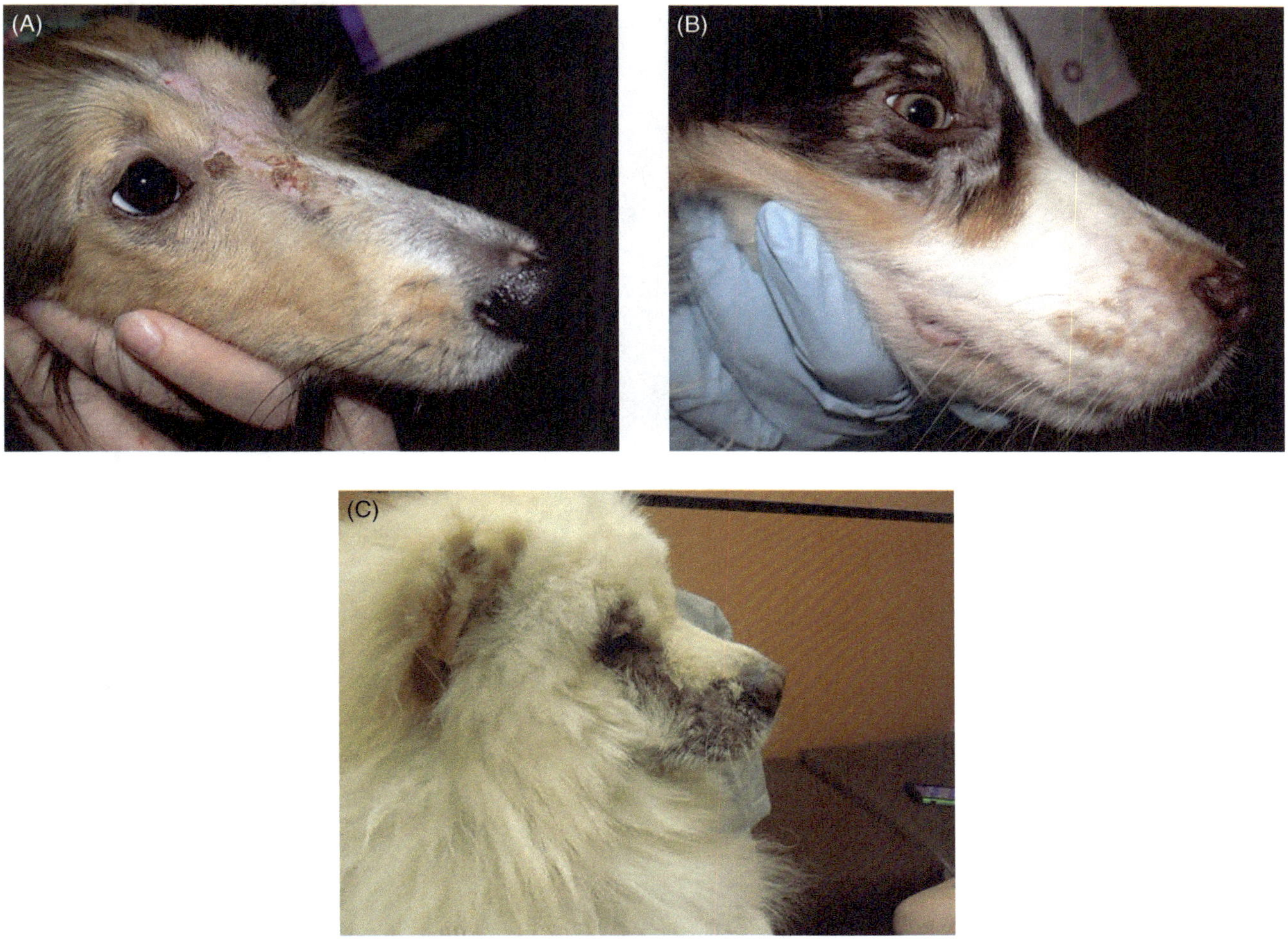

Figures 16.2A–C Dermatomyositis causing scarring alopecia with crusting in a young Sheltie, Australian Shepherd, and Chow.

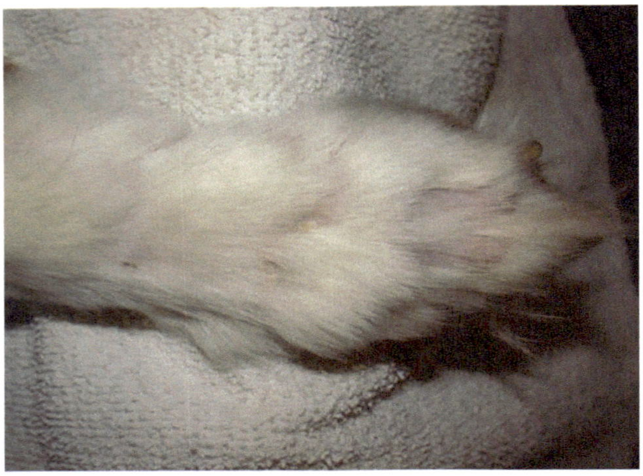

Figure 16.2D Alopecia and scarring on the distal limbs was also present in the Australian Shepherd.

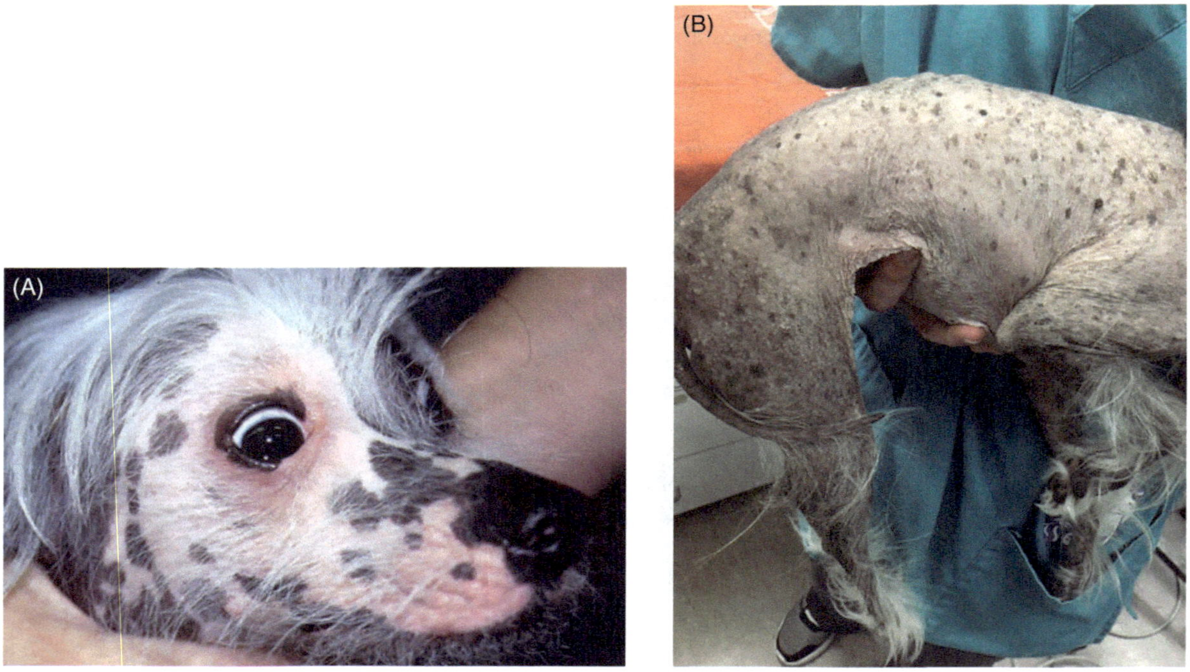

Figures 16.3A and B Two Chinese Crested dogs demonstrating typical congenital alopecia.

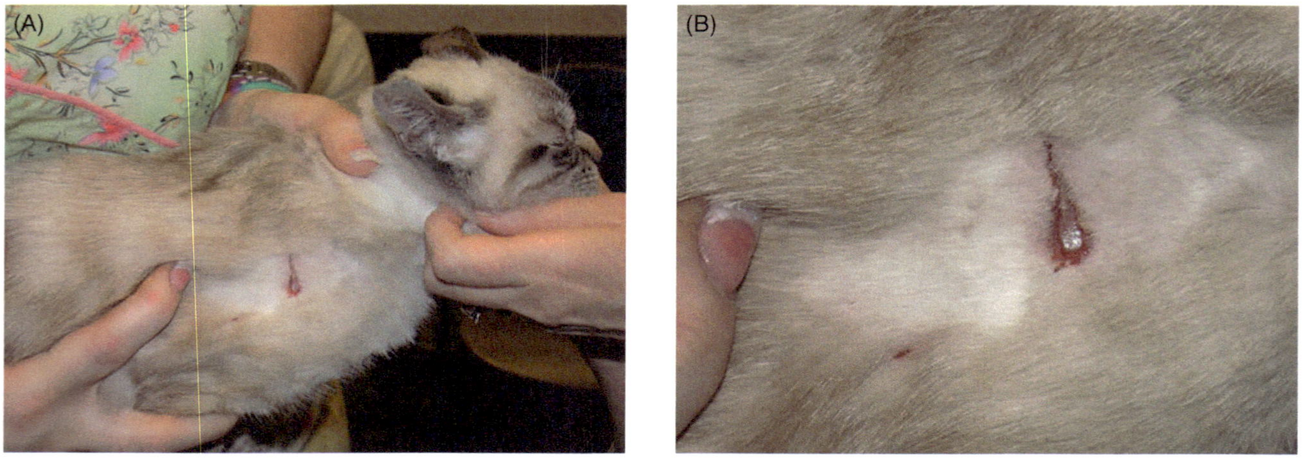

Figures 16.4A and B A young cat with easily torn skin due to cutaneous asthenia.

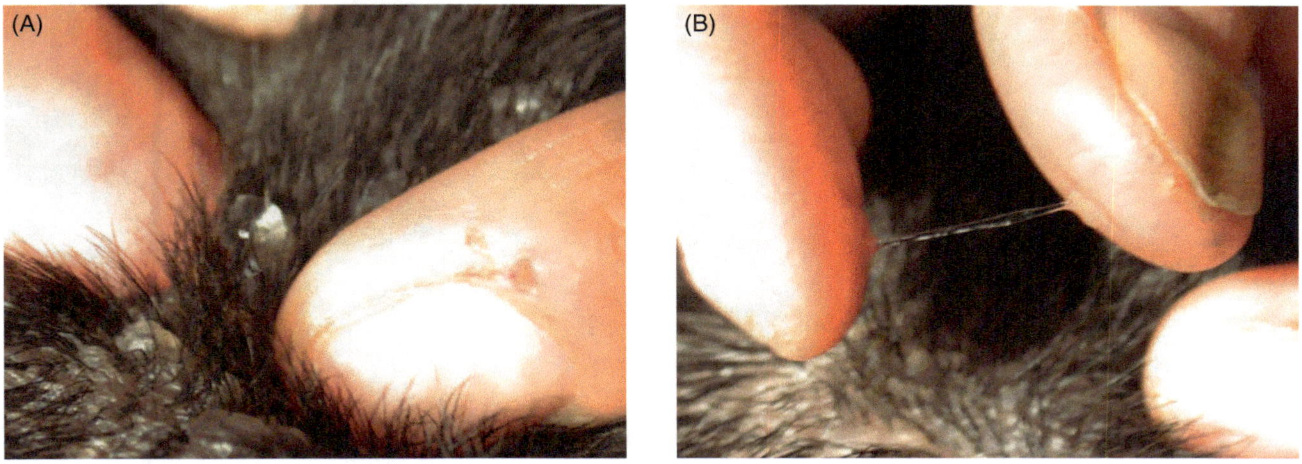

Figures 16.5A and B Mucinosis in a Shar-Pei.

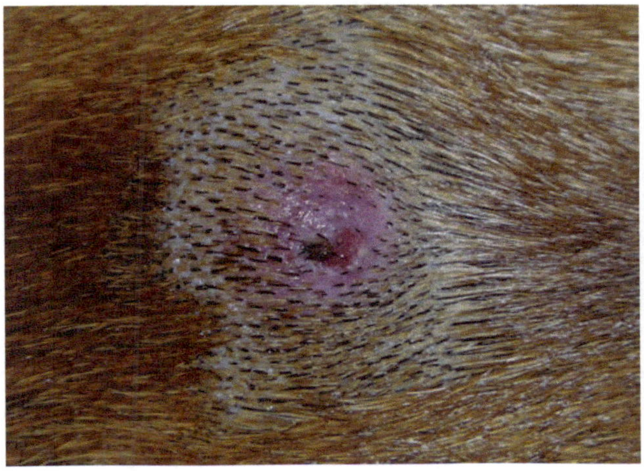

Figures 16.6A A dermoid sinus in a Rhodesian Ridgeback. *Source:* Image courtesy of VIN and Michael Goldman, DVM.

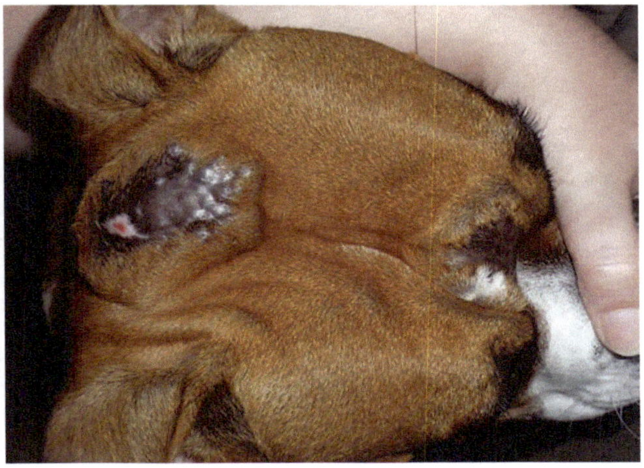

Figure 16.6B A dermoid cyst in a young Boxer dog. *Source:* Image courtesy of VIN and David Silver, DVM.

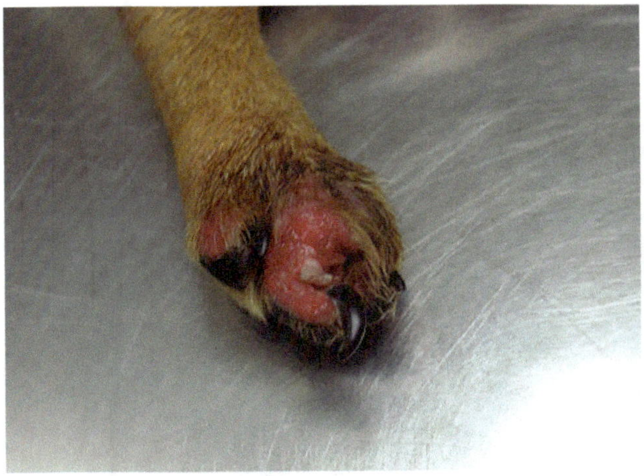

Figure 16.7 Acral mutilation in a four-month-old German Shepherd mix puppy. *Source:* Image courtesy of VIN and Steven Berry, DVM.

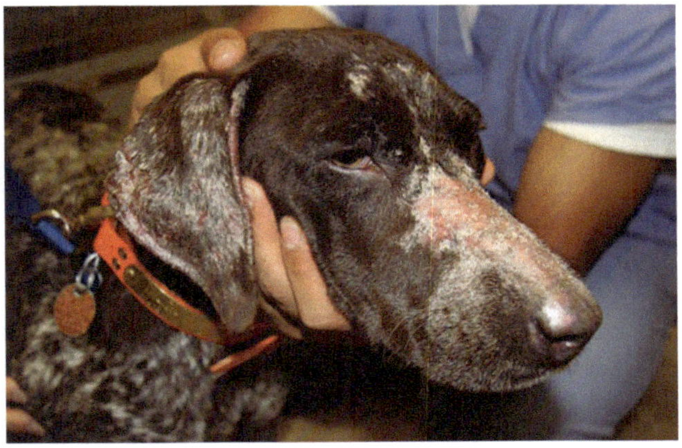

Figure 16.8A Alopecia and scaling on the muzzle and pinna of a German Shorthair Pointer with exfoliative cutaneous lupus erythematosus. *Source:* Image courtesy of Dr. William Miller, DACVD.

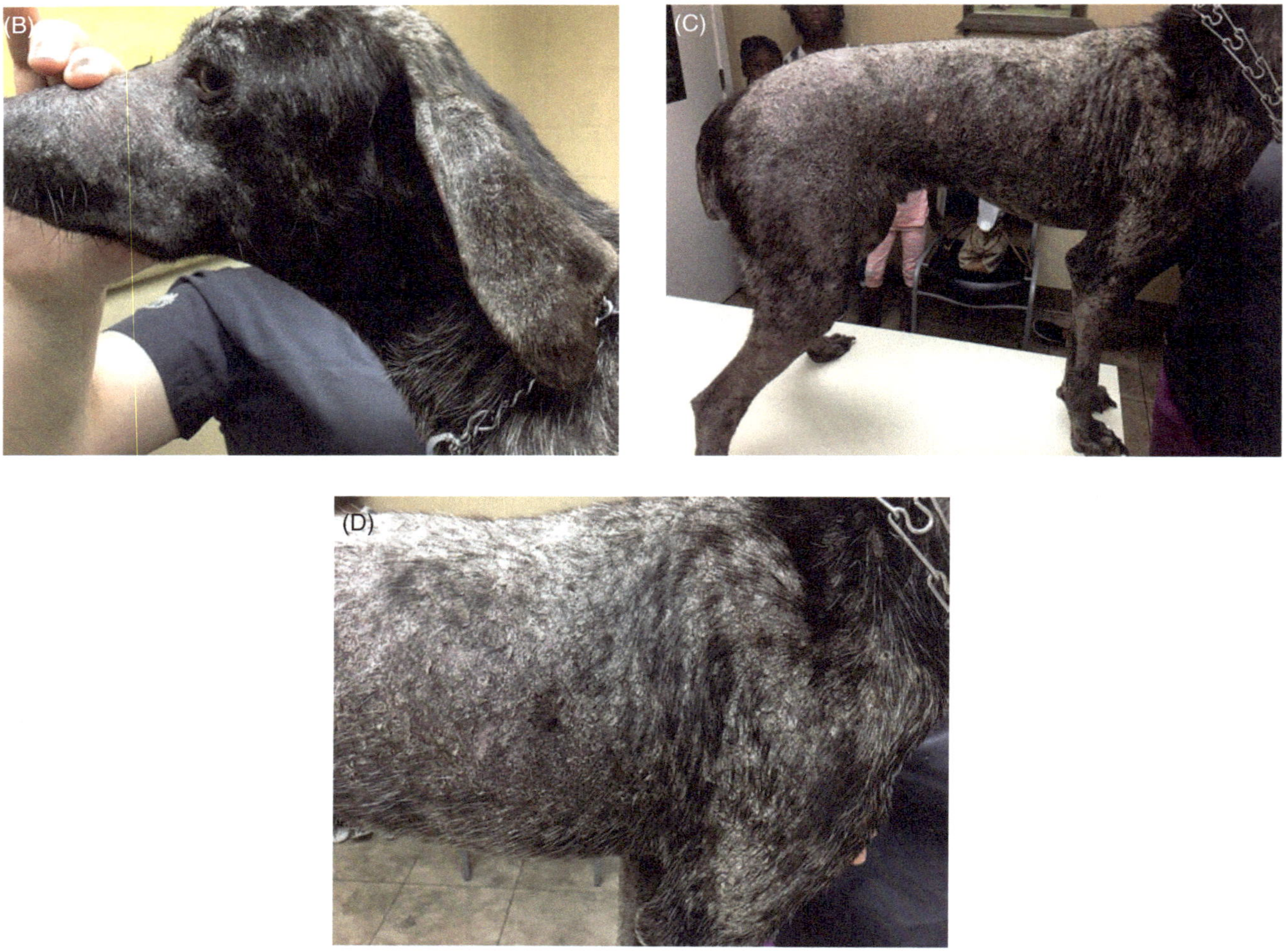

Figures 16.8B–D A German Shorthair Pointer with alopecia and marked adherent scaling on the face, ears, and trunk due to exfoliative cutaneous lupus erythematosus. *Source:* Images courtesy of Dr. Martha Friedman, DACVD.

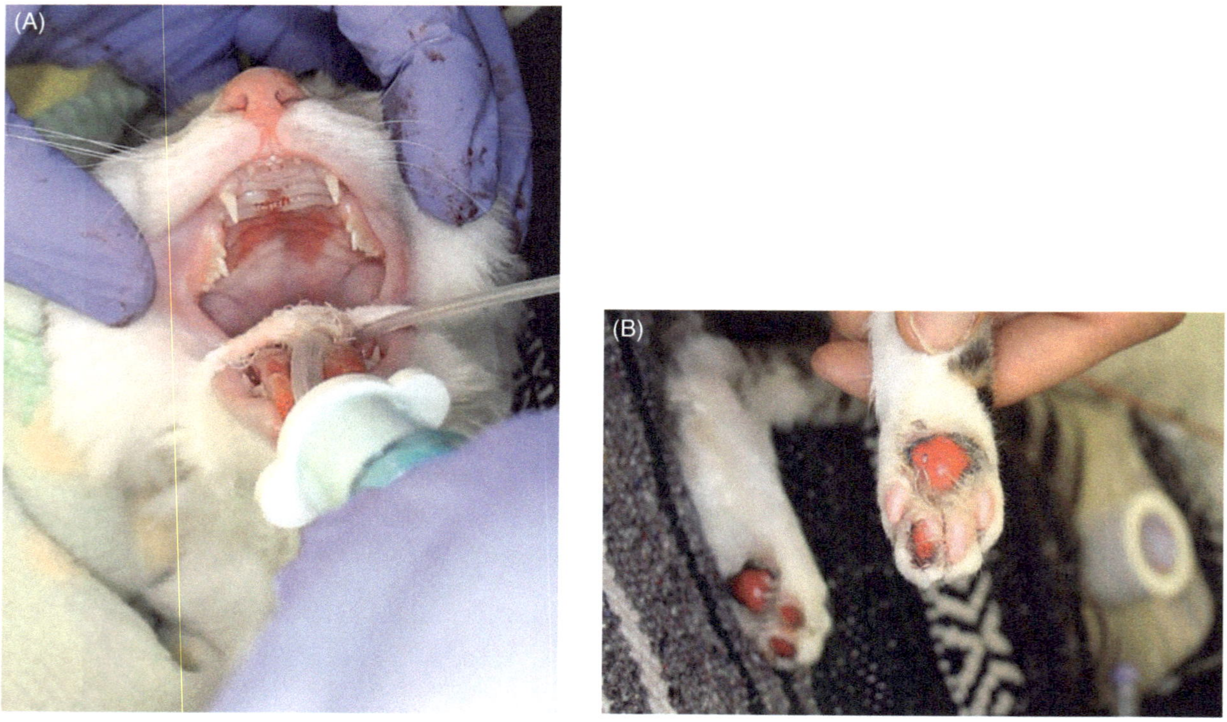

Figures 16.9A–B Epidermolysis bullosa in a three-month-old kitten, causing sloughing of paw pads and oral mucosa. *Source:* Images courtesy of Dr. Andrew Simpson, DACVD.

Further reading

Bardagí, M., Montoliu, P., Ferrer, L. et al. (2011). Acral mutilation syndrome in a miniature pinscher. *J. Comp. Pathol.* 144 (2–3): 235–238.

Barnett, K.C. (2006). Congenital keratoconjunctivitis sicca and ichthyosiform dermatosis in the cavalier King Charles spaniel. *J. Small Anim. Pract.* 47 (9): 524–528.

Bergvall, K. (2004). A novel ulcerative nasal dermatitis of Bengal cats. *Vet. Dermatol.* 15: 28.

Bellini, M.H., Caldini, E.T., Scapinelli, M.P. et al. (2009). Increased elastic microfibrils and thickening of fibroblastic nuclear lamina in canine cutaneous asthenia. *Vet. Dermatol.* 20: 139–143.

Bryden, S.L., White, S.D., Dunston, S.M. et al. (2005). Clinical, histopathological and immunological characteristics of exfoliative cutaneous lupus erythematosus in 25 German short-haired pointers. *Vet. Dermatol.* 16: 239–252.

Clark, L.A., Credille, K.M., Murphy, K.E., and Rees, C. (2005). Linkage of dermatomyositis in the Shetland Sheepdog to chromosome 35. *Vet. Dermatol.* 16: 392–394.

Docampo, M.J., Zanna, G., Fondevila, D. et al. (2011). Increased HAS2-driven hyaluronic acid synthesis in shar-pei dogs with hereditary cutaneous hyaluronosis (mucinosis). *Vet. Dermatol.* 22: 535–545.

Fleming, J.M., Platt, S.R., Kent, M. et al. (2011). Cervical dermoid sinus in a cat: case presentation and review of the literature. *J. Feline Med. Surg.* 13 (12): 992–996.

Hartley, C., Donaldson, D., Smith, K.C. et al. (2012). Congenital keratoconjunctivitis sicca and ichthyosiform dermatosis in 25 Cavalier King Charles Spaniel dogs – part I: clinical signs, histopathology, and inheritance. *Vet. Ophthalmol.* 15 (5): 315–326.

Mauldin, E.A. (2013). Canine ichthyosis and related disorders of cornification. *Vet. Clin. North Am. Small Anim. Pract.* 43 (1): 89–97.

McEwan, N.A., McNeil, P.E., Thompson, H., and McCandlish, I.A. (2000 Nov). Diagnostic features, confirmation and disease progression in 28 cases of lethal acrodermatitis of bull terriers. *J. Small Anim. Pract.* 41 (11): 501–507.

Mecklenburg, L. (2006). An overview on congenital alopecia in domestic animals. *Vet. Dermatol.* 17: 393–410.

Medeiros, G.X. and Riet-Correa, F. (2015). Epidermolysis bullosa in animals: a review. *Vet. Dermatol.* 26: 3–e2.

Pagé, N., Paradis, M., Lapointe, J.M., and Dunstan, R.W. (2003). Hereditary nasal parakeratosis in Labrador Retrievers. *Vet. Dermatol.* 14: 103–110.

Paradis, M. et al. (2005). Acral mutilation and analgesia in 13 French spaniels. *Vet. Dermatol.* 16 (2): 87–93.

17

Pigmentary dermatologic disorders

Jacquelyn Campbell, DVM, DACVD

Animal Allergy and Dermatology of Colorado, Colorado Springs, CO, USA

Author's note: The pigment of skin and hair depends on a multitude of factors including but not limited to genetic attributes, hormonal influence, UV exposure, inflammation, drug exposure, viral exposure, and nutrition. There are numerous varied clinical presentations of pigmentary changes to hair and skin that may not have an exact etiology determined and may resolve with observation. The table below highlights only some of the more commonly described conditions.

Clinical Atlas of Canine and Feline Dermatology, First Edition. Edited by Kimberly S. Coyner.

Companion website: www.wiley.com/go/coyner/dermatology

Table 17.1 Pigmentary dermatologic disorders.

Disease	Clinical signs	Diagnosis	Treatment
Lentigo (Canine) (Figures 17.1A and 17.1B) Occurs in mature dogs.	Flat, macular melanosis that is intensely black. Most commonly noted on ventrum; may be grouped or diffuse. Does not itch and of no concern to the pet. May need to be differentiated from raised pigmented tumors such as melanoma, papillomavirus induced lesions, or pigmented nevi.	History and clinical findings. Histopathology: Increased number of melanocytes and melanosomes. Typically, minimal to no structural changes within the epidermis.	Cosmetic, no treatment required.
Lentigo Simplex (Feline) (Figures 17.2A–17.2B; Chapter 2, Figure 2.2) Typically occurs in orange cats <1 year.	Asymptomatic flat, macular melanosis. Lesions start on lips and begin as tiny asymptomatic spots that gradually enlarge and increase in number. Nose, gingiva, and eyelids may be affected in addition to lips. Does not vary in intensity of pigment, well circumscribed, uniform, circular to coalescing.	History, signalment, clinical findings. Histopathology: Marked hypermelanosis, predominantly of basal layer of epithelium caused by increased melanocytes.	Cosmetic, no treatment required.
Acquired hormone-associated (Figures 17.3A–17.3E)	Diffuse hyperpigmentation as a result of metabolic or hormonal causes such as hypercortisolism, hypothyroidism, and sex hormone dermatosis.	History, clinical exam, and appropriate hematologic testing and endocrine testing.	Treatment of primary disease.
Acquired post-inflammatory hyperpigmentation (Figures 17.4A–17.4H) Common in dogs, and uncommon in cats.	The most common form of hyperpigmentation. Many diseases characterized by inflammation may undergo hyperpigmentation; often a sequela of underlying disease such as pyoderma, demodicosis, dermatophytosis, or hypersensitivity, especially atopic dermatitis. May have a lattice-like appearance and is commonly noted of glabrous skin of ventrum. Melanotrichia may also be observed after healing of deep inflammation.	History, clinical exam, and identification of underlying disease.	Identify and control underlying disease.

Table 17.1 Pigmentary dermatologic disorders (Continued)

Disease	Clinical signs	Diagnosis	Treatment
Vitiligo (Figures 17.5A–17.5C; Chapter 2, Figure 2.3; Chapter 3, Figures 3.8 and 3.23; Chapter 6, Figure 6.3) Uncommon with highest incidence in Belgian Tervurens, German Shepherds, Rottweilers, Dobermans, and Siamese cats.	Acquired disease of melanocyte destruction. Often symmetric macular areas of depigmentation of skin (leukoderma), or of hair (leukotrichia). Lesions typically affect nose, lips, face, and pawpads. Typically, lesions are not clinically inflammatory but transient erythema and scaling can be observed.	History, physical exam, and histopathology. Histopathology shows normal skin with absence of melanocytes. Transient inflammatory phase may be noted.	Cosmetic disease; no treatment documented as efficacious. In a case study of 4 canine vitiligo cases, L-phenylalanine (a precursor of melanin via tyrosine) 50 mg/kg/day PO for 6 months then twice a week for 4 months caused a reduction in depigmented areas within 2–6 months. Small number of cases may spontaneously resolve.
Nasal hypopigmentation "snow nose" "winter nose" (Figures 17.6A and 17.6B) Most commonly observed in Siberian Huskies, Golden Retrievers, Labrador Retrievers, Bernese Mountain dogs but can occur in any breed.	A common syndrome of seasonal lightening of the nasal planum; decrease in pigment of nasal planum typically seen in winter months. The normal nasal planum reticular pattern is preserved and there is no erosion or crusting to suggest immune-mediated disease.	History, physical exam.	No treatment necessary or effective.
Nasal depigmentation "Dudley nose" (Figure 17.7)	Dogs that have a tan or flesh colored nasal planum rather than black; congenital condition.	History, physical exam. Histopathology demonstrates absence of melanocytes with normal epidermis.	No treatment necessary or effective.
Acquired aurotrichia (Figure 17.8) Originally described in Miniature Schnauzers but can affect any breed.	Primary guard hairs turn from silver or black to gold. These gold hairs occur primarily in patches over dorsal thorax and abdomen. Periocular and pinnal involvement may occur.	History, signalment, physical exam.	No treatment documented. May resolve within 6–24 months; relapses may occur.
"Dalmatian bronzing" syndrome (Figure 17.9; Chapter 8, Figures 8.5E–8.5F) Occurs in Dalmatian dogs or any short-coated white dog.	Patchy brown haircoat discoloration usually associated with bacterial folliculitis and bacterial porphyrins production.	History, signalment, physical exam, skin cytology for infection.	No specific treatment for the brown discoloration is available; treat underlying bacterial skin infection.

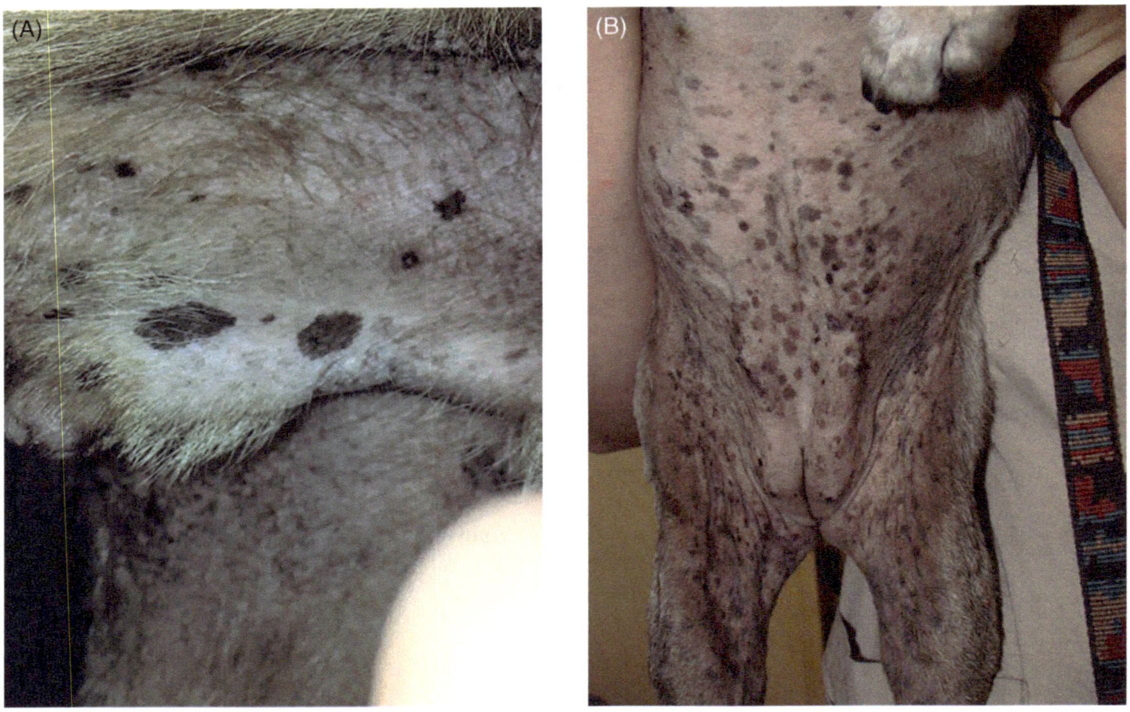

Figure 17.1A and B Canine lentigo; multiple, flat, black macules on the ventral trunk.

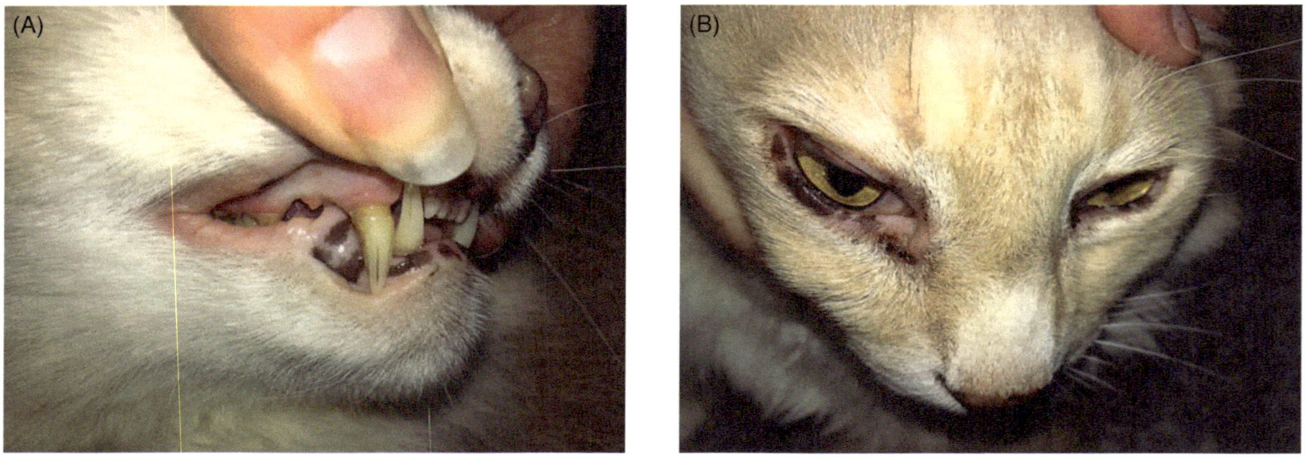

Figure 17.2A–B Feline lentigo simplex; multiple, flat, black macules on the lips and eyelids.

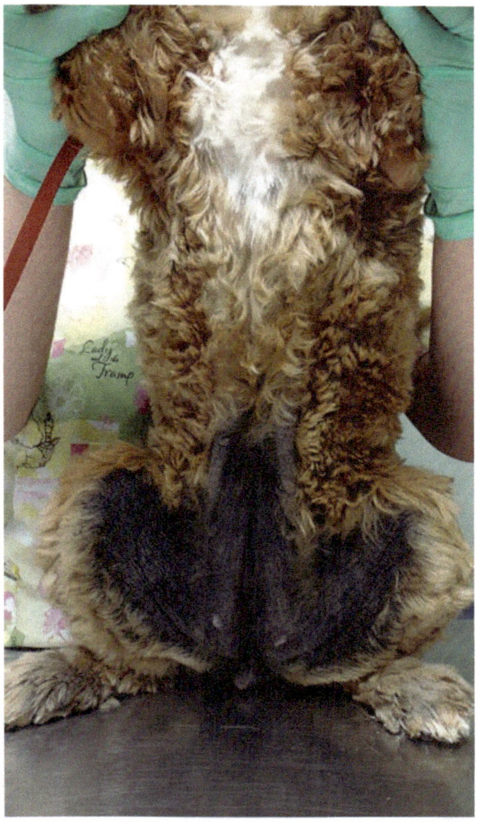

Figure 17.3A Inguinal hyperpigmentation due to hypothyroidism in a Cocker Spaniel.

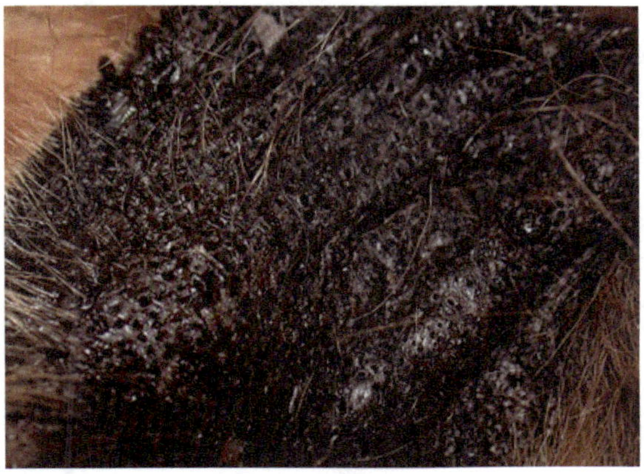

Figure 17.3B Marked inguinal hyperpigmentation and comedone formation in a Pekingese dog.

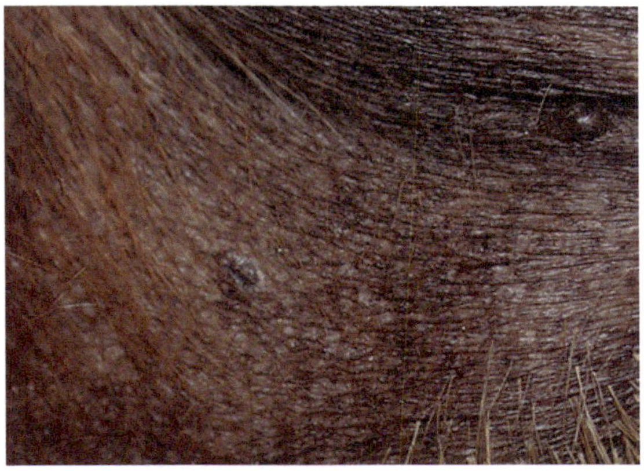

Figure 17.3C The same dog as in Fig. 17.3B; After thyroid supplementation, comedones have resolved and hyperpigmentation is improving.

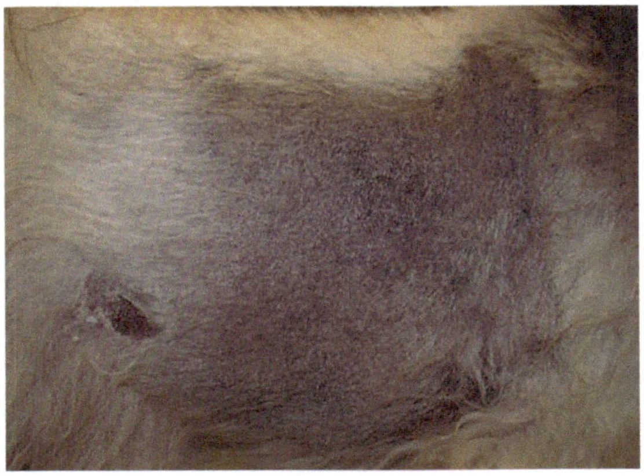

Figure 17.3D Truncal hyperpigmentation in a cushingoid Sheltie.

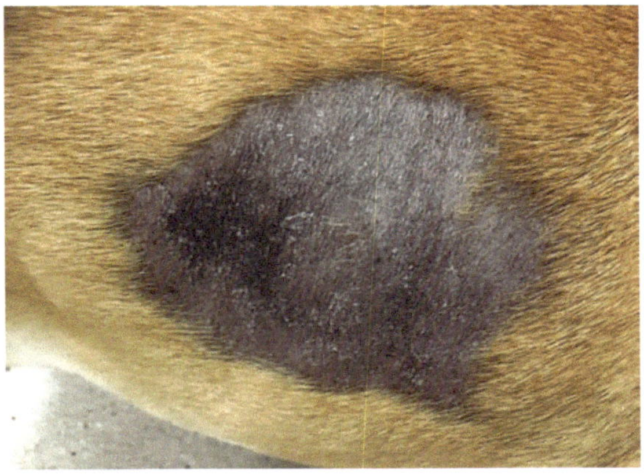

Figure 17.3E Alopecia and hyperpigmentation on the lateral trunk of an English Bulldog with both hypothyroidism and canine recurrent flank alopecia.

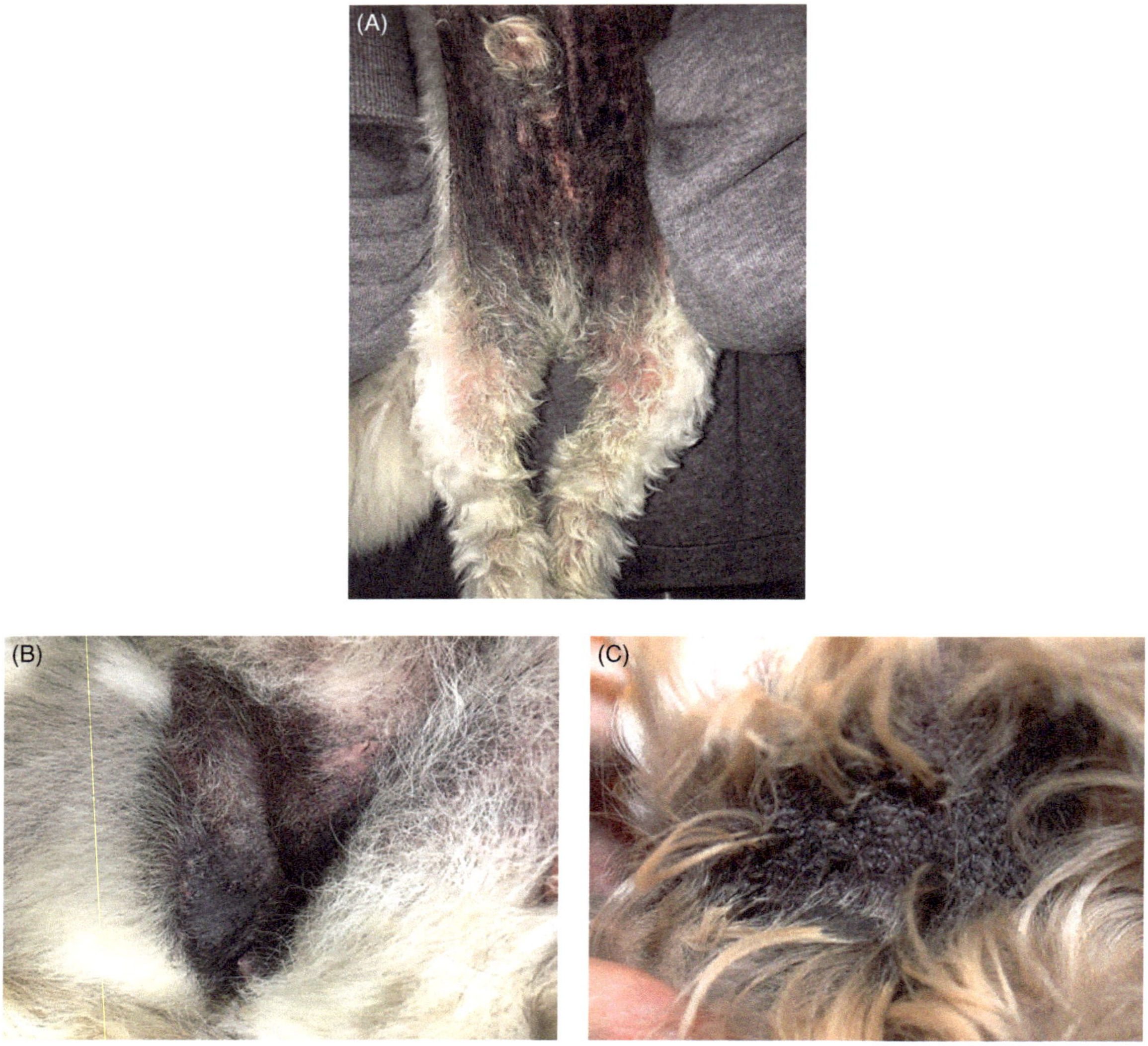

Figure 17.4A–C Post-inflammatory hyperpigmentation due to allergy and secondary bacterial pyoderma in several atopic dogs.

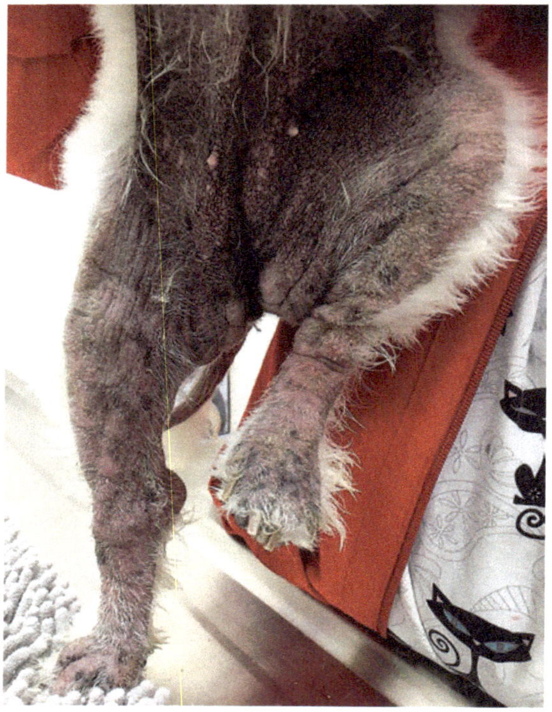

Figure 17.4D Severe bacterial and yeast skin infections caused lichenification and hyperpigmentation in this atopic Westie.

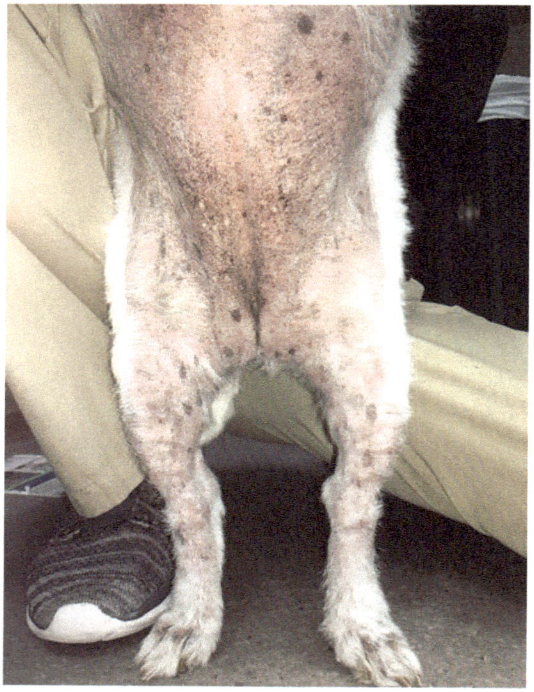

Figure 17.4E The same dog as in fig. 17.4D; After treatment of infections, lichenification has resolved and there is residual lattice hyperpigmentation due to atopy.

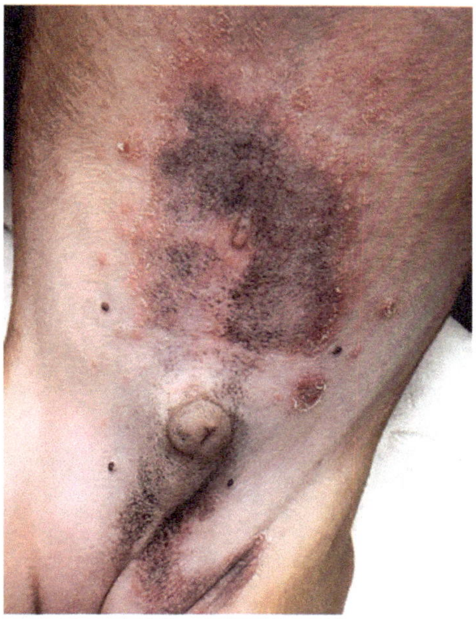

Figure 17.4F Patchy inguinal erythema and hyperpigmentation with peripheral scaling due to bacterial pyoderma.

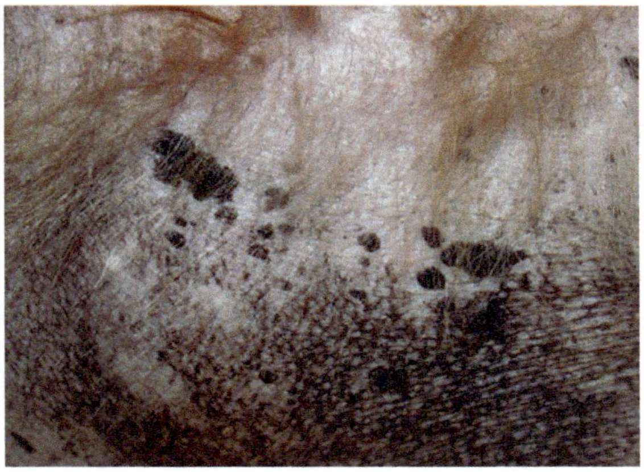

Figure 17.4G This atopic Yorkie had both lacey, inguinal post-inflammatory hyperpigmentation due to atopy as well as numerous small, raised, pigmented viral plaques which developed after treatment with oclacitinib.

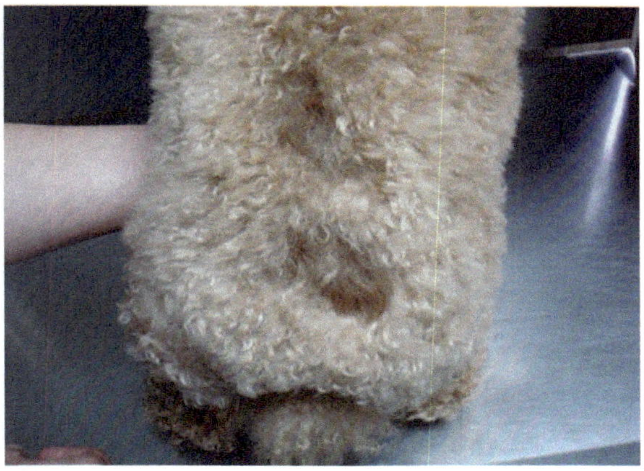

Figure 17.4H Patchy truncal melanotrichia in a Miniature Poodle; this can occur as a sequela to prior infection/inflammation, to sebaceous adenitis, or may be idiopathic in some mixed breed Poodles.

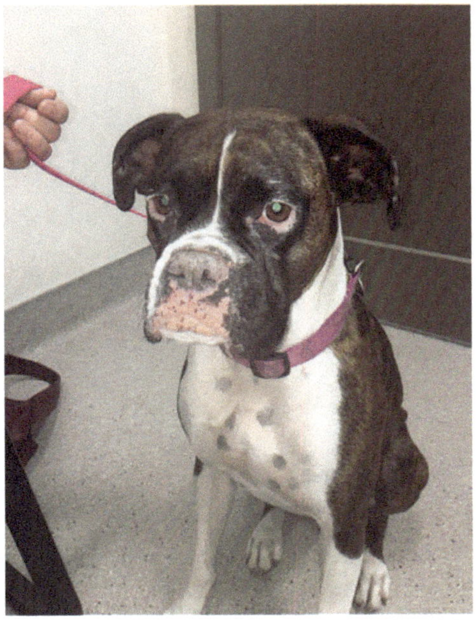

Figure 17.5A Patchy facial leukoderma in a Boxer with vitiligo.

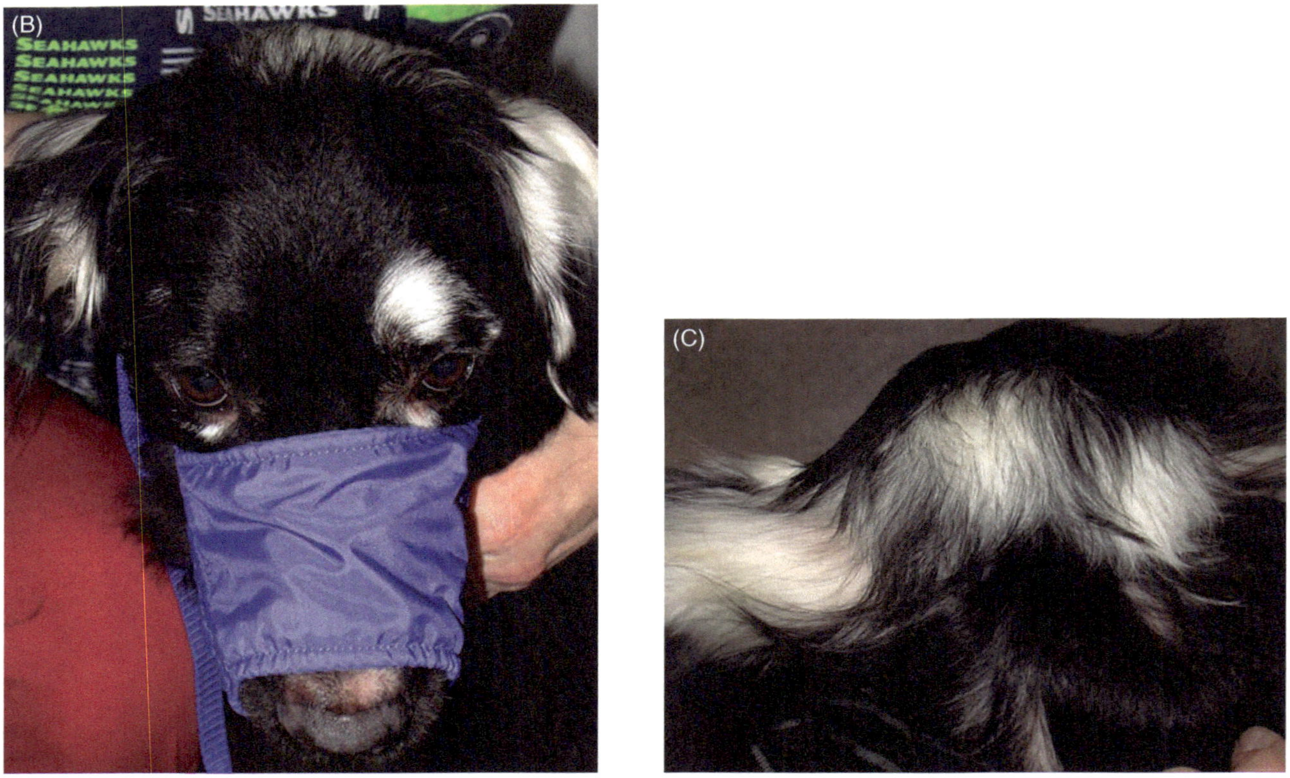

Figures 17.5B and C Multifocal leukotrichia due to vitiligo in a Shepherd mix.

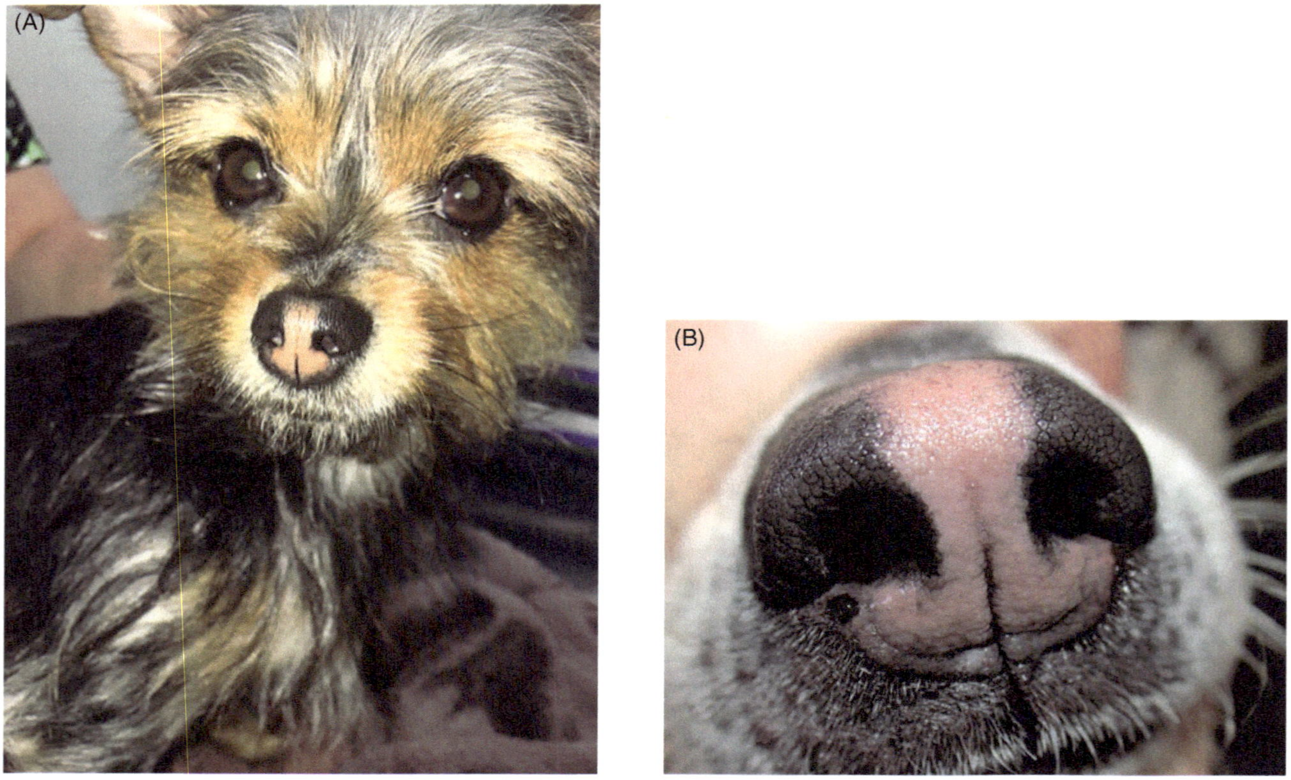

Figures 17.6A and B Snow nose causing a central strip of nasal hypopigmentation; note the normal reticular "nose print" is retained.

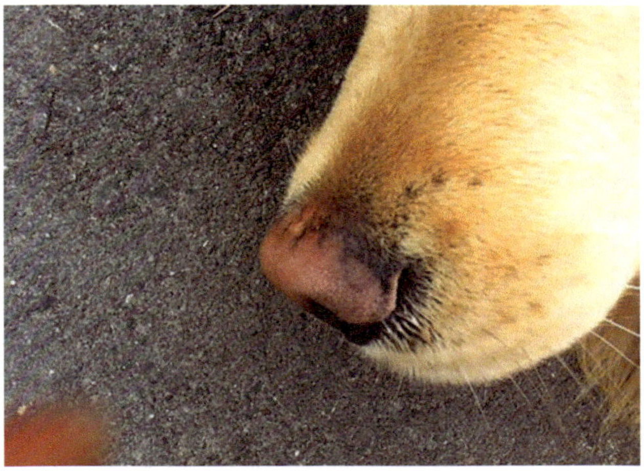

Figure 17.7 Dudley nose causing a tan rather than black nasal planum in a Labrador. *Source:* Image courtesy of VIN and Lisa Booth, DVM.

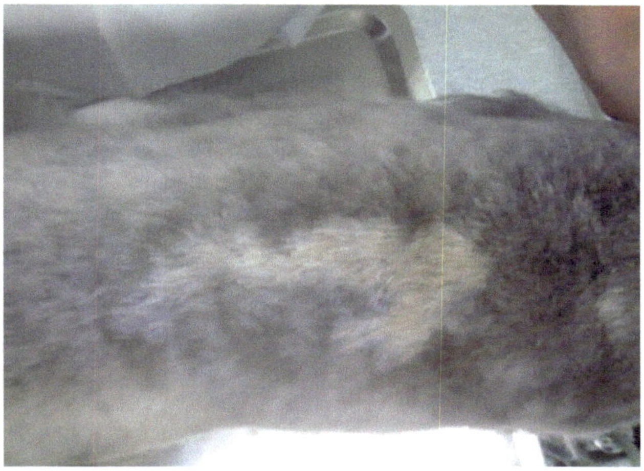

Figure 17.8 Aurotrichia in a Miniature Schnauzer. *Source:* Image courtesy of VIN and Marcella Ramos, DVM.

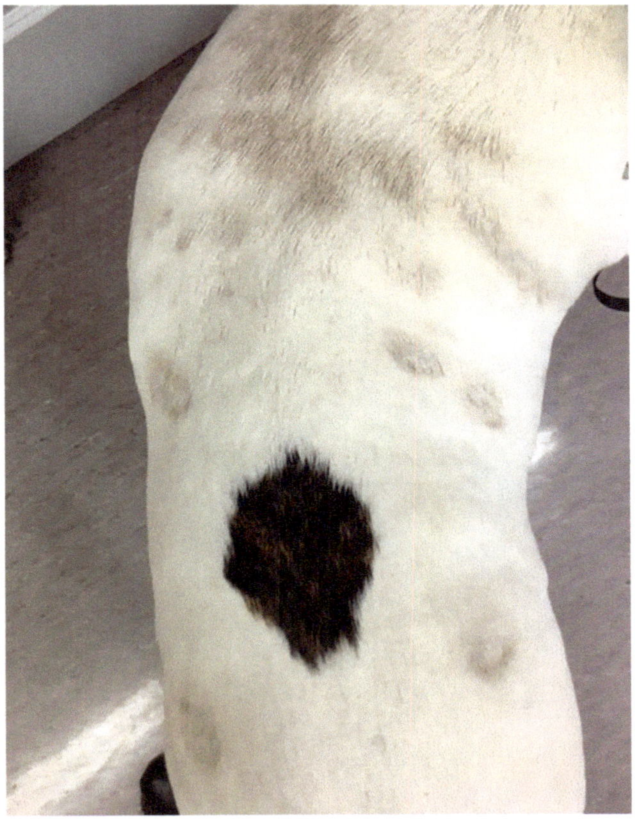

Figure 17.9 Brown discoloration of white fur due to bacterial folliculitis.

Further reading

Alhaidari, Z., Olivry, T., and Ortonne, J.P. (1999). Melanocytogenesis and melanogenesis: genetic regulation and comparative clinical diseases. *Vet. Dermatol.* 10: 3–16.

Coyner, K. (2012 January/February). Challenges and new developments in canine Pyoderma: disease overview and diagnosis. *Today's Veterinary Practice* 36–44.

Guaguère, E. and Muller, A. (2008). Efficacy of L-phenylalanine in the treatment of canine vitiligo: a preliminary report of 4 cases. 6th World Congress of Veterinary Dermatology, Hong Kong. *Vet. Dermatol.* 19 (suppl 1): 75.

Scott, D.W., Miller, W.H., and Griffin, C.E. (2013). *Muller & Kirk's Small Animal Dermatology*, 7e. Philadelphia: Elsevier.

Sulaimon, S.S. and Kitchell, B.E. (2003). The biology of melanocytes. *Vet. Dermatol.* 14: 57–65.

18

Environmental skin disorders

Kimberly S. Coyner, DVM, DACVD

Dermatology Clinic for Animals, Lacey, WA, USA

Clinical Atlas of Canine and Feline Dermatology, First Edition. Edited by Kimberly S. Coyner.

Companion website: www.wiley.com/go/coyner/dermatology

Table 18.1 Environmental skin disorders.

Disease	Clinical signs	Diagnosis	Prevention/Treatment
Solar dermatitis (Figures 18.1A–18.1G) Prolonged and repeated sun damage leads to keratinocyte proliferation, mutagenesis, atypia and premalignant actinic keratoses, which can progress to invasive squamous cell carcinoma. In dogs, solar dermatitis most commonly affects lightly skinned, short-coated breeds such as Pitbull and Staffordshire Bull Terriers, Bull Terriers, Boxers, Dalmatians, American Bulldogs, and Whippets. In cats, solar dermatitis most commonly affects non-pigmented skin on the ear pinnae, nose, and eyelids.	Cats: Early lesions present with non-pruritic erythema and fine scaling which progress to skin peeling and crusting; pinnal margins may be slightly curled or take on a scalloped appearance. Actinic keratosis or squamous cell carcinoma in situ can develop and appear as chronically crusted or eroded lesions. Dogs: Sun damage usually occurs on nonpigmented thinly haired areas such as the flank, inguinal and axillary areas, and the dorsal nose, but it can occur on the dorsal and lateral trunk and lateral legs as well as other areas. In dogs that prefer to lie on one side of their body, lesions may be worse on the more chronically sun-exposed side. Initial signs of actinic damage are erythematous scaly lesions, which may be tender. With chronic sun exposure, damaged areas become thickened and scarred with comedones, cysts, erosions, ulcers, crusts, and draining tracts. Secondary bacterial pyoderma is common. Actinic or solar keratoses can occur and appear as non-healing erythematous, scaly to crusty macules and plaques which represent focal areas of abnormal keratinocyte proliferation/differentiation which with time may progress to invasive squamous cell carcinoma. With chronic solar damage, sun-induced skin tumors such as squamous cell carcinoma, hemangioma, and cutaneous hemangiosarcoma may occur.	Consider signalment and clinical signs. Rule out other causes for scaly erythematous dermatitis or folliculitis (e.g. bacterial, *Demodex*, and dermatophyte infections). Biopsy/dermatopathology: Prior to biopsy, systemic antibiotics may be indicated for 2–3 weeks to ensure that secondary infection does not alter histopathologic interpretation. Early lesions: Nonspecific inflammation, fibrosis, epidermal hyperplasia with intraepidermal edema is seen, and vacuolated (sunburn cells) and apoptotic keratinocytes may be seen. Solar elastosis (linear bands of degenerated basophilic elastin accumulation arranged parallel to the skin surface) may also be present. In chronic cases, histologic examination may show follicular cysts, pyogranulomatous inflammation, and precancerous actinic keratosis or squamous cell carcinoma.	<u>Sun avoidance</u> Keep pet indoors during the day, especially between 9 a.m. and 3 p.m. Also avoid reflected sunlight (i.e. white concrete sidewalks or dog run flooring). If some sun exposure is unavoidable, then twice daily topical application of a waterproof, high SPF sunscreen that protects against UVA and UVB should be used. A dog sun suit is available at www.designerdogwear.com, or talented clients may be able to sew a sunsuit for their pets using sun-blocking fabric available for people. Tattooing is ineffective, as the tattoo ink is deposited in the dermis, which does not protect the epidermis; additionally, colorants absorb or reflect visible light but have no protection against ultraviolet rays. <u>Acute therapy</u> For mild acute cases of solar dermatitis, topical application of 1% hydrocortisone daily to BID for a week), or a 5–7 day course of oral anti-inflammatory prednisone may be helpful. <u>Therapy for chronic disease and actinic keratoses</u> *Systemic therapies* Carotenoids: To decrease sun damage, it has been reported in dogs that beta-carotene (30 mg orally BID for 30 days, then 30 mg/day for life) in combination with anti-inflammatory doses of oral glucocorticoids could be effective in early cases. In cats, beta-carotene and canthaxanthin (25 mg doses of active carotenoids) have been used orally with mixed success.

			Retinoids and Vitamin A: Skin damage may also be reduced by administering oral retinoids such as acitretin or isotretinoin 0.5–1 mg/kg PO q24h. Due to expense of retinoids and difficulty in obtaining them for veterinary use, oral vitamin A has been used anecdotally for canine solar dermatitis, suggested dosage of oral vitamin A for dogs is 800–1000 IU/kg PO daily for 3 months, then the frequency is reduced to three times weekly. Non-steroidal anti-inflammatories: Cyclooxygenase-2 (COX-2) expression has been detected in actinic keratosis and squamous cell carcinomas and administration of an oral NSAID can cause clinical and histopathological improvement. *Topical therapies* Imiquimod: Imiquimod applied three times weekly for actinic keratosis/SCC in situ. Potential side effects include erythema, crusting, alopecia, discomfort, hepatopathy if ingested. *Non-medical options* Depending on lesion location, actinic keratoses can also be potentially treated with surgery, cryotherapy, photodynamic therapy, or laser ablation.
Burns (Figures 18.2A–18.2I) Can be caused by strong chemicals, electric currents, solar and microwave radiation, and heat (fire, boiling liquids including hot garden hose water, heating pads, dryers, hot pavement). Burn injuries can be hidden by fur and not become evident for a week or more post injury when necrotic skin appears. Heating pad injury can be exacerbated by duration of exposure, fluid pooling, hypotension and concurrent systemic disease.	Clinical signs vary based on depth of burn injury in skin. Superficial (epidermis only): Erythematous desquamation, painful. Heals in 3–5 days via re-epithelialization. Partial thickness (epidermis, superficial to deep dermis): Erythematous, moist, +/– blisters and edema; black to yellow/white eschar formation if entire dermis involved. May be painful or have decreased sensation depending on depth. Milder burns heal in 1–2 weeks via re-epithelialization, deeper burns heal in 2–3 weeks, may need surgical intervention.	History, clinical signs. Biopsy: Gradually tapering coagulation necrosis (“outside–in”) of epidermis and deeper tissues confirm thermal or chemical burn.	Acute burns: Irrigate with cold tap water (59 °F) for 20 minutes (no ice). Wound care: Irrigation with antibacterial solution (chlorhexidene 1 : 40 dilution), debride necrotic tissue (daily hydrotherapy with handheld sprayer). Apply topical antimicrobial agents applied BID–TID, preferred topicals include silver sulfadiazine cream or mafenide acetate cream. Medical grade honey can be used initially, stop when granulation bed formed and change to non-adherent dressings.

(*Continued*)

Table 18.1 Environmental skin disorders (Continued)

Disease	Clinical signs	Diagnosis	Prevention/Treatment
Burns (cont.)	Full thickness (complete destruction of epidermis, dermis and SQ): Bloodless white eschar, hair easily plucked. Surgical intervention indicated, otherwise will heal by contraction and hypertrophic scarring/deformation. Animals with deep burns >20% skin surface will develop electrolyte imbalance and fluid loss, burns >50% skin surface are usually fatal. Necrosis of skin and damage to underlying vasculature sets patients up for secondary infection which systemic antibiotics cannot reach.		Silver impregnated wound dressings are available which can remain in place for 3–7 days on partial thickness burns for outpatient therapy. Conservative wound management with daily trimming of separating eschar edges appropriate for smaller, less extensive wounds and for unstable patients. Deep partial-thickness and full-thickness burns require eschar removal and topical antimicrobial treatment until wound closure or graft application possible. Monitor wound for local infection: Change in wound color/depth, increased exudate or pain, early separation of eschar. Systemic antibiotics are not effective in preventing infection due to impaired vasculature; use only if systemic infection present. Avoid steroids; pentoxifylline may help reduce hyperplastic scarring. Pain control essential: Opioids, benzodiazepines, +/– combination infusion with ketamine; manage fluid and electrolyte imbalances with fluids +/– colloids. Nutrition very important: Institute enteral feeding within 24–48 hours post injury, use nasogastric (NG) or E-tube (esophagostomy tube) if needed.

Radiant heat dermatitis (a.k.a. erythema ab igne, Figure 18.3) Results from prolonged and repetitive exposure to moderate heat sources such as lying near a stove, radiator, space heater, heat lamp, or on a kennel warming pad or electric blanket.	Variably shaped, often linear or lattice-like areas of hyperpigmentation and alopecia, often on trunk. May have areas of erythema or hyperpigmentation surrounding central hypopigmentation. May be scaly +/− crusted or focally eroded. Not pruritic or painful.	Clinical signs, history of exposure to local intense heat source such as stove, space heater, heat lamp. Biopsy: Atrophic hair follicles, fibrosis with eosinophilic, wavy, elastic fibrils in dermis.	Prevent exposure to heat source. Can lead to permanent scarring.
Frostbite (Figures 18.4A–18.4C) Occurs due to prolonged exposure to freezing temperatures. More common in debilitated animals or animals not acclimated to the cold. Wind, moisture/wetting and lack of shelter increase risk of frostbite.	Most commonly affects ear tips, digits, tail tip, and scrotum. Initially skin is pale and cool to touch; after thawing mild edema, erythema and discomfort +/− scaling occur. In severe cases, affected tissue becomes necrotic and sloughs; pinnal margins may curl. Scarring, alopecia, and leukotrichia may occur post healing.	Clinical signs, history.	Move patient to warm area and use warm (not hot) water to thaw affected areas. Healing will occur over days to weeks depending on severity; a short course of NSAIDs can reduce inflammation and discomfort and pentoxifylline may help increase circulation and improve tissue viability. In severe necrotic cases, amputation may be necessary.
Irritant contact dermatitis (ICD) (Figures 18.5A and 18.5B) A nonspecific inflammatory cutaneous reaction caused by direct contact with an irritating agent. Unlike allergic contact dermatitis, prior exposure and sensitization is not required; can affect multiple individuals living in the same household. Typical causes include caustic chemicals such as fertilizers, petrolatum based products, strong acids/alkalis, cleansers, solvents, insecticidal dips/collars/shampoos, and components of paints, carpets, and wood preservatives.	Lesions that develop from ICD typically develop only in the area of direct contact (unlike allergic contact dermatitis which may extend beyond the area of contact). Acute lesions include edema, erythema and papules; lesions can be painful (but not usually pruritic, in contrast to allergic contact dermatitis), and in severe cases necrosis and ulceration may occur. Chronic lesions can be scaly, lichenified, and fissured. Secondary bacterial and yeast infections can occur and increase inflammation and discomfort.	Clinical signs, history (including any recent environmental changes or new topical therapies), and response to removal from the irritant +/− re-exposure. Skin scrapings and cytology to rule out infectious causes of dermatitis. Biopsy: Acute lesions show epithelial cell damage +/− ulceration and intracellular vacuolation and edema with a mononuclear inflammatory infiltrate. Chronic lesions show epidermal hyperplasia and hyperkeratosis with increased dermal mononuclear cells.	Identify and remove irritant. Bathe with cool water, with or without a nonirritating shampoo to remove the irritant and soothe the skin. Topical corticosteroids can be used for localized lesions; in severe or generalized cases, systemic anti-inflammatory prednisone for 5–7 days may be helpful. Treat any secondary bacterial or yeast infections with appropriate topical or systemic antibacterial and antifungal medications.

(*Continued*)

Table 18.1 Environmental skin disorders (Continued)

Disease	Clinical signs	Diagnosis	Prevention/Treatment
Grass awns/burs (Figures 18.6A–E) Grass seeds (commonly known as foxtails) from *Hordeum jubatum* and similar grasses often become lodged between toes, in external ear canals or in the nasal cavity. Burdock (*Arctium*) burs often become trapped in fur in between toes.	Foxtails can cause interdigital granulomas and draining tracts, as well as acutely painful otitis and head shaking or explosive sneezing and nasal discharge. As foxtails migrate, they can carry in pathogenic bacteria such as *Nocardia* or *Actinomyces* and create chronic secondary, deep infection/draining tracts on the limbs and trunk. Foxtails can migrate to the lungs or abdomen, causing pyothorax and peritonitis. Burdock burs cause intense oral inflammation as the dogs try to remove the burs from their paws and coat; resultant lesions are 2–3 mm raised, white to pink papules to eroded plaques (granulomas) on the lips and dorsal tongue.	Clinical signs. Demonstration of plant awns on exploration of paw lesions or on otoscopic examination (though in chronic cases the plant awns have degraded or cannot be found due to migration or inflammatory and scar tissue). Cytology of draining tract exudate +/− tissue culture indicated if lesion is chronic or if bacteria are present on cytology despite empiric antibiotics. Biopsy: Foxtail-induced lesions: non-specific pyogranulomatous inflammation; plant material is occasionally found. Biopsy: Burdock induced lesions: pyogranulomatous to eosinophilic inflammation centered on plant material.	Exploration of draining tracts to identify and remove the plant awns, flush liberally with dilute chlorhexidine, +/− a 3–4 week course of systemic antibiotics for secondary infection; much longer courses of antibiotics needed for *Actinomyces* or *Nocardia* infections. For foxtails trapped in deep tissues, ultrasound may be helpful to locate lesions prior to surgical exploration. For burdock burs, debridement of granulomatous tissue/burrs using a scalpel blade or curette under general anesthesia is needed; aftercare includes soft to liquid foods for several days and oral antibiotics for 5 days. The procedure may need to be repeated more than once until the inflammation is resolved. Prevention: Careful inspection and combing of interdigital areas and coat to remove plant material after pet has been in areas containing seeded grasses or burdocks.
Post traumatic alopecia (Figure 18.7) Has been described in cats 3–4 weeks after road trauma, often in association with pelvic fractures. Suspected to be due to blunt force trauma causing shearing forces in the skin which damage subcutaneous and skin blood vessels, resulting in ischemia to overlying skin.	Hair loss begins on lumbar area or trunk 3–4 weeks post trauma; hairs are easily epilated and underlying skin is non-inflamed, often pale and shiny in appearance. Erosions or ulcers may develop. Not painful or pruritic, though cat may lick the affected area. Healing is slow and permanent scarring can result.	History, clinical findings. Skin biopsy: Ischemic changes with basal cell vacuolation and follicular/adnexal atrophy.	In mild cases, lesions slowly heal spontaneously. In severe cases with ulceration, wound care as for burns is needed.

Hygroma (Figure 18.8) A fluid-filled cyst which forms over boney prominences (elbows, hocks, ischia) due to repetitive trauma causes focal hemorrhage, necrosis, and inflammation.	Early lesions are soft to firm, fluid-filled cysts which contain straw colored or red tinged fluid. More chronic lesions can become scarred/fibrotic or inflamed with draining tracts if secondary infection occurs.	Clinical appearance/location. Aspirate/fluid cytology: Usually poorly cellular fluid containing scattered RBCs and inflammatory cells, purulent inflammation with bacteria may be present if secondary infection occurs. Biopsy (usually not necessary): Cystic spaces surrounded by granulation tissue.	Early lesions respond to padded bandages, donut bandages +/− orthotics such as Dogleggs® x 2–3 weeks. Severe lesions may require drainage or as a last resort surgery with prolonged post-operative wound care and bandaging to prevent dehiscence.
Pressure sore (decubitus ulcer) (Figures 18.9A and 18.9B) Results from prolonged pressure on bony prominences which compresses skin capillaries and causes skin ischemia. More common in older, large breed or heavy dogs.	Early lesions are erythematous to purplish skin discoloration which progresses to necrosis, exudation, and ulceration. Secondary bacterial infection is common.	Signalment, clinical signs. Cytology to identify secondary infection +/− culture if bacteria persist cytologically despite empiric antibiotics.	Prevention is important; recumbent animals should be provided with effective padding such as an eggcrate foam rubber pad and turned frequently or placed in slings; ensure bodily fluids do not accumulate to contribute to tissue maceration and inflammation. If a pressure sore develops, additional padding will be needed in the affected area in the form of soft bandages, donut bandages, and/or protective orthotics such as Dogleggs®. Frequent wound care is needed to cleanse wound bed and treat secondary infection; helpful topical products can include hydrocolloid dressings, sucralfate and silver containing dressings, mupirocin antibiotic ointment, honey, and collagen hydrolysate gel (Collasate®, PRN Pharmacal). Note: Preparation H hemorrhoid cream has been a recommended topical treatment in older references; the US formulation of this product has changed and does not contain the yeast extract (termed BioDyne) which stimulates wound healing. However at the time of this writing, the original Preparation H formula is available at some Canadian online pharmacies. Low level laser therapy may be helpful. In lesions with bone exposure, surgical closure is needed, but may dehisce unless animal is ambulatory.

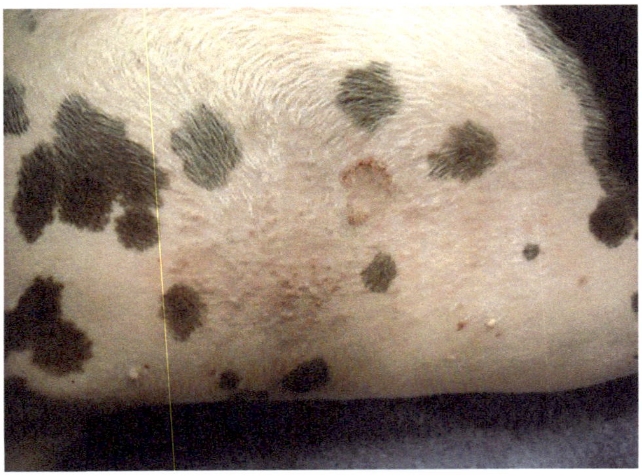

Figure 18.1A Truncal hypotrichosis, papules, comedones, and serpiginous crusts due to solar dermatitis.

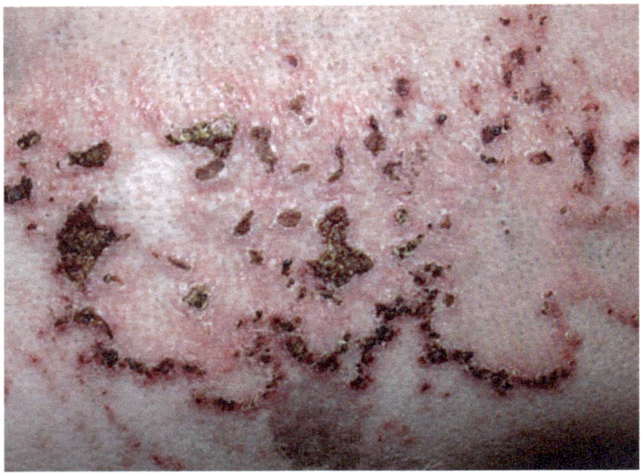

Figure 18.1B Erythema and crusts caused by solar dermatitis in a Pitbull.

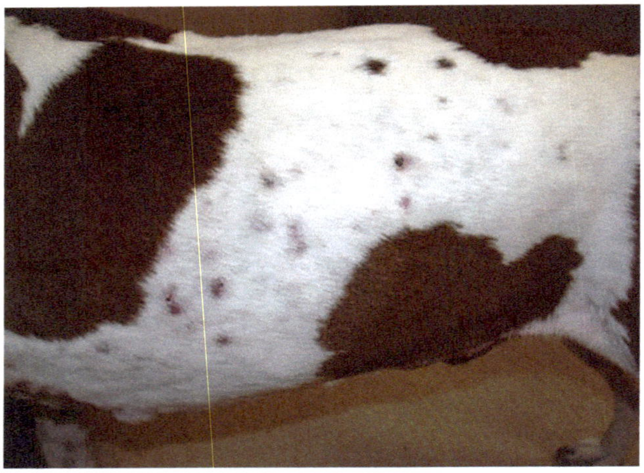

Figure 18.1C Raised, inflamed, cystic, crusted, truncal lesions due to solar dermatitis; note restriction of lesions to non-pigmented skin.

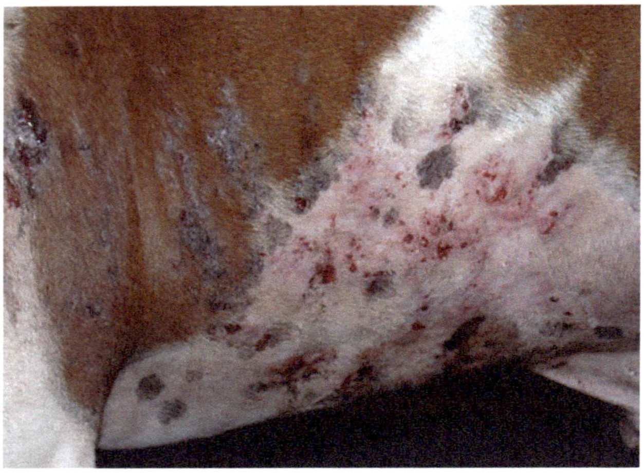

Figure 18.1D In this Pitbull with solar dermatitis, scarring and severe secondary deep pyoderma occurred and increased inflammation, causing draining tracts which affected both non-pigmented and pigmented skin.

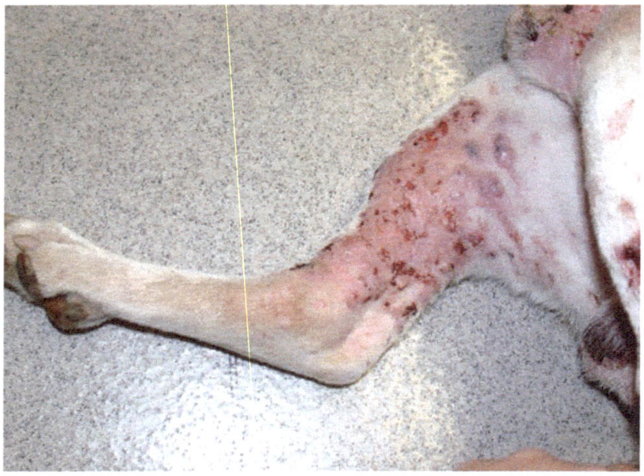

Figure 18.1E Erythema, scarring, crusts, and cystic lesions due to chronic sun damage.

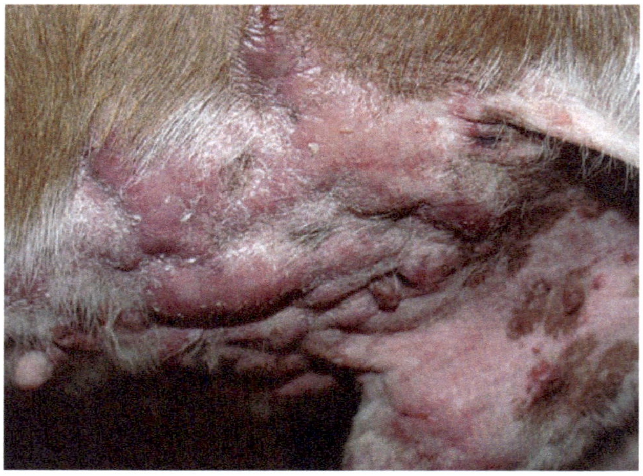

Figure 18.1F Inflamed, cystic, inguinal lesions due to chronic solar dermatitis.

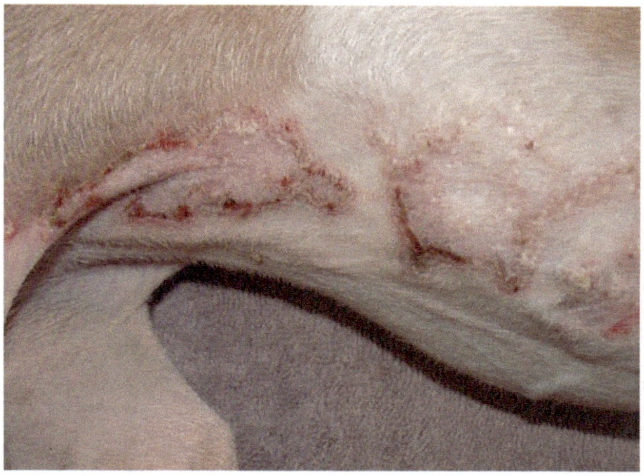

Figure 18.1G Serpiginous, scaly, inguinal lesions due to chronic sun damage and actinic keratoses in an Italian Greyhound.

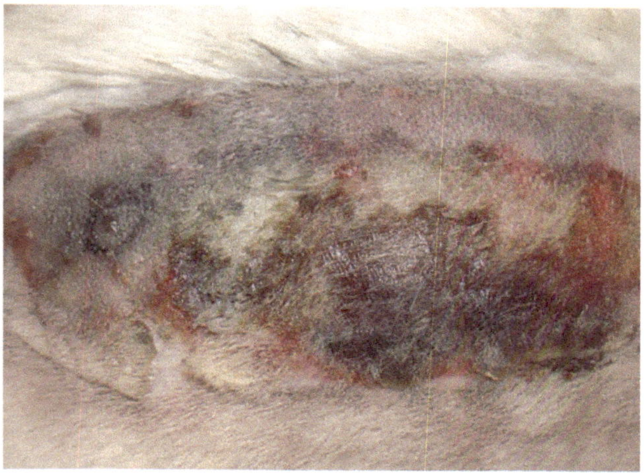

Figure 18.2A A thermal burn caused by a heating pad on the dorsal trunk of a dog.

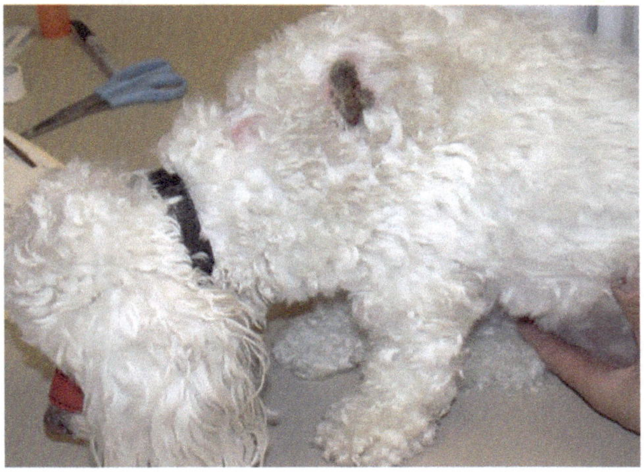

Figure 18.2B A thermal burn caused by a hot blow dryer on a Bichon.

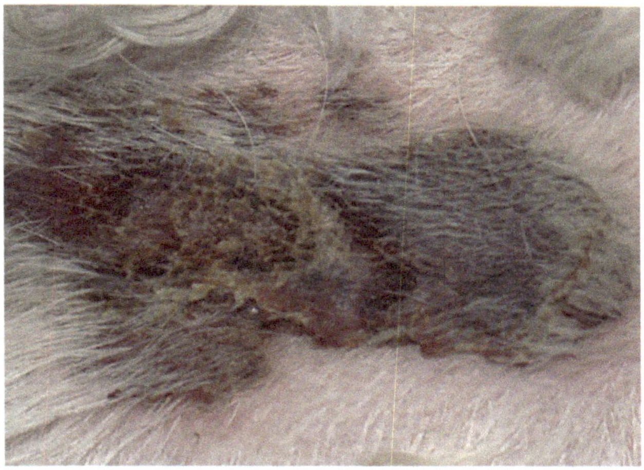

Figure 18.2C Close up view of thermal burn causing a focal necrotic eschar.

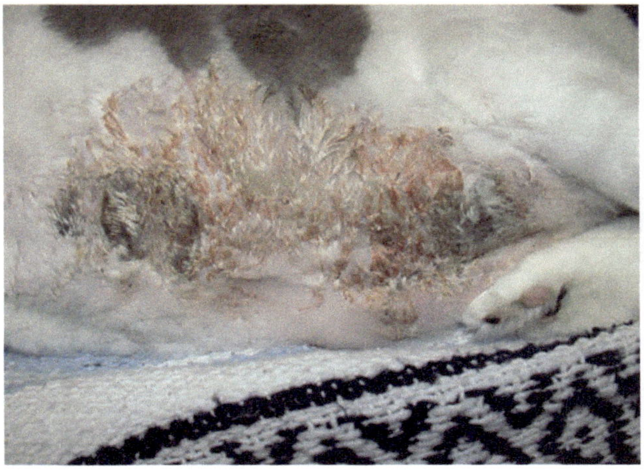

Figure 18.2D A thermal burn caused by a heating pad on the inguinal area of a cat. Superficial crusting and erythema developed several days after anesthesia.

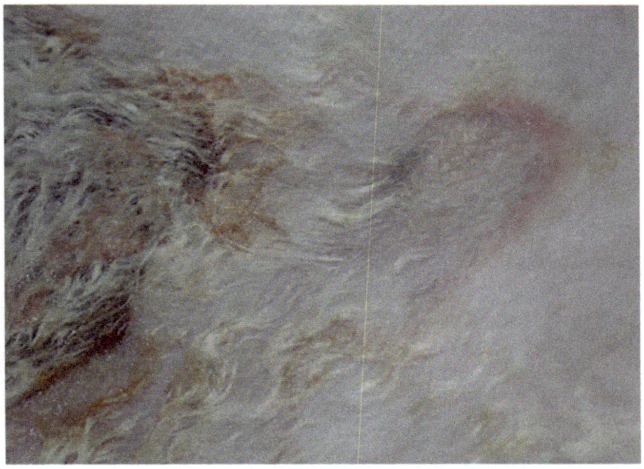

Figure 18.2E The margins of the superficial burn are visible as serpigenous areas of erythema and desquamation.

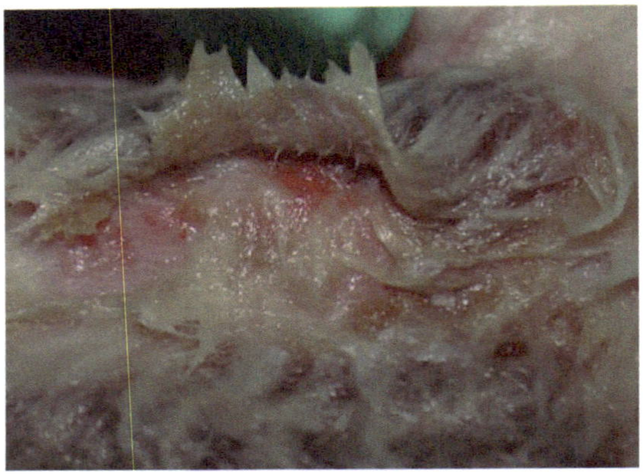

Figure 18.2F The central area of the lesion showed partial thickness burn when the overlying necrotic crust was moistened and lifted up to reveal underlying dermis.

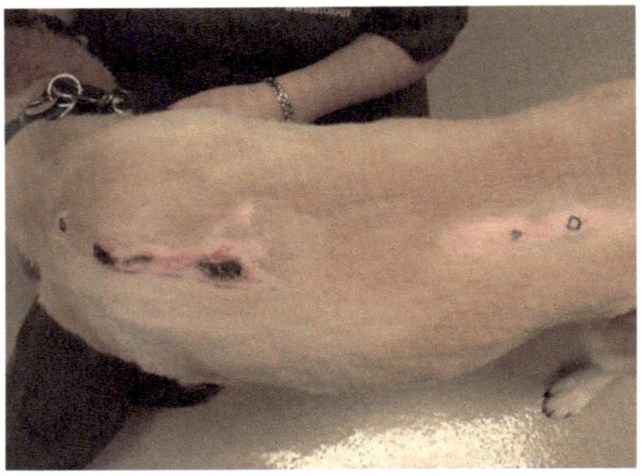

Figure 18.2G Solar-induced thermal burns in a dog which occurred after long hike in hot sunny weather; photos was taken 2 weeks after event occurred, note the exclusively dorsal distribution of crusts and scarring.

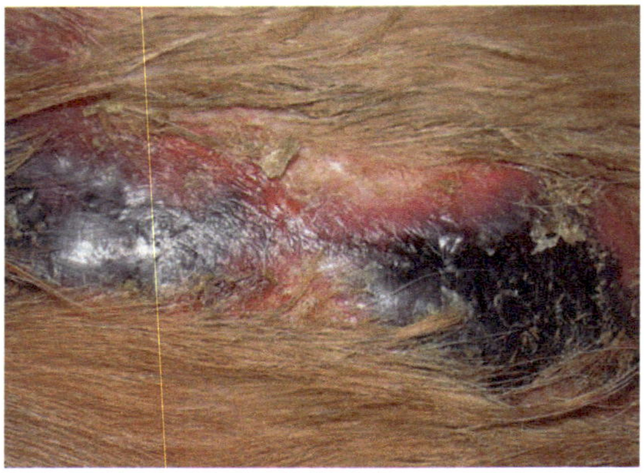

Figure 18.2H Solar induced thermal burns in this dog caused acute raised bullous blood filled lesions on the dorsal trunk.

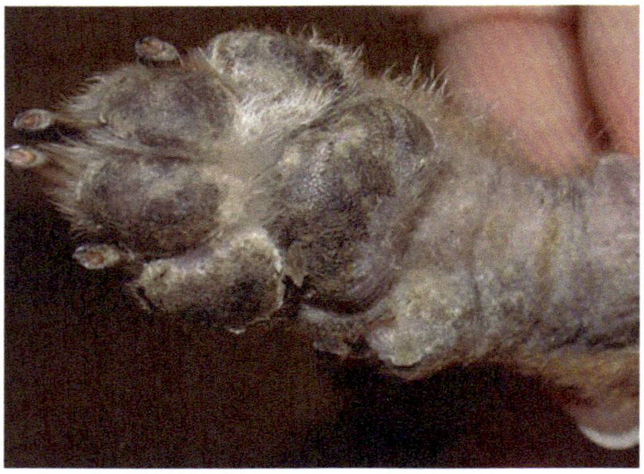

Figure 18.2I Thermal burns on the pawpads of a dog after walking on hot asphalt.

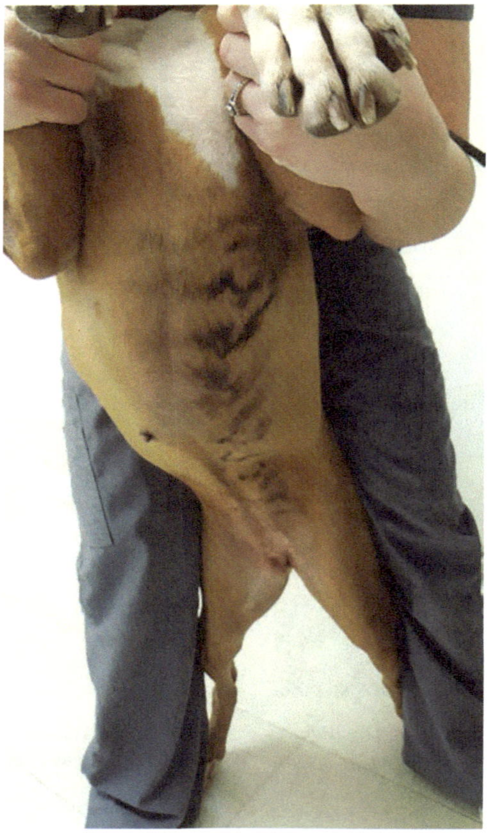

Figure 18.3 Erythema ab igne in a dog caused by sleeping next to a space heater for several weeks; lesions resolved when the space heater was removed. *Source:* Image courtesy of VIN and Sandra Marky, DVM.

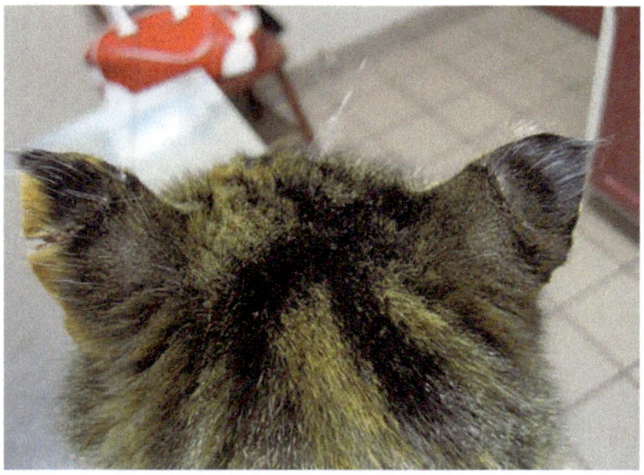

Figure 18.4A Frostbite causing distal pinnal necrosis in a cat. *Source:* Image courtesy of VIN and Tamara Goff, DVM.

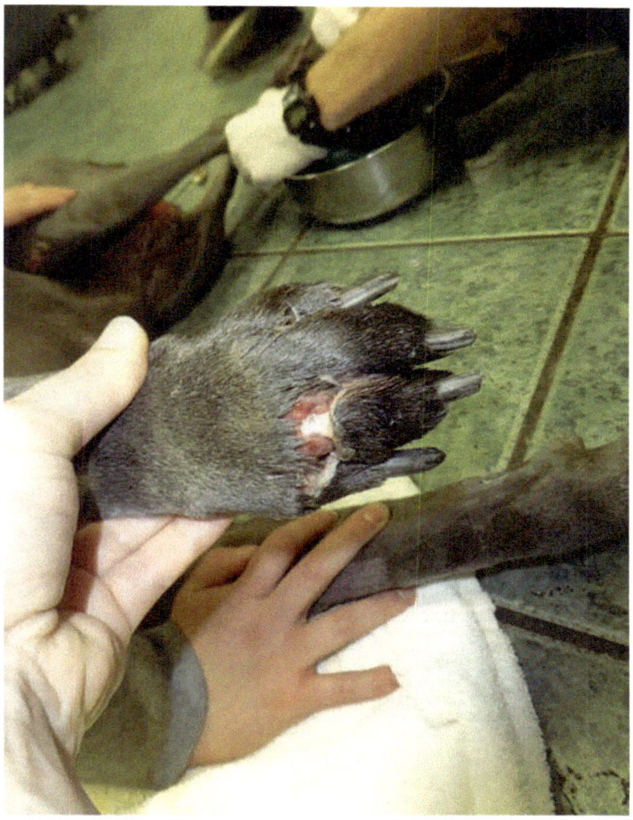

Figure 18.4B Frostbite caused toe necrosis in this dog; photo was taken 9 days post injury. 9 and 15 days post injury. *Source:* Images courtesy of VIN and Laura Carpenter, DVM.

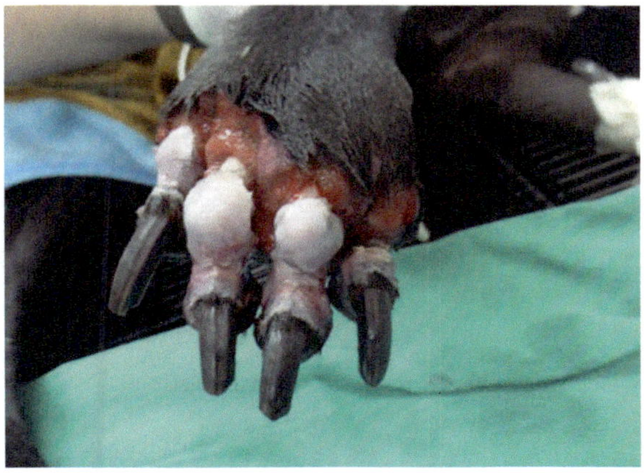

Figure 18.4C The same dog showing progressive frostbite induced toe necrosis 15 days post injury. *Source:* Images courtesy of VIN and Laura Carpenter, DVM.

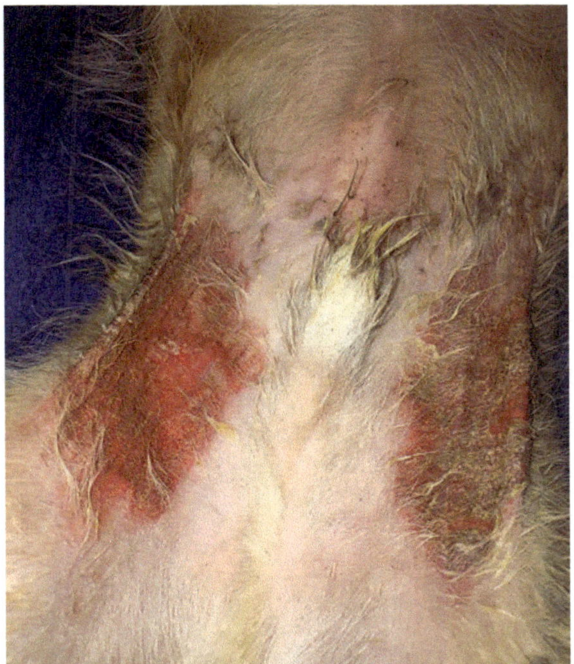

Figure 18.5A A dog with painful inguinal dermatitis caused by an irritant contact reaction to a chlorhexidene-based spray.

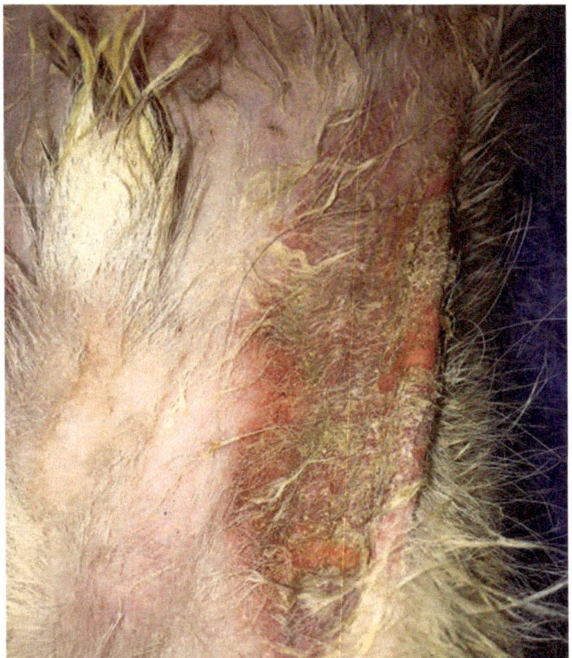

Figure 18.5B Close up of chlorhexidene induced irritant contact dermatitis; lesions were restricted to only where the spray was being applied.

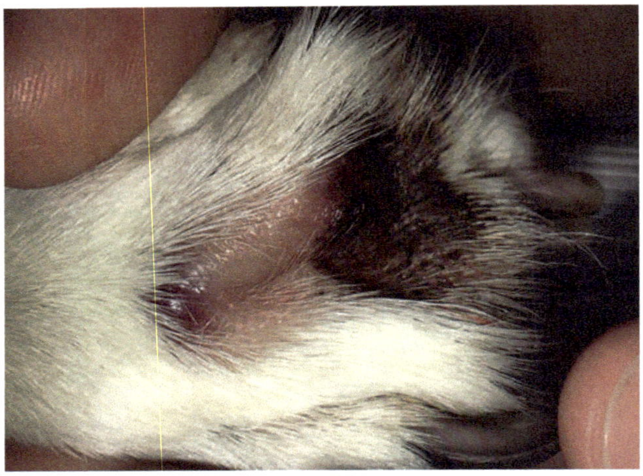

Figure 18.6A Focal interdigital swelling/inflammation and eventual draining tract due to a foxtail.

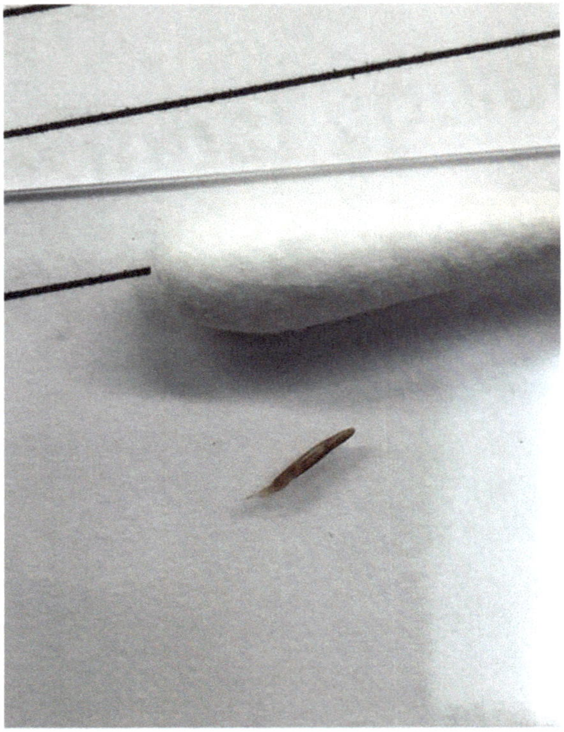

Figure 18.6B The tiny foxtail/grass seed after removal.

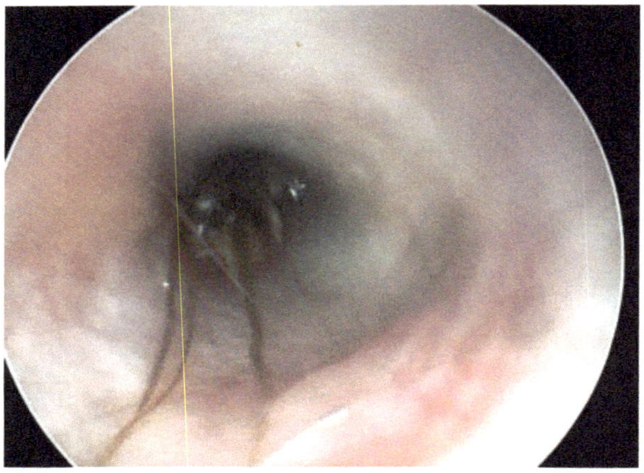

Figure 18.6C Foxtails in the proximal ear canal of a dog.

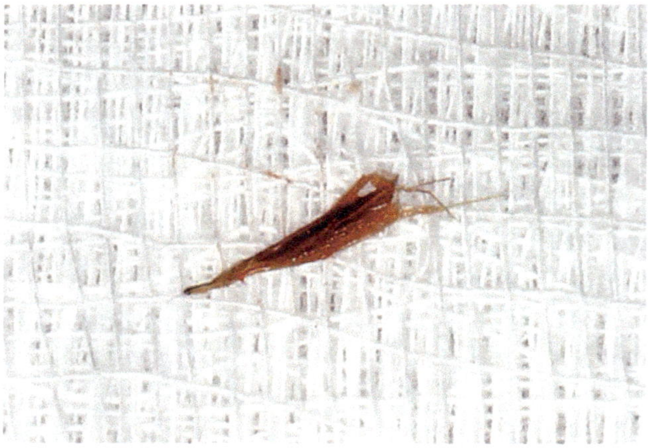

Figure 18.6D Close up of foxtail after removal from the ear canal.

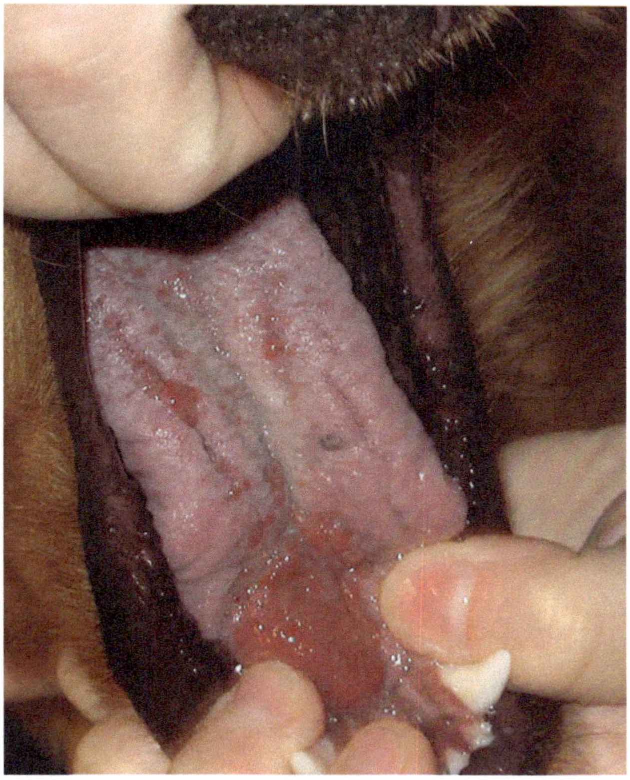

Figure 18.6E Burdock induced glossitis. *Source:* Image courtesy of VIN and Vicky Smith, DVM.

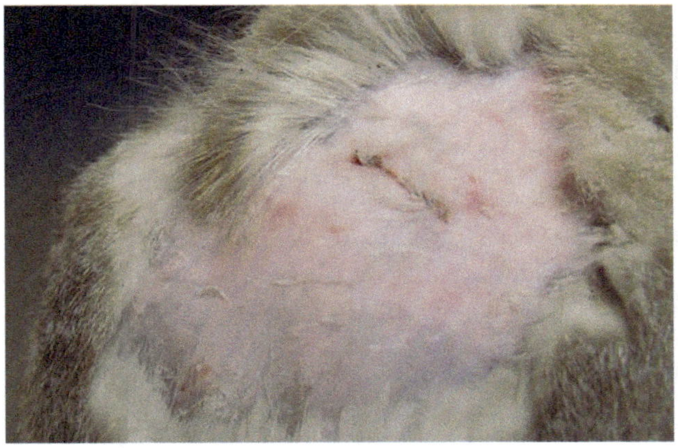

Figure 18.7 Easily epilated, traumatic-related alopecia in a cat which occurred three weeks after an unknown trauma to the hind end. *Source:* Image courtesy of VIN and Gary Old, DVM.

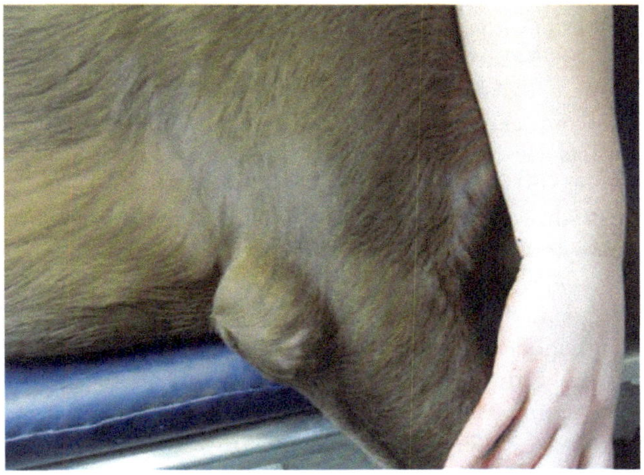

Figure 18.8 A hygroma on the elbow of a young, large breed dog. *Source:* Image courtesy of VIN and Cassandra Struke-Conrad, DVM.

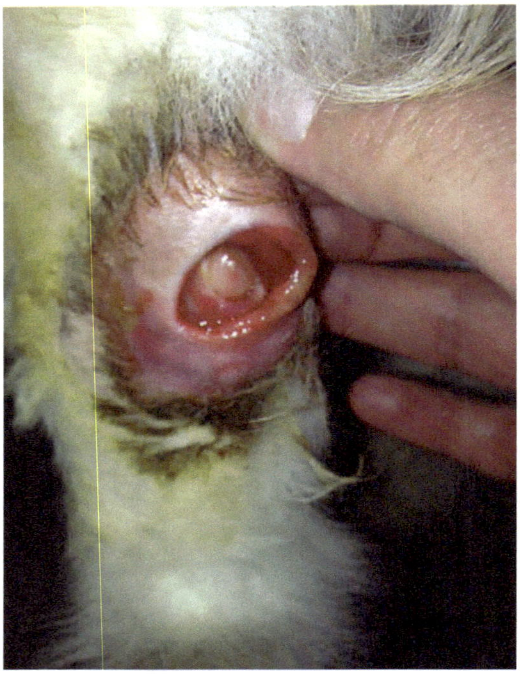

Figure 18.9A A deep decubital ulcer with bone exposure on the elbow of a geriatric dog. *Source:* Image courtesy of VIN and Andy Manoloff, DVM.

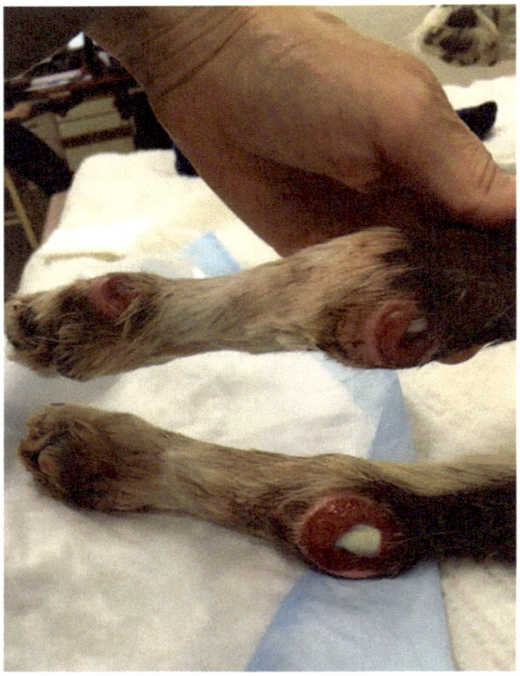

Figure 18.9B Deep decubitus ulcers on the hocks. *Source:* Image courtesy of VIN and Eric Stone, DVM.

Further reading

Alberts, D., Ranger-Moore, J., Einspahr, J. et al. (2004). Safety and efficacy of dose-intensive oral vitamin A in subjects with sun-damaged skin. *Clin. Cancer Res.* 10 (6): 1875–1880.

Albanese, F., Abramo, F., Caporali, C. et al. (2013). Clinical outcome and cyclo-oxygenase-2 expression in 5 dogs with solar dermatitis/actinic keratosis treated with firocoxib. *Vet. Dermatol.* 24 (6): 606–e147.

Amalsadvala, T. and Swaim, S.F. (2006). Management of hard-to-heal wounds. *Vet. Clin. Small Anim. Pract.* 36: 693–711.

Bardagi, M., Fondevila, D., and Ferrer, L. (2012). Immunohistochemical detection of COX-2 in feline and canine actinic keratoses and cutaneous squamous cell carcinoma. *J. Comp. Pathol.* 146 (1): 11–17.

Burrows, A.K. (2014). Actinic dermatoses and sun protection. In: *Kirk's Current Veterinary Therapy XV*, 480–482. St. Louis Mo: Elsevier.

Campbell, B.G. (2006). Dressings, bandages, and splints for wound management in dogs and cats. *Vet. Clin. North Am. Small Anim. Pract.* 36 (4): 759–791.

Declercq, J. (2004). Alopecia and dermatopathy of the lower back following pelvic fractures in three cats. *Vet. Dermatol.* 15 (1): 42–46.

Fahie, M.A. and Shettko, D. (2007). Evidence-based wound management: a systematic review of therapeutic agents to enhance granulation and epithelialization. *Vet. Clin. North Am. Small Anim. Pract.* 37 (3): 559–577.

Frantz, K. and Byers, C.G. (2011). Thermal injury. *Compend. Contin. Educ. Vet.* 33 (12): E1.

Gnudi, G., Volta, A., Bonazzi, M. et al. (2005). Ultrasonographic features of grass awn migration in the dog. *Vet. Radiol. Ultrasound* (5): 423–426.

Ho, K.K., Campbell, K.L., and Lavergne, S.N. (2015). Contact dermatitis: a comparative and translational review of the literature. *Vet. Dermatol.* 26 (5): 314–327, e66-7.

Hosgood, G. (2006). Stages of wound healing and their clinical relevance. *Vet. Clin. Small. Anim. Pract.* 36: 667–685.

Kimura, T. and Doi, K. (1994). Protective effects of sunscreens on sunburn and suntan reactions in cross-bred Mexican hairless dogs. *Vet. Dermatol.* 5: 175.

Klocke, E. (2014). CVC highlight: the hunt for grass awns. *Vet. Med.* http://veterinarymedicine.dvm360.com/cvc-highlight-hunt-grass-awns (accessed 14 February 2019).

Kunkle, G.A. (1988). Contact dermatitis. *Vet. Clin. North Am. Small Anim. Pract.* 18 (5): 1061–1068.

Miller, W.H., Griffin, C.E., and Campbell, K.L. (2013). *Muller and Kirk's Small Animal Dermatology*, 7e. St. Louis Mo: Elsevier.

Mathews, K.A. and Binnington, A.G. (2002). Wound management using honey. *Compendium Pract. Educ.* 24: 53–59.

Mathews, K.A. and Binnington, A.G. (2002). Wound management using sugar. *Compendium Pract. Educ.* 24: 41–49.

Olivry, T., Prélaud, P., Héripret, D., and Atlee, B.A. (1990). Allergic contact dermatitis in the dog. Principles and diagnosis. *Vet. Clin. North Am. Small Anim. Pract.* 20 (6): 1443–1456.

Pavletic, M.M. (2011). Use of commercially available foam pipe insulation as a protective device for wounds over the elbow joint area in five dogs. *J. Am. Vet. Med. Assoc.* 239 (9): 1225–1231.

Peters-Kennedy, J.P., Scott, D.W., and Miller, W.H. (2008). Case report: apparent clinical resolution of pinnal actinic keratoses and squamous cell carcinoma in a cat using topical imiquimod 5% cream. *J. Fel. Med. and Surg.* 10: 593–599.

Quist, E.M., Tanabe, M., Mansell, J.E., and Edwards, J.L. (2012). A case series of thermal scald injuries in dogs exposed to hot water from garden hoses (garden hose scalding syndrome). *Vet. Dermatol.* 23 (2): 162–166, e33.

Rosenkrantz, W.S. (1993). Solar dermatitis. In: *Current Veterinary Dermatology* (ed. C.E. Griffin, K.W. Kwochka, J.M. Macdonald, et al.), 309–315. St. Louis: Mosby-Year Book.

Schwartz, S.L., Schick, A.E., Lewis, T.P., and Loeffler, D. (2018). Dorsal thermal necrosis in dogs: a retrospective analysis of 16 cases in the southwestern USA (2009–2016). *Vet. Dermatol.* 29 (2): 139–e55.

Swaim, S.F. and Bohling, M.W. (2005). Bandaging and splinting canine elbow wounds. *Clinician's Brief* 21–24.

Swaim, S.F. and Henderson, R.A. (1997). *Small Animal Wound Management*, 2e. Baltimore: Williams and Wilkins.

Tchanque-Fossuo, C.N., Ho, D., Dahle, S.E. et al. (2016). A systematic review of low-level light therapy for treatment of diabetic foot ulcer. *Wound Repair Regen.* 24 (2): 418–426.

Thivierge, G. (1973). Granular stomatitis in dogs due to Burdock. *Can. Vet. Jour.* 14 (4): 96–97.

Vigani, A. and Culler, C.A. (2017). Systemic and local management of burn wounds. *Vet. Clin. North Am. Small Anim. Pract.* 47 (6): 1149–1163.

Walder, E.J. and Hargis, A.M. (2002). Chronic moderate heat dermatitis (erythema ab igne) in five dogs, three cats and one silvered langur. *Vet. Dermatol.* 13 (5): 283–292.

19

Skin tumors

Alexandra Gould, DVM[1,2]

[1] *Dermatology Clinic for Animals, Lacey, WA, USA*
[2] *Animal Allergy and Dermatology, Las Vegas, NV, USA*

Clinical Atlas of Canine and Feline Dermatology, First Edition. Edited by Kimberly S. Coyner.

Companion website: www.wiley.com/go/coyner/dermatology

Table 19.1 Benign and malignant skin tumors in dogs and cats.

Disease	Clinical signs	Diagnostics	Treatment
Squamous cell carcinoma (SCC) (Solar and Non-solar Origin) *Canine* (Figures 19.1–19.4) Older dogs (6–10 years). Non-solar: Predisposition for large or giant breed dogs, possibly with dark coats. Solar: Predisposition for short, light-colored coats.	Common locations: Non-solar: Trunk, limbs, scrotum, lips, anus, digits/clawbed Solar: Ventral abdomen, head. Variants: 1. Proliferative (papillary, cauliflower-like mass; can develop cutaneous horns). 2. Ulcerative (shallow ulcers that deepen over time). 3. Clawbed (single digit swollen/painful with misshapen or no claw). Often individual masses, but can multiply (especially in sunbathing dogs). Behavior varies by location: Cutaneous neoplasm: Metastasis rare. Digital SCC: Locally aggressive. Prevalence of distant metastasis to lymph nodes and lungs ranges from 5–25% of cases.	Biopsy Staging requires aspirate of draining lymph nodes and chest radiographs.	Local surgical excision, including digit amputation is often curative or prolongs survival times in case of digit masses. Local treatment options: Cryotherapy, Strontium-90 plesiotherapy (if superficial), topical imiquimod. Avoid sunlight to prevent further UV-induced SCC. Systemic treatments have no proven survival benefit, but options include: NSAIDs (such as piroxicam), toceranib phosphate, carboplatin, or mitoxantrone-based chemotherapy. Consider oncology consultation.
Squamous cell carcinoma (Solar and Non-solar Origin) *Feline* (Figures 19.5–19.7) Older cats (10–12 years) Solar: White cats at higher risk. Siamese cats and long-haired cats at decreased risk.	Common locations: Non-solar: Digit, thigh, neck. Solar: Pinna, nasal planum, eyelid, lips. Early lesion: Erythematous, crusted, sunken. Ears often thickened and curled at pinnal margins. Chronic lesion: Deep erosion or mass. Behavior: Slowly progressive, locally aggressive, metastasis unlikely.	Biopsy Staging requires aspirate of draining lymph nodes and chest radiographs.	Best option for pinnae, nasal planum, and eyelids: Surgical excision. Cryosurgery of small lesions, but masses can recur, especially in lesions larger than 5 mm. Nasal planum lesions can be treated with radiation or photodynamic therapy. Topical imiquimod helpful for early superficial lesions. Avoid sunlight or apply sunscreen to prevent further UV-induced SCC. Consider oncology consultation.
Bowenoid in situ carcinoma (Bowen's disease) *Feline* (Figures 19.8A and 19.8B) Middle-aged to older cats. Often related to papillomavirus infection.	Multifocal, well-circumscribed, hyperpigmented plaques and macules which may be ulcerated. Common locations: Face, neck, limbs.	Biopsy	Local surgical excision may be ineffective, as lesions can develop in other locations. Localized treatments: Topical imiquimod cream, Strontium-90 plesiotherapy (if superficial), and CO_2 laser ablation. Oncology consultation recommended if generalized lesions.

Basal cell carcinoma *Canine and feline* (Figures 19.9A–19.9F) Older animals: Dogs over 8 years. Cats over 10 years. More common in cats than dogs. Predisposed breeds: Siamese cats, Cocker Spaniel, Kerry Blue terrier, Shetland Sheepdog, Siberian Husky, English Springer Spaniel, Poodle. UV light exposure implicated in humans, but not proven in dogs.	Single lesions. Hardened plaques or umbilicated nodules, commonly with overlying crusts. Masses are often black or blue pigmented. Common locations: Cats: Nose, face, ears; less commonly trunk, neck, legs. Dogs: Trunk, rare only on glabrous skin. Low metastasis rate in cats, not documented in dogs.	Biopsy	Surgical excision, electrosurgery, cryosurgery; low risk of recurrence after removal.
Sebaceous gland tumors *Canine* (Figures 19.10–19.12) Occurs in older dogs. Nodular sebaceous hyperplasia: Predisposed breeds: Poodle, Cocker Spaniel, Manchester Terrier, Wheaten Terrier. Sebaceous adenoma: Predisposed breeds: Cocker Spaniel, Siberian Husky, Miniature Poodle, Coonhound, Samoyed, Beagle, Dachshund. Sebaceous adenocarcinoma: Predisposed breed: Cocker Spaniel.	Four forms of sebaceous gland tumor: Nodular sebaceous hyperplasia: Lesion: Solitary, yellow to white, firm, nodules or plaques that can appear wart-like but are more waxy than papillomas. Common locations: Limb, trunk, ears, face, eyelids. Sebaceous epithelioma: Lesion: Single or multiple frequently ulcerated, firm, nodular or plaque-like mass that are often hyperpigmented. Common locations: Eyelids, head, ears, dorsum. Behavior: Locally aggressive with rare distant metastasis. Sebaceous adenoma: Lesion: Single or multiple, yellow and pearly or hyperpigmented, dome-shaped or papillated masses. Common locations: Head most common, but can occur in any location. Sebaceous adenocarcinoma: Lesion: Single, firm, nodule that is often alopecic and ulcerated. Common locations: Head Behavior: Locally aggressive with rare distant metastasis.	Biopsy used to differentiate type of sebaceous gland tumor.	Removal methods include surgical excision, cryotherapy, CO_2 laser surgery, electrosurgery; recurrence is rare.

(Continued)

Table 19.1 Benign and malignant skin tumors in dogs and cats (Continued)

Disease	Clinical signs	Diagnostics	Treatment
Sebaceous gland tumor *Feline* Occurs in older cats Less common than in dogs. Sebaceous adenoma: Predisposed breed: Persian.	Lesion: Most commonly nodular sebaceous hyperplasia, but other sebaceous gland tumors can occur. Lesions appear identical to dog.	Same as dog.	Same as dog.
Follicular tumors *Canine* (Figures 19.13A–19.13D) Trichoepithelioma: Older dogs (8–9 years average). Predisposed breeds: Golden Retriever, Basset Hound, German Shepherd. Infundibular keratinizing acanthoma (intracutaneous cornifying epithelioma): Uncommon in dogs. Predisposed breeds: Norwegian Elkhound, Keeshond, German Shepherd dog, Terrier, Lhasa Apso, Pekingese, Yorkshire Terrier. Tricholemmoma: Predisposed breed: Afghan Hound. Trichoblastoma: Middle-aged dogs (6–9 years old). Predisposed breeds: Poodle, Cocker Spaniel, Kerry Blue Terrier, Bichon Friese, Cockapoo, Shetland Sheepdog, Siberian Husky. Pilomatrixoma (Pilomatricoma, Calcifying Epithelioma): Older dogs (average 8 years) Predisposed breeds: Kerry Blue Terrier, Miniature Poodle, Old English Sheepdog, Soft-coated Wheaten Terrier, Airedale Terrier, Bouviers des Flandres, Bichon Frise, Standard Schnauzer, Basset Hound.	Trichoepithelioma: Lesion: Single, solid or cystic, sometimes ulcerated and hyperpigmented masses. Common locations: Dorsal lumbar, lateral thoracic, limbs. Behavior: Rarely invade or metastasize. Infundibular keratinizing acanthoma: Lesion: Single or multiple, partially hairless nodules with central opening from which keratin may protrude. Common locations: Dorsal trunk. Behavior: Benign. Tricholemmoma: Lesion: Firm, non-ulcerated, ovoid nodule. Common locations: Head and neck. Behavior: Generally benign. Trichoblastoma: Lesion: Single (rarely multiple), firm, rounded or polypoid mass that can be ulcerated, hyperpigmented, or hairless. Common locations: Base of ear, head, neck. Behavior: Benign in most cases with rare metastasis. Pilomatrixoma: Lesion: Single (rarely multiple), firm or cystic, sometimes hyperpigmented and hairless, multilobular, rounded to plaque-like masses. Common locations: Shoulders, lateral thorax. Behavior: Rarely metastatic and invasive but can spread to lymph nodes, nervous system, lungs, bone.	Biopsy to differentiate types of hair follicle tumor.	Surgical excision, cryotherapy, electrosurgery, observation. Removal usually curative. Trichoblastoma may respond to chemotherapy. Oral retinoids are reported to help control multiple pilomatrixomas and infundibular keratinizing acanthomas.

Follicular tumors *Feline* <u>Trichoepithelioma:</u> Rare in cats. Occurs in cats older than 5 years. Predisposed breeds: Persians. <u>Tricholemmoma:</u> Rare in cats. <u>Trichoblastoma:</u> Older cats most commonly affected (average 9.9 years).	<u>Trichoepithelioma:</u> Same appearance and behavior as dog. Common locations: Head, limbs, tail. <u>Tricholemmoma</u>: Lesion: Small, rounded, hairless nodules that may be ulcerated when large. Behavior: Benign. <u>Trichoblastoma:</u> Lesion: Single, firm, pigmented, rounded nodule that is often hairless and ulcerated. Common locations: Limbs, neck, head, cranial trunk.	Same as dog.	Same as dog.
Dilated pore of Winer *Feline* Middle-aged cats (average 7.5 years).	Lesion: Single, firm, cyst-like structure protruding mass of dense keratin that can appear horn-like in some cases. Common locations: Cervical region, head. Behavior: Benign.	Biopsy	Surgical excision is curative.
Follicular cyst *Canine and feline* (Figures 19.14A–19.14D) Predisposed dog breeds: <u>Solitary cyst</u>: Boxer, Shih Tzu, Miniature Schnauzer, Old English Sheepdog. <u>Clustered cysts on head:</u> Boxer, Rhodesian Ridgeback.	Lesion: Usually single, firm nodules located in the dermis or subcutis, with intact epidermis that is tinted blue, white, or yellow by cyst contents. Pores can be present and keratin can protrude to form a horn shape in some cases. Cysts can sometimes rupture. Common locations: Variable, can include pressure points of large breed dogs, over surgical scars, in clusters along dorsal midline of head, interdigitally. Behavior: Benign, can contribute to recurrent interdigital dermatitis.	Biopsy Cytology: Abundant keratinized debris, sometimes mixed with inflammatory cells and bacteria.	Observation or complete surgical excision. Excision/laser ablation of ventral interdigital follicular cysts is reported to be curative in multiple cases. Manual evacuation is contraindicated, as cyst contents in the dermis or subcutis can lead to inflammatory response and secondary infection
Cutaneous horn *Canine and feline* (Figures 19.15A and 19.15B) Rare Associated with FeLV, papillomavirus, actinic keratosis, bowenoid in situ carcinoma, invasive squamous cell carcinoma, dilated pore of Winer, or infundibular keratinizing acanthoma.	Lesion: Protruding, cone-shaped or cylindrical mass of keratin. Behavior: Morphologic diagnosis, look for underlying associated lesions	Biopsy Immunohistochemistry and PCR for virus identification may be warranted.	Surgical excision with biopsy recommended for removal and identification of underlying lesion.

(*Continued*)

Table 19.1 Benign and malignant skin tumors in dogs and cats (Continued)

Disease	Clinical signs	Diagnostics	Treatment
Apocrine gland tumors *Canine* (Figures 19.16A and 19.16B) Epitrichial Sweat Gland Adenoma (Apocrine Secretory Adenoma): Older than 10 years. Predisposed breeds: Great Pyrenees, Chow, Malamute, Old English Sheepdog. Atrichial Sweat Gland Carcinoma: Extremely rare. Apocrine cyst: 6 years or older. Predisposed breeds: Old English Sheepdog, Weimaraner.	Epitrichial Sweat Gland Adenoma: Lesion: Solitary, well-circumscribed, firm or fluctuant, raised, hairless, often ulcerated mass. Masses can be blue or purple-tinged when cystic. Common locations: Neck, head, dorsal trunk. Behavior: Benign. Atrichial Sweat Gland Carcinoma: Lesion: Single, poorly defined swelling with ulceration and adjacent bone lysis. Common locations: Footpads and digit or distal leg. Behavior: Aggressive with local recurrence or rapid metastasis to draining lymph nodes and adjacent leg subcutaneous tissue. Apocrine Cyst: Lesion: Single (less often multiple) well-defined, firm or fluctuant nodules that are blue-tinted and contain clear material. Common locations: Head, legs, neck, dorsal trunk. Behavior: Non-neoplastic.	Biopsy for diagnosis. Atrichial sweat gland carcinoma biopsies cannot always predict biological behavior.	Epitrichial Sweat Gland Adenoma: Surgical excision, cryosurgery, observation. Atrichial Sweat Gland Carcinoma: Surgical excision should be considered, amputation of leg may be necessary. Apocrine Cyst: Surgical excision, observation without treatment.
Apocrine gland tumors *Feline* (Figure 19.17) Epitrichial Sweat Gland Adenoma: Older than 10 years. Predisposed breed: Siamese. Atrichial Sweat Gland Carcinoma: Extremely rare. Apocrine cyst: 6 years or older. Predisposed breed: Persian.	Epitrichial Sweat Gland Adenoma: Lesion: Same appearance as dog. Common locations: Head, pinna, neck, axilla, limb, tail. Atrichial Sweat Gland Carcinoma: Lesion: Single or multiple areas of lameness with swelling of affected areas that often ulcerates. Common locations: Footpads and digits. Behavior: Malignant in almost all cases, rapid progression, can metastasize to lungs. Apocrine cyst: Lesion: Single (less often multiple) well-defined, firm or fluctuant nodules that are dark brown to blue-tinted and contain red–brown material. Common location: Head. Behavior: Non-neoplastic.	Same as dog.	Same as dog.

Feline ceruminous (apocrine) cystomatosis (Figures 19.18A and 19.18B) Average age 8–9.5 years, but can occur in younger cats. Predisposed breeds: Abyssinian and Persian. Male predisposition. Can develop due to otitis externa, age-related changes, or sometimes are congenital.	Lesion: Multiple, small nodules or vesicles that are dark brown, blue, or black colored. Common locations: External ear canal, eyelids, lips, or inner pinnae/outer ear canals. Behavior: Benign, may cause or contribute to obstructive ceruminous otitis.	Biopsy.	CO_2 laser ablation is preferred method to remove nodules. Ablation of lesions with silver nitrate stick or trichloroacetic acid has been described.
Perianal gland tumors (Circumanal gland tumors, Hepatoid gland tumor) *Canine* (Figures 19.19A and 19.19B) Older dogs (11 years average). Intact male dogs are predisposed. Predisposed breeds: Cocker Spaniel, English Bulldog, Samoyed, Afghan, Dachshund, German Shepherd dog, Beagle, Siberian Husky, Shih Tzu, Lhasa Apso.	Lesion: Single or multiple, spherical to ovoid masses that become multinodular and ulcerated with growth. Can appear similar to nodular circumanal gland hyperplasia. Common locations: Adjacent to anus (most common), tail, perineum, prepuce, thigh, dorsal lumbosacral area. Behavior: Benign.	Location and cytology (sheets of mature, round hepatoid cells with abundant pink-blue cytoplasm) can be sufficient for diagnosis. Biopsy to definitively differentiate from adenocarcinoma.	Removal through surgical excision, cryosurgery, electrosurgery. Adenoma/hyperplasia treatment of choice: Male: Castration, with surgical excision only if recurrent or ulcerated masses. Female: Surgical excision necessary in all cases. Evaluate females and neutered males with recurrent lesions for hyperadrenocorticism.
Apocrine gland tumors of anal sac origin *Canine* Older dogs (10 years average). Females may be predisposed. Possible breed predisposition: German Shepherds, English Cocker Spaniel, Dachshund, Alaskan Malamute, English Springer Spaniel. Adenocarcinoma is most common tumor type.	Lesion: Palpable mass in anal sac (can be single or bilateral). Accompanying signs: Tenesmus, scooting, hypercalcemia, constipation, change in stool shape, perineal swelling. Behavior: Highly metastatic; spread to regional lymph nodes as well as lungs, spleen, liver, bones.	Biopsy Staging with thoracic radiographs, abdominal ultrasound +/− CT or MRI recommended to rule out metastasis. Chemistry panel recommended to screen for paraneoplastic hypercalcemia.	Surgery of primary tumor combined with removal of regional lymph nodes in cases of lymphadenopathy, recurrence is common. Radiation therapy may help control local disease and lymph node metastasis. Platinum chemotherapy may be helpful, but no definitive benefit established. Palliative options: Piroxicam, treatment for hypercalcemia. Recommend oncology consultation.

(*Continued*)

Table 19.1 Benign and malignant skin tumors in dogs and cats (Continued)

Disease	Clinical signs	Diagnostics	Treatment
Lipoma *Canine and feline* (Figures 19.20A and 19.20B) Dogs and cats >8 years. Predisposed breeds: Siamese cat Cocker Spaniel, Dachshund, Weimaraner, Doberman Pinscher, Miniature Schnauzer, Labrador Retriever, small Terriers. Obese female dogs may be predisposed.	Lesion: Single or multiple, well-circumscribed, variably sized, soft to rubbery masses that can be multilobulated. Common locations: Thorax, chest, abdomen, proximal limbs. Behavior: Benign.	Cytology: Acellular with many lipid droplets. Biopsy	Surgical excision or observation if small. Experimental treatment option: Dry liposuction for simple encapsulated lipomas.
Infiltrative Lipomas *Canine and feline* Rare Middle-aged to older patients more common. Females are predisposed. Predisposed breeds: Labrador Retriever, Standard Schnauzer, Doberman Pinscher.	Lesion: Poorly-circumscribed swellings in the deep subcutaneous and intramuscular tissues. Common locations: Deep tissue of neck, trunk, proximal legs. Behavior: Non-metastatic, but can be painful or impair movement depending upon location. Local recurrence can occur after removal.	Biopsy	Radical surgical excision +/− external beam radiation (often both are necessary).
Liposarcoma *Canine and feline* More common in dogs than cats. Affects older dogs (average 9–10 years). Predisposed breeds: Shetland Sheepdogs, Beagles.	Lesion: Variably sized and circumscribed, soft masses that usually affect subcutaneous tissue. With secondary dermal involvement, overlying skin is thickened and hairless. Common locations: Shoulder, thorax, axilla, tail base, hip, proximal legs. Rarely located in internal organs. Behavior: Locally invasive. Distant metastasis is rare, but has been reported to spread to lungs, liver, and bone. Best prognosis with wide excision, may recur after surgery.	Biopsy necessary to differentiate from lipoma.	Surgical excision necessary; wide margins recommended to reduce recurrence.

Mast cell tumor *Canine* (Figures 19.21A–19.21F) Average age 8 years, but Chinese Shar-Pei at 4 years or younger. Predisposed breeds: Boston Terrier, Boxer, English Bulldog, Bull Terrier, Fox Terrier, Staffordshire Terrier, Labrador Retriever, Dachshund, Beagle, Pug, Golden Retriever, Weimaraner, Chinese Shar-Pei, Rhodesian Ridgeback.	Lesion: Alopecic, solitary to multiple, erythematous and edematous, nodular or pedunculated and variably circumscribed and ulcerated if large. Common locations: Trunk, extremities, head. Location predilections can vary by breed: Hindleg: Boxers, Boston Terrier, Pug, English Setter, American Staffordshire Terrier. Tail: Rhodesian Ridgeback. Head: English Setter. Behavior: Consider all potentially malignant; histopathologic grading needed. Generally locally invasive. Grade 1 and 2 tumors often cured with surgical excision. 12 to 18 months survival with treatment in metastatic cases.	Fine needle aspirate cytology for diagnosis, but not grading or biologic behavior: variably differentiated round cells with metachromatic staining granules in cytoplasm and extracellular space. Biopsy to determine histologic grade. Staging tests: FNA or biopsy of regional lymph nodes, abdominal ultrasound with spleen or liver aspirate when enlarged, if grade III tumor, or if lymph node metastasis and systemic signs present.	Recommendations based upon tumor stage, location, and grade. Surgical excision: 2 cm margins and fascial plane or wider. Revision surgery may be needed if incomplete resection. Adjunctive treatment following incomplete resection: Radiation therapy, systemic chemotherapy (corticosteroids, vinblastine, toceranib phosphate, and other tyrosine kinase inhibitors). Metastatic disease treatment: Systemic chemotherapy with possible surgical debulking and palliative radiation therapy. Consider antihistamines, H2 blockers. Consider oncology consultation.
Mast cell tumor *Feline* (Figures 19.22A and 19.22B) Average age 9–11 years. Predisposed breed: Siamese.	Lesion: Frequently multiple, occasionally single. Firm to soft, tan papules, nodules, or plaques that are occasionally ulcerated and pruritic. Common locations: Head and neck. Behavior: Mainly benign with low rate of recurrence at same site and possible occurrence at new sites Multiple masses may be secondary to visceral lesions (spleen, alimentary tract).	Biopsy for diagnosis, but grading does not correlate reliably with prognosis in cats. Staging is recommended for all cats with multiple cutaneous masses (CBC, Chemistry panel, coagulation profile, bone marrow aspirate, thoracic radiographs, abdominal ultrasound and radiographs).	Surgical resection or cryotherapy of single masses (Scott et al., 2013) Consider H_1 or H_2 blockers. Alternatives to surgery: Strontium-90 irradiation, chemotherapy with lomustine, toceranib phosphate. Oncology consultation recommended in cases of multiple cutaneous masses and concern for visceral mast cell tumors.
Fibroma *Canine and feline* Older dogs and cats. Predisposed breeds: Boxer, Boston Terrier, Doberman Pinscher, Golden Retriever, Fox Terrier.	Lesion: Solitary, single, fluctuant, rubbery or firm, polypoid, dome-shaped, or ovoid mass; can be pedunculated. Mass can be hyperpigmented and pin-feathered in dogs. Common locations: Head, legs. Behavior: Non-metastatic but can be locally aggressive.	Biopsy	Observation if slow-growing and not uncomfortable. Surgical excision, cryotherapy, or electrosurgery if removal is required.
Dermatofibroma *Canine and feline* Dogs and cats younger than 5 years old.	Lesion: Single, well-demarcated, firm, small, alopecic nodule. Common location: Head. Behavior: Non-metastatic and non-invasive.	Biopsy	Observation or removal (surgical excision, cryosurgery.) Surgical excision is curative.

(*Continued*)

Table 19.1 Benign and malignant skin tumors in dogs and cats (Continued)

Disease	Clinical signs	Diagnostics	Treatment
Nodular dermatofibrosis *Canine* (Figures 19.23A and 19.23B) Predisposed breeds: German Shepherd dogs. Mean age of diagnosis: 6.4 years.	Lesion: Multiple, firm, 2–5 mm diameter subcutaneous nodules that are non-pruritic Common locations: Limbs, head. Behavior: Nodules are benign, but they are cutaneous markers for renal cystadenocarcinomas or uterine leiomyomas. Renal dysfunction signs usually develop within 3–5 years of cutaneous nodule development.	Biopsy Abdominal ultrasound to evaluate kidneys and uterus.	Surgical excision, or cryosurgery to remove cutaneous masses. Management of renal disease is important for extending survival.
Acrochordon **(Skin tag)** *Canine and feline* (Figures 19.24A and 19.24B) More common in dogs than cats.	Lesion: Single or multiple, polypoid or narrow, small masses; a proliferative response to chronic friction. Epidermis can be thickened, hairless, or darkly pigmented and sometimes eroded or ulcerated. Common locations: Trunk, pressure points on legs and sternum. Behavior: Benign.	Biopsy	Surgical excision is curative.
Mammary tumors *Canine* (Figure 19.25) Commonly affects older female dogs that are sexually intact or were spayed late in life.	Lesion: General presentation: One or more discrete masses palpable in mammary glands that may be of varying size, fixed or freely movable, sometimes ulcerated. Can be accompanied by enlarged lymph nodes. Inflammatory carcinoma: Acute presentation of edematous, red, and firm mammary glands that may have palpable cutaneous nodules or mammary masses. Types of tumors: Carcinoma (multiple histologic forms), inflammatory carcinoma, squamous cell carcinoma, sarcoma (e.g. osteosarcoma, chondrosarcoma, fibrosarcoma, hemangiosarcoma), benign forms (e.g. adenoma, fibroadenoma, myoepithelioma), hyperplasia. Behavior: Variable, likely <50% metastasis. Inflammatory carcinoma shows high mortality rate, mean survival time of 60 days. Poor prognostic factors: Large tumor size, skin ulceration, lymph node metastasis, high histologic grade, vascular or lymphatic invasion, diagnosis of sarcoma (worse prognosis than carcinoma).	Biopsy Primary tumor fine needle aspirate helps distinguish benign and malignant tumors. Additional staging recommended: 3-view chest x-rays, regional lymph node aspirate.	Spay prior to first estrus reduces risk of tumor development. Wide surgical excision can be curative for single tumors, consider complete mastectomy for multiple tumors. Adjuvant chemotherapy and NSAIDs (piroxicam) recommended in cases of inflammatory carcinomas. Recommend referral to veterinary oncologist.

Mammary tumors *Feline* (Figures 19.26A–19.26C) Older females 10–12 years old, no difference between intact and spayed cats. Predisposed breed: Siamese cats.	Lesion: Single to multiple masses in mammary glands, usually 2–3 cm diameter. Types of tumors: Adenocarcinomas most common. Benign forms occur (e.g. duct papilloma, adenoma, fibroadenoma) along with non-neoplastic lesions (e.g. cysts, focal fibrosis, non-inflammatory hyperplasia). Behavior: Locally aggressive, over 80% metastasis to nodes, liver, lungs. Prognosis guarded to poor, average survival time if untreated is 12 months. Poor prognostic factors: Tumor size over 3 cm, lymphatic invasion, higher clinical stage and histologic grade, increased proliferation markers.	Biopsy Additional staging recommendations: 3-view chest x-rays, regional lymph node aspirate, abdominal ultrasound.	Unilateral or bilateral mastectomy using 2–3 cm margins, with lymph node removal. Doxorubicin-based chemotherapy and NSAIDs can be helpful. Recommend consultation with veterinary oncologist.
Hemangioma *Canine* (Figures 19.27A–19.27D) Adult to older dogs (9 years average age). Predisposed breeds: Boxer, Golden Retriever, German Shepherd dog, English Springer Spaniel, Airedale Terrier, Whippet, Dalmatian, Beagle, American Staffordshire Terrier, Basset Hound, Saluki, Bloodhound, English Pointer.	Lesion: Well-circumscribed, blue to red/black pigmentation, ovoid or discoid mass. Solar-induced masses are often multiple, ulcerated, and less well-demarcated with frequent hemorrhage. Common locations: Head, trunk, extremities, ventrum of dogs with lightly pigmented, sparse hairs associated with solar-induced lesions. Behavior: Benign but large lesions can cause hematologic abnormalities/disseminated intravascular coagulation due to their vascular nature.	Biopsy for diagnosis.	Surgical excision, cryosurgery, electrosurgery, observation.
Hemangioma *Feline* Older (10 years). Possible predominance in male cats (studies equivocal).	Lesion: Single, firm to fluctuant, round, blue to red/black color. Common locations: No site predilection. Behavior: Slow growing, but can spontaneously bleed in some cases.	Same as dog.	Same as dog.

(Continued)

Table 19.1 Benign and malignant skin tumors in dogs and cats (Continued)

Disease	Clinical signs	Diagnostics	Treatment
Hemangiosarcoma *Canine* (Figures 19.28A and 19.28B) Older dogs (9–10 years old). Predisposed breeds: (subcutaneous hemangiosarcoma)German Shepherd dogs, Golden Retrievers, Bernese Mountain dogs, Boxers. Cutaneous solar-induced hemangiosarcoma predisposed in short-haired, light skinned dog breeds: Whippet, Dalmatian, Beagle, Greyhound, American Staffordshire Terrier, Basset Hound, Saluki, English Pointer.	Lesions: Subcutaneous (SC) hemangiosarcoma: Single lesion, poorly circumscribed, large, soft masses with dark red or blue-black coloration Solar-induced cutaneous hemangiosarcoma: Multiple lesions, variably circumscribed, small (2 cm), red to dark blue plaques or nodules Shared features: Alopecia, thick skin, hemorrhage, ulceration. Common locations: SC hemangiosarcoma: Trunk, extremities. Solar-induced hemangiosarcoma: Lightly haired ventral areas. Behavior: Cutaneous hemangiosarcomas are often not aggressive and can be effectively treated with surgical excision. SC hemangiosarcoma: Highly invasive and malignant, with common metastasis.	Biopsy for identification. Staging recommended when tumors identified to rule out metastasic visceral hemangiosarcoma: CBC/ Chemistry panel, urinalysis, thoracic radiographs, echocardiogram, abdominal ultrasound.	Cutaneous hemangiosarcomas are often not aggressive and can be effectively treated with surgical excision. Radical surgical excision recommended for cutaneous hemangiosarcomas (often including limb amputation), but recurrence is common. Post-operative chemotherapy (vincristine, doxorubicin, cyclophosphamide) can improve survival in SC hemangiosarcomas. Recommend consultation with veterinary oncologist.
Hemangiosarcoma *Feline* (Figure 19.29) Older cats (12.5 years mean). White cats predisposed to superficial hemangiosarcoma.	Lesion: Single, poorly circumscribed, red to blue-black plaques/nodules (dermal) or soft (SC) masses with hairless, thick skin, hemorrhage, ulceration. Common locations: Head and pinna of white-haired cats, limbs, inguinal, axillary regions. Behavior: Fast growing, with variable metastasis, frequent local recurrence.	Biopsy	Radical surgical excision recommended, recurrence common. Amputation can be curative on distal limbs and digits. Recommend consultation with veterinary oncologist.
Cutaneous progressive angiomatosis *Canine and feline* (Figures 19.30A–19.30D) Young to middle-aged dogs and cats most commonly affected. May be triggered by *Bartonella* infection (bacillary angiomatosis) in some cases.	Lesion: Dark red macules, patches, plaques, or nodules with irregular margins that periodically develop hemorrhage after irritation. Common locations: Usually unilateral limb involvement of the digits and feet. Can include face, tongue, neck, axillary region. Behavior: No reported metastasis. Progressive in all locations, but destructive when involving the digits. Spontaneous regression is not documented in dogs and cats.	Partially blanch with diascopy. Biopsy Screen for Bartonellosis.	Wide surgical excision or amputation most commonly recommended. Photocoagulation via Nd:YAG laser has reportedly been helpful.

Hemangiopericytoma *Canine* (Figures 19.31A and 19.31C) Dogs aged 7–10 years. Predisposed breeds: German Shepherd dog, Boxer, Cocker Spaniel, Springer Spaniel, Irish Setter, Siberian Husky, Fox Terrier, Collie, Beagle.	Lesion: Single, multilobulated mass of variable appearance (often fatty, firm, or soft, white to red colored). Common locations: Limbs (stifle and elbow most common). Behavior: Rarely metastatic but locally invasive.	Biopsy	Aggressive surgical excision or amputation of limb recommended. Radiation therapy improves local control if excision is impossible. Recommend consultation with veterinary oncologist.
Lymphangioma *Canine and feline* Dogs and cats often young or present at birth. May develop after trauma.	Lesion: Large (up to 18 cm), fluctuant, poorly circumscribed swellings, which are spongy when touched and often leak lymph. Common locations: Ventral midline and limbs. Behavior: Usually benign but can recur.	Biopsy	Surgical excision recommended, but can recur without complete resection.
Lymphangiosarcoma *Canine* All ages reported. Large breed dogs over-represented.	Lesion: Single, diffuse, fluctuant swelling up to 20 cm diameter. Associated with pitting edema, lymph drainage, and ulceration. Common locations: Limbs, ventral areas (abdomen, cervical region, and thorax). Behavior: Malignant, metastasis to local lymph nodes common at time of diagnosis.	Biopsy Staging is necessary (bloodwork, urinalysis, regional lymph node palpation, thoracic radiographs, abdominal ultrasound).	Surgical excision or amputation if possible, combined with chemotherapy. Doxorubicin, metronomic cyclophosphamide, and carboplatin have been reported to either slow recurrence or rarely induce remission. Recurrence common. Recommend consultation with veterinary oncologist.
Lymphangiosarcoma *Feline* (Figures 19.32A–19.32C) Adult and geriatric cats. No definitive gender predisposition.	Lesion: Diffuse plaque, edematous, ulcerated, or cystic mass. Overlying skin is spongy, red to purple-tinged and leaking lymph. Common locations: Caudal abdomen, ventral abdomen most common. Behavior: Malignant, rapidly growing, metastasis seems rare.	Same as dog.	Recurrence common. Surgical excision can be performed, many cats euthanized within months of surgery.
Fibrosarcoma *Canine* (Figure 19.33A) Rare, occurs in older dogs. Predisposed breeds: Doberman Pinscher, Cocker Spaniel, Golden Retriever.	Lesion: Single, irregular and nodular, commonly infiltrating, subcutaneous firm mass that ranges in size from 1–15 cm diameter and is poorly demarcated; alopecia and ulceration common. Common locations: Limbs, trunk. Behavior: Low rate of metastasis but some cases will grow to large sizes precluding excision.	Biopsy	Complete surgical resection is often curative; may involve amputation if extremities involved. Radiation therapy can prevent local recurrence if complete excision is impossible. Recommend consultation with veterinary oncologist.

(*Continued*)

Table 19.1 Benign and malignant skin tumors in dogs and cats (Continued)

Disease	Clinical signs	Diagnostics	Treatment
Fibrosarcoma *Feline* (Figures 19.33B and 19.33C) Feline Sarcoma Virus (FeSV)-induced tumors occur in younger cats (mean age: 3 years old). Older cats (12 years or more) are not FeSV-induced. Feline injection site sarcomas associated with vaccines or other foreign substances, microchip implantation, and trauma.	Lesions: Same appearance as dogs. Single lesion in older cats, multicentric if FeSV-induced. Common locations: Trunk, distal limbs, pinnae, digits. Behavior: Non-FeSV-induced tumors are locally infiltrative and commonly recur. FeSV-associated tumors show rapid spread and metastasis is more common (regional lymph nodes and lungs). Feline injection site sarcomas are highly locally aggressive, rarely metastasize, and often recur after marginal excision. Prognosis: Worst prognosis on head, back, or limbs with mitotic index of 6 or more. Survival time of injection site fibrosarcomas is 6 months with only radical surgery. Postoperative radiation prolongs survival time by hundreds of days.	Biopsy Staging: CT or MRI to determine tumor size, complete bloodwork, 3-view chest x-rays, lymph node palpation, abdominal ultrasound.	Radical surgical excision recommended. Radiotherapy recommended pre-operatively to reduce metastatic seeding or postoperatively to prolong survival. Adjunctive chemotherapy for injection site sarcomas has debatable efficacy, though doxorubicin has been found to prolong survival.
Cutaneous epitheliotropic lymphoma (Mycosis fungoides, Epitheliotropic T cell lymphoma) *Canine and feline* (Figures 19.34A–19.34K) Older dogs and cats. Potential breed predilection in Golden Retrievers.	Lesion: Widespread skin erythema, developing into plaques, scaled patches, ulcerations, and nodules (single or multiple). Variable pruritus (more common in dogs). Erythematous, ulcerated oral mucosa. Depigmentation of lips, nasal planum, and philtrum. Common locations: Dog: Trunk, head, paw pads, face, mucocutaneous junctions, gingiva, palate, tongue. Cat: Face, eyelids, mucocutaneous junctions, elbow, trunk. Behavior: Slowly progressive despite treatment. Metastasis to lymph nodes or other organs is more common in dogs than cats. Prognosis poor, survival time is generally weeks to months, but may be more variable in cats.	Biopsy For tumor staging: Lymph node biopsy or aspirate, thoracic radiography, abdominal ultrasound.	Systemic chemotherapy most common recommendation (lomustine is most commonly reported in dogs). Whole body radiation treatment induced remission for 18 months in one canine case. Adjunctive treatments: Systemic retinoids, interferons, linoleic acid. Recommend veterinary oncology consultation.

Cutaneous non-epitheliotropic lymphoma *Canine and feline* (Figures 19.35A–19.35C) Most common form of cutaneous lymphoma in cats. Predisposed dog breeds: Weimaraner, Boxer, Saint Bernard, Basset Hound, Irish Setter, Cocker Spaniel, German Shepherd, Golden Retriever, Scottish Terrier.	Lesion: Single or multiple, infiltrative plaques or nodules in the dermal or subcutaneous space. Oral cavity not commonly affected. Lymphadenopathy and ulcers are common. Location: Any body site. Behavior: Generally rapid progression and metastasis to draining lymph nodes.	Same as epitheliotropic T cell lymphoma.	Cutaneous excision rarely reported as curative in dogs. Reported treatments: Glucocorticoids, lomustine, surgery, electron beam radiation, vincristine with cyclophosphamide, intravenous and local fibronectin. Lomustine reported to resolve skin lesions in one cat, but poor response to CHOP-based protocol (vincristine, doxorubicin, cyclophosphamide, prednisolone) was reported in one cat with previous traumatic fracture and metal implant. Recommend veterinary oncology consultation.
Feline cutaneous lymphocytosis (Figures 19.36A–19.36D) Rarely reported condition. Mean age: 12–13 years. Spayed females overrepresented.	Lesion: Single, hairless, variably sized, crusted, ulcerated or excoriated and erythematous mass of varying size. Pruritus common. Common locations: Thorax, but can affect all other body sites. Behavior: Acute onset with slowly progressing, waxing and waning lesions and rare systemic signs (anorexia, weight loss); may be reactive or a low grade indolent lymphoma in some cats.	Biopsy Bloodwork is non-diagnostic.	Variable response to surgical excision and topical or systemic corticosteroids. Chlorambucil and lomustine improve response in some cats. Spontaneous remission rare.
Plasmacytoma *Canine* (Figures 19.37A–19.37E) Average affected age of dogs: 10 years. Potential male predisposition. Potential predisposed breeds: Cocker Spaniel, Airedale Terrier, Kerry Blue Terrier, Scottish Terrier, Standard Poodle.	Lesion: Firm, raised, dermal mass, less than 2 cm diameter, sparsely haired or alopecic, rare ulceration. Common locations: Dog: pinnae, lips, digits, chin, oral cavity, legs and trunk, paws, mucosa. Behavior: Benign, rarely recur.	Biopsy	Surgical excision is treatment of choice. Megavoltage radiation therapy can improve local disease control.
Plasmacytoma *Feline* Affects older cats. Potential male predisposition.	Lesion: Same as dog. Common locations: Paws, thorax, neck, shoulder, tail, metatarsus, lip, chin, oral cavity. Behavior: Benign.	Biopsy	Surgical excision is treatment of choice.

(*Continued*)

Table 19.1 Benign and malignant skin tumors in dogs and cats (Continued)

Disease	Clinical signs	Diagnostics	Treatment
Melanocytoma *Canine and feline* (Figures 19.38A–19.38G) Average affected age in cats and dogs: 9 years. Dogs with dark pigmented skin are predisposed to melanocytic tumors. Higher incidence in female cats.	Lesion: Dermal and intraepidermal locations. Single, well-circumscribed, blue, brown, or black colored, hairless nodules of varying shapes (plaque-like, rounded, papular). Common locations: Cats: pinnae Dogs: trunk, head (eyelids, muzzle). Less commonly on extremities, especially between digits (usually dermal melanocytomas). Behavior: Benign, malignant transformation can rarely occur.	Biopsy	Surgical excision is recommended, as benign behavior cannot be predicted based on clinical or histopathological appearance alone.
Malignant melanoma *Canine* (Figures 19.39A–19.39E) Mean age: 9 years. Predisposed breeds: Scottish Terrier, Airedale, Boston Terrier, Cocker Spaniel, Springer Spaniel, Boxer, Golden Retriever, Irish Setter, Irish Terrier, Miniature Schnauzer, Doberman Pinscher, Chihuahua, Chow. Predisposed breeds to nailbed melanomas: Schnauzers, Scottish Terrier, Irish Setter.	Lesion: Single, variably circumscribed, variably shaped (plaque, rounded, polyp-like), variably colored (gray, brown, black, or amelanotic), variably sized (0.5–10 cm). Common locations: Lips, eyelids, legs, nailbeds. Behavior: Nailbed, mucocutaneous junctions, and oral mucosa melanomas show more malignant behavior; recurrence after surgery and metastasis possible to lymph nodes and lungs. Prognosis: Digital melanomas have 12 month median survival time after surgery, cutaneous melanomas have median survival time of almost 2 years.	Biopsy	Radical surgical excision or radiation therapy recommended. Carboplatin combined with piroxicam did not significantly extend survival time in oral, cutaneous, or digital melanomas in one study, but the medications were well tolerated. Adjunctive treatments: Oncept (xenogenic tyrosinase vaccine), mitoxantrone. Recommend veterinary oncology consultation.
Malignant melanoma *Feline* (Figures 19.40A–19.40C) Mean age: 10–11 years. Cats with melanoma of the pinnae are often younger than 10 years old.	Lesion: Single, variably circumscribed, variably shaped (rounded, plaque, polyp-like), brown to black colored, variable size (0.5–5 cm). Common locations: Head is most common (including pinnae), oral cavity (lip, gingiva), thorax, tail. Behavior: Can metastasize to lymph nodes and lungs; non-pigmented melanomas may be associated with worse prognosis; median survival time for pigmented tumors was 179 days versus 71 days for amelanotic tumors.	Biopsy	Surgical resection recommended and may prolong survival time. Xenogenic tyrosinase DNA vaccine (Oncept) found to be safely administered to cats, but no data on efficacy yet available. Recommend veterinary oncology consultation.

Canine cutaneous histiocytoma (Figures 19.41A–19.41C) Young dogs, usually <3 years. Predisposed breeds: Boxer, Dachshund, Cocker Spaniel, Great Dane, Shetland Sheepdog, Bull Terrier.	Lesion: Single, dome-shaped nodule or plaque with associated lesion, alopecia, and ulceration; non-painful lymphadenopathy can be present. Common locations: Head (most common, including pinnae), limbs. Behavior: Benign, usually fast growing but spontaneously regresses.	Biopsy can show high mitotic index despite benign behavior.	Spontaneous regression commonly occurs within 1–2 months of development. Persistent lesions can be treated with surgical or electrosurgical excision or cryotherapy.
Canine reactive cutaneous histiocytosis (Figures 19.42A–19.42J) Middle-aged to older dogs. Possible male predilection. Golden Retrievers may be over-represented.	Lesion: Multiple cutaneous and subcutaneous nodules (up to 4 cm diameter), crusts or depigmentation with rare overlying ulceration. Lesions may spontaneously regress then reappear elsewhere. Common locations: Skin: Face, ears, nose, neck, trunk, extremities, foot pads, perineum, scrotum. Involves draining lymph nodes. Behavior: Non-neoplastic, rapidly growing with waxing and waning behavior and possibility of spontaneous remission.	Biopsy: select early lesions with intact skin surface.	Treatments that have been found to induce remission include: tetracycline/niacinamide, glucocorticoids at immunosuppressive doses, cyclosporine, and azathioprine. Patients can relapse without long-term maintenance therapy.
Canine systemic histiocytosis Dogs 2–8 years old. Predisposed breeds: Bernese Mountain Dog Irish Wolfhound, Rottweiler, Golden Retriever, Labrador Retriever.	Cutaneous lesions identical to cutaneous histiocytosis, but ulceration of nodules is common. Associated clinical signs: Weight loss, anorexia, conjunctivitis, stertor. Common locations: Skin: scrotum, nose, eyelids most common. Internal organs: regional lymph nodes, lung, spleen, liver, bone marrow. Behavior: Non-neoplastic, associated with waxing and waning behavior, majority of cases are slowly progressive.	Biopsy needed for diagnosis and to rule out infectious etiology. CBC: Anemia, monocytosis, lymphopenia.	Long-term immune suppression by a combination of medications often necessary and some patients may fail to respond: cyclosporine, leflunomide, azathioprine, doxorubicin. Ophthalmic cyclosporine drops used to treat ocular lesions.
Feline progressive histiocytosis (Figures 19.43A–19.43F) Affects middle-aged to older cats. Females more often affected.	Lesions: Single or multiple intradermal papules, nodules, or plaques that are hairless, sometimes ulcerated, firm, non-pruritic, and non-painful. Common locations: Feet, legs, face. Behavior: Slowly progressive, lesions can wax and wane. Can spread to lymph nodes, lungs, kidney, spleen, liver. Poor long-term prognosis because treatments have not been effective.	Biopsy findings change with chronicity (histiocytes become less differentiated over time). Rule out infectious agents early in disease using special stains on biopsy.	Poor long-term response to high dose glucocorticoids or chemotherapeutics. Surgical excision of solitary or a low number of lesions can be attempted, but recurrence can occur at surgery sites and new lesions develop in other locations.

(*Continued*)

Table 19.1 Benign and malignant skin tumors in dogs and cats (Continued)

Disease	Clinical signs	Diagnostics	Treatment
Canine cutaneous langerhans cell histiocytosis Predisposed breeds: Shar-Pei.	Lesions: Multiple (can develop hundreds), masses resemble cutaneous histiocytomas. Common locations: Can involve draining lymph nodes. Behavior: Can take up to 10 months to regress and develop ulcerations that negatively impact quality of life, leading to euthanasia. Much worse prognosis if involves lymph nodes. Systemic spread is rapid and euthanasia usually necessary. Most often involves peripheral lymph nodes and lungs, but other organs can be affected.	Biopsy	CCNU effective in most cases, but response is temporary. No response noted to cyclosporine or levamisole.
Collagenous hamartoma (Collagenous nevus) *Canine* Middle-aged or older dogs.	Lesion: Single, small (<1 cm), dome-shaped, firm, alopecic nodule. Common locations: Head, neck, proximal legs. Behavior: Benign, non-invasive.	Biopsy	Surgical excision or observation.
Calcinosis circumscripta *Canine and feline* Figures 19.44A–19.44D) Dogs, usually over 2 years old. Rare in cats. Predisposed breeds: Large breeds, especially German Shepherds, Rottweiler, Labrador Retriever.	Lesion: Usually single, 0.5–3 cm, rounded, firm, white nodule to cystic mass that develops ulceration and discharge of white gritty material with chronicity. Common locations: Near pressure points and bony prominences (lateral metatarsi, phalanges, elbow, dorsal aspects of fourth to sixth cervical vertebrae), the tongue, or footpads. Behavior: Benign, single lesions are associated with localized trauma; multiple lesions can be associated with chronic renal failure.	Biopsy Radiography shows soft tissue mineralization.	Surgical excision for localized lesions.

Transmissible venereal tumor *Canine* (Figures 19.45A–19.45C) Sexually intact young adult dogs.	Lesion: Cauliflower-like, pedunculated, papillary, or nodular shape. Masses are vascularized and friable. Nasal masses develop epistaxis, sneezing, or facial deformity. External genitalia masses increase risk of ascending urinary tract infection. Common locations: Nose or external genitalia. Male: base of glans penis. Female: caudal to vagina or in vestibule. Behavior: Usually transmitted during coitus. May spontaneously regress. Metastasis is rare (0–5%); central nervous system or eye can be affected. Prognosis overall good to excellent.	Biopsy Cytology can be definitive; round to oval cells with multiple clear cytoplasmic vacuoles, often containing mitotic figures.	High rate of spontaneous regression. Surgery shows low efficacy, high recurrence rate, and can cause damage to nearby tissues. Vincristine is drug of choice for therapy; better response may be seen alone, instead of in combination with other chemotherapeutics. Sterilization of dogs important for eradication in endemic areas.
Feline lung-digit syndrome (Metastatic Pulmonary Carcinoma) (Figures 19.46A and 19.46B) Elderly cats most commonly affected (average age 12 years old). Most often associated with bronchial and bronchioalveolar adenocarcinoma.	Lesion: Presentation for lameness or painful paws. Swelling of distal digit, ulcerated digit or clawbed, purulent discharge, fixed exsheathment, deviation of claw, loss of claw. Rarely display respiratory or non-specific systemic signs, i.e. weight loss, lethargy, dyspnea, anorexia, pyrexia, cough. Common locations: Usually multiple digits, often multiple paws. Third phalanx of weight-bearing digits most commonly affected. Not yet recognized in dew claws. Behavior: Metastasis to digits is most commonly reported, but can also metastasize to muscle, skin, eye, vertebrae, and aortic trifurcation. Prognosis grave. Median survival time of 67 days after presentation. Majority of cats euthanized due to poor prognosis and poor quality of life.	Radiography: Digits: osteolysis of third phalanx +/− invasion into intra-articular space and osteolysis of second phalanx. Thorax: evaluate for pulmonary neoplasm, CT scan more sensitive. Full digit amputation and biopsy is gold standard for diagnosis, but mass fine needle aspirate and wedge biopsy can be diagnostic in some cases. True confirmation of lung-digit syndrome requires identification of same tumor type on biopsy of digit and pulmonary neoplasm.	No effective treatment demonstrated. Digit amputation is not palliative; metastasis will continue to spread.

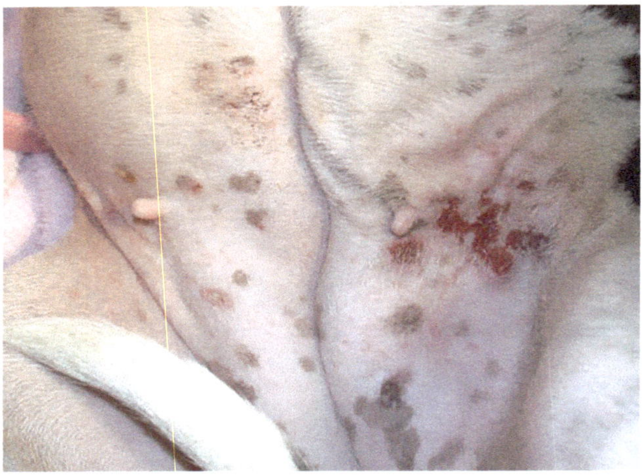

Figure 19.1A Ulcerated inguinal lesions due to solar-induced squamous cell carcinoma in a Pitbull dog.

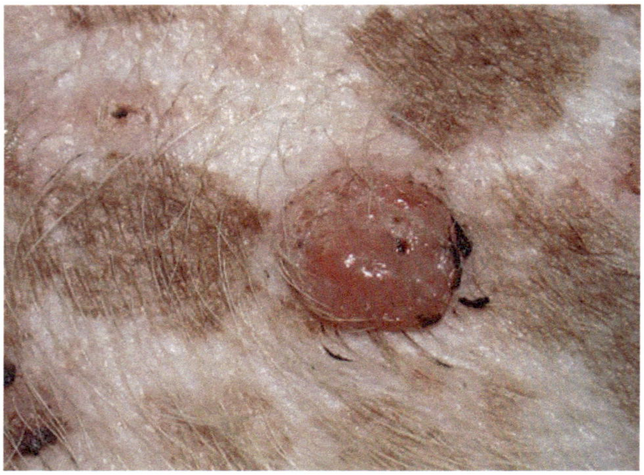

Figure 19.1B A raised, round, eroded mass, which was also a sun-induced squamous cell carcinoma.

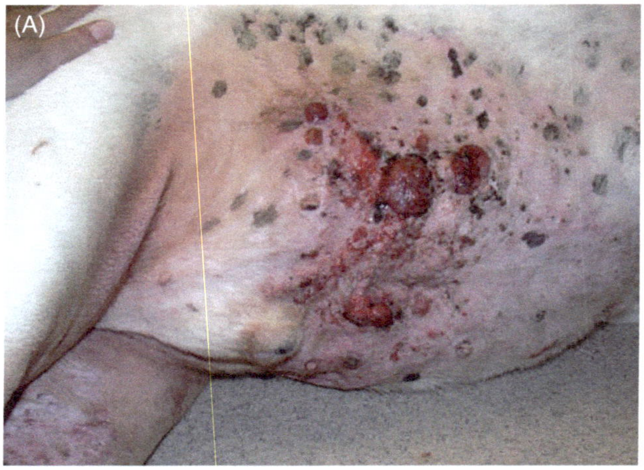

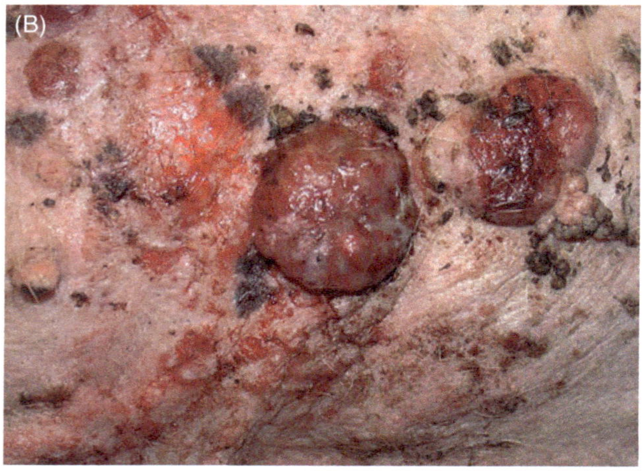

Figures 19.2A and B Severe solar dermatitis and multiple squamous cell carcinomas in an American Bulldog.

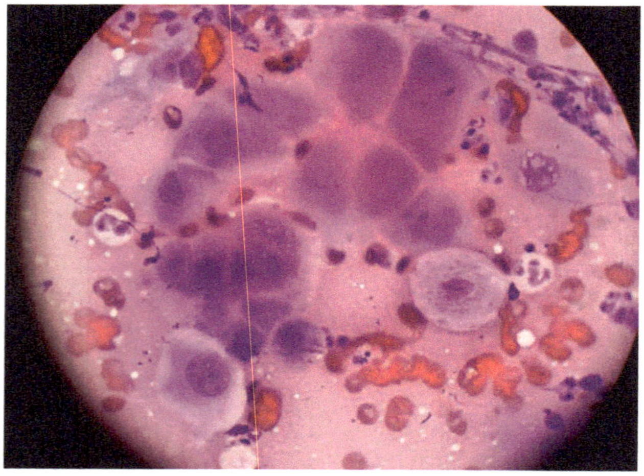

Figure 19.3 Fine needle aspirate for cytology showed large, bizarre epithelial cells, some with retained nuclei. 100x

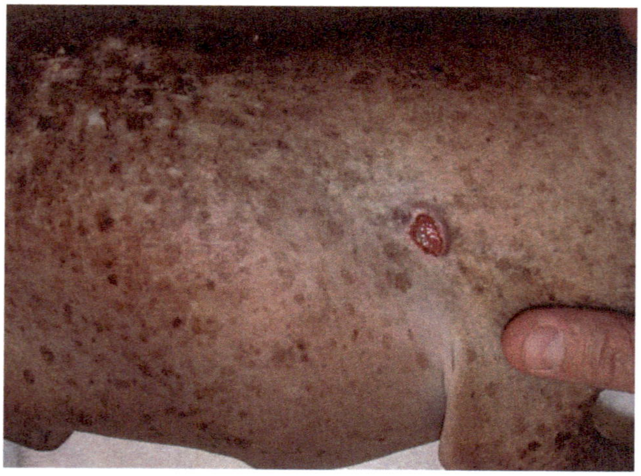

Figure 19.4A An ulcerative truncal lesion caused by squamous cell carcinoma in a Chinese Crested dog with a history of chronic sun exposure.

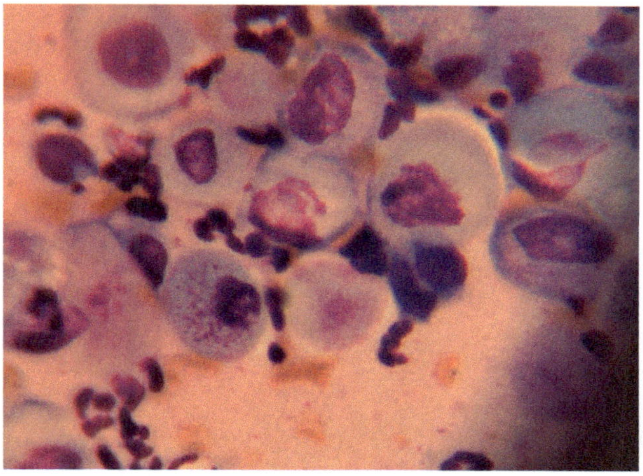

Figure 19.4B Impression smear of the surface of the ulcerated lesion showed atypical epithelial cells. 100x

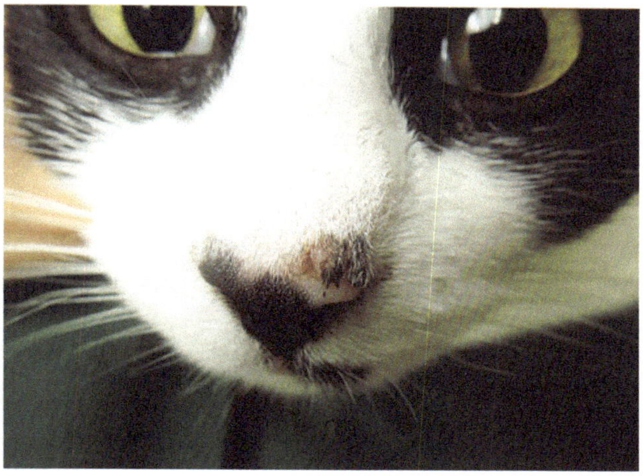

Figure 19.5 Solar-induced squamous cell carcinoma in situ on the nose of a cat.

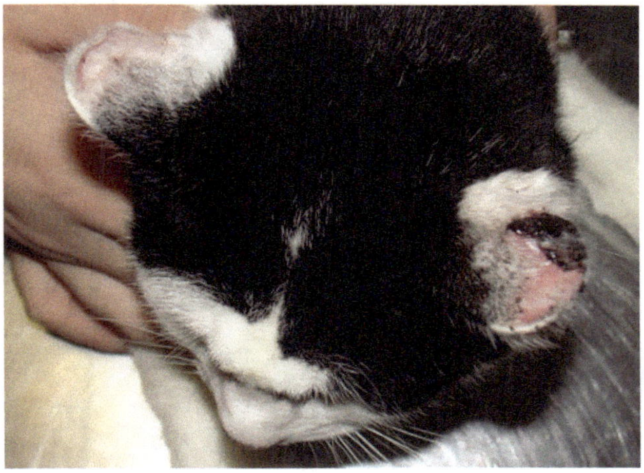

Figure 19.6A A cat with pinnal solar dermatosis and squamous cell carcinoma.

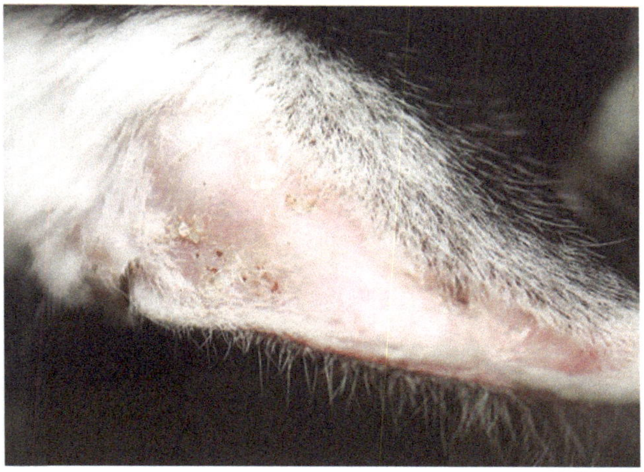

Figure 19.6B Solar-induced squamous cell carcinoma in situ causing small, non-healing crusts and erosions.

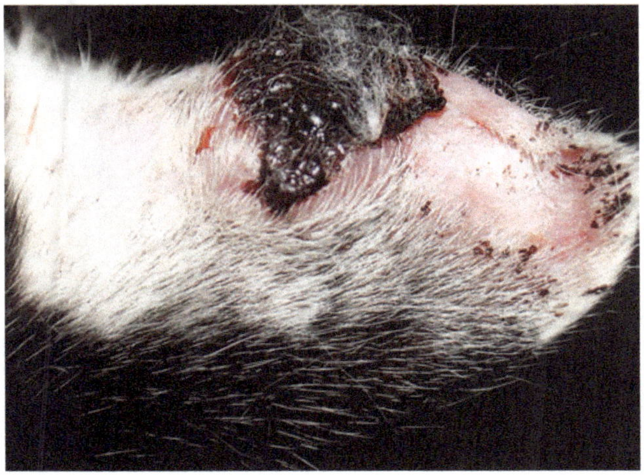

Figure 19.6C On the opposite ear, a large, ulcerated mass had developed which was a squamous cell carcinoma.

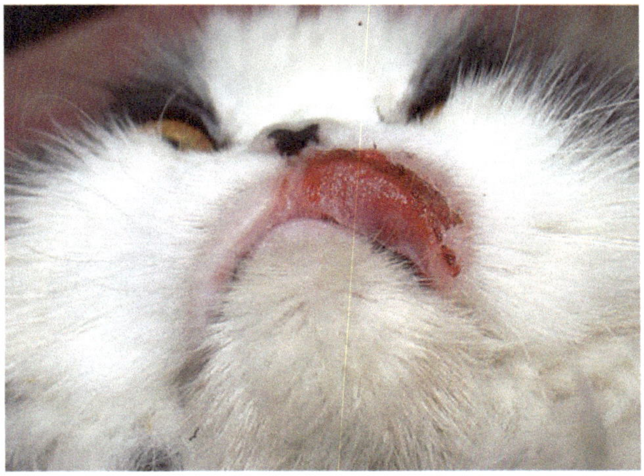

Figure 19.7 A cat with a chronically thickened, ulcerated lip which did not respond to steroids for suspected indolent ulcer; biopsy revealed squamous cell carcinoma.

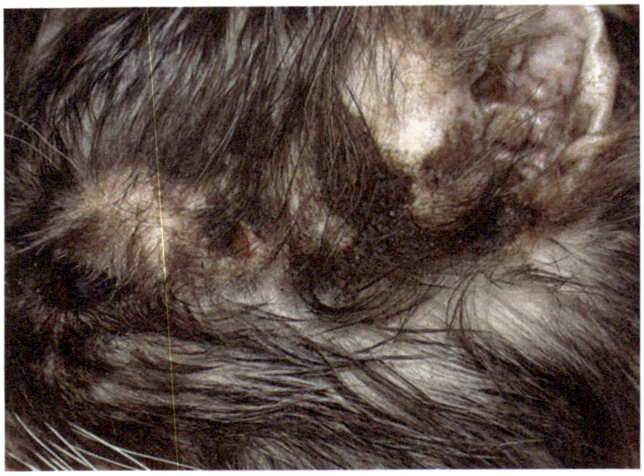

Figure 19.8A Irregular pigmented and lichenified plaques with erosions caused by Bowen's disease (viral induced squamous cell carcinoma in situ) on the temporal area of a cat.

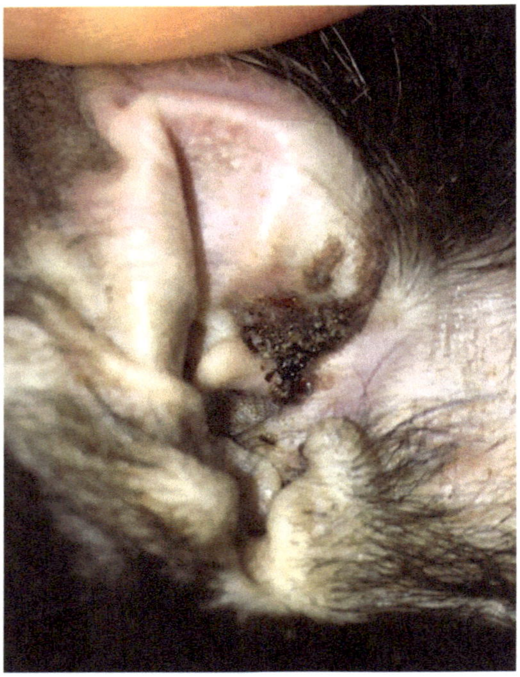

Figure 19.8B A chronically crusted, pigmented plaque on the inner ear pinna caused by Bowen's disease.

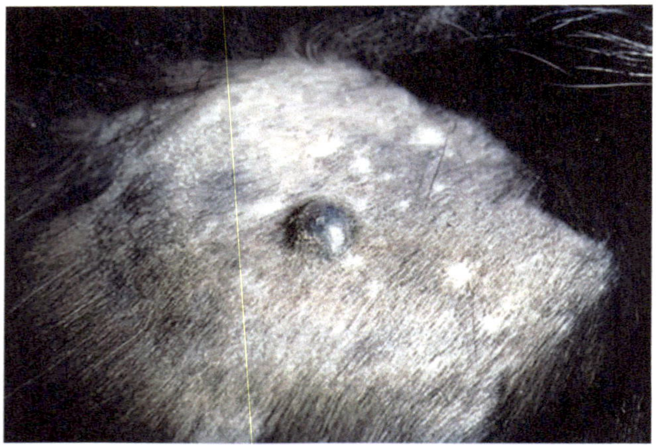

Figure 19.9A A raised, smooth, dark gray, dermal mass on the trunk of a dog; biopsy revealed basal cell tumor. *Source:* Image courtesy of Dr. William Miller, DACVD.

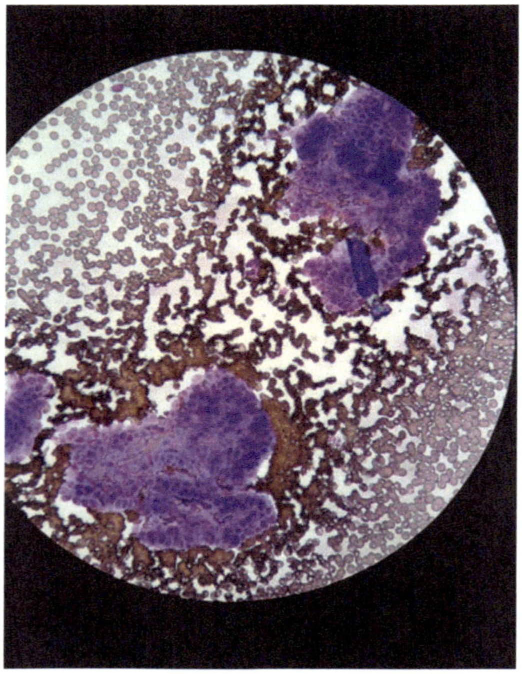

Figure 19.9B Aspirate of a basal cell tumor for cytology shows clumps of monomorphic, basaloid epithelial cells. 4x. *Source:* Image courtesy of VIN and Jennifer Beckwith, DVM.

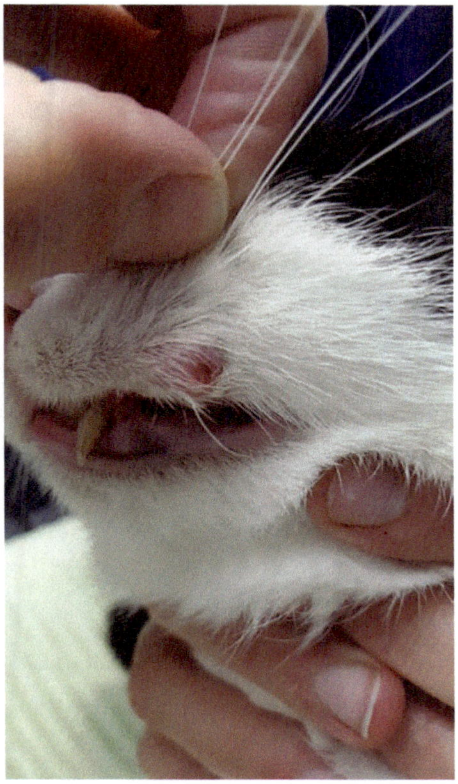

Figure 19.9C A pink, eroded, basal cell tumor on the upper lip of a cat. *Source:* Image courtesy of VIN and Cheryl Matuszewski, DVM.

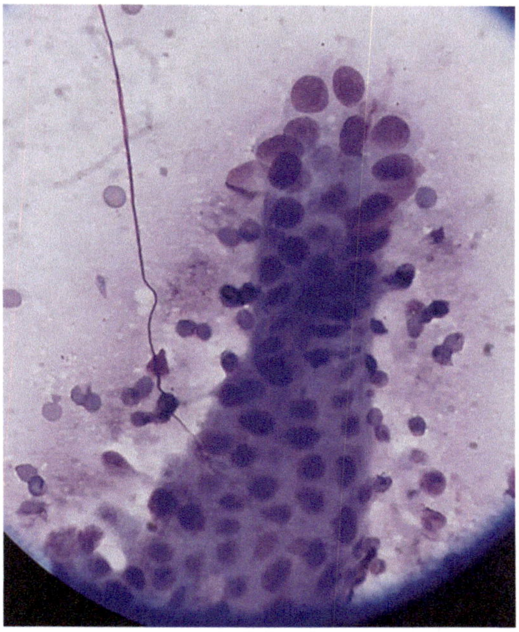

Figure 19.9D Aspirate for cytology showed clumps of monomorphic, basaloid epithelial cells. 10x. *Source:* Image courtesy of VIN and Cheryl Matuszewski, DVM.

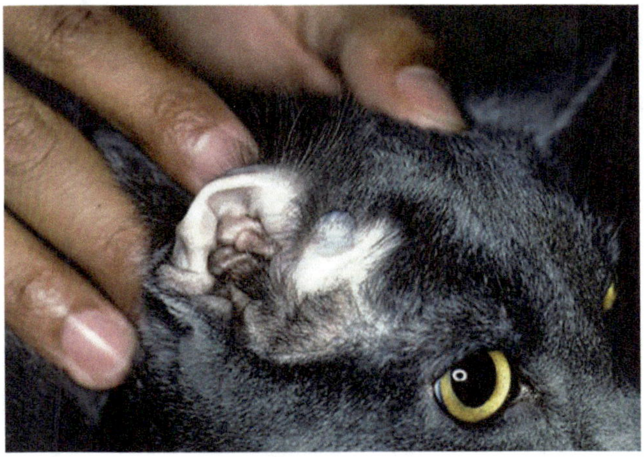

Figure 19.9E A raised, smooth, dark gray, basal cell tumor on the head of an older cat. *Source:* Image courtesy of Dr. William Miller, DACVD.

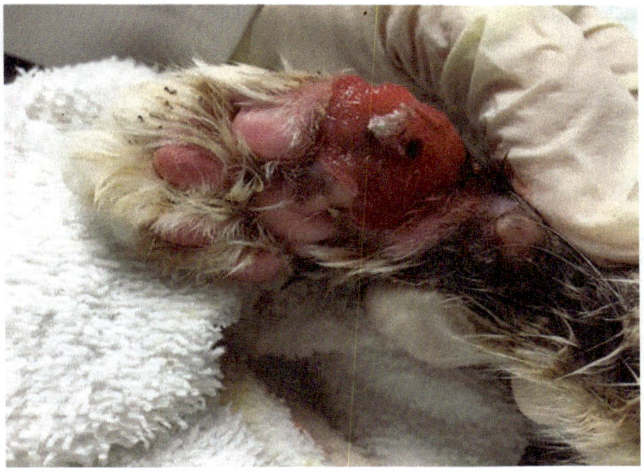

Figure 19.9F A large, ulcerated, basal cell tumor on the paw of an older cat. *Source:* Image courtesy of VIN and Karen Dowd-Martin, DVM.

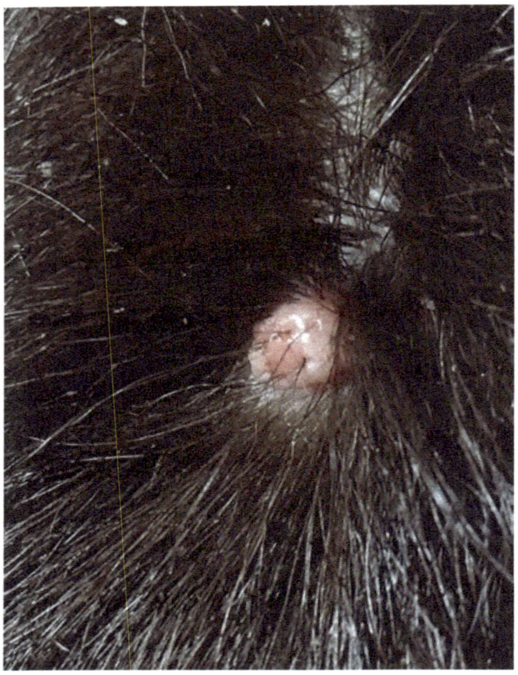

Figure 19.10A A small, raised, pink, lobulated, dermal mass on a dog due to sebaceous gland adenoma.

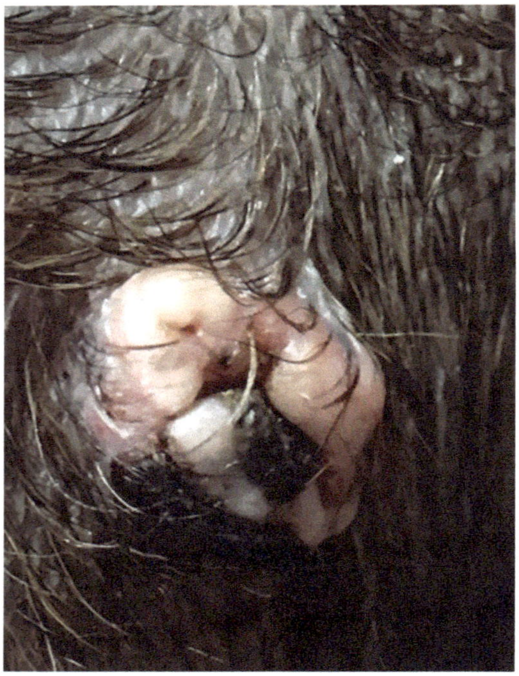

Figure 19.10B A larger sebaceous gland adenoma with typical oily secretions.

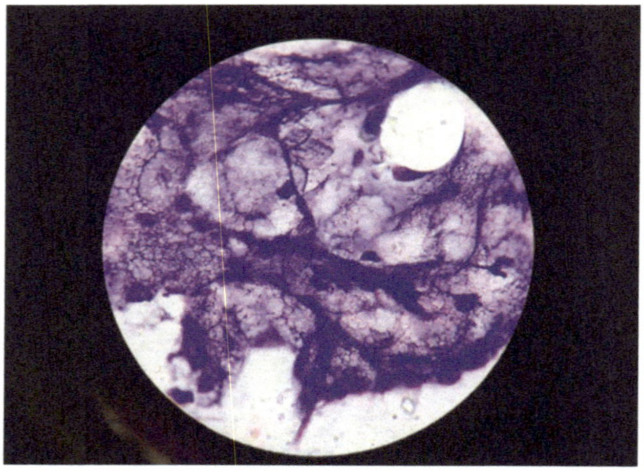

Figure 19.10C Fine needle aspirate for cytology showed typical bland sebaceous gland cells. 10x

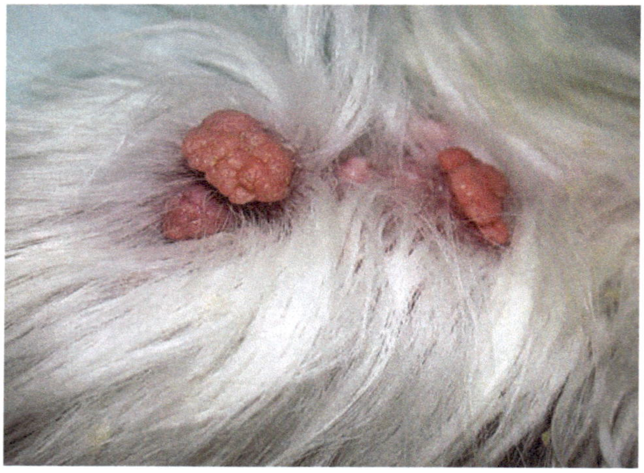

Figure 19.11 Multiple benign, sebaceous gland tumors in a dog which could be mistaken for papillomas.

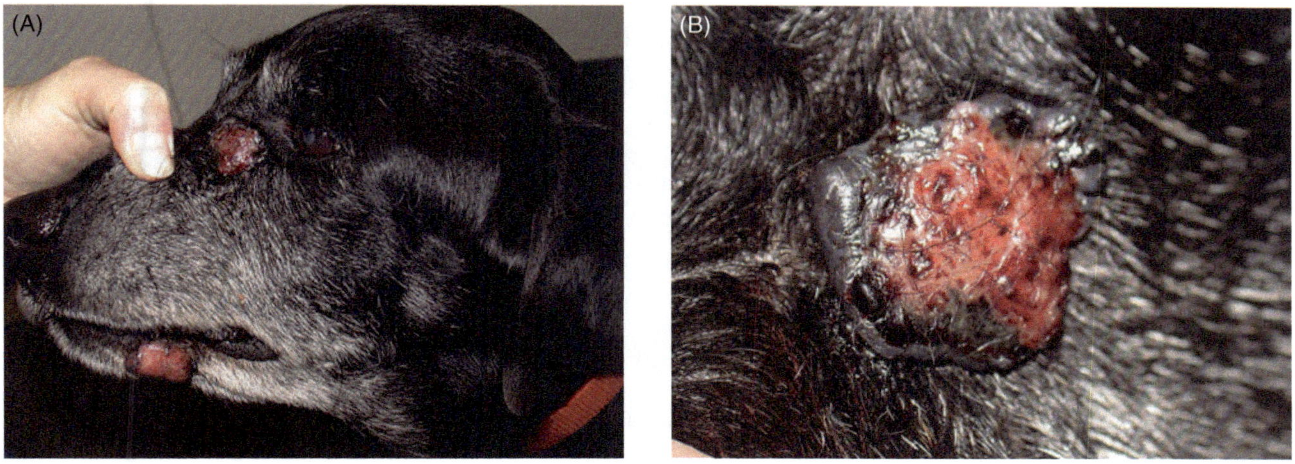

Figures 19.12A and B Raised, erosive masses on the face of an older dog caused by sebaceous epitheliomas.

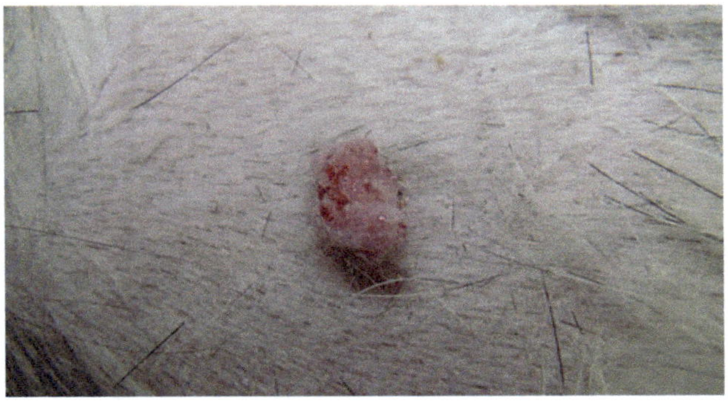

Figure 19.13A An exophytic mass on an Elkhound due to infundibular keratinizing acanthomas.

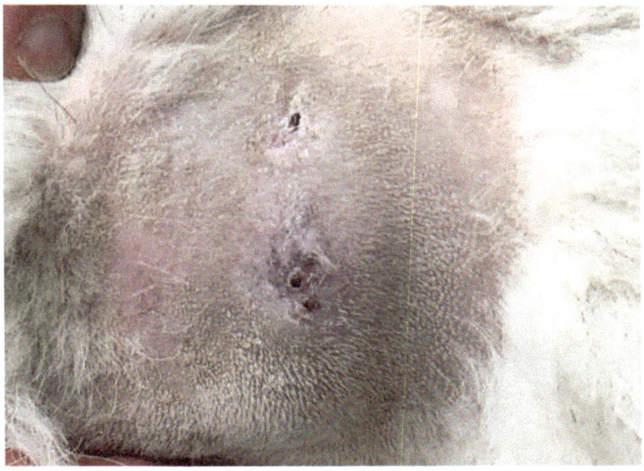

Figure 19.13B Larger dermal cysts with central pores also due to infundibular keratinizing acanthomas.

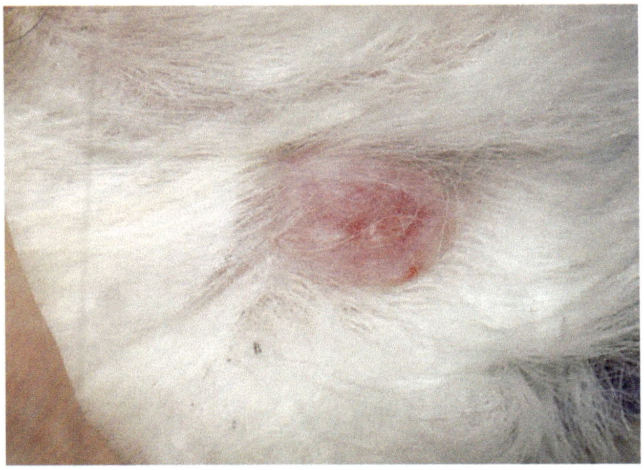

Figure 19.13C An alopecic, raised, dermal mass caused by a trichoblastoma.

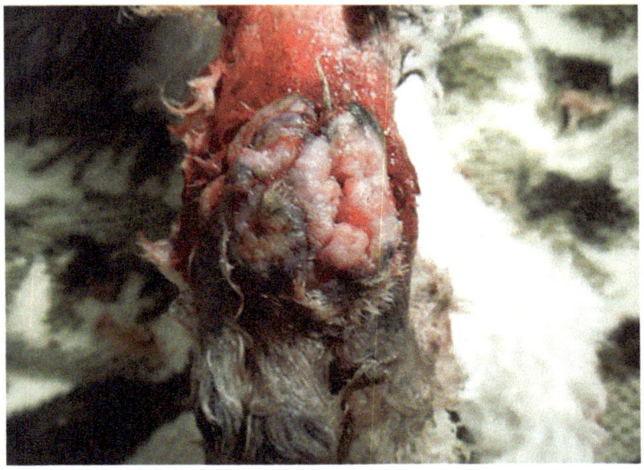

Figure 19.13D A large pilomatricoma on the paw of a dog.

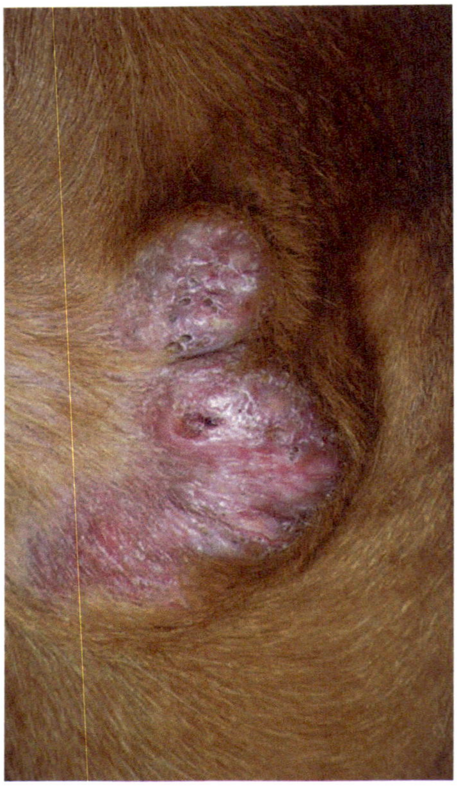

Figure 19.14A Firm, raised follicular, cysts and comedones induced by chronic friction on the lateral elbow of a large breed dog.

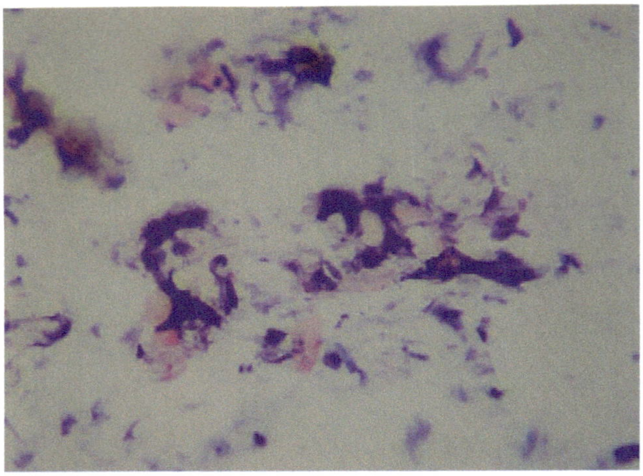

Figure 19.14B Aspirate of follicular cysts for cytology showed typical amorphous keratin and follicular debris. 4x

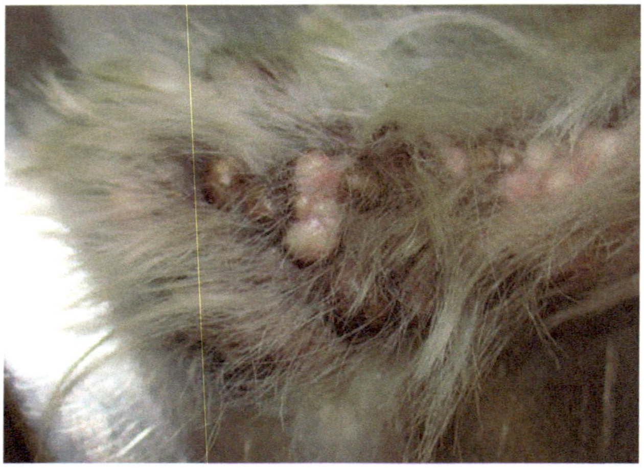

Figure 19.14C Follicular cysts on the paw of a Chinese Crested dog.

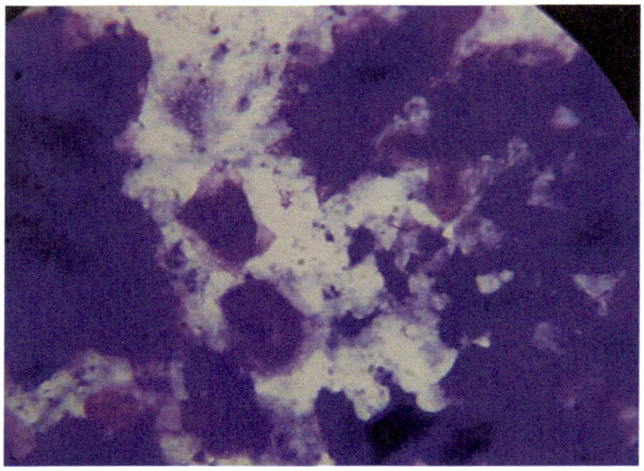

Figure 19.14D Aspirate of follicular cysts for cytology showed typical amorphous keratin and follicular debris. 10x

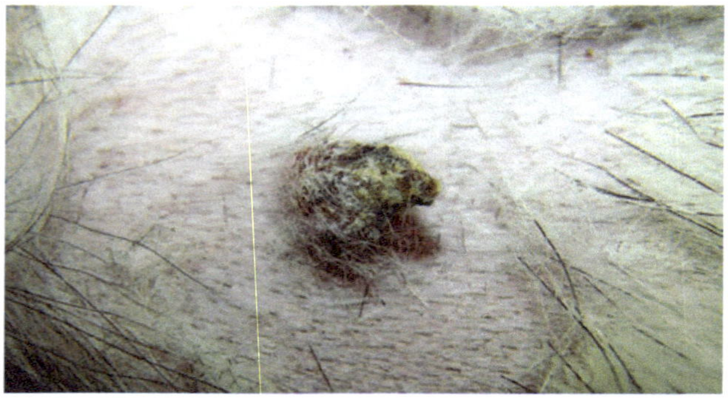

Figure 19.15A A cutaneous horn overlying an infundibular keratinizing acanthoma.

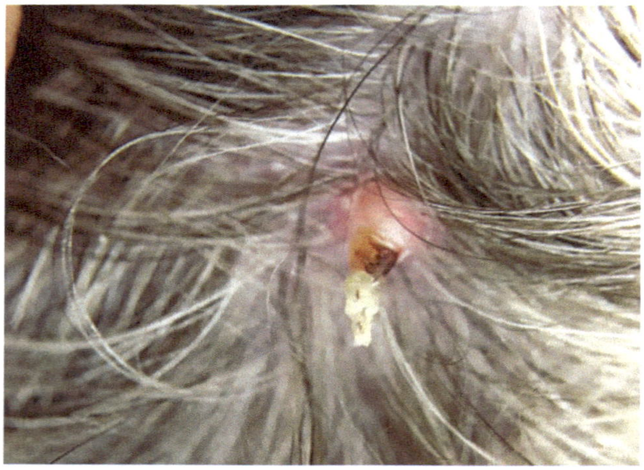

Figure 19.15B A small cutaneous horn on top of a small epithelial tumor.

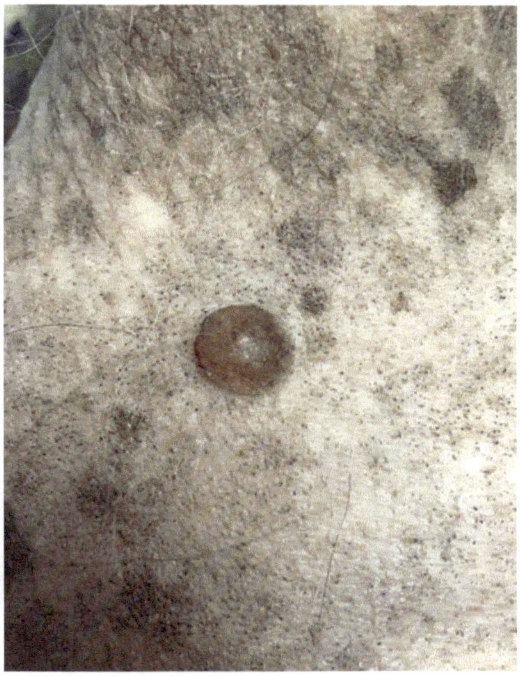

Figure 19.16A A raised, round, cystic, dermal mass caused by an apocrine cyst on a Chinese Crested dog.

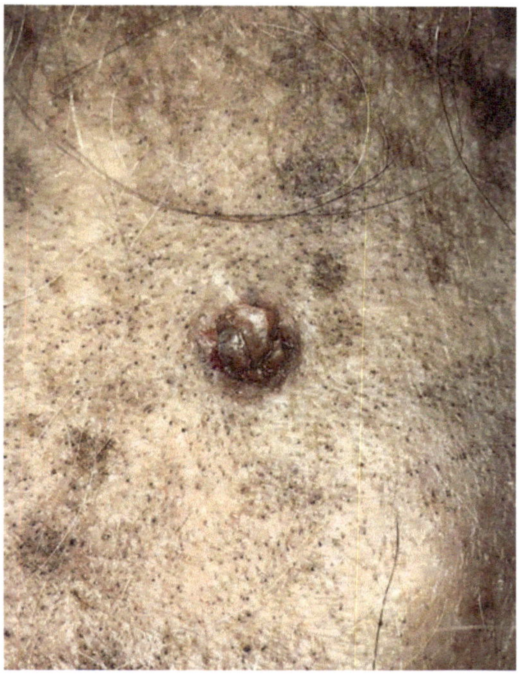

Figure 19.16B When the mass was aspirated a small amount of clear fluid was obtained and the mass collapsed.

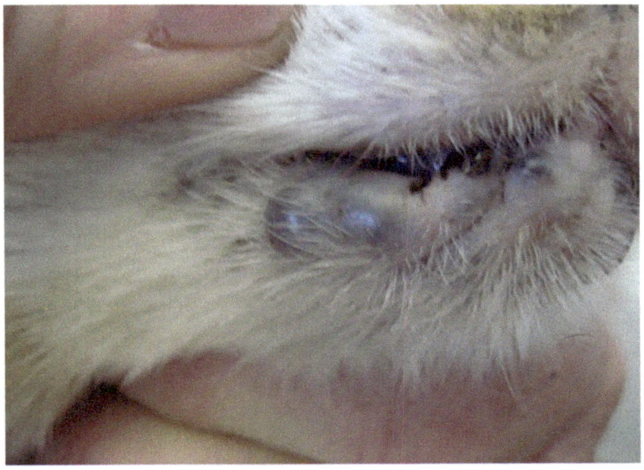

Figure 19.17 Multiple, raised, dark gray, apocrine cysts on the lower lip of a cat. *Source:* Image courtesy of VIN and Daniel Hall, DVM.

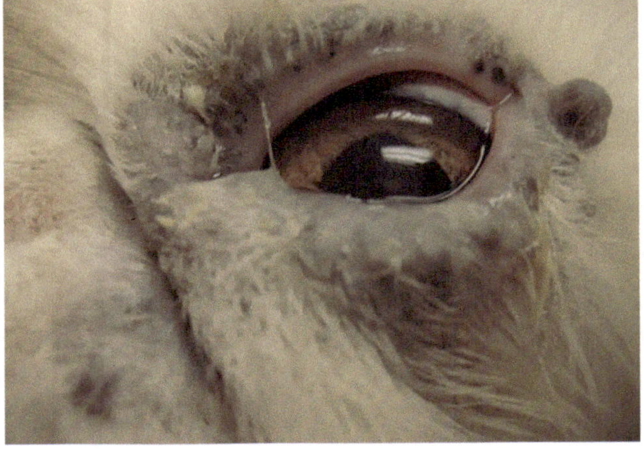

Figure 19.18A Multiple, raised, gray, cystic, dermal masses on the eyelid of a Persian due to feline apocrine cystomatosis. *Source:* Image courtesy of VIN and Mike Bloomer, DVM.

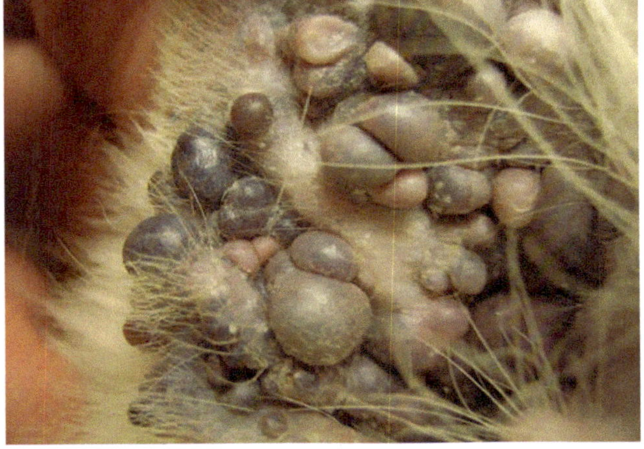

Figure 19.18B In the same Persian cat, ear canals were obstructed by similar blue-gray, firm, cystic masses. *Source:* Image courtesy of VIN and Mike Bloomer, DVM.

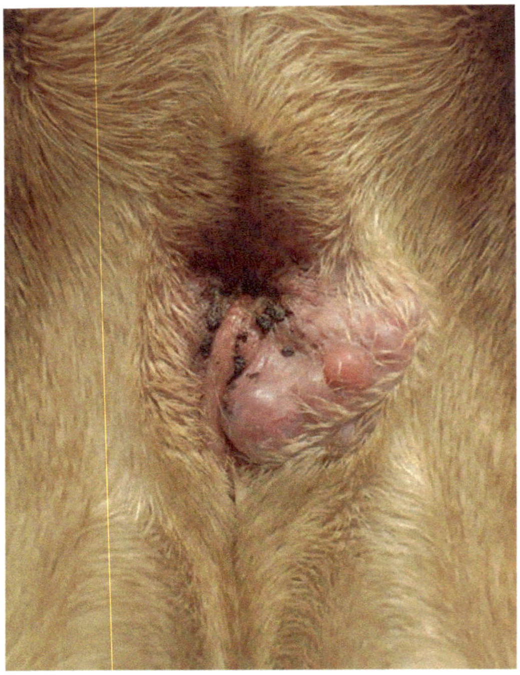

Figure 19.19A Raised, firm, alopecic, pink masses caused by perianal adenomas. *Source:* Image courtesy of VIN and Stephen Skinner, DVM.

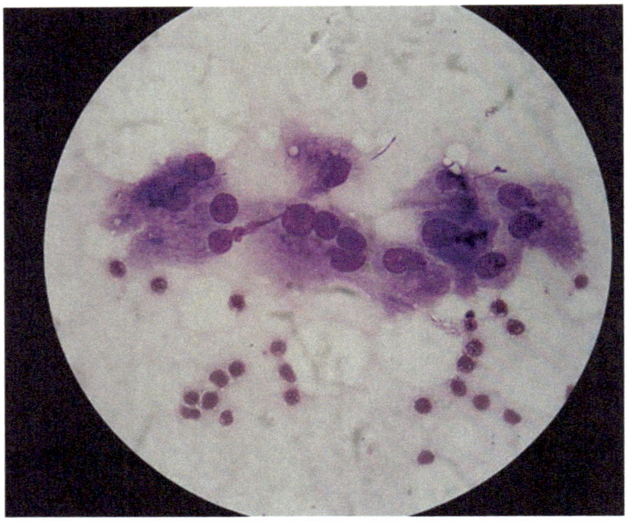

Figure 19.19B Aspirate and cytology of a perianal adenoma showing clumps of hepatoid epithelial cells. 100x. *Source:* Image courtesy of VIN and Sharon Regev, DVM.

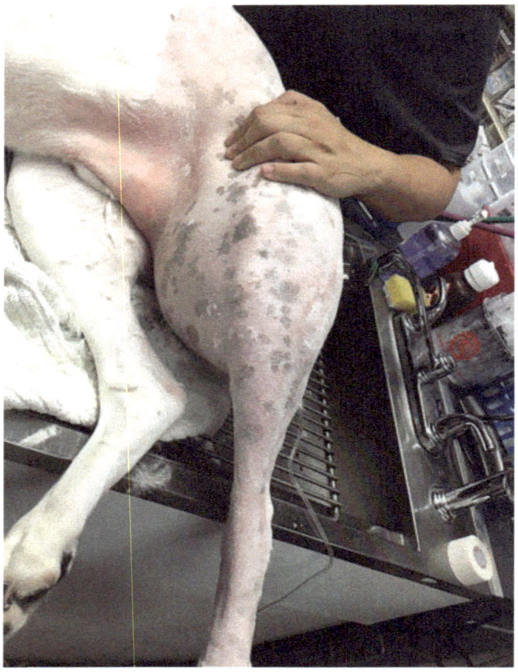

Figure 19.20A A large, soft, subcutaneous mass on the medial thigh of a dog caused by a lipoma.

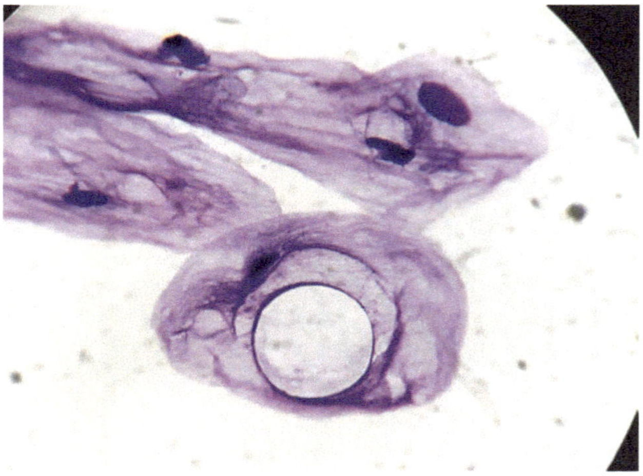

Figure 19.20B Aspirate and cytology of a lipoma demonstrating clumps of delicate, thin-walled lipocytes. 100x

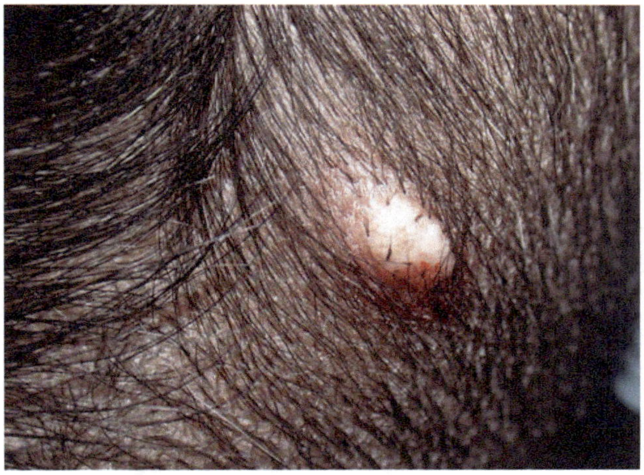

Figure 19.21A This small, pink, dermal mass was found on aspirate to be a mast cell tumor.

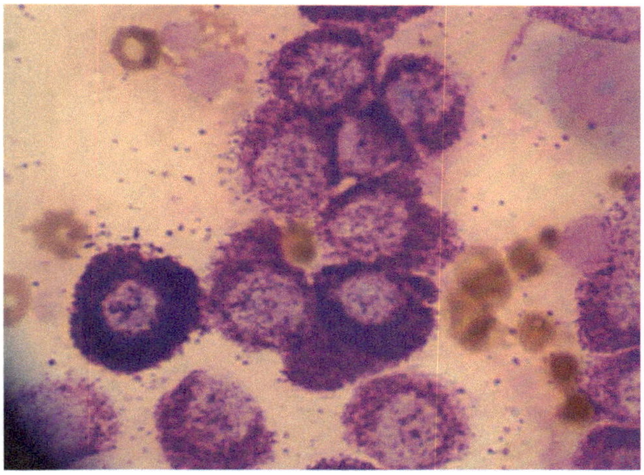

Figure 19.21B Aspirate of the tumor showed numerous, well granulated, mast cells. 100x with digital zoom.

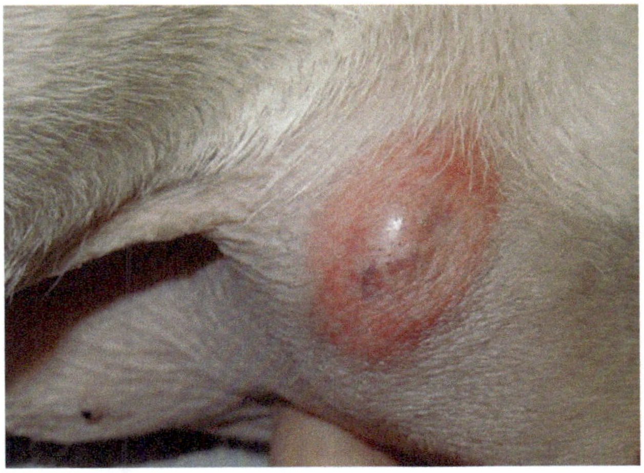

Figure 19.21C An erythematous, slightly raised plaque on the groin of a Pug caused by a mast cell tumor.

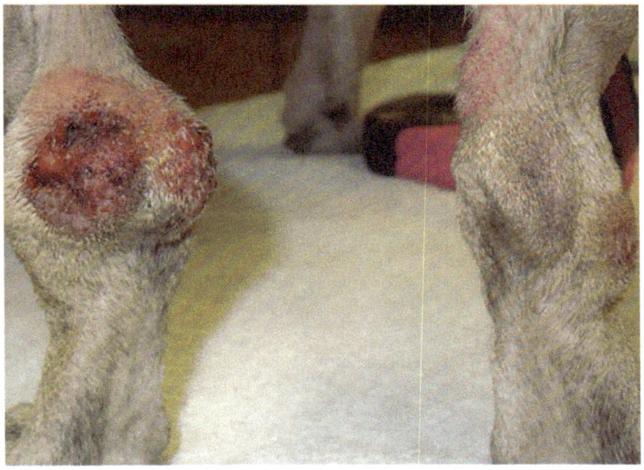

Figure 19.21D The same dog had numerous other large, often crusted and eroded mast cell tumors.

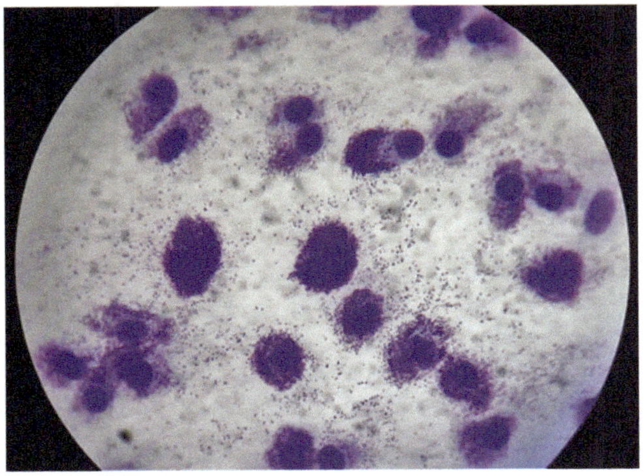

Figure 19.21E Mast cell tumor cytology. 100x

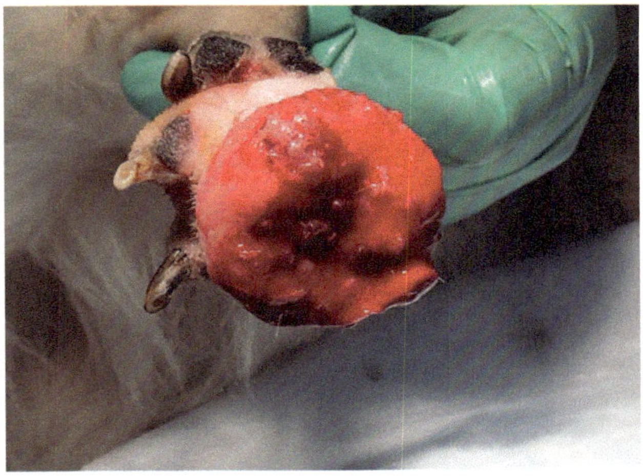

Figure 19.21F A large, ulcerated, mast cell tumor between the toes of a dog.

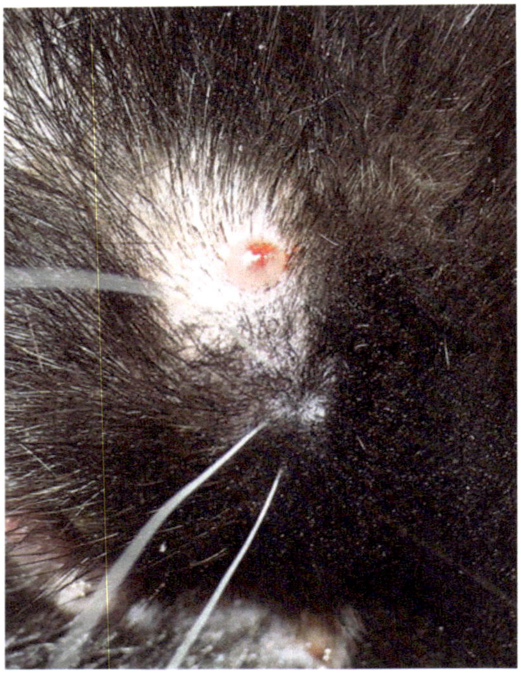

Figure 19.22A A small, pink, raised, dermal mass on the temporal area of a cat due to a mast cell tumor.

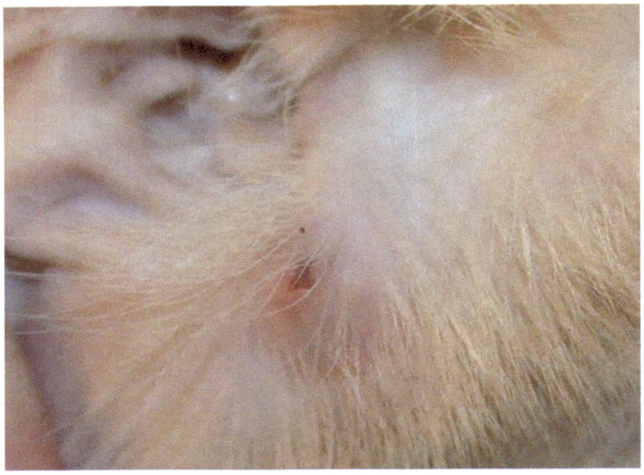

Figure 19.22B A mast cell tumor on the proximal pinna of a cat causing a raised, slightly eroded, dermal mass.

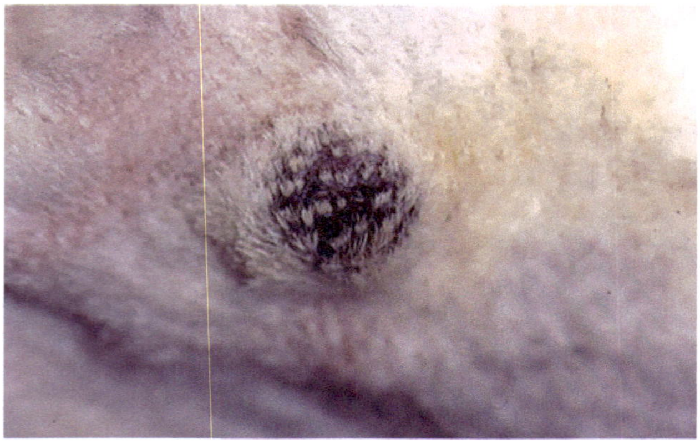

Figure 19.23A Nodular dermatofibrosis in a German Shepherd dog causing multiple, raised, firm, dermal masses. *Source:* Image courtesy of Dr. Michele Rosenbaum, DACVD.

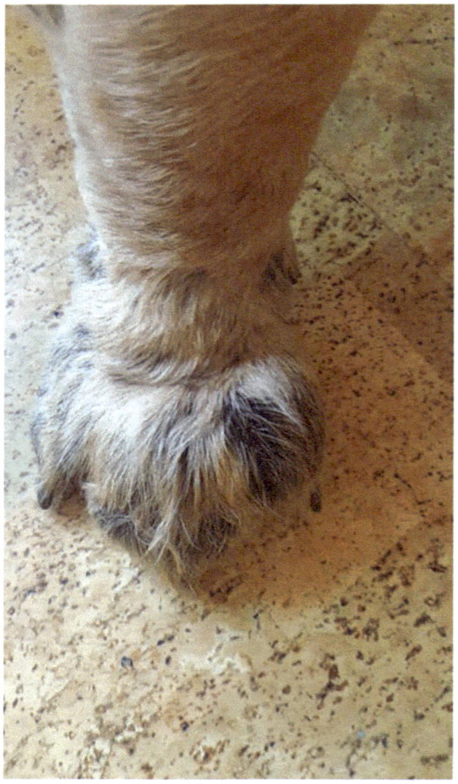

Figure 19.23B Multiple, rubbery, dark masses on the paws of a German Shepherd with nodular dermatofibrosis. *Source:* Image courtesy of Dr. Amy Shumaker, DACVD.

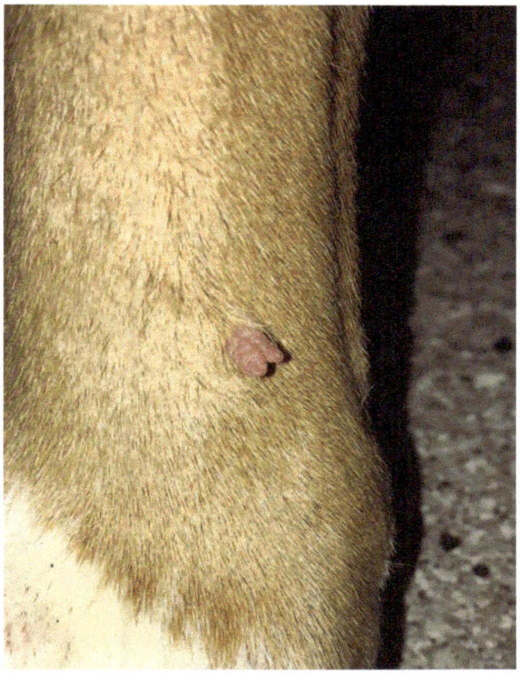

Figure 19.24A A small, pedunculated, pink skin tag.

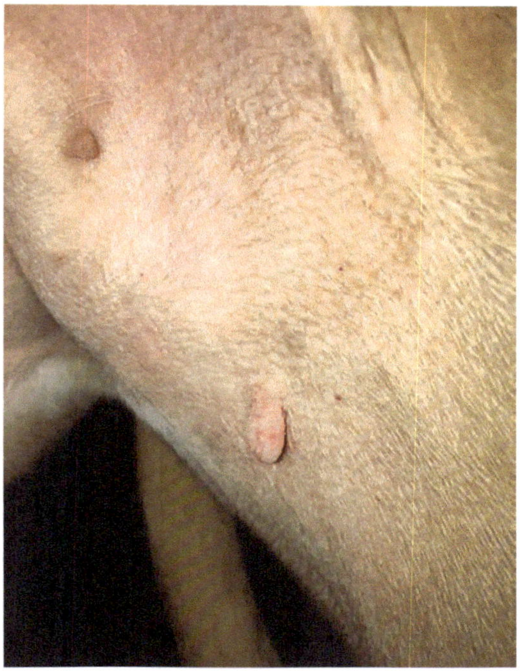

Figure 19.24B The same dog had similar skin tags elsewhere.

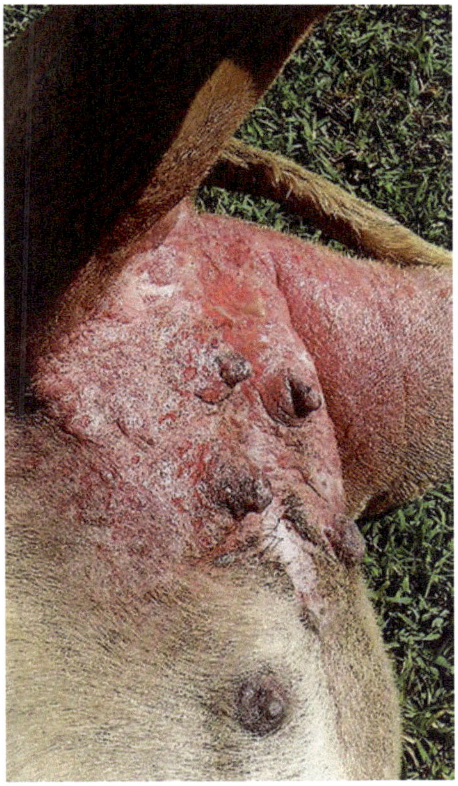

Figure 19.25 Inflammatory mammary carcinoma in a dog causing acutely progressive, painful, erosive, inguinal dermatitis. *Source:* Image courtesy of VIN and Steve Denley, BVSc.

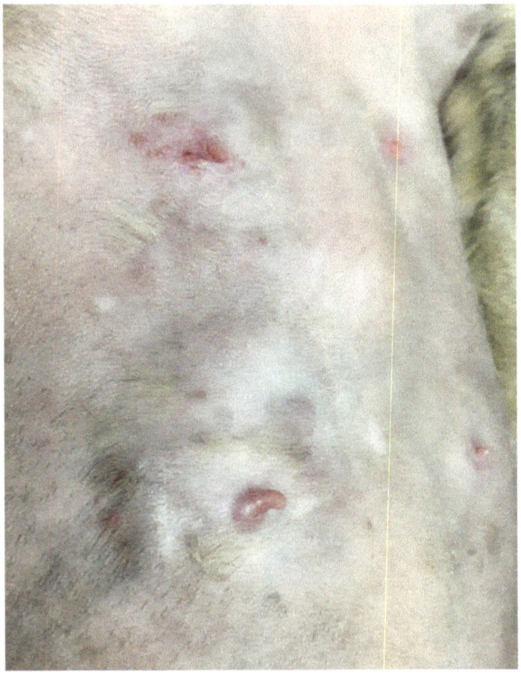

Figure 19.26A Raised, firm, mammary masses in a cat, which were found on histopathology to be mammary adenocarcinoma.

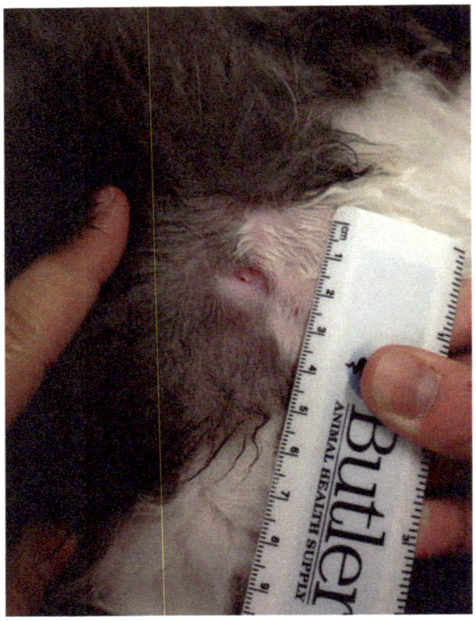

Figure 19.26B In this cat with mammary adenocarcinoma, draining tracts were present in addition to nodules. *Source:* Photo courtesy of VIN and Sharon Nath, DVM.

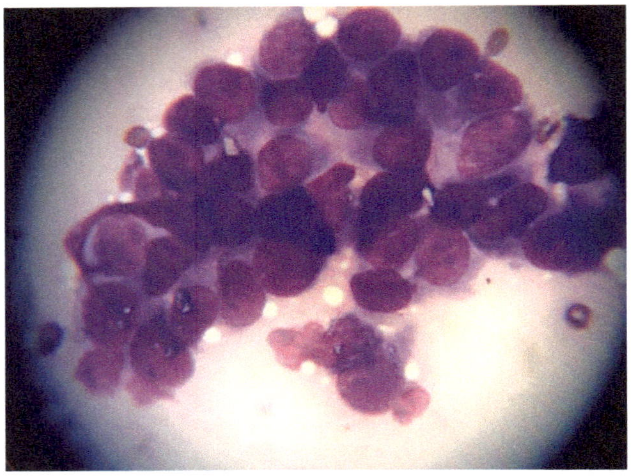

Figure 19.26C Cytology of mammary carcinoma. 100x. *Source:* Image courtesy of VIN and Sharon Nath, DVM.

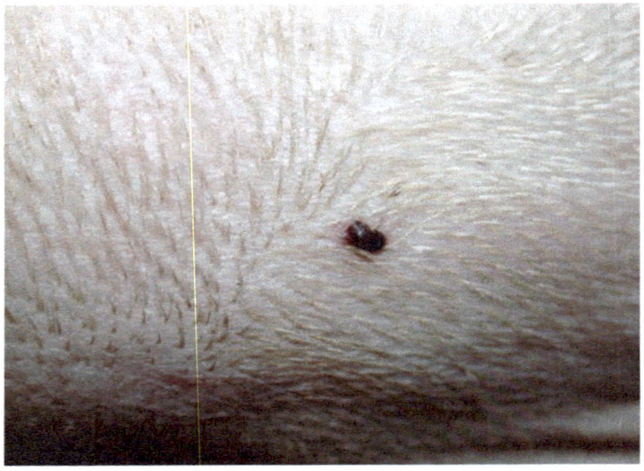

Figure 19.27A A small, dark red, dermal mass caused by a solar-induced hemangioma.

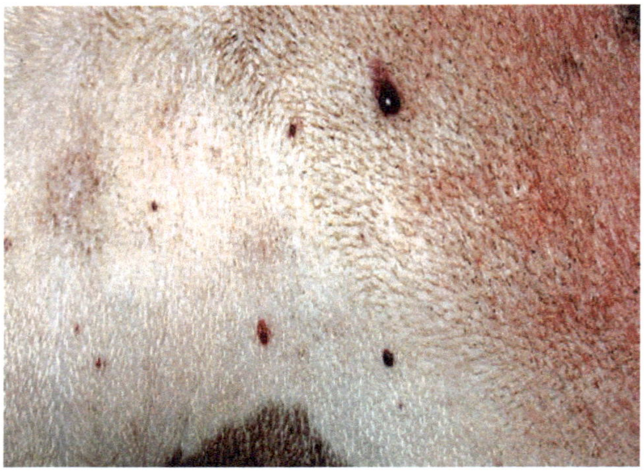

Figure 19.27B Numerous hemangiomas and solar dermatitis on a Pitbull dog.

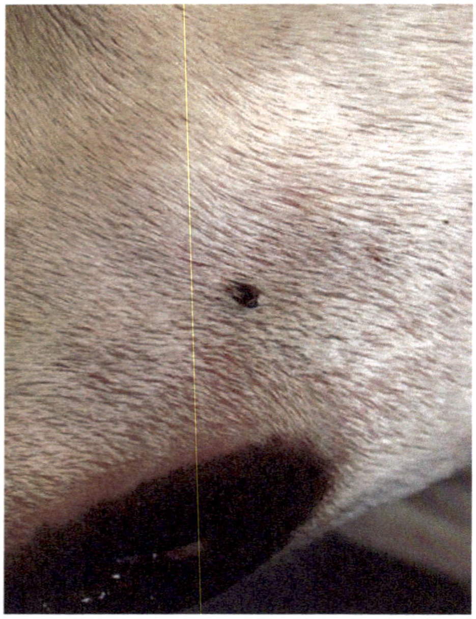

Figure 19.27C The hemangioma on this Pitbull was slightly pedunculated.

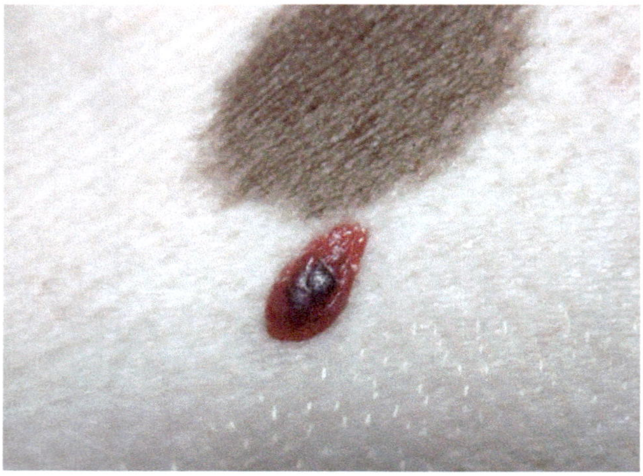

Figure 19.27D A larger hemangioma also due to chronic sun exposure.

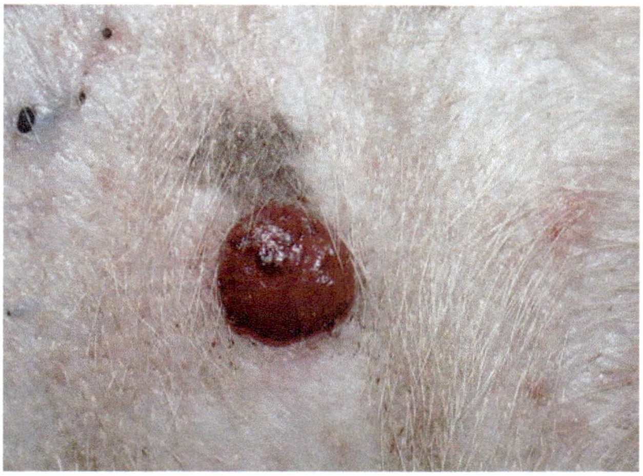

Figure 19.28A A dermal hemangiosarcoma due to chronic sun damage on a Pitbull; note the comedones and scaly actinic keratosis surrounding the mass.

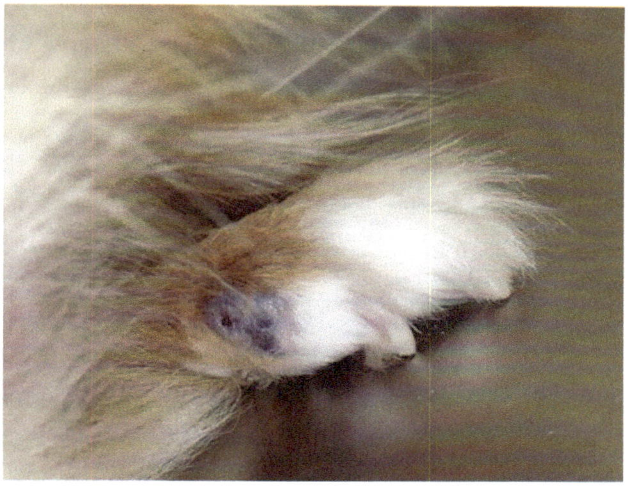

Figure 19.28B Cutaneous hemangiosarcoma on a dog, not associated with sun exposure. *Source:* Image courtesy of VIN and Charlotte Leong, DVM.

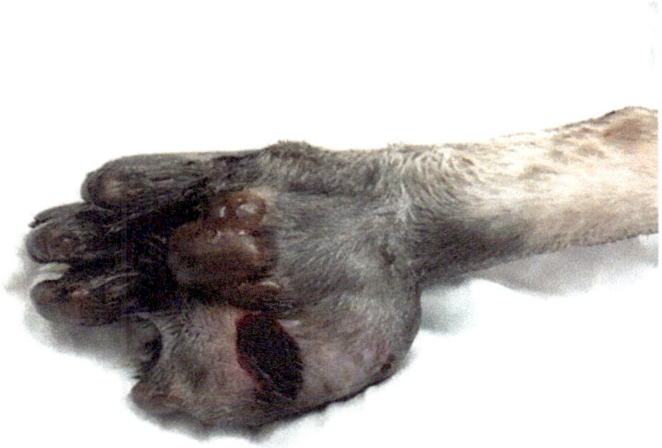

Figure 19.29 A cutaneous hemangiosarcoma on the paw of a cat. *Source:* Image courtesy of Dr. Eric Hoots, DACVS.

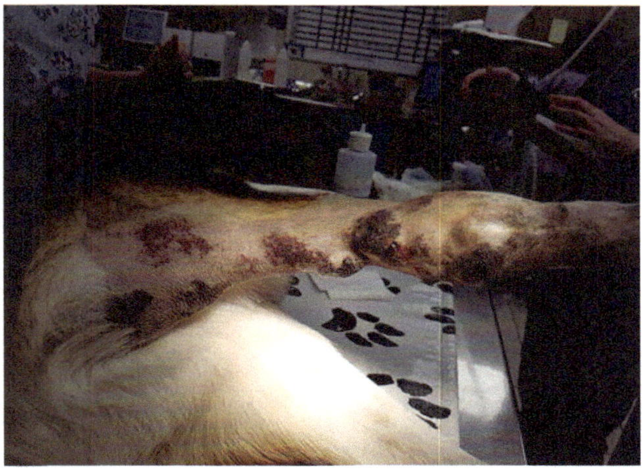

Figure 19.30A Intradermal to raised, blood-filled plaques caused by cutaneous angiomatosis in a young Golden Retriever. *Source:* Image courtesy of VIN and Karyn Jones, DVM.

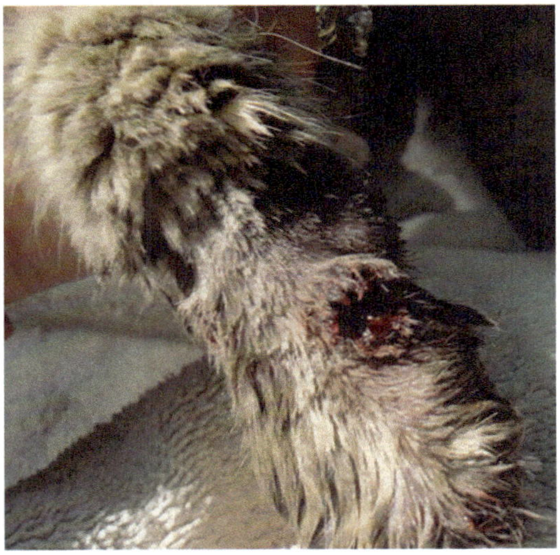

Figure 19.30B A chronic, non-healing, bleeding paw wound on a cat with cutaneous angiomatosis. *Source:* Image courtesy of VIN and Peter Gaveras, DVM.

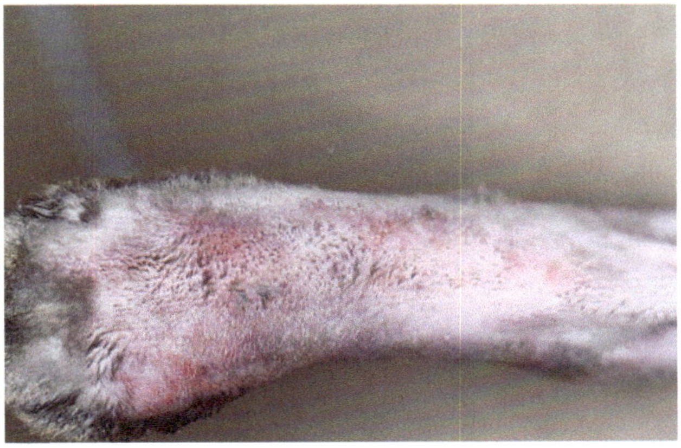

Figure 19.30C Cutaneous angiomatosis in this cat was characterized by indistinct, slightly raised, red dermal lesions on a paw. *Source:* Image courtesy of VIN and Howard Gittelman, DVM.

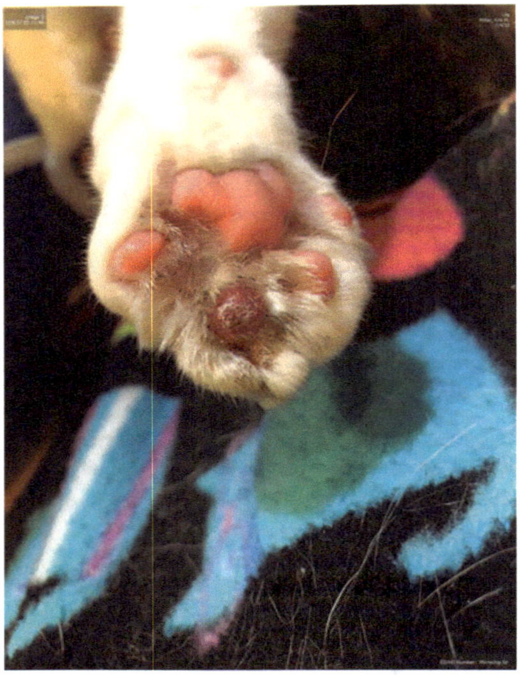

Figure 19.30D Angiomatosis causing a bleeding, crusted wound on the paw pad of a cat. *Source:* Image courtesy of VIN and Jillian Kindermann, DVM.

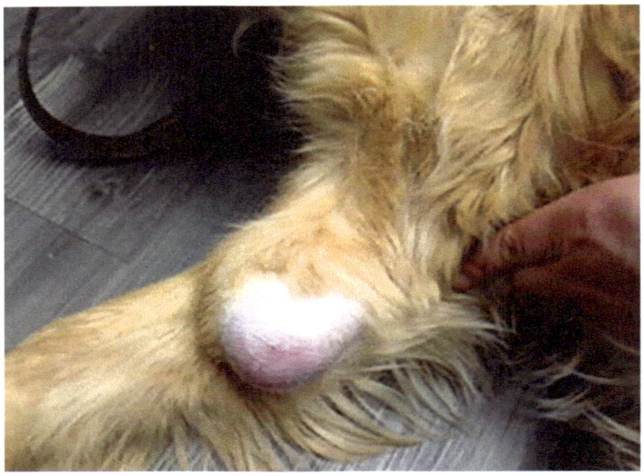

Figure 19.31A A large, firm mass on the leg of a dog due to a hemangiopericytoma. *Source:* Image courtesy of VIN and Marie North, DVM.

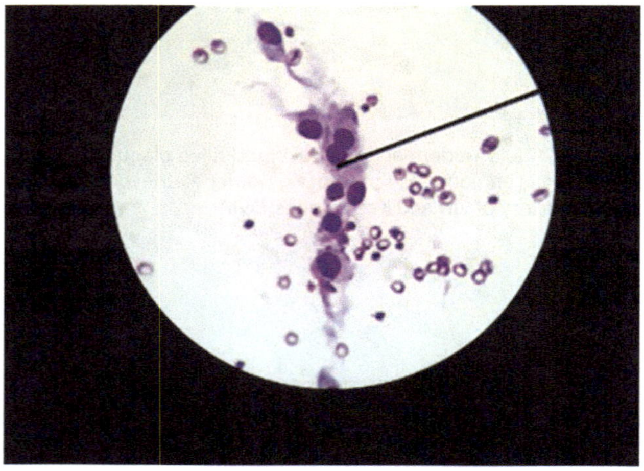

Figure 19.31B Fine needle aspirate of the hemangiopericytoma demonstrating spindle cells. 100x. *Source:* Image courtesy of VIN and Marie North, DVM.

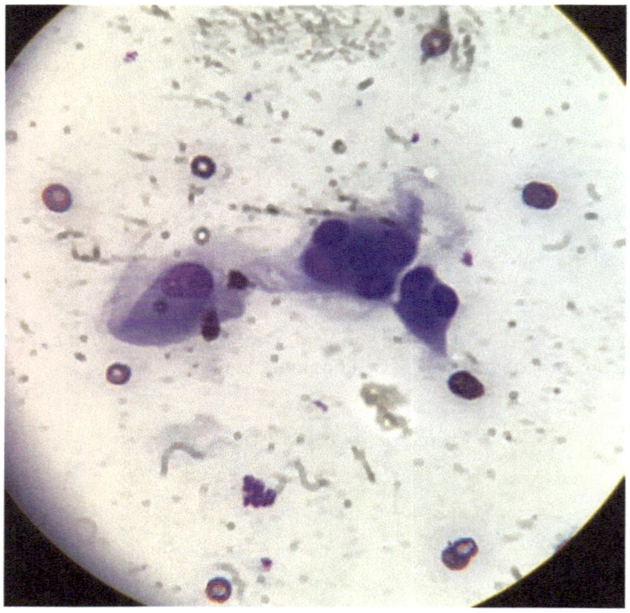

Figure 19.31C Multi-nucleate spindle cells on cytology of a hemangiopericytoma. 100x. *Source:* Image courtesy of VIN and Lisa Boals, DVM.

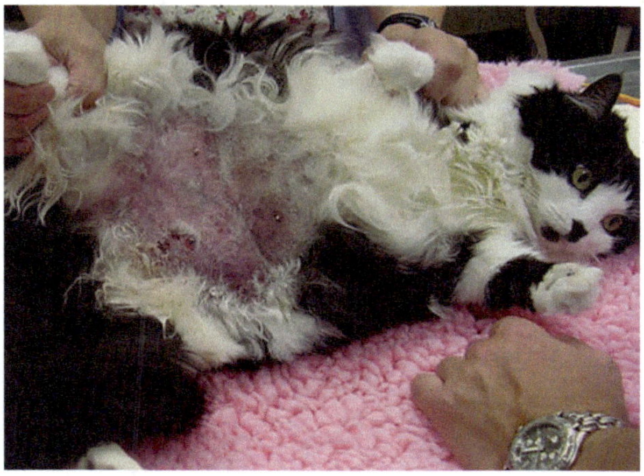

Figure 19.32A Diffuse, inguinal bruising in a cat caused by lymphangiosarcoma.

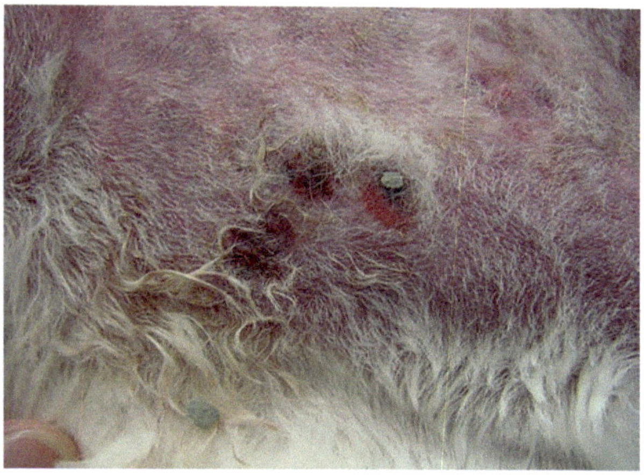

Figure 19.32B In the same cat close examination revealed small draining tracts which oozed serosanguinous fluid.

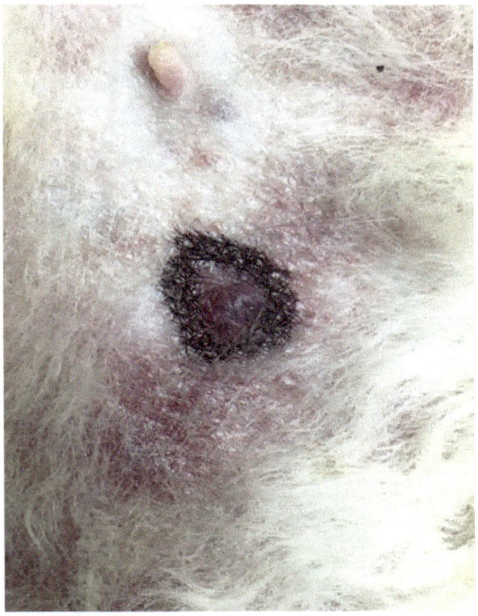

Figure 19.32C Feline lymphangiosarcoma causing irregular bruising and vesicles on the groin of a cat; the sharpie marking is used to designate a biopsy site.

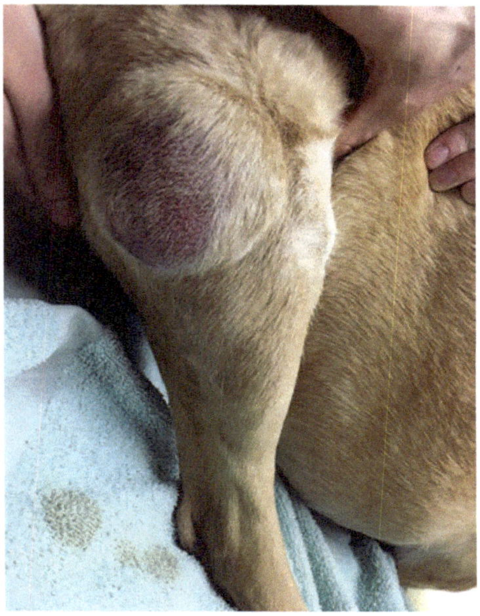

Figure 19.33A A large mass caused by fibrosarcoma on the thigh of a dog.

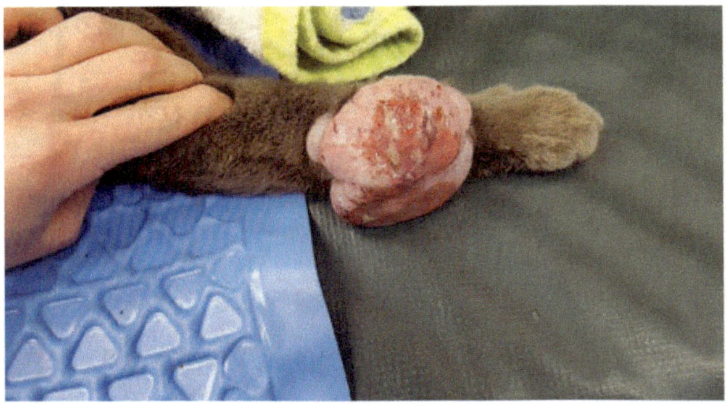

Figure 19.33B A large, alopecic, ulcerated mass on a cat's leg which was revealed on biopsy to be a fibrosarcoma. *Source:* Image courtesy of VIN and Julianne Fisher, DVM.

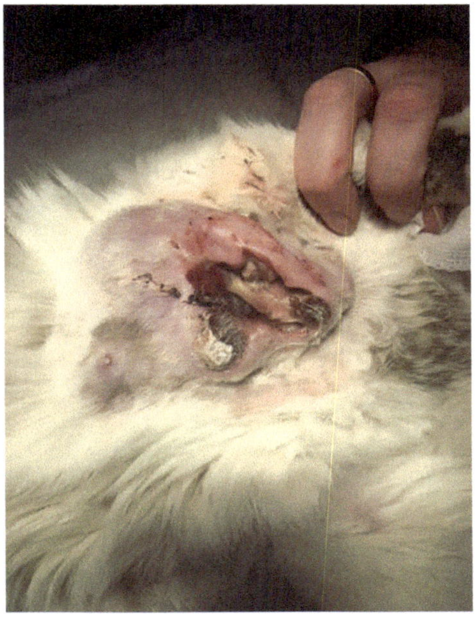

Figure 19.33C A large, necrotic fibrosarcoma on the abdomen of a cat. *Source:* Image courtesy of VIN and Janet Edson, DVM.

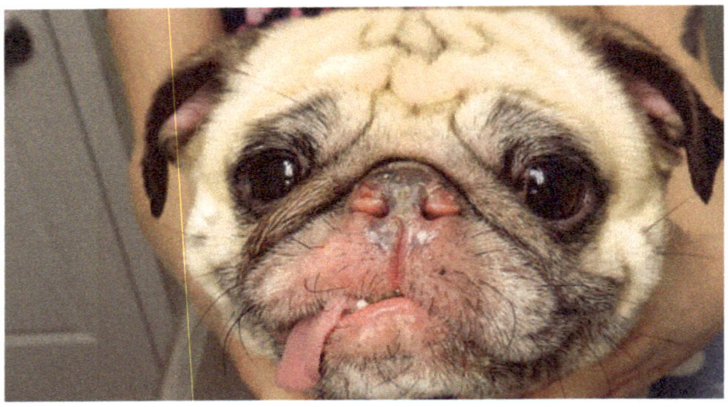

Figure 19.34A A Pug with facial and nasal depigmentation due to cutaneous epitheliotropic lymphoma.

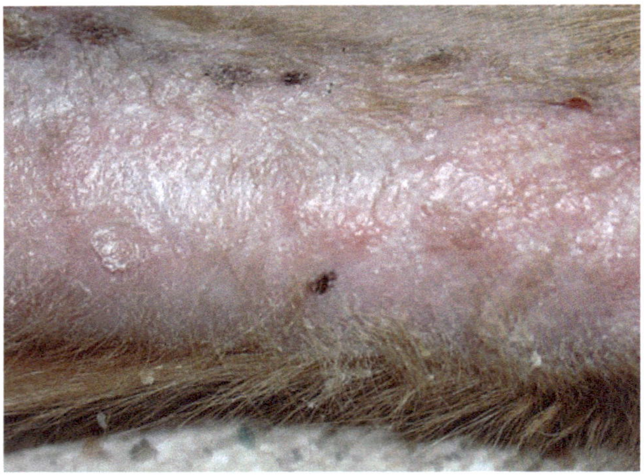

Figure 19.34B Alopecia erythema and exfoliative scaling due to cutaneous epitheliotropic lymphoma.

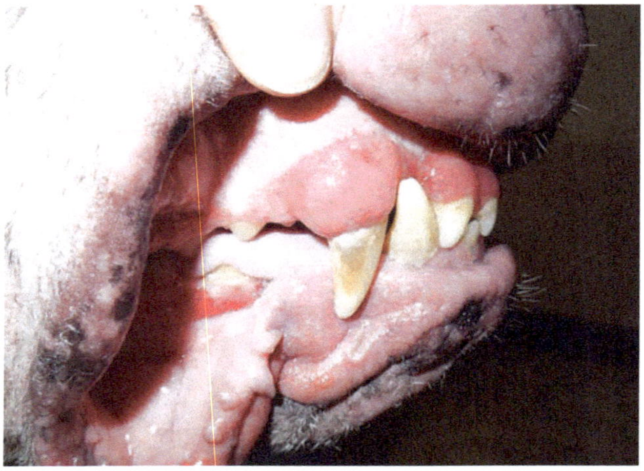

Figure 19.34C In this dog with epitheliotropic lymphoma, oral involvement was demonstrated by marked gingival hyperemia.

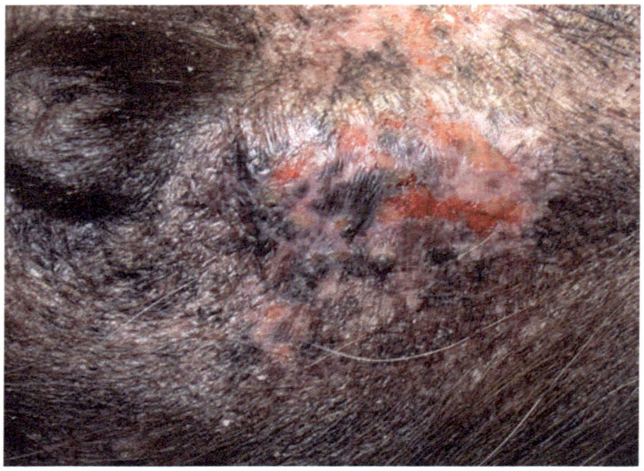

Figure 19.34D Patchy depigmentation and hyperpigmentation with erosions on the inguinal area in a dog with epitheliotropic lymphoma.

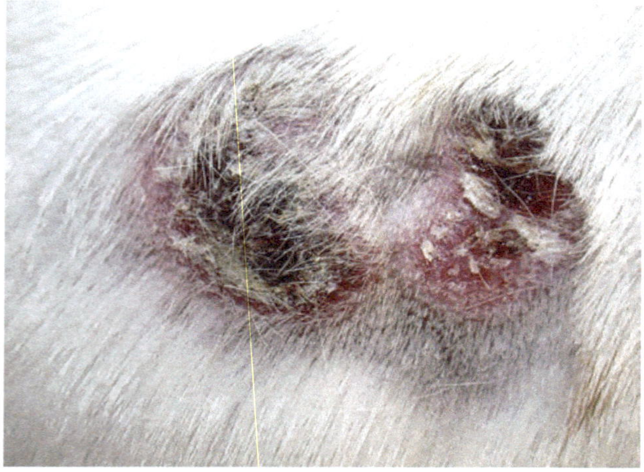

Figure 19.34E A Bulldog with epitheliotropic lymphoma characterized by C-shaped erythematous crusted truncal plaques.

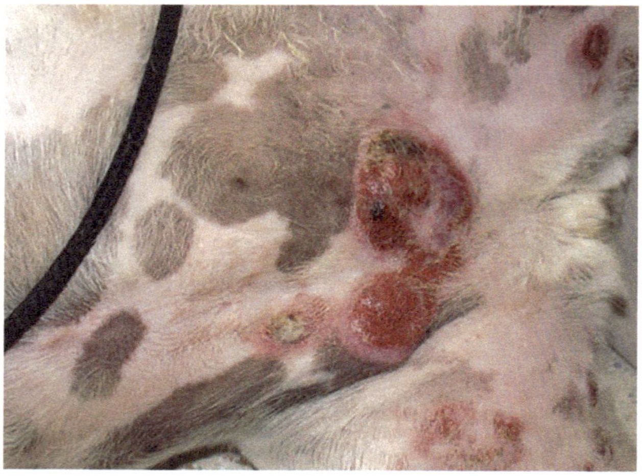

Figure 19.34F The inguinal plaques of the same dog as Figure 19.34E.

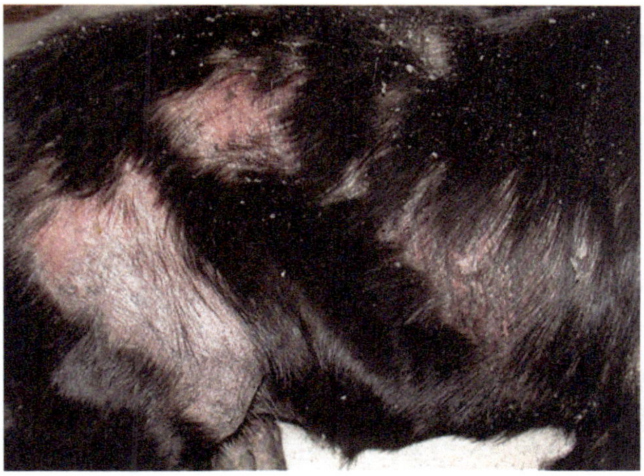

Figure 19.34G Generalized, patchy hypotrichosis, erythema, and exfoliative scaling in an elderly Labrador with cutaneous epitheliotropic lymphoma.

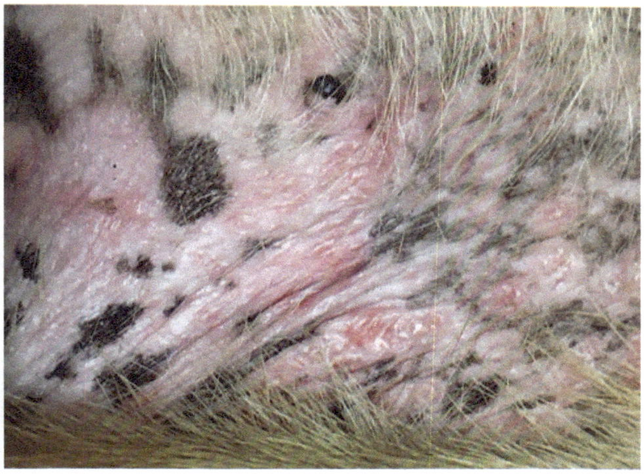

Figure 19.34H Patchy depigmentation and hyperpigmentation with erythema on the inguinal area in a dog with epitheliotropic lymphoma.

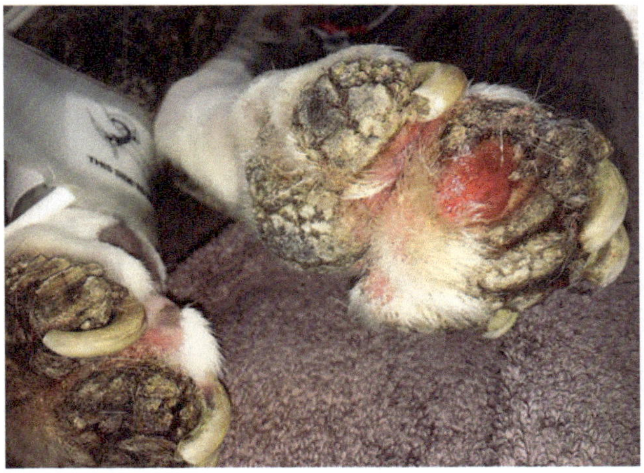

Figure 19.34I Marked paw pad crusting and ulceration in a dog caused by cutaneous epitheliotropic lymphoma.

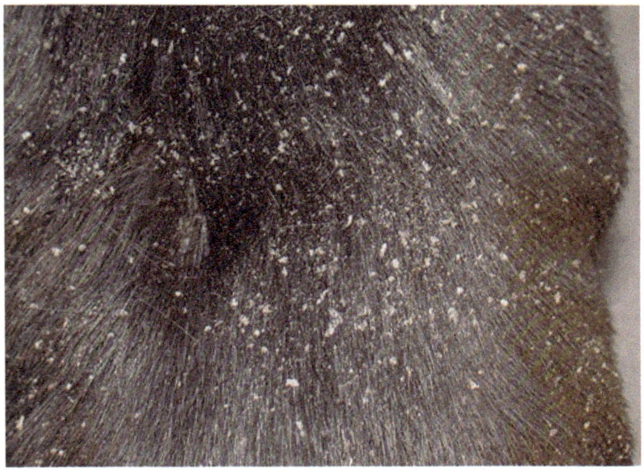

Figure 19.34J Marked exfoliative scaling due to cutaneous epitheliotropic lymphoma.

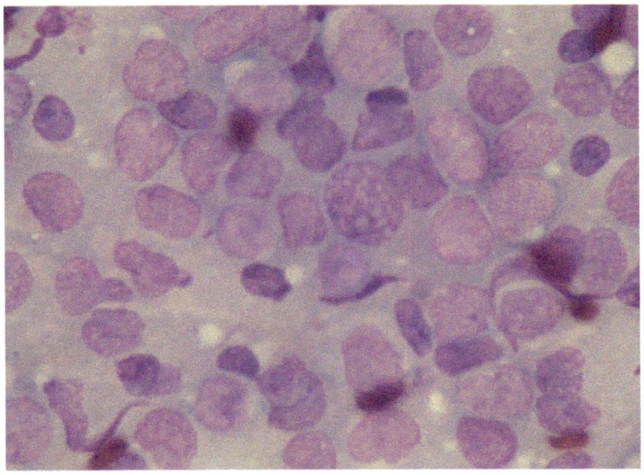

Figure 19.34K Cytology of the eroded surface showed neoplastic lymphocytes. 100x

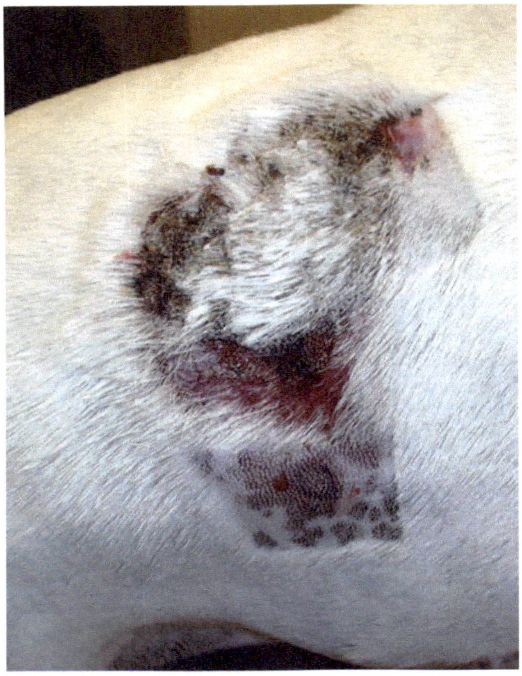

Figure 19.35A A large eroded and crusted plaque on the lateral thorax of a boxer caused by cutaneous non-epitheliotropic lymphoma.

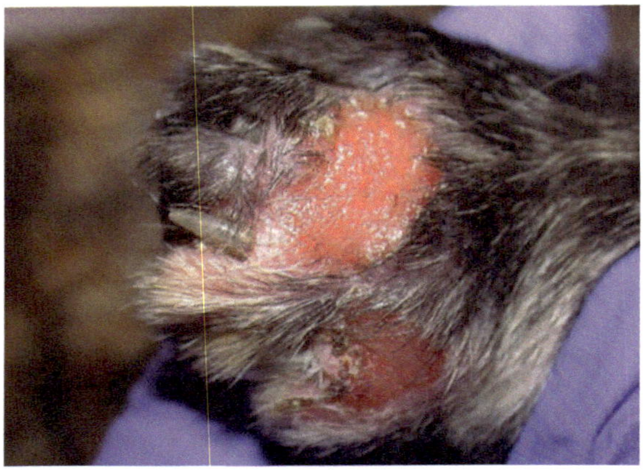

Figure 19.35B Chronic ulcerated digital lesions in a cat caused by cutaneous non-epitheliotropic lymphoma.

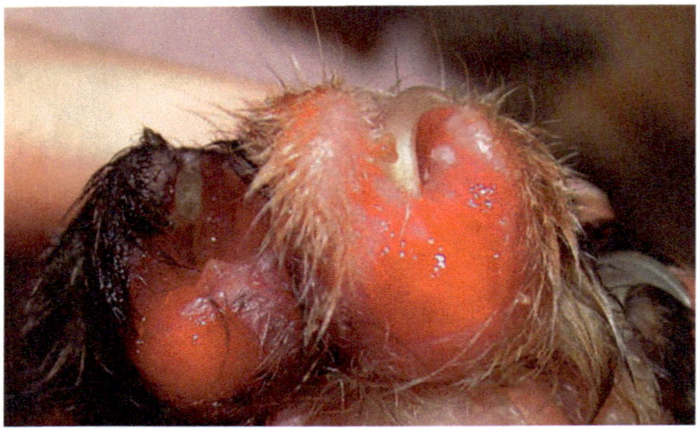

Figure 19.35C Chronic ulcerated digital lesions in a cat caused by cutaneous non-epitheliotropic lymphoma.

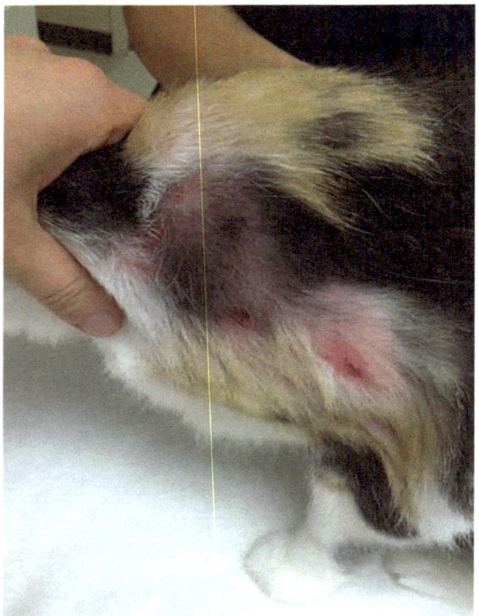

Figure 19.36A Patchy alopecia, erythema and erosions in a cat caused by cutaneous lymphocytosis. *Source:* Image courtesy of Dr. Megan Solc.

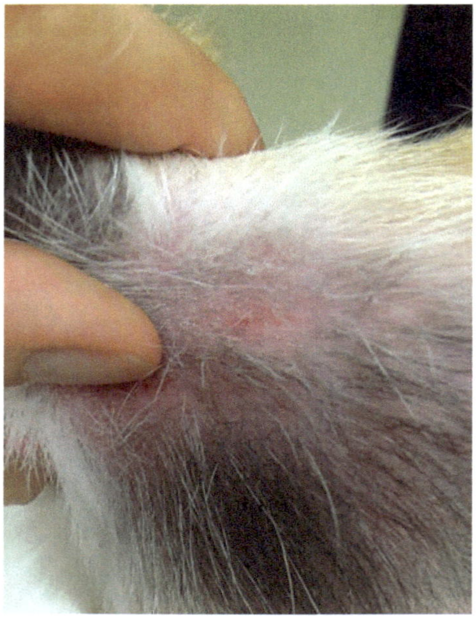

Figure 19.36B Hypotrichosis erythema and scaling caused by cutaneous lymphocytosis. *Source:* Image courtesy of Dr. Megan Solc.

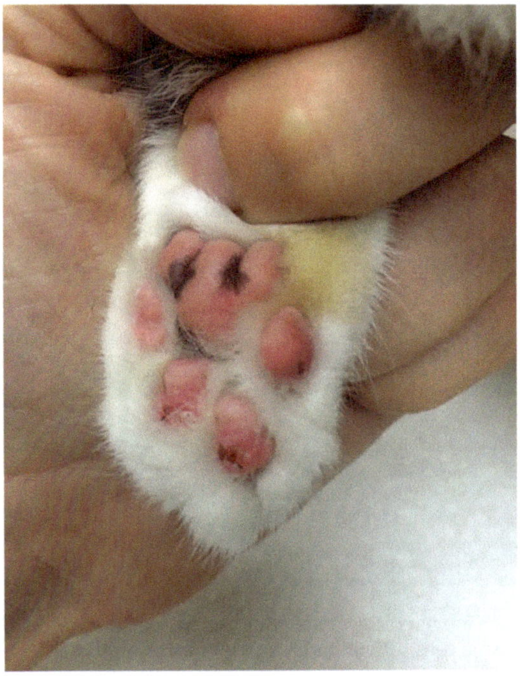

Figure 19.36C Focally crusted and inflamed paw pads in the same cat as 19.36A. *Source:* Image courtesy of Dr. Megan Solc.

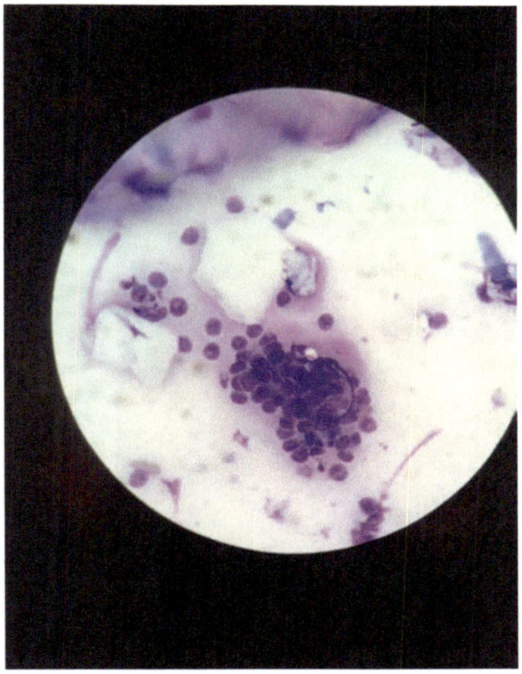

Figure 19.36D Surface cytology demonstrates numerous small lymphocytes. 100x. *Source:* Image courtesy of Dr. Megan Solc.

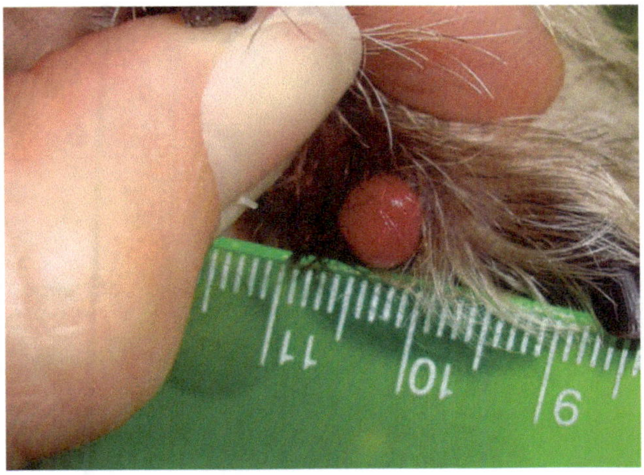

Figure 19.37A A red, raised mass on the toe of a dog caused by a plasmacytoma. *Source:* Image courtesy of VIN and Jillian Kindermann, DVM.

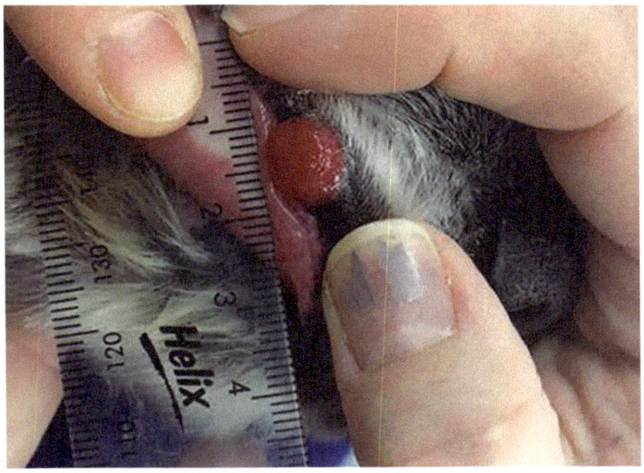

Figure 19.37B A similar plasmacytoma on the lip of a dog. *Source:* Image courtesy of VIN and Kathryn Hahn, DVM.

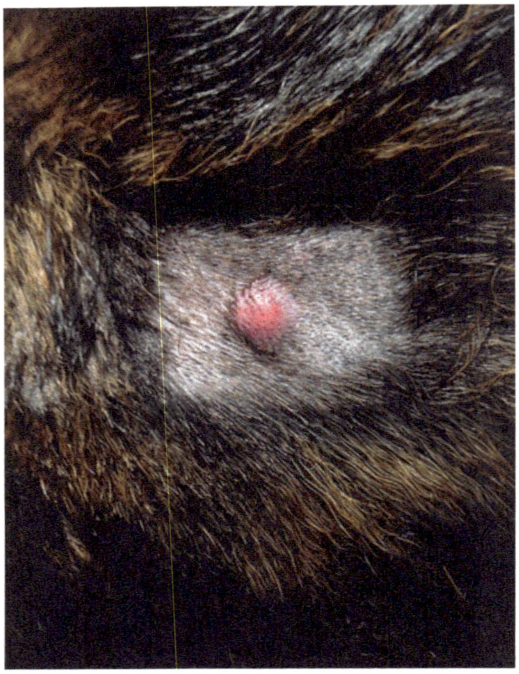

Figure 19.37C A pink, raised, round mass on the thorax of a dog due to a plasmacytoma. *Source:* Image courtesy of VIN and Katie Dull, DVM.

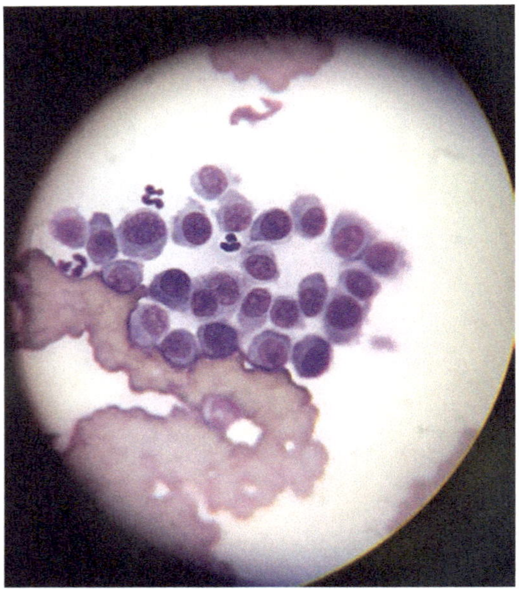

Figure 19.37D Fine needle aspirate and cytology demonstrates numerous plasma cells. 100x. *Source:* Image courtesy of VIN and Brittney Shaw, DVM.

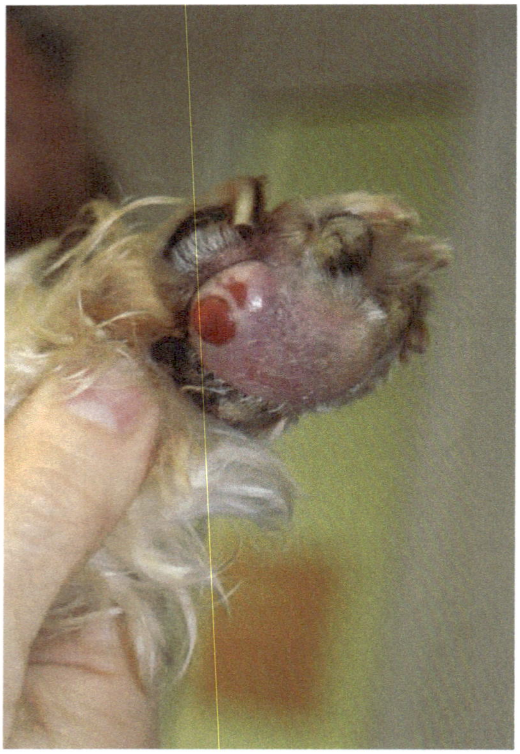

Figure 19.37E A large, ulcerated plasmacytoma on the paw of a dog. *Source:* Image courtesy of VIN and Kathryn Hahn, DVM.

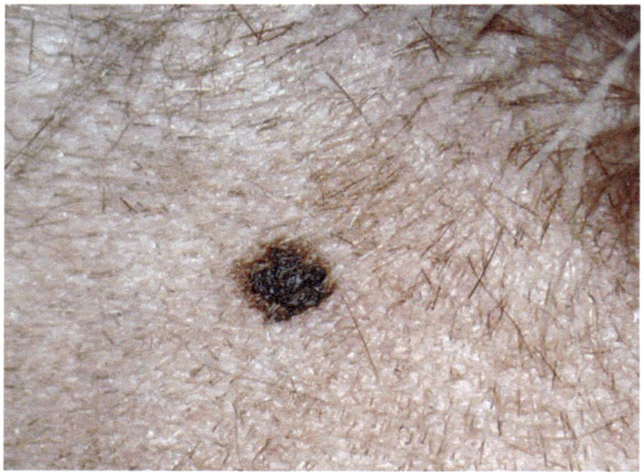

Figure 19.38A A slightly raised, pigmented dermal mass caused by a melanocytoma.

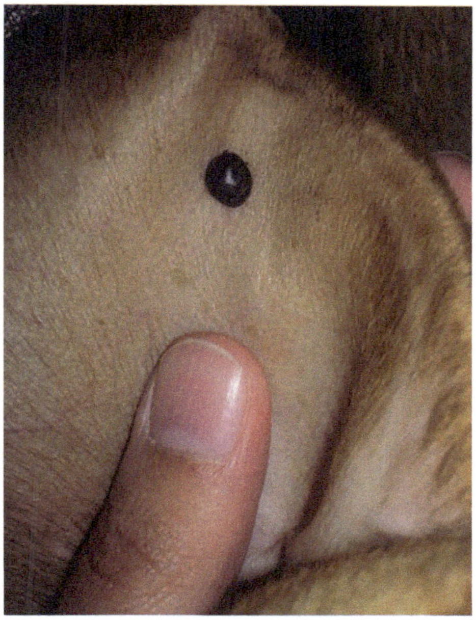

Figure 19.38B This round, raised, black, pinnal mass was also a melanocytoma. *Source:* Image courtesy of VIN and Kelly Green, DVM.

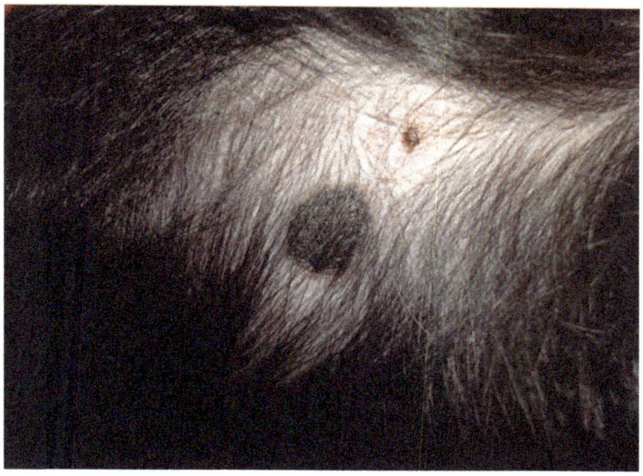

Figure 19.38C Canine melanocytoma. *Source:* Image courtesy of VIN and Joanne Gonzalez, DVM.

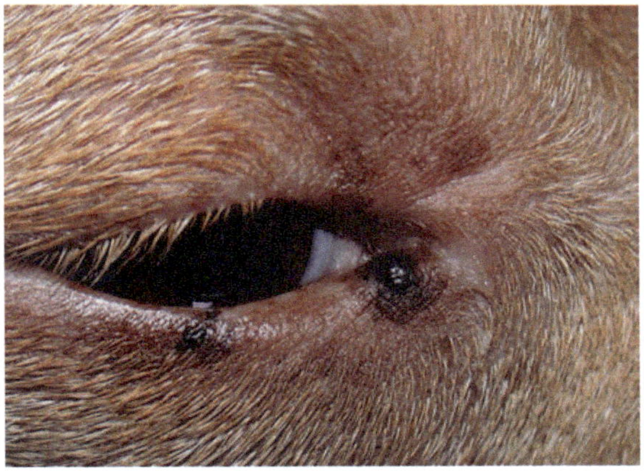

Figure 19.38D A slightly raised melanocytoma on the eyelid of a dog.

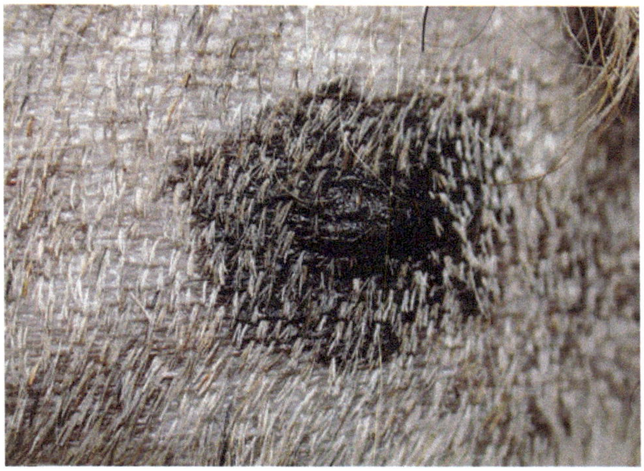

Figure 19.38E Close-up of a melanocytoma.

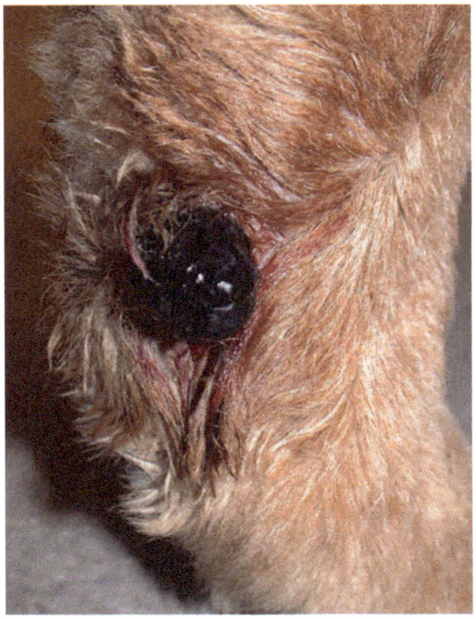

Figure 19.38F A large, pedunculated melanocytoma on the leg of an elderly dog.

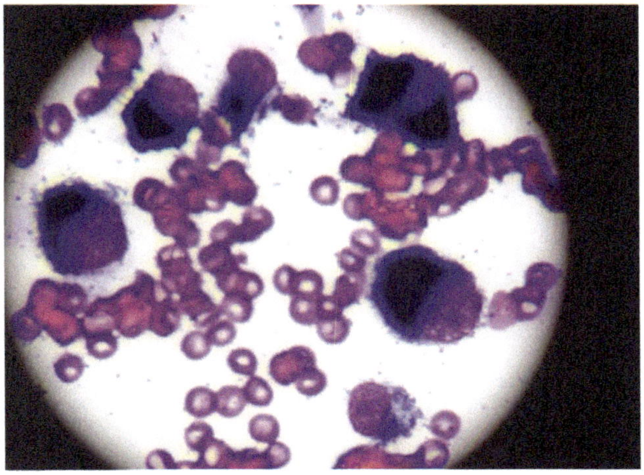

Figure 19.38G Cytology of the mass in Figure 19.38F revealed numerous well-granulated melanocytes. 100x

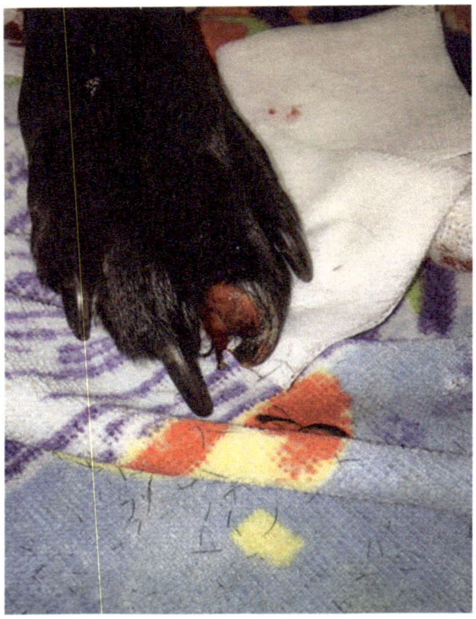

Figure 19.39A A malignant melanoma on the claw bed of a Labrador. *Source:* Image courtesy of VIN and Mark Terry, DVM.

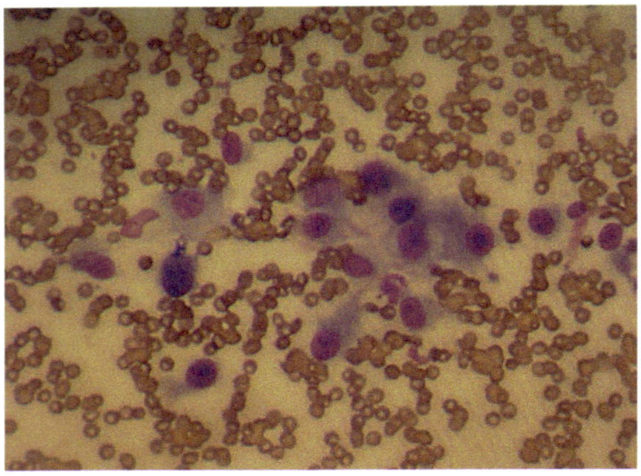

Figure 19.39B Fine needle aspirate for cytology revealed poorly differentiated melanocytes. 100x. *Source:* Image courtesy of VIN and Mark Terry, DVM.

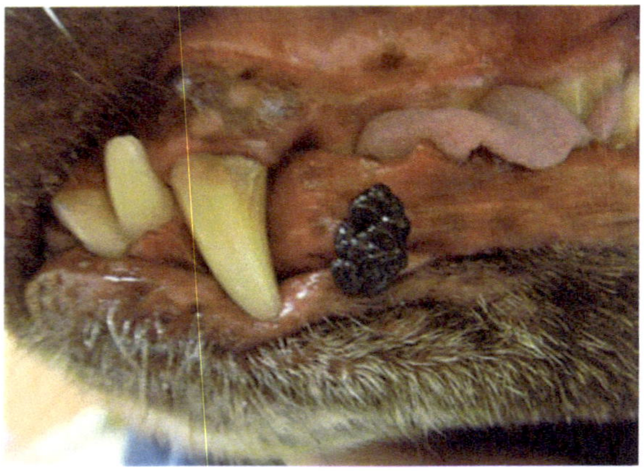

Figure 19.39C A malignant melanoma on the lip of a dog. *Source:* Image courtesy of VIN and Michael Goldmann, DVM.

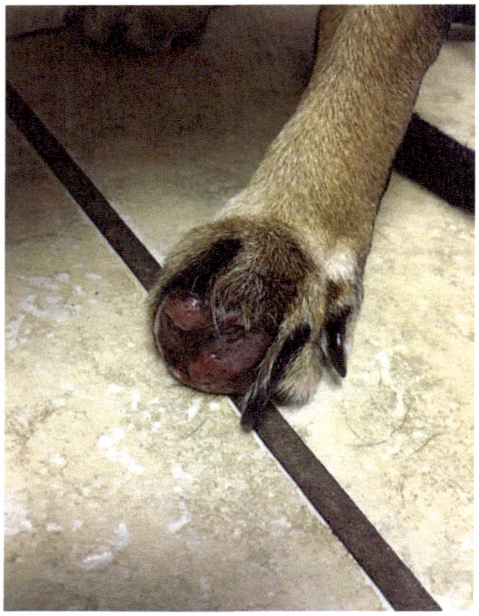

Figure 19.39D A large, malignant melanoma on the toe of a dog. *Source:* Image courtesy of VIN and Jennie Yarborough, DVM.

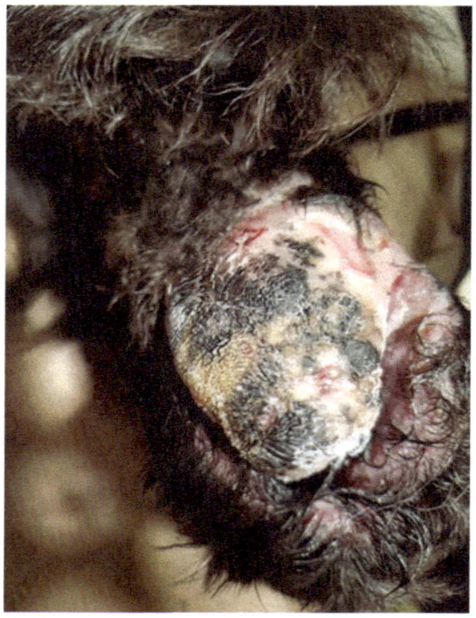

Figure 19.39E Amelanotic melanoma causing swelling, depigmentation, and erosion on the metacarpal pad of a dog. *Source:* Image courtesy of Dr. Amy Shumaker, DACVD.

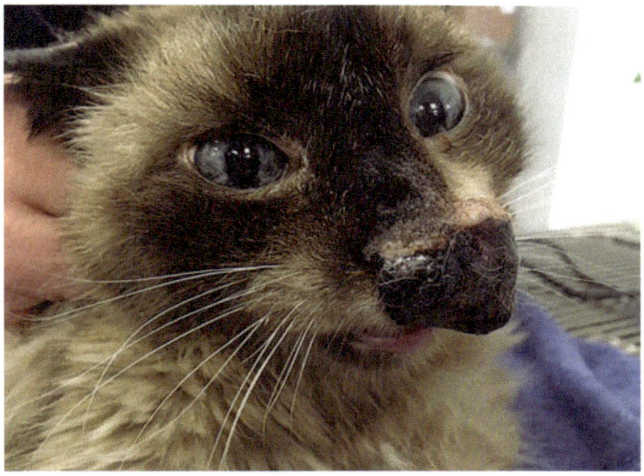

Figure 19.40A A large, malignant melanoma on the nasal planum of a cat. *Source:* Image courtesy of VIN and Adam Boardman, DVM.

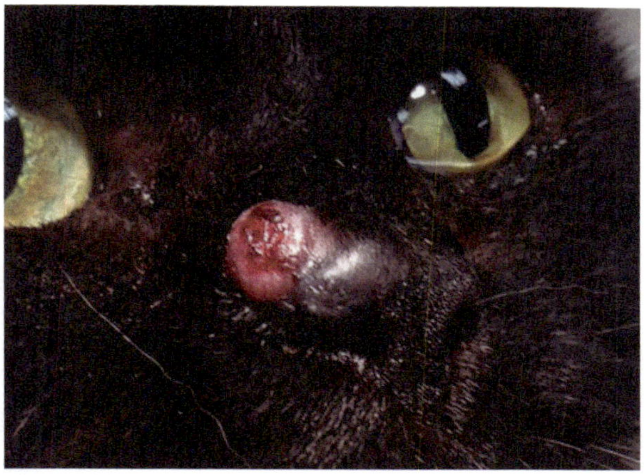

Figure 19.40B A raised, eroded mass on the nose of a cat caused by malignant melanoma. *Source:* Image courtesy of VIN and Karen Fischer, DVM.

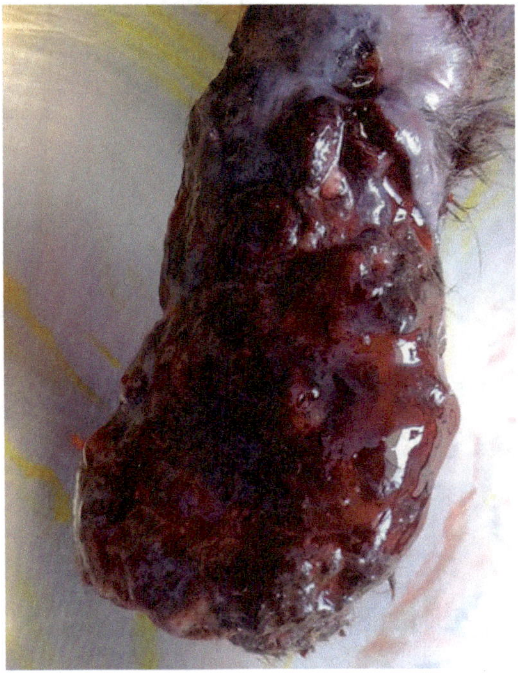

Figure 19.40C A malignant melanoma encompassing the paw of a cat. *Source:* Image courtesy of VIN and Paul Arora, DVM.

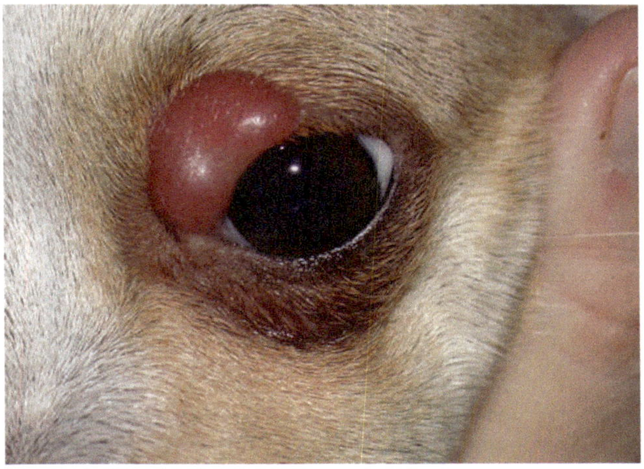

Figure 19.41A A large, red, raised mass on the eyelid of a young Chihuahua which was a histiocytoma.

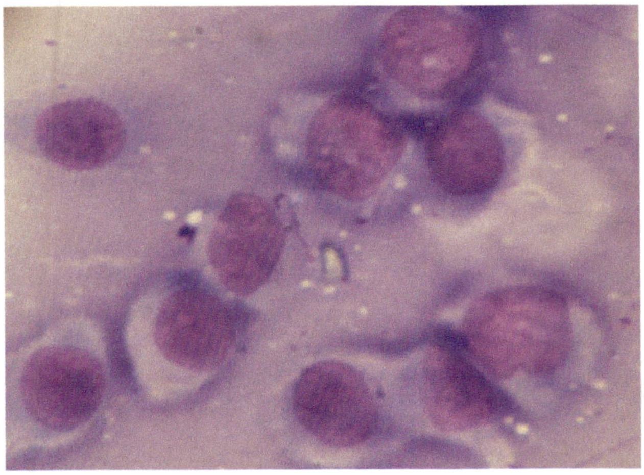

Figure 19.41B Aspirate for cytology demonstrating typical histiocytic round cells with abundant light blue, slightly granular, and slightly vesiculated cytoplasm and large, open, sometimes indented nuclei. 100x with digital zoom.

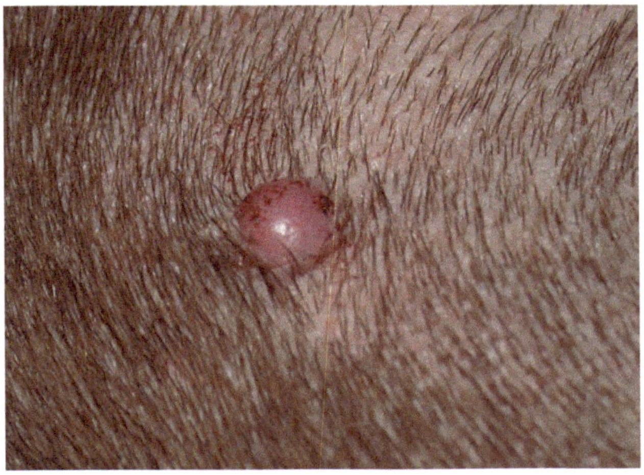

Figure 19.41C A pink, raised mass or "button" tumor typical for a histiocytoma.

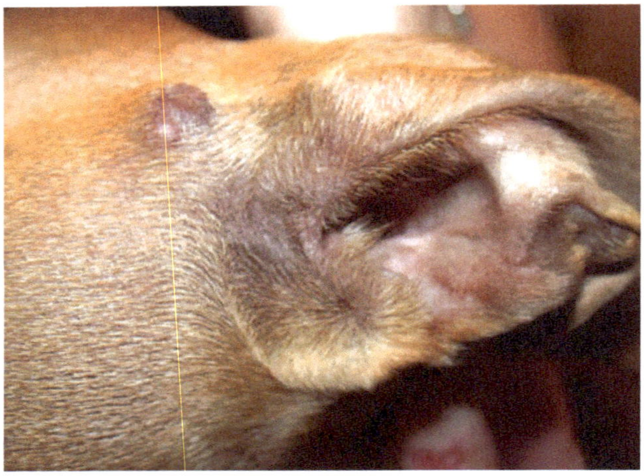

Figure 19.42A A raised mass on the ear of a dog with cutaneous reactive histiocytosis.

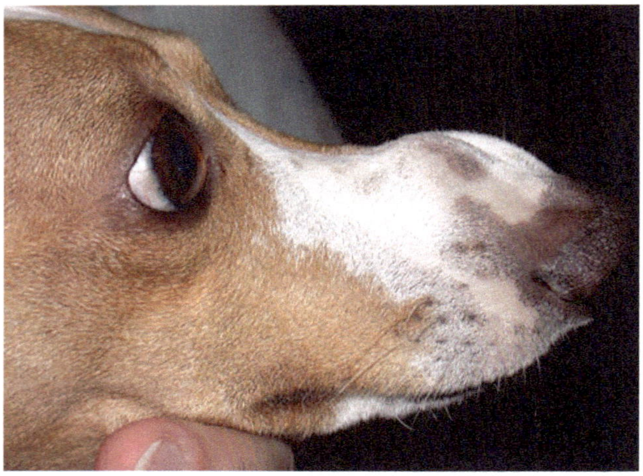

Figure 19.42B The same dog had a large nasal swelling caused by histiocytosis.

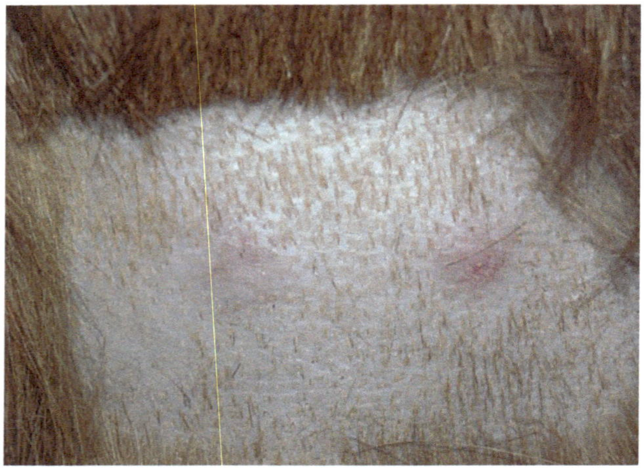

Figure 19.42C A Golden Retriever with cutaneous reactive histiocytosis; numerous, slightly pink, dermal masses were present all over the trunk.

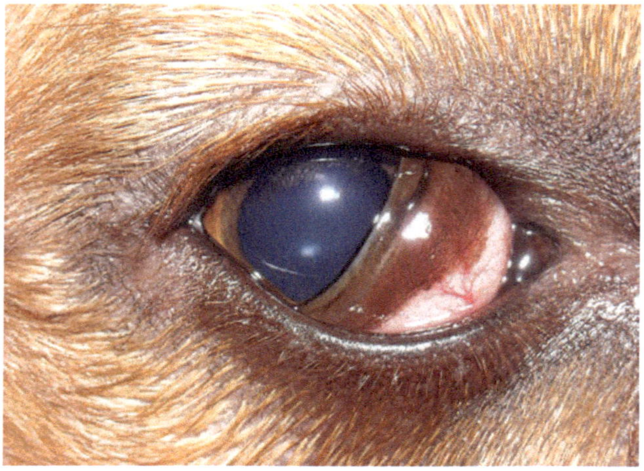

Figure 19.42D The same dog as in 19.42C; the third eyelid conjunctiva was involved.

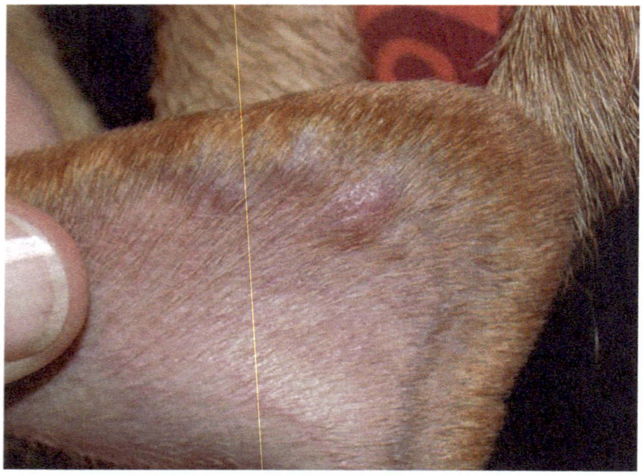

Figure 19.42E Raised, pink, dermal masses on the pinna caused by histiocytosis.

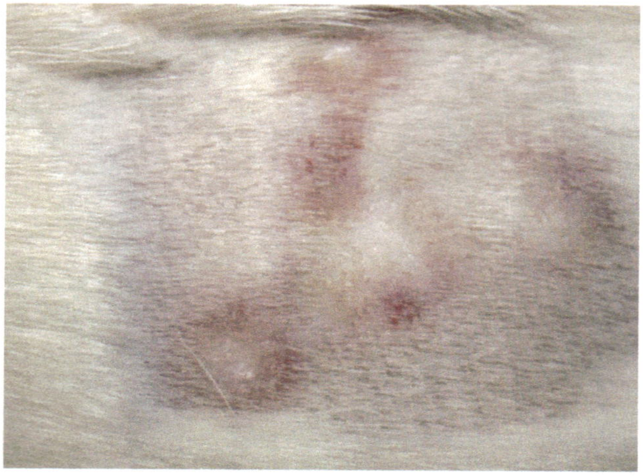

Figure 19.42F Irregular, erythematous plaques on the trunk of a Labrador with reactive histiocytosis.

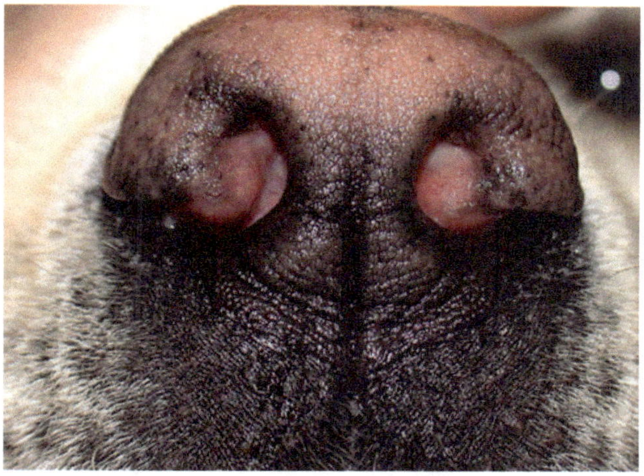

Figure 19.42G The same dog as in 19.42F; swelling involved the inner nares, causing strained stertorous breathing.

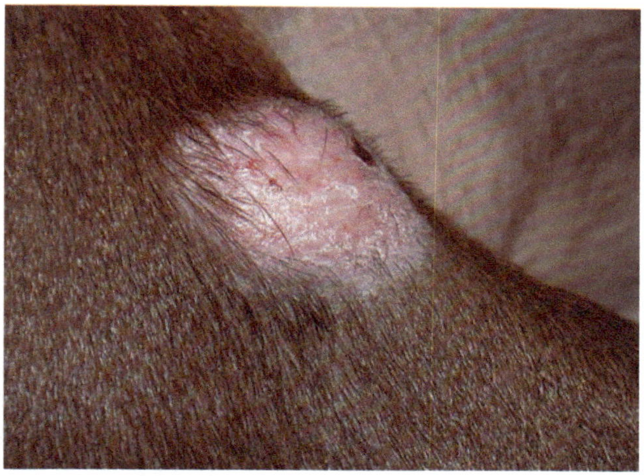

Figure 19.42H A pink, raised mass on the limb of a dog with cutaneous histiocytosis.

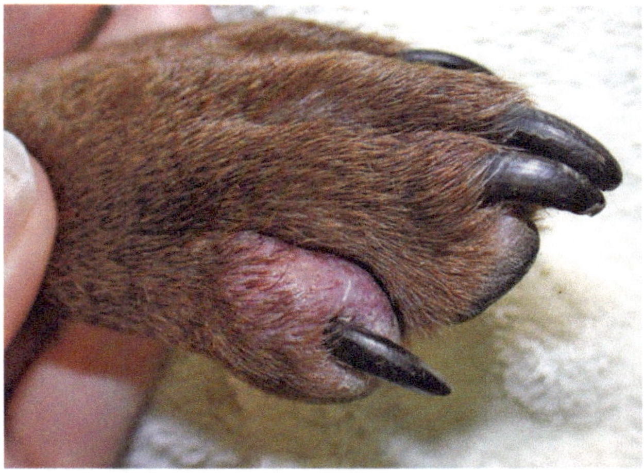

Figure 19.42I The same dog showing involvement of the toe.

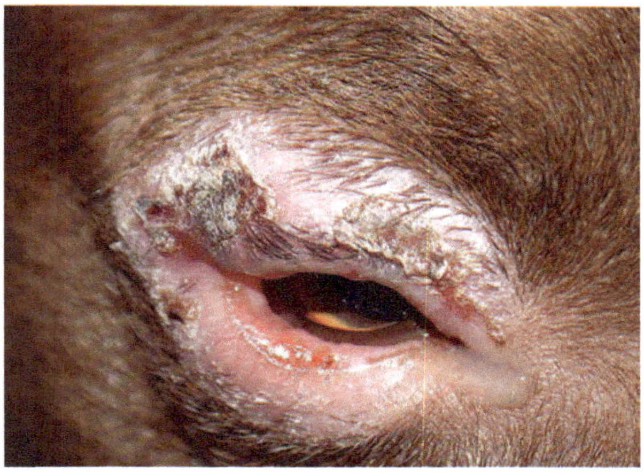

Figure 19.42J This dog also had severe eyelid swelling caused by histiocytosis.

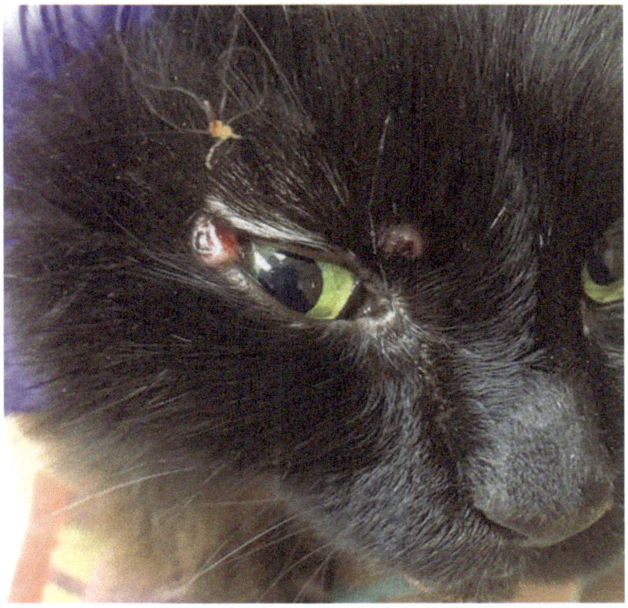

Figure 19.43A Ulcerated, crusted, pink masses on the face of a cat due to feline progressive histiocytosis. *Source:* Image courtesy of Dr. Megan Solc.

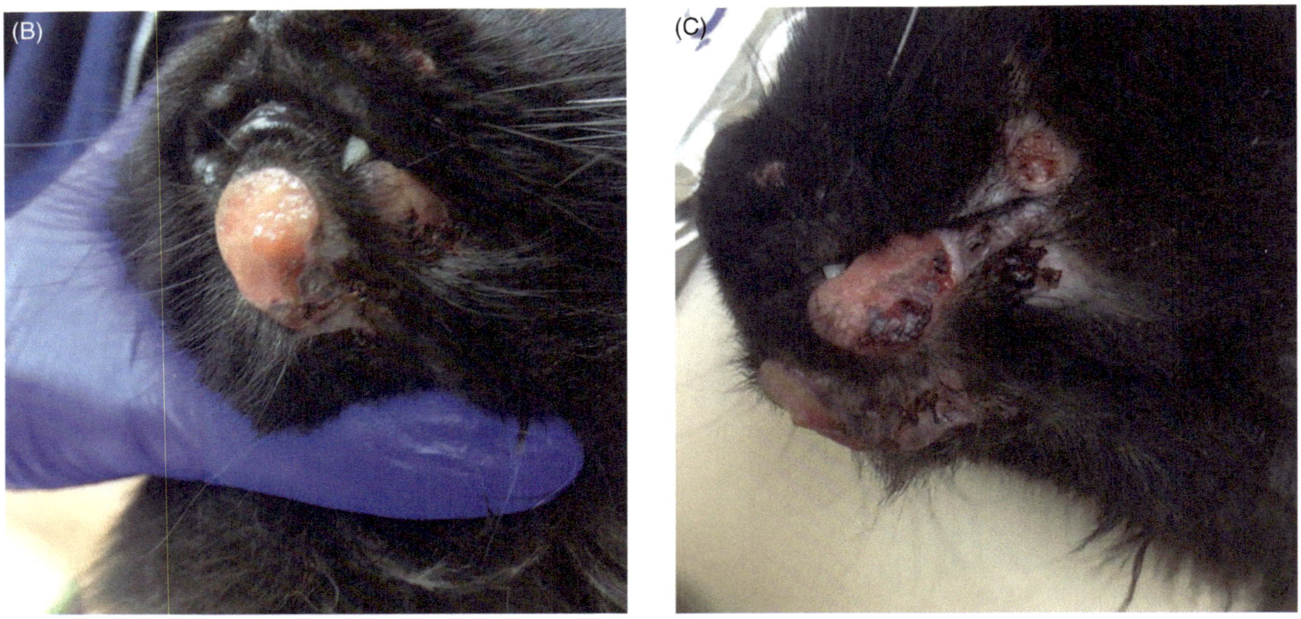

Figures 19.43B and C The same cat as in 19.43A; large, erosive masses were also present on the chin and lips. *Source:* Image courtesy of Dr. Megan Solc.

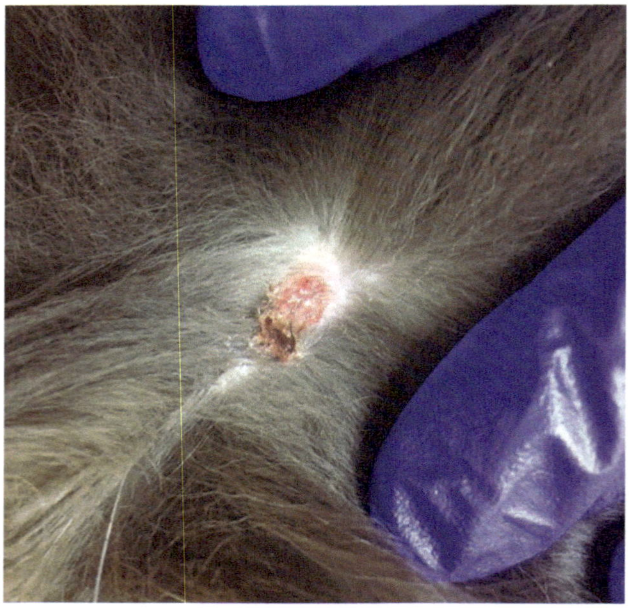

Figure 19.43D Smaller masses were present on the trunk as well. *Source:* Image courtesy of Dr. Megan Solc.

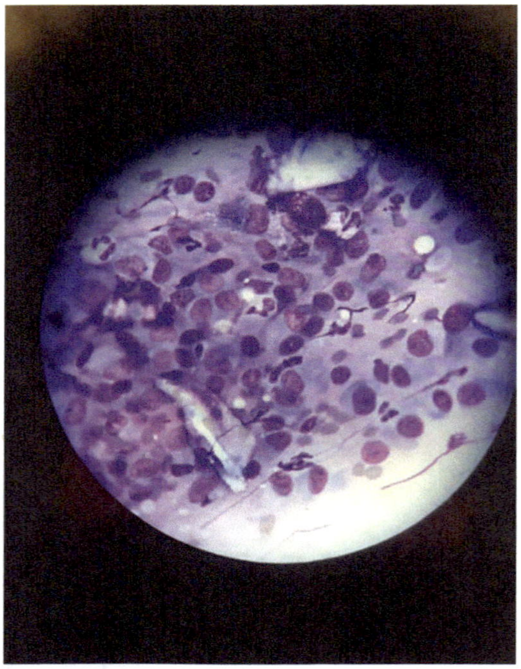

Figure 19.43E Cytology revealed atypical histiocytic cells. 100x. *Source:* Image courtesy of Dr. Megan Solc.

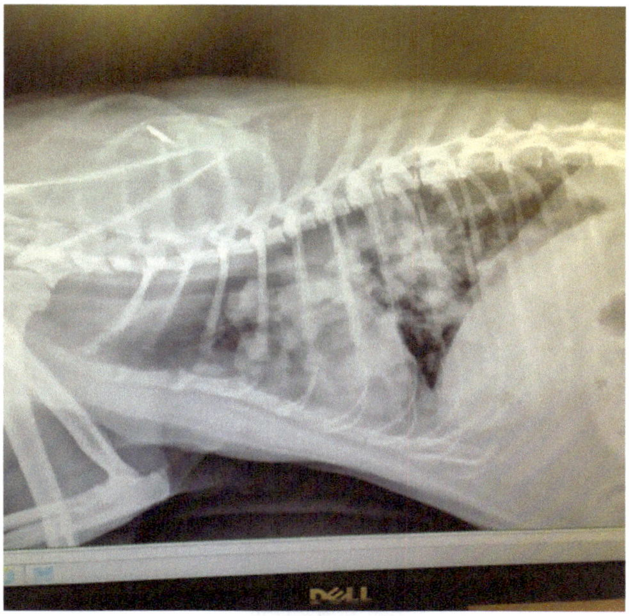

Figure 19.43F Thoracic radiographs revealed extensive lung involvement. *Source:* Photo courtesy of Dr. Megan Solc.

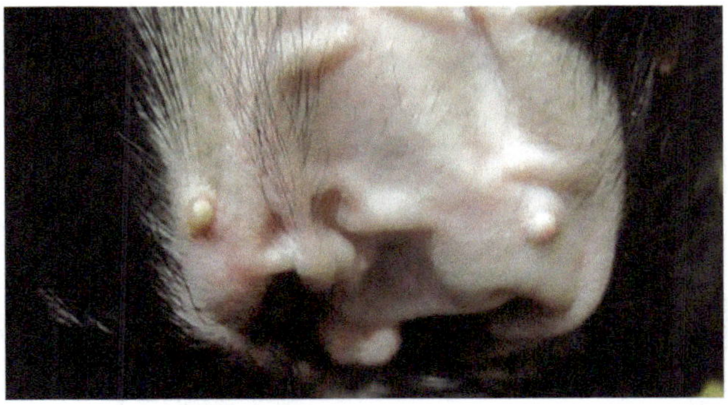

Figure 19.44A Raised, white, firm, pinnal masses on a puppy due to calcinosis circumscripta. *Source:* Image courtesy of VIN and Shawn Seibel, DVM.

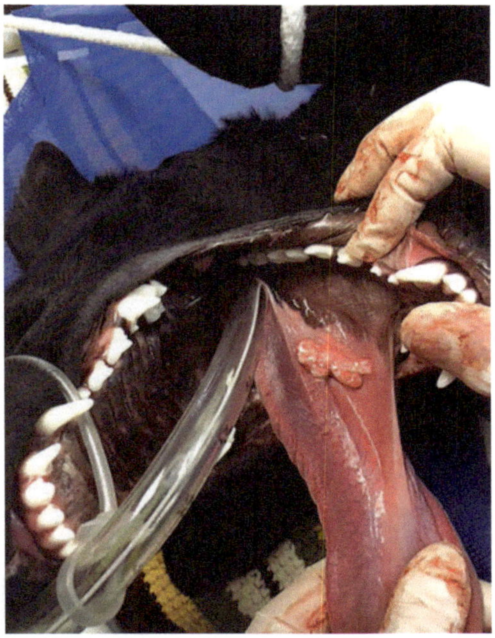

Figure 19.44B Calcinosis circumscripta on the ventral tongue. *Source:* Image courtesy of VIN and Peter Jennings, DVM.

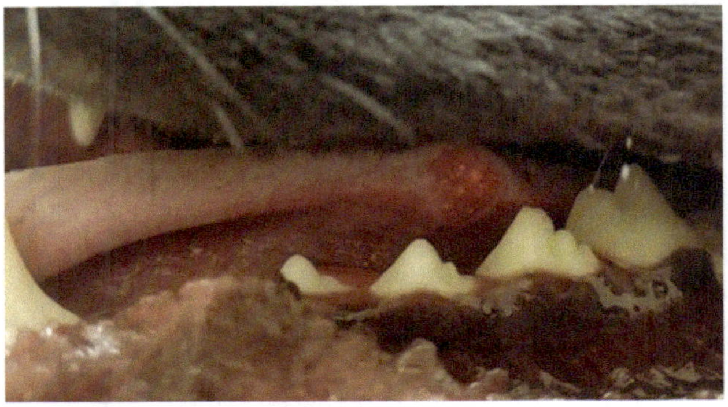

Figure 19.44C A raised, gritty mass caused by calcinosis circumscripta on the tongue of a young dog. *Source:* Image courtesy of VIN and Brett Bower, DVM.

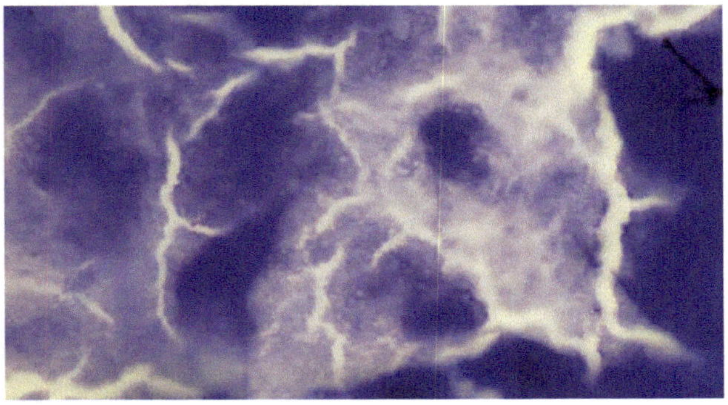

Figure 19.44D Fine needle aspirate for cytology of calcinosis circumscripta shows amorphous, basophilic, crystalline material. 10x. *Source:* Image courtesy of VIN and Shawn Seibel, DVM.

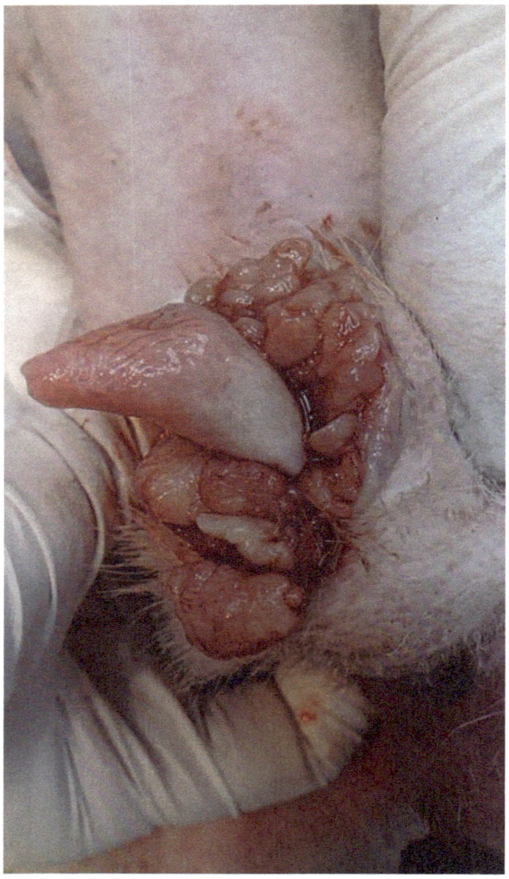

Figure 19.45A Transmissible venereal tumor in the prepuce of a dog. *Source:* Image courtesy of VIN and Wen Yu Theng, DVM.

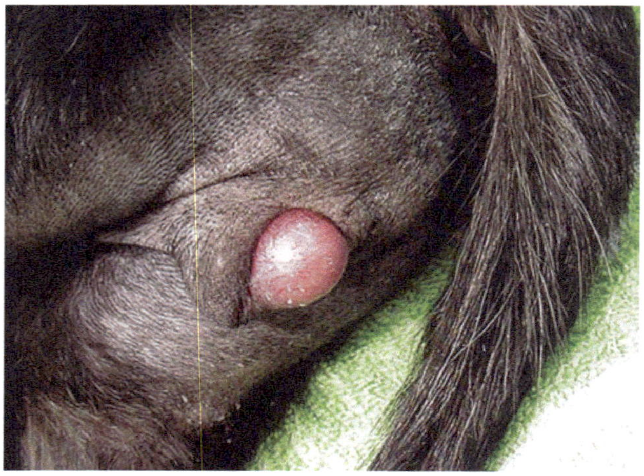

Figure 19.45B A smooth, pink, vaginal mass caused by a transmissible venereal tumor. *Source:* Image courtesy of VIN and Joshua Winston, DVM.

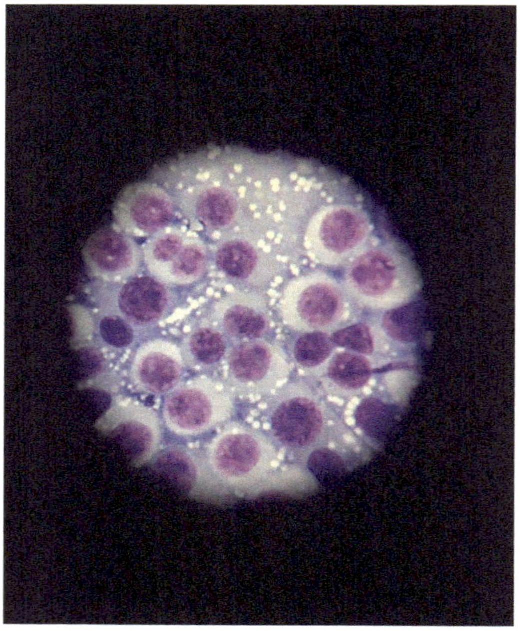

Figure 19.45C Cytology of a transmissible venereal tumor demonstrating round cells, occasional bi-nucleate cells and basophilic background. 100x. *Source:* Image courtesy of VIN and Mariah Coakley, DVM.

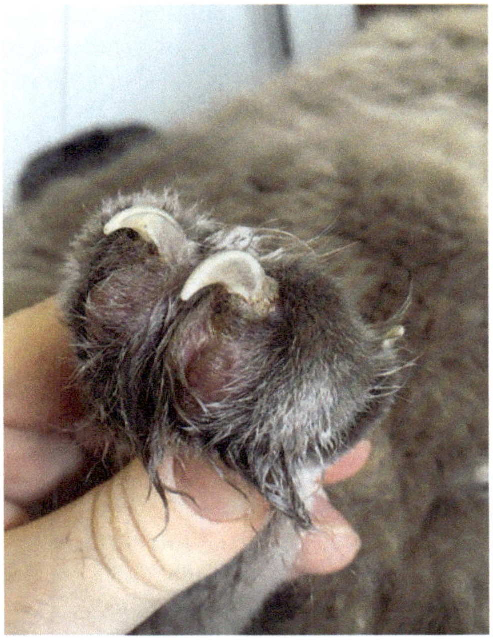

Figure 19.46A A cat with feline lung digit syndrome demonstrating swelling and crusting on multiple nailbeds. *Source:* Image courtesy of VIN and Shannon Donovan, DVM.

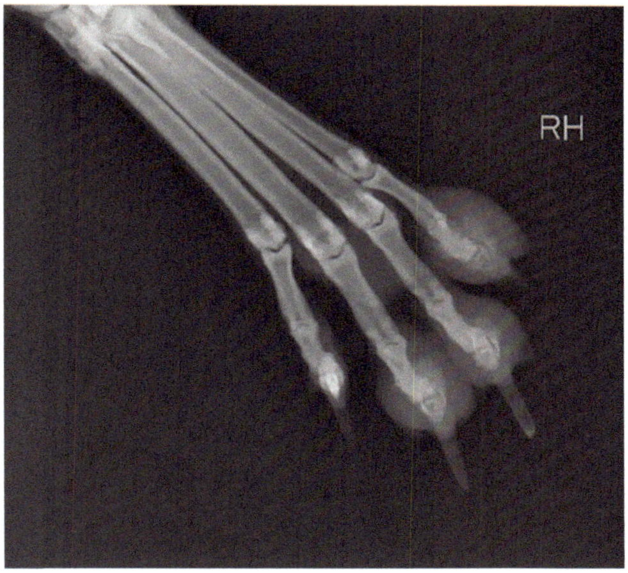

Figure 19.46B Radiograph of the cat's paw shows soft tissue swelling and bony reaction to the neoplasia. *Source:* Image courtesy of VIN and Shannon Donovan, DVM.

References and further reading

Abramo, F., Pratesi, F., Cantile, C. et al. (1999). Survey of canine and feline follicular tumours and tumour-like lesions in central Italy. *J. Small Anim. Pract.* 40: 479–481.

Adedeji, A., Affolter, V., and Christopher, M. (2017). Cytologic features of cutaneous follicular tumors and cysts in dogs. *Vet. Clin. Pathol.* 46 (1): 143–150.

Affolter, V. and Moore, P. (2006). Feline progressive histiocytosis. *Vet. Pathol.* 43: 646–655.

Baer, K., Patnaik, A., Gilbertson, S., and Hurvitz, A. (1989). Cutaneous plasmacytomas in dogs: a morphologic and immunohistochemical study. *Veterinary Pathology* 26: 216–221.

Baez, J., Hendrick, M., Shofer, F. et al. (2004). Liposarcomas in dogs: 56 cases (1989–2000). *Journal of the American Veterinary Medical Association* 224 (6): 887–891.

Belluco, S., Brisebard, E., Watrelot, D. et al. (2013). Digital squamous cell carcinoma in dogs: epidemiological, histological, and immunohistochemical study. *Veterinary Pathology* 50 (6): 1078–1082.

Bennet, P., DeNicola, D., Bonney, P. et al. (2002). Canine anal sac adenocarcinomas: clinical presentation and response to therapy. *Journal of Veterinary Internal Medicine* 16: 100–104.

Biller, B., Berg, J., Garret, L. et al. (2016). 2016 AAHA oncology guidelines for dogs and cats. *Journal of the American Animal Hospital Association* 52: 181–204.

Brockley, L., Cooper, M., and Bennett, P. (2013). Malignant melanoma in 63 dogs (2001–2011): the effect of carboplatin chemotherapy on survival. *New Zealand Veterinary Journal* 61 (1): 25–31.

Campos, A., Cogliati, B., Guerra, J., and Matera, J. (2014). Multiple trichoblastomas in a dog. *Veterinary Dermatology* 25: 48–e19.

Chamel, G., Abadie, J., Albaric, O. et al. (2017). Non-ocular melanomas in cats: a retrospective study of 30 cases. *Journal of Feline Medicine and Surgery* 19 (4): 351–357.

Chan, C., Frimberger, A., and Moore, A. (2018). Clinical outcome and prognosis of dogs with histopathological features consistent with epitheliotropic lymphoma: a retrospective study of 148 cases (2003–2015). *Veterinary Dermatology* 29: 154–e59.

Corriveau, L. (2012). Use of a carbon dioxide laser to treat ceruminous gland hyperplasia in a cat. *Journal of Feline Medicine and Surgery* 14 (6): 413–416.

Curran, K., Halsey, C., and Worley, D. (2014). Lymphangiosarcoma in 12 dogs: a case series (1998–2013). *Veterinary and Comparative Oncology* 14 (2): 181–190.

Duclos, D. (2016). Lasers in veterinary dermatology. *Veterinary Clinics of North America: Small Animal Practice* 36: 15–37.

Duclos, D., Hargis, A., and Hanley, P. (2008). Pathogenesis of canine interdigital palmar and plantar comedones and follicular cysts, and their response to laser surgery. *Veterinary Dermatology* 19: 134–141.

Falk, E., Lange, C., Jennings, S., and Ferrer, L. (2017). Two cutaneous horns associated with canine papillomavirus type 1 infection in a pit bull dog. *Veterinary Dermatology* 28: 420–421.

Fontaine, J., Heimann, M., and Day, M. (2010). Canine cutaneous epitheliotropic T-cell lymphoma: a review of 30 cases. *Veterinary Dermatology* 21: 267–275.

Fontaine, J., Heimann, M., and Day, M. (2011). Cutaneous epitheliotropic T-cell lymphoma in the cat: a review of literature and five new cases. *Veterinary Dermatology* 22: 454–461.

Fuentealba, I., Illanes, O., and Haines, D. (2000). Eccrine adenocarcinoma of the footpads in 2 cats. *Canadian Veterinary Journal* 41: 401–403.

Ganguly, B., Das, U., and Das, A. (2013). Canine transmissible venereal tumour: a review. *Veterinary and Comparative Oncology* 14 (1): 1–12.

Gimenez, F., Hecht, S., Craig, L., and Legendre, A. (2010). Early detection, aggressive therapy optimizing the management of feline mammary masses. *Journal of Feline Medicine and Surgery* 12: 214–224.

Goldfinch, N. and Argyle, D. (2012). Feline lung-digit syndrome: unusual metastatic patterns of primary lung tumours in cats. *Journal of Feline Medicine and Surgery* 14: 202–208.

Goldschmidt, M. and Goldschmidt, K. (2017). Squamous cell carcinoma. In: *Tumors in Domestic Animals* (ed. D. Meuten). Ames: Wiley.

Goldschmidt, M., Pena, L., Rasotto, R., and Zappulli, V. (2011). Classification and grading of canine mammary tumors. *Veterinary Pathology* 48 (1): 117–131.

Gottfried, S., Popovitch, C., Goldschmidt, M., and Schelling, C. (2000). Metastatic digital carcinoma in the cat: a retrospective study of 36 cats (1992-1998). *Journal of the American Animal Hospital Association* 36: 501–509.

Graves, G., Bjorling, D., and Mahaffey, E. (1988). Canine hemangiopericytoma: 23 cases (1967–1984). *Journal of the American Veterinary Medical Association* 192 (1): 99–102.

Gross, T., Ihrke, P., Walder, E., and Affolter, V. (2005a). Basal cell carcinoma. In: *Skin Diseases of the Dog and Cat. Clinical and Histopathological Diagnosis*, 2e. Oxford: Blackwell Science.

Gross, T., Ihrke, P., Walder, E., and Affolter, V. (2005b). Sebaceous tumors. In: *Skin Diseases of the Dog and Cat. Clinical and Histopathological Diagnosis*, 2e. Oxford: Blackwell Science.

Gross, T., Ihrke, P., Walder, E., and Affolter, V. (2005c). Follicular tumors. In: *Skin Diseases of the Dog and Cat. Clinical and Histopathological Diagnosis*, 2e. Oxford: Blackwell Science.

Gross, T., Ihrke, P., Walder, E., and Affolter, V. (2005d). Cutaneous horn of the feline pawpad. In: *Skin Diseases of the Dog and Cat. Clinical and Histopathological Diagnosis*, 2e. Oxford: Blackwell Science.

Gross, T., Ihrke, P., Walder, E., and Affolter, V. (2005e). Sweat gland tumors. In: *Skin Diseases of the Dog and Cat. Clinical and Histopathological Diagnosis*, 2e. Oxford: Blackwell Science.

Gross, T., Ihrke, P., Walder, E., and Affolter, V. (2005f). Nodular perianal gland hyperplasia and perianal gland adenoma. In: *Skin Diseases of the Dog and Cat. Clinical and Histopathological Diagnosis*, 2e. Oxford: Blackwell Science.

Gross, T., Ihrke, P., Walder, E., and Affolter, V. (2005g). Lipocytic tumors. In: *Skin Diseases of the Dog and Cat. Clinical and Histopathological Diagnosis.* Oxford: Blackwell Science.

Gross, T., Ihrke, P., Walder, E., and Affolter, V. (2005h). Mast cell tumors. In: *Skin Diseases of the Dog and Cat. Clinical and Histopathological Diagnosis*, 2e. Oxford: Blackwell Science.

Gross, T., Ihrke, P., Walder, E., and Affolter, V. (2005i). Fibrous tumors. In: *Skin Diseases of the Dog and Cat. Clinical and Histopathological Diagnosis*, 2e. Oxford: Blackwell Science.

Gross, T., Ihrke, P., Walder, E., and Affolter, V. (2005j). Vascular tumors. In: *Skin Diseases of the Dog and Cat. Clinical and Histopathological Diagnosis*, 2e. Oxford: Blackwell Science.

Gross, T., Ihrke, P., Walder, E., and Affolter, V. (2005k). Perivascular tumors. In: *Skin Diseases of the Dog and Cat. Clinical and Histopathological Diagnosis*, 2e. Oxford: Blackwell Science.

Gross, T., Ihrke, P., Walder, E., and Affolter, V. (2005l). Lymphocytic tumors. In: *Skin Diseases of the Dog and Cat. Clinical and Histopathological Diagnosis*, 2e. Oxford: Blackwell Science.

Gross, T., Ihrke, P., Walder, E., and Affolter, V. (2005m). Melanocytoma. In: *Skin Diseases of the Dog and Cat. Clinical and Histopathological Diagnosis*, 2e. Oxford: Blackwell Science.

Gross, T., Ihrke, P., Walder, E., and Affolter, V. (2005n). Melanoma. In: *Skin Diseases of the Dog and Cat. Clinical and Histopathological Diagnosis*, 2e. Oxford: Blackwell Science.

Gross, T., Ihrke, P., Walder, E., and Affolter, V. (2005o). Canine cutaneous histiocytoma. In: *Skin Diseases of the Dog and Cat. Clinical and Histopathological Diagnosis*, 2e. Oxford: Blackwell Science.

Gross, T., Ihrke, P., Walder, E., and Affolter, V. (2005p). Reactive histiocytosis. In: *Skin Diseases of the Dog and Cat. Clinical and Histopathological Diagnosis*, 2e. Oxford: Blackwell Science.

Gross, T., Ihrke, P., Walder, E., and Affolter, V. (2005q). Calcinosis circumscripta. In: *Skin Diseases of the Dog and Cat. Clinical and Histopathological Diagnosis*, 2e. Oxford: Blackwell Science.

Hammer, A., Couto, C., Filppi, J. et al. (1991). Efficacy and toxicity of VAC chemotherapy (vincristine, doxorubicin, cyclophosphamide) in dogs with hemangiosarcoma. *Journal of Veterinary Internal Medicine* 5: 160–166.

Hargis, A., Ihrke, P., Spangler, W., and Stannard, A. (1992). A retrospective clinicopathologic study of 212 dogs with cutaneous hemangiomas and hemangiosarcomas. *Veterinary Pathology* 29: 316–328.

Hendrick, M. (2002). Fibrosarcoma. In: *Tumors in Domestic Animals,* 5e (ed. D. Meuten). Ames: Wiley.

Hendrick, M. (2017a). Canine hemangiopericytoma. In: *Tumors in Domestic Animals,* 5e (ed. D. Meuten). Ames: Wiley.

Hendrick, M. (2017b). Lymphangioma and lymphangiosarcoma. In: *Tumors in Domestic Animals,* 5e (ed. D. Meuten). Ames: Wiley.

Henry, C. and Herrera, C. (2013). Mast cell tumors in cats: clinical update and possible new treatment avenues. *Journal of Feline Medicine and Surgery* 15: 41–47.

Hinrichs, U., Puhl, S., Rutteman, G. et al. (1999). Lymphangiosarcomas in cats: a retrospective study of 12 cases. *Veterinary Pathology* 36: 164–167.

Hunt, G., Wong, J., and Kuan, S. (2011). Liposuction for removal of lipomas in 20 dogs. *Journal of Small Animal Practice* 52: 419–425.

Iwamoto, K., Bennett, L., Norman, A. et al. (1992). Linoleate produces remission in canine mycosis fungoides. *Cancer Letters* 64 (1): 17–22.

Javanbakht, J., Tavassoli, A., Sasani, F. et al. (2013). An overall assessment of circumanal gland adenoma in a terrier mix breed dog. *Asian Pacific Journal of Tropical Biomedicine* 3 (7): 580–583.

Jegatheeson, S., Wayne, J., and Brockley, L. (2018). Cutaneous non-epitheliotropic T-cell lymphoma associated with a fracture site in a cat. *Journal of Feline Medicine and Surgery Open Reports* 4 (1): 1–6.

Komori, S., Nakamura, S., Takahashi, K., and Takagawa, M. (2005). Use of lomustine to treat cutaneous nonepitheliotropic lymphoma in a cat. *Journal of the American Veterinary Medical Association* 226 (2): 237–239.

Kusters, A., Peperkamp, K., and Hazewinkel, H. (1999). Atrichial sweat gland adenocarcinoma in the dog. *Veterinary Dermatology* 10: 51–54.

Luther, P., Scott, D., and Buerger, R. (1989). The dilated pore of winer – an overlooked cutaneous lesion of cats. *Journal of Comparative Pathology* 101: 375–379.

de M Souza, C., Toledo-Piza, E., Amorin, R. et al. (2009). Inflammatory mammary carcinoma in 12 dogs: clinical features, cyclooxygenase-2 expression, and response to piroxicam treatment. *Canadian Veterinary Journal* 50: 506–510.

Marcinowska, A., Warland, J., Brearly, M., and Dobson, J. (2013). A novel approach to treatment of lymphangiosarcoma in a boxer dog. *Journal of Small Animal Practice* 54: 334–337.

Marconato, L., Romanelli, G., Stefanello, D., and Giacoboni, C. (2009). Prognostic factors for dogs with mammary inflammatory carcinoma: 43 cases (2003–2008). *Journal of the American Veterinary Medical Association* 235: 967–972.

Mikiewicz, M., Otrocka-Domagala, I., Pazdzior-Czapula, K., and Gesek, M. (2016). Morphology and immunoreactivity of canine and feline extramedullary plasmacytomas. *Polish Journal of Veterinary Sciences* 19 (2): 345–352.

Miller, M., Nelson, S., Turk, J. et al. (1991). Cutaneous neoplasia in 340 cats. *Veterinary Pathology* 28: 389–395.

Miller, M., Ramos, J., and Kreeger, J. (1992). Cutaneous vascular neoplasia in 15 cats: clinical, morphologic, and immunohistochemical studies. *Veterinary Pathology* 29: 329–336.

Mills, S., Musil, K., Davies, J., and Hendrick, S. (2015). Prognostic value of histologic grading for feline mammary carcinoma: a retrospective survival analysis. *Veterinary Pathology* 52 (2): 238–249.

Moe, L. and Lium, B. (1997). Hereditary multifocal renal cystadeno-carcinomas and nodular dermatofibromas in 51 German shepherd dogs. *Journal of Small Animal Practice* 38: 498–505.

Moore, P. (2014). A review of histocytic diseases of dogs and cats. *Veterinary Pathology* 51 (1): 167–184.

Moriello, K. and Diesel, A. (2014). Question 224. In: *Small Animal Dermatology, Volume 2: Advanced Cases: Self-Assessment Color Review.* Boca Raton: CRC Press.

Munday, J., Gibson, I., and French, A. (2011). Papillomaviral DNA and increased p16 CDKN2A protein are frequently present within feline cutaneous squamous cell carcinoma in ultraviolet-protected skin. *Veterinary Dermatology* 22: 360–366.

Munday, J., Kiupel, M., French, A. et al. (2007). Detection of papillomaviral sequences in feline bowenoid in situ carcinoma using consensus primers. *Veterinary Dermatology* 18: 241–245.

Murphy, S. (2013). Cutaneous squamous cell carcinoma in the cat: current understanding and treatment approaches. *Journal of Feline Medicine and Surgery* 15: 401–407.

Palmeiro, B., Morris, D., Goldschmidt, M., and Mauldin, E. (2007). Cutaneous reactive histiocytosis in dogs: a retrospective evaluation of 32 cases. *Veterinary Dermatology* 18: 332–340.

Pariser, M. and Gram, D. (2014). Feline cutaneous lymphocytosis: case report and summary of the literature. *Journal of Feline Medicine and Surgery* 16: 758–763.

Peavy, G., Walder, E., Nelson, J., and Rosenberg, M. (2001). Use of laser photocoagulation for treatment of cutaneous angiomatosis in one dog and two cats. *Journal of the American Veterinary Medical Association* 219 (8): 1094–1097.

Porcellato, I., Menchetti, L., Brachelente, C., and Sforna, M. (2017). Feline injection-site sarcoma: matrix remodeling and prognosis. *Veterinary Pathology* 54 (2): 204–211.

Potanas, C., Padgett, S., and Gamblin, R. (2015). Surgical excision of anal sac apocrine gland adenocarcinomas with and without adjunctive chemotherapy in dogs: 42 cases (2005–2011). *Journal of the American Veterinary Medical Association* 246: 877–884.

Rees, C. and Goldschmidt, M. (1998). Cutaneous horn and squamous cell carcinoma in situ (Bowen's disease) in a cat. *Journal of the American Animal Hospital Association* 34: 485–486.

Santoro, D., Kubicek, L., Lu, B. et al. (2017). Total skin electron therapy as treatment for epitheliotropic lymphoma in a dog. *Veterinary Dermatology* 28: 246–e65.

Sarbu, L., Kitchell, B., and Bergman, P. (2017). Safety of administering the canine melanoma DNA vaccine (Oncept) to cats with malignant melanoma – a retrospective study. *Journal of Feline Medicine and Surgery* 19 (2): 224–230.

Scott, D. and Anderson, W. (1991). Canine hair follicle neoplasms: a retrospective analysis of 80 cases (1986–1987). *Veterinary Dermatology* 2: 143–150.

Scott, D., Miller, W., and Griffin, C. (2013). Neoplastic and non-neoplastic tumors. In: *Muller and Kirks Small Animal Dermatology*, 7e, 774–843. St. Louis: Elsevier.

Sorenmo, K., Rasotto, R., Zappulli, V., and Goldschmidt, M. (2011). Development, anatomy, histology, lymphatic drainage, clinical features, and cell differentiation markers of canine mammary gland neoplasms. *Veterinary Pathology* 48 (1): 85–97.

Strakova, A. and Murchison, E. (2014). The changing global distribution and prevalence of canine transmissible venereal tumour. *BMC Veterinary Research* 10 (168): 1–10.

Tafti, A., Hanna, P., and Bourque, A. (2005). Calcinosis circumscripta in the dog: a retrospective pathological study. *Journal of Veterinary Medicine. A, Physiology, Pathology, Clinical Medicine* 52: 13–17.

Thomson, M. (2007). Squamous cell carcinoma of the nasal planum in cats and dogs. *Clinical Techniques in Small Animal Practice* 22: 42–45.

Thrift, E., Greenwell, C., Turner, A.L. et al. (2017). Metastatic pulmonary carcinomas in cats ('feline lung-digit syndrome'): further variations on a theme. *Journal of Feline Medicine and Surgery Open Reports* 3 (1): 1–8.

Toma, S. and Noli, C. (2005). Isotretinoin in the treatment of multiple benign pilomatrixomas in a mixed-breed dog. *Veterinary Dermatology* 16: 346–350.

Ward, H., Fox, L., Calderwood-Mays, M. et al. (1994). Cutaneous hemangiosarcoma in 25 dogs: a retrospective study. *Journal of Veterinary Internal Medicine* 8 (5): 345–348.

White, S., Rosychuk, R., Scott, K. et al. (1993). Use of isotretinoin and etretinate for the treatment of benign cutaneous neoplasia and cutaneous lymphoma in dogs. *Journal of the American Veterinary Medical Association* 202 (3): 387–391.

Wilhelm, S., Degorce-Rubiales, F., Godson, D., and Favrot, C. (2016). Clinical, histological and immunohistochemical study of feline viral plaques and bowenoid in situ carcinomas. *Veterinary Dermatology* 17: 424–431.

Yager, J., Best, S., Maggi, R. et al. (2010). Bacillary angiomatosis in an immunosuppressed dog. *Veterinary Dermatology* 21: 420–428.

Yang, S., Liu, C., Hsu, C. et al. (2007). Use of chemical ablation with trichloroacetic acid to treat eyelid apocrine hidrocystomas in a cat. *Journal of the American Veterinary Medical Association* 230 (8): 1170–1173.

Zabielska-Koczywas, K., Wojtalewicz, A., and Lechowski, R. (2017). Current knowledge on feline injection-site sarcoma treatment. *Acta Veterinaria Scandinavica* 59 (47): 2–7.

Zappulli, V., Rasotto, R., Caliari, D. et al. (2015). Prognostic evaluation of feline mammary carcinomas: a review of the literature. *Veterinary Pathology* 52 (1): 46–60.

20

Dermatology formulary

Anthea Schick, DVM, DACVD[1,2]

[1] *Dermatology for Animals, Gilbert, AZ, USA*
[2] *Dermatology for Animals, Scottsdale, AZ, USA*

Disclaimer

Due to continual changes and new developments in medical knowledge and medication doses/recommendations, readers are recommended to consult current drug books/literature and manufacturer recommendations prior to prescribing therapy.

Clinical Atlas of Canine and Feline Dermatology, First Edition. Edited by Kimberly S. Coyner.

Companion website: www.wiley.com/go/coyner/dermatology

Table 20.1 Systemic antibiotics.

Drug	Indications	Dose	Side effects/Comments
Amoxicillin/Clavulanic Acid	Bacterial skin and soft tissue infections.	Dogs: 13.75 mg/kg PO q12h, or 20–25 mg/kg PO q12h. Cats: 62.5 mg per cat PO q12h or 10–20 mg/kg PO q12h.	Anorexia, vomiting, diarrhea.
Azithromycin	Bacterial skin and soft tissue infections, oral papillomatosis, cyclosporine-induced gingival overgrowth, *Mycobacteria* infections.	Dogs: 5–10 mg/kg PO q24h. Cats: 7–15 mg/kg PO q24h.	Anorexia, vomiting, diarrhea, abdominal pain.
Cefadroxil	Bacterial skin and soft tissue infections.	Dogs: 22–35 mg/kg PO q12h. Cats: 22–35 mg/kg PO q24h.	Anorexia, vomiting, diarrhea, lethargy.
Cefovecin sodium	Bacterial skin and soft tissue infections.	Dogs and cats: 8 mg/kg SC q14 days; per package insert do not exceed 2 injections.	Anorexia, vomiting, diarrhea, lethargy, mild injection site reactions.
Cefpodoxime proxetil	Bacterial skin and soft tissue infections.	Dogs and cats: 5–10 mg/kg PO q24h.	Anorexia, vomiting, diarrhea.
Cephalexin	Bacterial skin and soft tissue infections.	Dogs and cats: 22–30 mg/kg PO q12h.	Anorexia, vomiting, diarrhea.
Chloramphenicol	Bacterial skin and soft tissue infections.	Dogs: 40–60 mg/kg PO q8h. Cats: 20-30 mg/kg or 50 mg per cat PO q12h.	Anorexia, vomiting, diarrhea, depression, weakness, weight loss, neurotoxicity, rare myelosuppression Monitor: Baseline CBC then q 3–4 weeks.
Ciprofloxacin	Bacterial skin and soft tissue infections.	Dogs: Not recommended due to poor GI absorption; 25 mg/kg PO q24h. Cats: 20 mg/kg PO q24h.	Anorexia, vomiting, diarrhea, permanent cartilage damage in growing animals. NOT to be used growing animals.
Clarithromycin	Bacterial skin and soft tissue infections.	Dogs: 5–10 mg/kg PO q12h. Cats: 7.5 mg/kg PO q12h.	Anorexia, vomiting, diarrhea, generalized or pinnal erythema in cats and orange staining of the skin.

Clindamycin	Bacterial skin and soft tissue infections.	Dogs: 11 mg/kg PO q12h. Cats: 11–33 mg/kg PO q24h for skin disease.	Anorexia, vomiting, diarrhea, colitis (dogs), esophageal stricture (cats).
Clofazimine	Skin and soft tissue infections caused by *Mycobacteria*. Clofazimine is currently unavailable in the US except with individual patient FDA compassionate use approval.	Dogs: 4–12 mg/kg PO q24h. Cats: 25–50 mg per cat PO q24–48h or 8 mg/kg PO q24h.	Vomiting, diarrhea, skin, eye, and body fluid orange-brown discoloration, hepatic and renal abnormalities. Monitor: Baseline chemistry panel then q 4 weeks.
Difloxacin HCl	Bacterial skin and soft tissue infections.	Dogs: 5–10 mg/kg PO q24h. Unknown in cats.	Anorexia, vomiting, diarrhea, cartilage damage in young animals. NOT to be used in growing animals.
Doxycycline	Bacterial skin and soft tissue infections. Combined with niacinamide: Various sterile immune-mediated skin diseases.	Dogs and Cats: 5 mg/kg PO q12h or 10 mg/kg PO q24h.	Anorexia, vomiting, diarrhea, liver enzyme elevation (rare), esophageal stricture (cats). Follow dose with 15–30ml water. Bone and dental abnormalities are much less likely than with other tetracyclines, but use with caution in pregnant and juvenile animals. Compounded liquid doxycycline has been shown to contain effective amounts of drug for only one week.
Enrofloxacin	Bacterial skin and soft tissue infections.	Dogs: 5–20 mg/kg PO q24h (recommend at least 10 mg/kg for skin infections). Cats: 5 mg/kg PO q24h.	Anorexia, vomiting, diarrhea, elevated liver enzymes, permanent cartilage damage in growing animals, ocular toxicity (cats). NOT to be used growing animals.
Erythromycin	Bacterial skin and soft tissue infections.	Dogs and Cats: 10–20 mg/kg PO q8h or 15–25 mg/kg PO q12h.	Anorexia, vomiting.
Imipenem	Used as a last resort to treat serious gram-negative infections based on culture, when multi-drug resistant bacteria are documented to be susceptible to imipenem.	Dogs and Cats: 5–10 mg/kg IV q6–8h.	GI effects (vomiting, anorexia, diarrhea), CNS toxicity (seizures, tremors), rare increases in renal/liver values.
Lincomycin HCl	Bacterial skin and soft tissue infections.	Dogs and cats: 15 mg/kg PO q8h or 22 mg/kg PO q12h.	Vomiting and diarrhea. Caution: resistance occurs easily.
Marbofloxacin	Bacterial skin and soft tissue infections.	Dogs and cats: 2.75–5.5 mg/kg PO q24h.	Anorexia, vomiting, diarrhea. NOT to be used growing animals.

(Continued)

Table 20.1 Systemic antibiotics (Continued)

Drug	Indications	Dose	Side effects/Comments
Meropenem	Reserved as last resort drug for treatment of multidrug-resistant infections caused by Enterobacteriaceae or *Pseudomonas aeruginosa*.	8.5 mg/kg q12h SC or q8h IV.	Occasional GI upset, occasional hair loss at site of injection. Reduce dose with renal disease.
Minocycline HCl	Skin and soft tissue infections, including those caused by *Mycobacteria*. Combined with niacinamide: Sterile immune-mediated skin diseases.	Dogs and cats: 5–10 mg/kg PO or IV q12h; up to 25 mg/kg q12h for Actinomycosis/Nocardiosis. Give with small amount canned food, dry food inhibits antibiotic absorption.	Anorexia, vomiting and nausea, liver enzyme elevation (rare).
Orbifloxacin	Bacterial skin and soft tissue infections.	Dogs and cats: 2.5–7.5 mg/kg PO q24h.	Nausea, anorexia, vomiting, diarrhea, lethargy. NOT to be used growing animals.
Ormetoprim + sulfadimethoxine	Bacterial skin and soft tissue infections (Dogs).	Dogs: 55 mg/kg PO on first day, then 27.5 mg/kg PO q24h.	Fever, thrombocytopenia, hepatopathy, keratoconjunctivitis sicca, neutropenia, hemolytic anemia, crystalluria, arthropathy, uveitis, eruptions, urticaria, angioedema, proteinuria, hypothyroidism, diarrhea, vomiting, anorexia, seizures. Monitor: Schirmer tear tests, baseline then weekly. Monitor CBC q2 weeks with long-term therapy.
Pradofloxacin	Bacterial skin and soft tissue infections.	Dogs: Not approved for use in dogs in the US due to concern of bone marrow toxicity. In Europe: 3–4.5 mg/kg PO q24h. Cats: Oral suspension: 5–7.5 mg/kg PO once daily. Oral tablets: 3–4.5 mg/kg PO once daily.	Nausea, anorexia, vomiting, diarrhea, lethargy. NOT to be used growing animals. Monitor CBC regularly with long-term use, discontinue if leukopenia occurs.

Rifampin	Bacterial skin and soft tissue infections including those caused by *Mycobacteria*	Dogs: Deep or resistant pyoderma: 5–10 mg/kg PO q24h. Mycobacterial infections: 10–15 mg/kg PO q24h always combined with at least one other antibiotic appropriate for mycobacteria. Cats: Mycobacterial infections: 10–20 mg/kg PO q24h.	Allergic reactions (cats), hepatopathy, pancreatitis, red-orange discoloration of body fluids/secretions and mucous membranes, thrombocytopenia, hemolytic anemia, anorexia, vomiting, diarrhea, and death. Give on an empty stomach. Monitor: Liver values q 2 weeks.
Sulfadiazine/ sulfamethoxazole + trimethoprim	Bacterial skin and soft tissue infections.	Skin or soft tissue infections: 30 mg/kg PO q24h or 15 mg/kg PO q12h. Nocardiosis: 45–60 mg/kg PO q12h (more concern with serious side effects at this dose). Cats: 15 mg/kg PO q12h.	Fever, thrombocytopenia, hepatopathy, keratoconjunctivitis sicca (dogs), neutropenia, hemolytic anemia, crystalluria, arthropathy, uveitis, eruptions, urticaria, angioedema, proteinuria, facial palsy, hypothyroidism, diarrhea, vomiting, anorexia, seizures. Monitor: Schirmer tear tests, baseline then weekly. CBC every 2 weeks with long-term therapy.
Tetracycline HCl	Bacterial skin and soft tissue infections. Combined with niacinamide: Various sterile immune-mediated skin diseases.	Dogs and cats: Infections: 22 mg/kg PO q8h. Dog: Immune mediated disorders: 250 mg PO q8–12h for dogs <10 kg and 500 mg PO q8–12h for dogs >10 kg.	Anorexia, vomiting, diarrhea, renal damage, tooth discoloration. NOT to be used in pregnant or young animals.
Ticarcillin disodium + clavulanate potassium	Otitis externa and/or media caused by resistant *Pseudomonas*.	Dogs and cats: 15–25 mg/kg IV/IM/SQ q8h. As an otic solution, dilute injectable formulation as directed by manufacturer, draw into 2.0 ml aliquots and freeze. Thaw one aliquot daily and instill 0.5 ml into affected ear q12h.	Diarrhea and allergic reactions. Drug is inconsistently available.

Table 20.2 Systemic antifungals.

Drug	Indications	Dose	Comments
Amphotericin B-liposomal formulation	Leishmaniasis, pythiosis, systemic mycoses.	Dogs: 1–3.3 mg/kg IV over 2 hours. Give q48h for 4 weeks or until cumulative dose of 24–30 mg/kg dependent on patient response and drug toxicity (note doses are much higher than conventional amphotericin B). Cats: 1 mg/kg slowly IV q48h for 4 weeks or until cumulative dose of 12 mg/kg.	Nephrotoxic, check CBC/Chemistry panel and UA monitor pretreatment and at least weekly thereafter during therapy.
Caspofungin acetate	Deep infections caused by *Aspergillus*, *Candida*, and *Sporothrix*.	Dogs and cats: 0.5–2 mg/kg q24h IV infused over 1 hour. Suggested maximum daily dose 50 mg total extrapolated from humans.	Side effects unknown; rarely used.
Fluconazole	Systemic mycoses. Less effective treatment option than other azoles for dermatophytosis, *Malassezia* dermatitis.	Dogs: 5–10 mg/kg PO q12–24h. Cats: 50 mg per cat PO q12–24h or 5–10 mg/kg PO q24h.	Increased liver enzymes. Renal excretion, reduce dose or avoid with renal disease. Avoid compounded drugs, especially liquid formulations due to poor manufacturing accuracy.
Griseofulvin	Dermatophytosis. Use only if other more effective treatments are unavailable.	Dogs: Microsize: 25 mg/kg PO q12h or 50 mg/kg PO q24h. Ultramicrosize: 5–10 mg/kg PO q24h or divided q12. Cats: Microsize: 25 mg/kg PO q12h. Ultramicrosize: 5–10 mg/kg PO q24h.	Anorexia, vomiting, diarrhea, hepatotoxicity, myelosuppression. NOT to be used in pregnant animals. Caution in cats. Monitor: Baseline CBC then q 2–3 weeks in cats.
Itraconazole	Systemic mycoses dermatophytosis, *Malassezia* dermatitis.	Dogs and cats: 5–10 mg/kg PO q24h. Pulse dosing for feline dermatophytosis: 5–10 mg/kg PO q24h on an alternating week schedule until 2 negative DTMs 1–2 weeks apart.	Anorexia, weight loss, vomiting, hepatotoxicity, vasculitis-dogs (rare). Monitor: monthly ALT (alanine aminotransferase). Do not use compounded itraconazole as it has very poor bioavailability compared with generic and brand name formulations.
Ketoconazole	Systemic mycoses dermatophytosis, *Malassezia* dermatitis.	Systemic mycosis: 5–10 mg/kg PO q12h or 15–20 mg/kg q12h with CNS involvement. Dermatophytosis: 5–10 mg/kg PO q24h. *Malassezia* dermatitis: 5–10 mg/kg PO q24h.	Anorexia, vomiting, diarrhea, reversible lightening of hair coat (rare), hepatotoxicity. Monitor: Liver enzymes. Caution in cats.
Posaconazole	Systemic mycoses (Cats).	Dogs: 5–10 mg/kg PO q12–24h. Cats: 5–7.5 mg/kg PO q24h or divided into two doses per day.	Pruritus, hepatopathy (little information is known).
Terbinafine Hydrochloride	Systemic mycoses dermatophytosis, *Malassezia* dermatitis.	Dogs and cats: Dermatophytosis and systemic mycoses: 30–40 mg/kg PO q24h. *Malassezia* dermatitis: 30 mg/kg PO q24h.	Anorexia, vomiting, lethargy, lymphopenia, elevated liver values (ALP, ALT). Monitor: Baseline liver enzymes and during therapy with long-term use.
Voriconazole	Systemic mycoses (Dogs).	Dogs: 4–5 mg/kg PO q12h. Cats: 5 mg/kg PO q12–24h.	Unknown in animals, avoid with liver disease.

Table 20.3 Systemic antiviral/antiprotozoal medications.

Drug	Indications	Dose	Comments/Side effects
Allopurinol	Leishmaniasis	Dogs: 15–30 mg/kg PO q12h. Cats: 20 mg/kg PO q24h.	Vomiting, diarrhea, nausea, pruritus, myelosuppression. Monitor hepatic/renal function and for xanthine urolithiasis.
Famciclovir	Herpes viral dermatitis.	Cats: typical dose is 125 mg PO BID in adult cats, or up to 40–90 mg/kg PO BID–TID.	Possible renal side effects. Monitor: Chemistry/urinalysis in long-term use.
Meglumine antimoniate	Leishmaniasis.	Dogs: 100 mg/kg SC q24h or 50–75 mg/kg SC q12h for 30–40 days combined with allopurinol at 15–30 mg/kg PO q12h.	Anorexia, vomiting, nausea, lethargy, liver enzyme elevation.

Table 20.4 Antihistamines.

Drug	Indications	Dose	Comments/Side effects
Amitriptyline HCl	Behavior disorders, neurogenic pain, and psychogenic and pruritic/allergic conditions.	Dogs: 1–3 mg/kg PO q12h. Cats: 0.5–1 mg/kg PO q12–24h or 5–10 mg per cat PO.	Sedation, constipation, urinary retention.
Cetirizine HCl.	Pruritic/allergic skin conditions.	Dogs: 1 mg/kg or 10–20 mg per dog PO q12–24h. Cats: 1 mg/kg or 5 mg per cat PO q12–24h.	Sedation, transient vomiting, hypersalivation.
Chlorpheniramine maleate	Pruritic/allergic skin conditions.	Dogs: 4–8 mg per dog (max. dose of 0.5 mg/kg) PO q8–12h. Cats: 2–4 mg per cat PO q8–12h.	Lethargy, paradoxical excitement (cats).
Clemastine fumarate	Pruritic/allergic skin conditions.	Dogs: 0.05–1.5 mg/kg PO q12h (not recommended due to poor bioavailability). Cats: 0.34–0.68 mg per cat PO q12h.	Sedation, dry mouth, paradoxical hyperactivity, diarrhea (cats).
Clomipramine HCl	Behavior disorders.	Dogs: 2–4 mg/kg PO q24h or divided q12h. Cats: 0.25–1 mg/kg PO q24h,	Anorexia, vomiting, diarrhea, lethargy, liver enzyme elevations, and anticholinergic effects. Start a lower dose and slowly increase to effect; taper off slowly to discontinue.
Cyproheptadine HCl	Pruritic/allergic skin conditions.	Dogs: 0.5–2 mg/kg PO q8–12h. Cats: 2–4 mg per cat PO q12–24h.	Lethargy, sedation, dry mouth, paradoxical excitement (cats). Little evidence to support antipruritic efficacy.

(*Continued*)

Table 20.4 Antihistamines (Continued)

Drug	Indications	Dose	Comments/Side effects
Diphenhydramine HCl	Pruritic/allergic skin conditions.	Dogs and cats: 2–4 mg/kg PO q8–12h.	Lethargy, dry mouth, urinary retention, paradoxical excitement (cats).
Doxepin HCl	Pruritic/allergic skin conditions, behavior disorders, neurogenic pain, and psychogenic dermatoses.	Dogs: 0.5–3 mg/kg PO q12h. Cats: 0.5–1 mg/kg PO q12–24h.	Cardiac arrhythmias, hyperexcitability, diarrhea, vomiting, lethargy/sedation, polyphagia. Start a lower dose and slowly increase to effect; taper off slowly to discontinue.
Fexofenadine HCl	Pruritic/allergic skin conditions.	Dogs: 2–5 mg/kg PO q12–24h. Cats: 10–15 mg per cat PO q12–24h.	None reported.
Hydroxyzine HCl/ pamoate	Pruritic/allergic skin conditions.	Dogs: 2 mg/kg PO q12h. Cats: 5–10 mg per cat q12h.	Sedation, dry mouth.
Loratadine	Pruritic/allergic skin conditions.	Dogs: 0.25–1 mg/kg PO q24h. Cats: 0.5 mg/kg PO q24h	None reported.

Table 20.5 Systemic glucocorticoids.

Drug	Indications	Dose	Comments/Side effects
Dexamethasone	Allergic dermatoses, Immune-mediated diseases. 8–10 times more potent than prednisone and has 48 hours duration of effect.	Dogs: Anti-inflammatory: 0.07–0.15 mg/kg PO q24h or divided q12h to effect then taper off. Immunosuppression: 0.1–0.2 mg/kg PO q12–24h, taper to 0.05–0.1 mg/kg PO q48–72h. Low dose dexamethasone suppression test: 0.01 mg/kg IV, obtain serum samples for cortisol measurement prior to injection and 4 and 8 hours post injection. High dose dexamethasone suppression test: 0.1 mg/kg IV, same sampling protocol as for low dose Cats: Anti-inflammatory: 0.125–0.25 mg/kg PO q24h or divided q12h to effect then taper off Immunosuppression: 0.2 mg/kg PO q12–24h, taper to 0.05–0.1 mg/kg PO q 2–5 days	Polyuria, polydipsia and polyphagia, weight gain, panting, vomiting, diarrhea, elevated liver enzymes (ALP), pancreatitis, diabetes mellitus, muscle atrophy, skin and coat changes, behavioral changes, heart failure (cats). Monitor: Immunosuppressive doses; baseline CBC/Chemistry panel/Urinalysis then q 2–4 weeks.
Methylprednisolone/ methylprednisolone acetate	Allergic dermatoses, immune-mediated diseases.	Dogs: Anti-inflammatory disorders: 0.8–1.0 mg/kg PO q24h to effect then taper to 0.2–0.4 mg/kg PO q48h/try to taper off. Immunosuppression: 0.8–1.5 mg/kg PO q12h, taper to q 0.4–0.8 mg/kg PO q48h. Cats: Anti-inflammatory disorders: 2 mg/kg PO q24h to effect then taper to 0.8 mg/kg PO q48h/try to taper off. Immunosuppression: 4 mg/kg PO q24h, taper to 0.8–1.8 mg/kg PO q48–72h Long lasting injection: Anti-inflammatory or immunosuppression: 10–20 mg per cat SC or IM (not recommended except as last resort due to risk of side effects such as diabetes and heart failure).	Polyuria, polydipsia and polyphagia, weight gain, panting, vomiting, diarrhea, elevated liver enzymes (ALP), pancreatitis, diabetes mellitus, muscle atrophy, skin and coat changes, skin and urinary tract infections, heart failure (cats) Monitor: Immunosuppressive doses: Baseline CBC/Chemistry panel/Urinalysis then q2–4 weeks.
Prednisone/ prednisolone	Allergic dermatoses, immune-mediated diseases.	Dogs: Anti-inflammatory: 0.5–1.0 mg/kg PO q24h to effect then taper to 0.25–0.5 mg/kg PO q48h/try to taper off. Immunosuppression: 2.2 mg/kg PO q24h, taper to 0.5–1 mg/kg PO q48h. Cats (*use prednisolone only*): Anti-inflammatory: 2.2 mg/kg PO q24h to effect then taper to 1 mg/kg PO q48h/try to taper off. Immunosuppression (*use prednisolone only*): 4.4 mg/kg PO q24h, taper to 0.8–1.8 mg/kg PO q48–72h.	Polyuria, polydipsia and polyphagia, weight gain, panting, vomiting, diarrhea, elevated liver enzymes (ALP), pancreatitis, diabetes mellitus, muscle atrophy, skin and coat changes, urinary tract infections, heart failure (cats). Monitor: Immunosuppressive doses: Baseline CBC/Chemistry panel/Urinalysis then q 2–4 weeks.

(*Continued*)

Table 20.5 Systemic glucocorticoids (Continued)

Drug	Indications	Dose	Comments/Side effects
Triamcinolone acetonide	Allergic dermatoses, immune-mediated diseases.	Dogs: Anti-inflammatory: 0.11 mg/kg PO q24h then taper to 0.05–0.1 mg/kg PO q48–72hr/ try to taper off. Immunosuppression: 0.4–0.6 mg/kg PO q24h, taper to 0.1–0.2 mg/kg PO q48–72h. Cats: Anti-inflammatory: 0.09–0.26 mg/kg PO q 24h; taper to 0.08 mg/kg PO q48–72h/try to taper off. Immunosuppression: 0.6–2 mg/kg PO q24h, taper to 0.6–1 mg/kg PO q 2–7 days. For injectable product (package insert): 0.11–0.22 mg/kg SC or IM for inflammatory or allergic disorders, and 0.22 mg/kg SC or IM for dermatological disorders. Effects generally persist for 7–15 days; *due to risk of side effects such as diabetes, long-acting steroids are not recommended unless oral steroids cannot be administered.* For intralesional injection: Usual dose is 1.2–1.8 mg; inject around lesion at 0.5–2.5 cm intervals. Do not exceed 0.6 mg at any one site or 6 mg total dose.	Polyuria, polydipsia and polyphagia, weight gain, panting, vomiting, diarrhea, elevated liver enzymes (ALP), pancreatitis, diabetes mellitus, muscle atrophy, skin and coat changes, urinary tract infections, heart failure (cats). Monitor: Immunosuppressive doses: Baseline CBC/Chemistry panel/Urinalysis then q 2–4 weeks.
Trimeprazine tartrate + prednisolone *Temaril P*®	Allergic dermatoses, (Dogs). Each tablet contains 5 mg trimeprazine and 2 mg prednisolone.	Dogs (package insert): Up to 10 lb: ½ tablet PO q12h. 11–20 lb: 1 tablet PO q12h. 21–40 lb: 2 tablets PO q12h. Over 40 lb: 3 tablets PO q 12h Give to effect then taper to lowest effective alternate day dose based on prednisolone dose of 0.25–0.5 mg/kg PO q 48h, or taper off if possible.	Sedation, lethargy, hypotension, tremors, weakness, restless, polyuria, polydipsia, polyphagia, panting, vomiting, diarrhea, muscle wasting, thin skin, hair loss, calcinosis cutis, skin and urinary tract infections, elevated liver enzymes. Monitor: Baseline: CBC/Chemistry panel/ Urinalysis then q 6–12 months.

Table 20.6 Non-steroidal immunomodulating and immunosuppressive drugs.

Drug	Indications	Dose	Comments/Side effects
Azathioprine	Immune-mediated skin diseases (pemphigus complex, blistering diseases, discoid lupus erythematosus, cutaneous vasculitis, sterile pyogranulomatous disorders, uveodermatologic syndrome).	Dogs: 1.5–2.5 mg/kg PO q24h until remission, then reduce to q48h. DO NOT USE IN CATS	Diarrhea, myelosuppression. Monitor: Baseline CBC/Chemistry panel then CBC q 2–3 weeks for the first 3–4 months, Chemistry q 2–3 months.
Chlorambucil	Immune-mediated skin diseases (pemphigus complex, blistering diseases, cutaneous vasculitis) and lymphocyte, mast cell, and plasma cell malignancies.	Dogs: 0.1–0.2 mg/kg PO q24h to effect then taper to q48h. Cats: 0.1–0.2 mg/kg PO q24h; usually ½ of a 2 mg tablet once daily for larger cats. Alternate dosing schedule: 2 mg PO q48h for cats >4 kg and 2 mg PO q72h for cats <4 kg.	Myelosuppression, vomiting, diarrhea, anorexia. Monitor: Baseline CBC and platelet count then qo weekly or monthly for the first 3 months, then q 3–4 months.
Colchicine	Canine cutaneous amyloidosis, Shar-Pei fever and acute neutrophilic vasculitis, epidermolysis bullosa acquisita.	Dogs: 0.01–0.03 mg/kg PO q24h. DO NOT USE IN CATS	Nausea, anorexia, vomiting, diarrhea, liver enzyme elevation, myelosuppression. Monitor: Baseline CBC then q 2–4 weeks.
Cyclophosphamide	Neoplastic disease, immune-mediated diseases.	Dogs: 50 mg/m^2 PO q48h or q24h for 4 consecutive days per week. Cats: 2–2.5 mg/kg PO q24h 4 days per week.	Myelosuppression (usually 7–14 days into treatment), hepatotoxicity, nephrotoxicity, cardiotoxicity. Oncologist consultation recommended. Monitor: Baseline CBC and urinalysis, repeat after 10–14 days of treatment, then q monthly.
Cyclosporine	Atopic dermatitis, perianal fistulas, sebaceous adenitis, sterile nodular dermatoses, vasculitis and many other immune-mediated diseases.	Dogs: 5 mg/kg PO q24h. Cats: 7 mg/kg PO q24h.	Vomiting, diarrhea and anorexia, hirsutism, lethargy, gingival overgrowth, viral papillomas, urinary tract infection, weight loss (cats). Numerous drug interactions; refer to drug book. Monitor: Baseline CBC/Chemistry panel/ Urinalysis then q 6–12 months.

(*Continued*)

Table 20.6 Non-steroidal immunomodulating and immunosuppressive drugs (Continued)

Drug	Indications	Dose	Comments/Side effects
Dapsone	Skin and soft tissue infections caused by *Mycobacteria*, immune-mediated diseases refractory to other treatments; brown recluse spider bites.	Dogs: 1 mg/kg PO q8h until remission then 1 mg/kg q12–24h or twice weekly as maintenance. DO NOT USE IN CATS	Liver enzyme elevations, myelosuppression, vomiting, diarrhea and anorexia. Monitor: Baseline CBC/Chemistry/Urinalysis q 2–3 weeks during first 4 months then q 3–4 months.
Immunoglobulin, human intravenous (hIVIG)	Immune-mediated diseases (drug reactions, erythema multiforme, severe auto-immune diseases).	Dogs and cats: 0.5–1.5 g/kg IV in 5–6% infused over 4–12 hours.	Vomiting, allergic reactions. Monitor: CBC/Chemistry panel/Urinalysis and TPRs with blood pressures during infusion.
Interferon alpha, recombinant human	Immunostimulant-viral infections, T cell lymphoma.	Dogs: 1.5–2 million units (MU)/m^2 SC of alpha-2a, 3 times weekly or 20 000 IU PO q24h. Cats: 30 units per cat PO q24h on alternate weeks or 60–300 units per cat PO or SC q24h for 30 consecutive days or on alternate weeks.	PO side effects: Vomiting, nausea. SC side effects: Allergic reactions, fever, lethargy.
Interferon omega Recombinant feline	Labeled (in Europe) for treating FeLV & FIV in cats and Parvo in dogs; has also been used to treat herpesvirus dermatitis and calicivirus stomatitis in cats and canine atopic dermatitis. Not commercially available in USA.	Dogs (extra-label for atopic dermatitis):Per injection: Dogs: 8–15 kg = 1 million units; 15–29 kg = 2 million units; 29–40 kg = 3 million units; 29–40 kg = 4 million units. In one study, dogs were dosed SC on days: 0, 3, 7, 14, 21, 35, 56, 90, 120, and 150. Cats: One cat with herpesvirus dermatitis responded well to 6 injections administered over 23 days of 1.5 million units (MU)/kg of rFeIFN-ω, in 4 treatments half the interferon dose was injected perilesionally and intradermally and the other half subcutaneously; the other 2 treatments were SQ only. Stomatitis/calicivirus positive: Daily oromucosal treatment with 0.1 MU of rFeIFN-ω was as effective as daily oral steroids in one case series of 36 cats. *For treatment of FeLV or FIV* as labeled (extra-label in USA): 1 million units/kg SC once daily for 5 days. Three separate 5-day treatments performed at day 0, day 14, and day 60.	Potential adverse effects: Fever, vomiting, diarrhea, lethargy. Increases in liver enzymes and bone marrow suppression have been seen.

Leflunomide	Systemic and cutaneous reactive histiocytosis, pemphigus complex.	Dogs: 3–4 mg/kg PO q24h to effect then taper to lowest effective dose/frequency. Cats: 2–3 mg/kg PO q24h to effect then taper to lowest effective dose/frequency.	Vomiting, anemia, and lymphopenia. Monitor: liver enzymes, CBC.
Levamisole HCl	Idiopathic recurrent pyoderma, systemic lupus erythematosus, eosinophilic granuloma (cats).	Dogs and cats: 2.5–5 mg/kg PO q48h.	Vomiting, diarrhea, anorexia, lethargy, salivation, tremors, cutaneous drug reaction, blood dyscrasias.
Lomustine	Epitheliotropic and non-epitheliotropic lymphoma, mast cell tumor, histiocytic sarcoma.	Dogs: 50–90 mg/m^2 PO q 21–28 days. Cats: 50–60 mg/m^2 PO q 21–42 days or 10 mg per cat.	Myelosuppression (neutropenia and thrombocytopenia) with nadir occurring 7–21 days after treatment. Monitor: Liver enzymes and CBC before each dose and 7–10 days after dose. Oncologist consultation recommended.
Masitinib mesylate	Mast cell tumor (Dogs).	Dogs: 12.5 mg/kg PO q24h (may need to reduce dose if toxicity occurs).	Anorexia, vomiting, diarrhea, lethargy, proteinuria, low albumin, myelosuppression. Monitor: Albumin levels and urinalysis q 2 weeks, CBC and chemistry q 4 weeks. Oncologist consultation recommended.
Mycophenolate mofetil	Immune-mediated diseases, most commonly pemphigus foliaceus (Dogs).	Dogs: 20–40 mg/kg/day PO divided into three doses.	Anorexia, vomiting, diarrhea, lethargy. Monitor: CBC/Chemistry panel pre-treatment, at 3–4 weeks then q4–6 months.
Pentoxifylline	Various inflammatory and immune-mediated skin conditions (dermatomyositis, vasculitis, erythema multiforme, discoid lupus erythematosus, symmetric lupoid onychodystrophy, acral lick dermatitis, sterile panniculitis, interdigital furunculosis).	Dogs: 10–30 mg/kg PO q8–12h. Cats: 100 mg PO q12h.	Vomiting, diarrhea, anorexia. Use cautiously with severe hepatic or renal impairment or bleeding risk.
Piroxicam	Oral and cutaneous squamous cell carcinomas, nasal carcinoma, mammary adenocarcinoma, and transmissible venereal tumor.	Dogs: 0.3 mg/kg PO q24–48h. Cats: 0.3 mg/kg PO q48–72h.	GI ulceration, renal damage. Monitor: Liver and renal values with long-term use.

(*Continued*)

Table 20.6 Non-steroidal immunomodulating and immunosuppressive drugs (Continued)

Drug	Indications	Dose	Comments/Side effects
Staphage lysate	Canine recurrent pyoderma caused by *Staphylococcus* (Dogs).	Dogs: 0.5 ml SC twice weekly for a 10–14 weeks then 0.5–1 ml once every 2–4 weeks.	Pain, erythema, swelling, and pruritus at injection site. Rare: Vomiting, diarrhea, weakness, fever, and lethargy.
Sulfasalazine	Immune-mediated skin diseases (vasculitis) (Dogs).	Dogs: 20–40 mg/kg PO q8h or 15–22 mg/kg PO q8–12h.	Anorexia, vomiting allergic reactions, keratoconjunctivitis sicca, ataxia, depression, clinical signs of hypothyroidism, anemia, leukopenia, hepatopathy, orange-yellow discoloration of urine or skin. Monitor: Schirmer's tear tests; baseline then weekly. CBC–biweekly with long-term therapy.
Toceranib phosphate	Mast cell tumor (Dogs).	Dogs: Induction dose: 3.25 mg/kg PO every other day (or three times weekly). Many oncologists recommend a lower dose of 2.5–2.75 mg/kg every other day or Mon/Weds/Fri.	Anorexia, vomiting, diarrhea, hematochezia or hemorrhagic diarrhea, lethargy, lameness/skeletal pain. Monitor: For the first 6 weeks: CBC weekly, chemistry panel and urinalysis monthly. Oncologist consultation recommended.

Table 20.7 Behavior modifying medications/analgesics.

Drug	Indications	Dose	Comments/Side effects
Amitriptyline HCl	Behavior disorders, neurogenic pain, and psychogenic dermatoses, pruritic/allergic conditions.	Dogs: 1–3 mg/kg PO q12h. Cats: 0.5–1 mg/kg PO q24h or 5–10 mg per cat PO q24h.	Sedation, constipation, urinary retention. Start a lower dose and slowly increase to effect; taper off slowly to discontinue.
Clonazepam	Self-mutilation, compulsive disorders, acral lick granulomas, hyperesthesia.	Dogs: 0.1–1 mg/kg PO q12h. Cats: 0.025–0.2 mg/kg PO q12–24h.	Sedation, ataxia, hepatic necrosis (cats). Monitor: Liver values in cats. Start a lower dose and slowly increase to effect; taper off slowly to discontinue.
Clomipramine HCl	Behavior disorders.	Dogs: 2–4 mg/kg PO q24h or divided q12h. Cats: 0.25–1 mg/kg PO q24h.	Anorexia, vomiting, diarrhea, lethargy, liver enzyme elevations, and anticholinergic effects. Start a lower dose and slowly increase to effect; taper off slowly to discontinue.
Diazepam	Self-mutilation, compulsive disorders, acral lick granulomas, hyperesthesia.	Dogs: 0.5–2.2 mg/kg PO q12–24h. Cats: 0.2–0.5 mg/kg PO q12–24h.	Sedation, ataxia, polyphagia, hepatic necrosis (cats). Monitor: Liver values in cats.
Doxepin HCl	Behavior disorders, neurogenic pain, psychogenic dermatoses, pruritic/allergic conditions.	Dogs: 0.5–3 mg/kg q12h Cats: 0.5–1 mg/kg PO q12–24h.	Cardiac arrhythmias, hyperexcitability, diarrhea, vomiting, lethargy/sedation, polyphagia. Start a lower dose and slowly increase to effect; taper off slowly to discontinue.
Fluoxetine hydrochloride	Behavior disorders, psychogenic dermatoses, hyperesthesia.	Dogs: 1–2 mg/kg PO q24h. Cats: 0.5–2 mg/kg PO q24h.	Lethargy, anorexia, vomiting, diarrhea, tremors, anxiety, irritability. Start a lower dose and slowly increase to effect; taper off slowly to discontinue.
Gabapentin	Neurogenic pain/pruritus.	Dogs: 5–15 mg/kg PO q12h. Cats: Suggested initial dosages range from 3 mg/kg PO q24h titrated upwards to 5–10 mg/kg PO q12h to effect.	Sedation, ataxia.
Lorazepam	Self-mutilation, compulsive disorders, acral lick granulomas, hyperesthesia.	Dogs: 0.025–0.2 mg/kg PO q12–24h. Cats: 0.025–0.08 mg/kg PO q12–24h.	Polyphagia, paradoxical excitement, vocalization, aggression, anxiety. Monitor: Liver enzymes in cats.
Paroxetine hydrochloride	Behavior disorders, psychogenic dermatoses, hyperesthesia.	Dogs: 0.5–2 mg/kg PO q24h. Cats: 0.5–1 mg/kg PO q12–24h.	Lethargy, anorexia, vomiting, diarrhea, tremors, anxiety, irritability. Start a lower dose and slowly increase to effect; taper off slowly to discontinue.

Table 20.8 Systemic antiparasitic drugs.

Drug	Indications	Dose	Comments/Side effects
Afoxolaner	Flea and tick control (Dogs).	Dogs: Minimum dosage of 2.5 mg/kg PO q 4 weeks.	Anorexia, vomiting, diarrhea, seborrhea, lethargy.
Doramectin	Demodicosis, sarcoptic mange, notoedric mange.	Dogs: Demodicosis: 0.6 mg/kg SC or PO once weekly. Sarcoptic mange: 0.2–0.3 mg/kg SC once weekly. Cats: Demodicosis: 0.4–0.6 mg/kg SC once weekly. Notoedric mange: 0.2–0.3 mg/kg SC q 1–2 weeks for 2–3 treatments.	Hypersalivation, mydriasis, blindness, lethargy, tremors, ataxia and pain or swelling at the injection site. Check heartworm status prior to use. Caution in Collies/herding breeds.
Fluralaner	Flea control, ticks, demodicosis, sarcoptic mange.	Dogs: Minimum dose of 25 mg/kg PO q 12 weeks (dosed on body weight range) or topical minimum dose of 25 mg/kg (dosed on body weight range). Cats: Topical minimum dose of 40 mg/kg (dosed on body weight range).	Anorexia, vomiting, diarrhea.
Ivermectin	Demodicosis, sarcoptic mange, notoedric mange, cheyletiellosis, *Otodectes*, nasal mites.	Demodicosis: 0.3–0.6 mg/kg PO q24h until one month beyond negative skin scraping. Sarcoptic mange, notoedric mange, cheyletiellosis: 0.2–0.4 mg/kg PO or SC every 2 weeks for 3 doses. *Otodectes*: 0.3 mg/kg SC every 2 weeks for 3 treatments or topically (Acarexx® 0.01% ivermectin otic suspension) 0.5 ml per ear for 1–2 treatments. Nasal mites: 0.3 mg/kg SC every 1–2 weeks for 2–3 doses.	Hypersalivation, mydriasis, blindness, lethargy, weakness/ tremors, ataxia, depression, anorexia, vomiting and diarrhea, injection site pain or swelling. Do not use in Collies, herding breeds or ivermectin-sensitive breeds with ABCB1–1 (MDR1) allele mutation. Check heartworm status prior to use.
Milbemycin oxime	Demodicosis, sarcoptic mange, cheyletiellosis, nasal mites.	Demodicosis: 0.5–2 mg/kg PO q24h. Sarcoptic mange and cheyletiellosis: 2 mg/kg PO weekly for 3–8 weeks. Nasal mites: 0.5–1 mg/kg PO once weekly for two doses.	Lethargy, vomiting, ataxia, trembling. Check heartworm status prior to use.
Moxidectin	Demodicosis, sarcoptic mange, *Otodectes*.	Dogs: Demodicosis: 0.2–0.4 mg/kg PO q24h until one month beyond negative skin scraping. Topical moxidectin (Advantage Multi®) q1–2 weeks until one month beyond negative skin scraping (helpful in mild cases). Sarcoptic mange: 0.2–0.25 mg/kg PO or SC weekly for 3–6 weeks. Topical moxidectin (Advantage Multi) q30d × 2tx. *Otodectes*: 0.2 mg/kg PO or SC twice 10 days apart. Cats: *Otodectes:* 0.2 mg/kg SC. *Demodex*: Topical moxidectin (Advantage Multi) q1–2 weeks until one month beyond negative skin scraping.	Urticaria, angioedema, erythema, restless, ataxia, lethargy, anorexia, vomiting. Caution in ivermectin sensitive animals. Check heartworm status prior to use.

Table 20.8 Systemic antiparasitic drugs (Continued)

Drug	Indications	Dose	Comments/Side effects
Nitenpyram	Flea control, maggot removal.	Dogs: 11.4 mg tablet PO q24h (dogs 1–11.4 kg or 2–25 lb), 57 mg tablet PO q24h (dogs 11.5–56.8 kg or 25.1–125 lb). Cats: 11.4 mg tablet PO q24h (cats 1–11.4 kg or 2–25 lb).	None reported.
Sarolaner	Flea control, ticks, demodicosis, sarcoptic mange (Dogs).	Minimum dose of 2 mg/kg PO q 4 weeks (dosed on body weight range).	Anorexia, vomiting, diarrhea.
Selamectin	Flea control, sarcoptic mange, notoedric mange, cheyletiellosis, *Otodectes*, lice, *Dermacentor variabilis* ticks, heartworm, hookworm, and roundworm prevention.	Dogs and cats: Flea control: 6 mg/kg topically monthly. Lice: 6 mg/kg topically, one dose. *Otodectes*: 6–12 mg/kg topically q 2 weeks for two doses. Cheyletiellosis: 6–12 mg/kg topically q 2 weeks for three treatments. Sarcoptic or notoedric mange: 6–12 mg/kg topically q 2 weeks for 3–4 doses. Ticks: 6 mg/kg topically q 4 weeks.	Pruritus, erythema, and alopecia at application site. Check heartworm status prior to use.
Spinosad +/− milbemycin oxime	Spinosad: Flea control, (dogs and cats). Spinosad with milbemycin oxime: Flea control, heartworm prevention, and hookworm, roundworm, and whipworm treatment and control (Dogs).	Dogs and cats: Spinosad minimum dosage of 30 mg/kg spinosad (50 mg/kg for cats). PO with food q 4 weeks (dosed on body weight range). Dogs: Spinosad with milbemycin oxime minimum dosage of 30 mg/kg spinosad and 0.5 mg/kg milbemycin. PO with food q 4 weeks (dosed on body weight range).	Anorexia, vomiting, lethargy, diarrhea. Do not combine with ivermectin due to neurologic toxicity.

Table 20.9 Topical antiparasitics.

Active ingredient	Targeted parasites	Formulation	Comments
Amitraz	*Demodex, Sarcoptes*, Fleas and Ticks (Collar).	Concentrated solution, collar.	May cause sedation, ataxia, bradycardia, vomiting, diarrhea, hypothermia, and a transient hyperglycemia. Rarely, seizures have been reported. Topical effects can include edema, erythema, and pruritus. Do not use with other MAO inhibitors, or in cats. Prescription only.
Dinotefuran Combination with pyriproxyfen or permethrin	Fleas, ticks and mosquitoes (with permethrin).	Spot-on solution.	Permethrin containing products are NOT to be used in CATS or dogs that are in contact with cats.
Fipronil ± combination with methoprene	Fleas, ticks, lice, chiggers, *Sarcoptes Cheyletiella*, and *Otodectes*.	Spray, spot-on solution.	Do not bathe within 48hr after application.
Fluralaner	Fleas, ticks.	Spot-on solution.	Effective extra-label for mites including *Demodex*.
Imidacloprid Combination with pyriproxyfen, permethrin, moxidectin	Fleas and lice (imidacloprid and pyriproxyfen). Fleas, ticks, lice, flies and mosquitoes (imidacloprid, permethrin, and pyriproxyfen). Heartworms, fleas, hookworms, roundworms, whipworms, *Demodex*, *Sarcoptes*, and *Cheyletiella* (imidacloprid and moxidectin).	Spot-on solution.	Hypersalivation if oral exposure. Permethrin containing products are NOT to be used in CATS or dogs that are in contact with cats.
Lime sulfur	Antifungal keratolytic, keratoplastic, antiparasitic, and antipruritic.	Concentrate	Avoid contact with eyes or mucus membranes. Stains skin, hair, clothes, jewelry. Strong sulfur odor.
Methoprene (insect growth regulator) Combination with permethrin, phenothrin	Fleas	Spot-on solution.	Permethrin or phenothrin-containing products are NOT to be used in CATS or dogs that are in contact with cats.
Picaridin	Mosquitos, flies, fleas, ticks, and chiggers (repellent).	Spray, wipes.	
Pyrethrin Combination with methoprene, permethrin, piperonyl, pyriproxyfen	Fleas, lice, ticks, and *Cheyletiella*.	Shampoo, spray, dust, solution, dip.	Permethrin or phenothrin-containing products are NOT to be used in CATS or dogs that are in contact with cats.
Pyriproxyfen **(insect growth regulator)** **Combination with pyrethrin, tetramethin, permethrin, piperonyl, imidacloprid**	Fleas	Shampoo, spot-on solution, spray, fogger.	Permethrin or phenothrin-containing products are NOT to be used in CATS or dogs that are in contact with cats.
Rotenone	*Demodex*	Ointment	
Spinetoram	Fleas	Spot-on solution.	Cats only. May cause skin irritation, local alopecia.

Table 20.10 Nutritional supplements/vitamins/retinoids.

Drug	Indications	Dose	Side effects/comments
Acitretin	Color dilution alopecia, Schnauzer comedo syndrome, lamellar ichthyosis, actinic keratoses, epitheliotropic lymphoma, intracutaneous cornifying epitheliomas, idiopathic seborrhea.	Dogs: 0.5–3 mg/kg PO once daily. Cats: 3 mg/kg or one 10 mg capsule PO once daily.	Teratogenic in humans. Keratoconjunctivitis sicca, anorexia, vomiting, diarrhea, lethargy, behavioral changes, joint pain/stiffness, pruritus, skin eruptions, polydipsia; adverse effects more common in cats. Monitor: Baseline liver values and Schirmer tear tests (dogs) then q 1–2 months, limit UV exposure.
Isotretinoin	Sebaceous adenitis, vitamin A responsive dermatosis, sebaceous adenomas, solar/actinic dermatosis, infundibular keratinizing acanthomas (multiple keratoacanthomas or intracutaneous cornifying epitheliomas), ichthyosis.	Dogs: Keratinization disorders and follicular tumors: 1 mg/kg PO q 12–24h. Cutaneous epitheliotropic lymphoma: 3–4 mg/kg PO once daily or divided twice daily. Cats: *Feline acne*: 5–10 mg per cat PO once daily. *Epitheliotropic lymphoma*: 10 mg per cat once daily.	Teratogenic in humans. Keratoconjunctivitis sicca, anorexia, vomiting, diarrhea, lethargy, behavioral changes, joint pain/stiffness, pruritus, skin eruptions, polydipsia; adverse effects more common in cats. Monitor: Baseline liver values and Schirmer tear tests (dogs) then q 1–2 months, limit UV exposure.
Niacinamide	Combined with doxycycline: various sterile immune-mediated skin diseases.	Dogs: ≤10 kg, give 250 mg PO q8h, >10 kg, give 500 mg PO q8h.	Anorexia, vomiting, diarrhea, increased liver enzymes (rare), implicated in seizures.
Omega-3 Fatty Acids **Eicosapentaenoic acid (EPA)** **Alpha linolenic acid** **Docosahexaenoic acid (DHA)**	Allergic and inflammatory dermatoses.	Dogs and cats: 180 mg EPA/10 lb.	Anorexia, vomiting, diarrhea. Contraindicated with pancreatitis, coagulopathy.
Omega-6 fatty acids **Linoleic acid**	Seborrhea sicca, cutaneous epitheliotropic lymphoma (Dogs).	Dogs: Topical spot on products containing fatty acids and plant derived oils as directed by product manufacturer. Cutaneous epitheliotropic lymphoma: 3 ml/kg safflower oil PO twice weekly.	Oral: Anorexia, vomiting, diarrhea, weight gain.
Vitamin A	Sebaceous adenitis, vitamin A-responsive dermatosis, primary seborrhea, other keratinization disorders (Dogs).	Dogs: 1000 IU/kg PO q24h.	(High doses) hepatopathy, anorexia, vomiting, constipation, lethargy, skin and hair changes.
Vitamin E	Various immune-mediated skin diseases (discoid lupus erythematosus, dermatomyositis), pansteatitis (cats).	Dogs: 400–800 IU per dog PO q12h. Cats: 10 mg PO q24h.	None known.
Zinc	Zinc-responsive dermatosis, superficial necrolytic dermatitis.	Dogs: Zinc methionine, zinc sulfate, or zinc gluconate; dose on elemental zinc content of supplement: 2–3 mg/kg/day with food.	Anorexia, nausea, vomiting.

Table 20.11 Non-glucocorticoid hormones.

Drug	Indications	Dose	Side effects/monitoring
Calcitriol	Primary idiopathic seborrhea (Dogs).	Dogs: 10 ng/kg (0.01 mcg/kg) PO q24h.	Hypercalcemia. Monitor: Baseline calcium and phosphate levels then monthly during treatment.
Corticotropin (ACTH gel)	For diagnosis of hyperadrenocorticism.	ACTH stimulation test. Dogs: 2.2 IU/kg IM with serum cortisol measured pre- and 2 hours post-injection. Cats: 2.2 IU/kg IM with serum cortisol measured pre- and 1 and 2 hours post-injection.	For testing use, none.
Cosyntropin (Cortrosyn)	For diagnosis of hyperadrenocorticism	Dogs: 5mcg/kg IV (or 250 mcg per dog IM, IV) with serum cortisol measured pre- and 1 hour post injection. Cats: 5mcg/kg IV (or 125 mcg/cat) with serum cortisol measured pre- and 1 hour post injection.	
Levothyroxine sodium	Hypothyroidism	Dogs: 0.02 mg/kg PO q12-24h on an empty stomach. Cats: 0.05–0.1 mg per cat PO q24h.	Panting, polyuria, polydipsia, polyphagia, weight loss, nervousness, excitability, and tachycardia. Dogs with concurrent cardiac disease: Start with lower levothyroxine dose of 0.005 mg/kg BID and increase dose by 0.005 mg every 2 weeks to 0.02 mg/kg BID.
Lignans	Use in treatment of excess adrenal activity. Lignan has phytoestrogenic activity, and competes with estradiol for tissue estrogen receptors, with less biological effect. Also inhibits aromatase enzyme (lowers estradiol). Available as flax hull (SDG) lignan or HMR lignan.	Suggested doses (Clinical Endocrinology Service/College of Veterinary Medicine/ University of Tennessee): SDG lignan: 2 mg/kg/day; HMR lignan: 10–40 mg/day for small to large dogs.	Available online or at vitamin stores.
Megestrol acetate	Feline atopy (refractory, last resort).	Cats: Initial dose of 2.5–5 mg per cat q48h × 1–3 weeks then reduce to 2.5–5 mg every 7–14 days.	Pyometra, estrus postponement, acromegaly, mammary gland hyperplasia, diabetes mellitus, lethargy, polyuria/polydipsia, polyphagia, weight gain, hepatopathy, adrenocortical suppression, alopecia, cutaneous atrophy, poor wound healing. Monitor: Blood glucose, liver values, and body weight regularly.

Melatonin	Alopecia X, pattern baldness, canine recurrent flank alopecia, color dilution alopecia.	Dogs: 3–12 mg (depending on dog size) PO q12h. Implant: 8 mg (dogs <9 kg), 12 mg (dogs 9–18 kg), and 18 mg (dogs >18 kg).	OTC supplement; *ensure it does not contain xylitol, a sweetener toxic to dogs.* Melatonin may cause sedation (rare), and impair fertility of intact animals. Melatonin implants are contraindicated in pregnant or juvenile animals; sterile abscesses can occur.
Methyltestosterone	Alopecia X.	Dogs: 1 mg/kg (maximum dose 30 mg) PO q24h until hair regrowth is noted then 1 mg/kg q48h for 2 months, followed by 1 mg/kg twice weekly for 2 months, then once weekly for maintenance.	Aggression, hepatopathy, clitoral hypertrophy, vaginal discharge, prostatic hyperplasia, seborrhea oleosa. Monitor: liver values.
Misoprostol	Atopic dermatitis (Dogs).	Dogs: 5 mcg/kg PO q8h.	Vomiting, diarrhea.
Mitotane (o,p'-DDD)	Hyperadrenocorticism(HAC)	Induction dose: 30–50 mg/kg PO divided twice daily for 5–10 days or when post-ACTH cortisol level is between 1–5mcg/dl. Maintenance dose: 35–50 mg/kg PO per week divided in 2–3 doses.	*Hypoadrenocorticism:* Lethargy, depression, ataxia, anorexia, vomiting, and/or diarrhea. Monitoring: Perform ACTH stimulation test at 5–10 days or sooner if side effects occur. Goal is to have basal and post-ACTH cortisol between 1–5 mcg/dl. If basal and post-ACTH cortisol <1 mcg/dl, temporarily stop mitotane and supplement with glucocorticoids until cortisol normal (2 weeks to months). If post-ACTH cortisol is above normal, continue daily mitotane and recheck ACTH stimulation tests at 5–10 day intervals until serum cortisol is between 1–5 mcg/dl. Monitor maintenance therapy with ACTH stimulation test after 1 month of maintenance treatment and then every 3 months.
Selegiline HCl	Pituitary-dependent hyperadrenocorticism, canine cognitive disorders (Dogs).	Dogs: Start with 1 mg/kg PO q24h. If no response is noted after 2 months increase the dose to 2 mg/kg PO q24h.	Anorexia, vomiting, diarrhea, central nervous system signs (rare).
Trilostane	Hyperadrenocorticism (HAC).	Dogs: HAC: 2–5 mg/kg/day PO q24h or 0.21–1.1 mg/ kg PO q12h. Alopecia X: 2 mg/kg PO q12–24h. Cats: 15–30 mg per cat PO q12–24h.	*Hypoadrenocorticism:* Lethargy, anorexia, vomiting, diarrhea, increased potassium. Monitoring: Check ACTH stimulation and electrolytes after 14 days at this dose, adjust dose according to package insert to a goal post-ACTH serum cortisol of 1.45–9.1 mcg/dl. Recheck ACTH stimulation test 14 days after every dose alteration then q 3 months.

Table 20.12 Topical non-steroidal antipruritic therapies.

Active ingredient	Properties	Formulation	Comments
Aluminum acetate solution	Astringent, soothing, antipruritic, antiseptic/antimicrobial effects.	Soak (powder packs and tablets), solution.	Also known as Burow's Solution.
Benzocaine	Anesthetic, antipruritic.	Spray, solution, gel, paste.	
Calamine	Soothing, antipruritic.	Solution	Calamine is a combination of zinc oxide and ferric oxide.
Camphor	Anesthetic, antipruritic.	Lotion	
Ceramides	Soothing, moisturizing.	Spray, foam, spot-on.	Ceramides include phytosphingosine.
Colloidal oatmeal	Anti-inflammatory, antipruritic.	Spray, soak, shampoo, conditioner, lotion.	
Dimethyl sulfoxide (DMSO)	Anti-inflammatory, antipruritic.	Solution, gel, cream.	May cause irritation. Also increases penetration/absorption of other medications when mixed.
Diphenhydramine hydrochloride	Anti-inflammatory properties, mild analgesic properties.	Spray, shampoo, conditioner, lotion, cream, gel.	
Essential oils	Soothing, moisturizing, antiseptic.	Spray, shampoo, conditioner, lotion, foam, spot-on, balm, wipes.	Caution in cats with non-veterinary formulations.
Fatty acids	Soothing, moisturizing, antiseborrheic.	Spray, foam, spot-on.	
Hamamelis	Astringent, soothing, antipruritic, antiseptic/antimicrobial effects.	Solution	Also known as witch hazel.
Lidocaine	Anesthetic, antipruritic.	Spray, lotion, cream, gel.	
Menthol	Analgesic, soothing.	Spray, solution, balm.	
Pimecrolimus	Anti-inflammatory, immunosuppressive.	Cream	May cause irritation. Prescription only.
Pramoxine	Antipruritic, anesthetic.	Spray, shampoo, conditioner, lotion, cream, gel.	
Tacrolimus	Anti-inflammatory, immunosuppressive.	Ointment	May cause irritation. Prescription only.
Zinc gluconate	Antipruritic, antiseptic/antimicrobial effects.	Solution, spray.	

Table 20.13 Topical glucocorticoids.

Active ingredient	Properties	Formulation	Comments
Betamethasone	Medium to high potency depending on modification.	Spray, cream, lotion, ointment, gel.	Often mixed into combination products. Can be absorbed systemically. Long-term use can cause skin atrophy, milia, comedones, and poor wound healing.
Dexamethasone	Low potency.	Lotion	Combination otic product.
Hydrocortisone	Low to medium potency depending on modification.	Solution, shampoo, spray, cream, lotion, gel, wipes.	Often mixed into combination products. Less likely to be absorbed systemically and less likely to cause skin changes with long-term use.
Isoflupredone acetate	High potency.	Ointment, powder.	Often mixed into combination products. Can be absorbed systemically. Long-term use can cause skin atrophy, milia, comedones, and poor wound healing.
Mometasone furoate monohydrate	High potency.	Suspension (otic), cream, ointment, lotion.	Combination otic product.
Triamcinolone acetonide	Medium potency.	Spray, cream, ointment, lotion, spray.	Often mixed into combination products. Can be absorbed systemically. Long-term use can cause skin atrophy, milia, comedones, and poor wound healing.

Table 20.14 Topical antimicrobials/otics.

Active ingredient	Properties	Formulation	Comments
Acetic acid/boric acid	Antibacterial, antifungal, ceruminolytic, keratolytic, keratoplastic, astringent.	Shampoo, spray, wipes.	Acetic acid is the main ingredient in vinegar, some products may have a slightly vinegar odor.
Bacitracin	Antibacterial	Ointment	Combination ophthalmic product.
Benzoyl peroxide	Antimicrobial (especially antibacterial), keratolytic, comedolytic ("follicular flushing"), and degreasing actions.	Shampoo, lotion, cream, gel.	Avoid contact with eyes or mucus membranes. Can be drying to the skin. Can bleach hair and fabrics.
Chlorhexidine gluconate	Antibacterial, antifungal (at higher concentrations).	Solution, scrub, shampoo, conditioner, rinse, spray, leave-on spray, otic flush, foam, wipes.	Many combination products available. Irritant reactions may occur.
Chloroxylenol	Antibacterial	Shampoo, scrub, spray, wipes.	
Clindamycin	Antibacterial	Solution, lotion, gel, wipes, foam.	Used for feline acne.
Clotrimazole	Antifungal	Solution, suspension, ointment, cream, lotion.	Many combination products available.
Ethyl lactate	Antibacterial, keratoplastic, antiseborrheic.	Shampoo	
Fusidic acid	Antibacterial	Ointment, cream, gel.	Often mixed into combination products. Can cause irritant reactions.

(*Continued*)

Table 20.14 Topical antimicrobials/otics (Continued)

Active ingredient	Properties	Formulation	Comments
Gentamicin sulfate	Antibacterial	Spray, ointment, cream, suspension.	Often mixed into combination products, many otic products can cause ototoxicity. Can cause irritant reactions.
Hypochlorous acid	Antibacterial	Solution, spray, gel, flush.	Very safe.
Ketoconazole	Antifungal	Shampoo, conditioner, spray, otic flush, cream, wipes.	
Lime sulfur	Antifungal keratolytic, keratoplastic, antiparasitic, and antipruritic.	Concentrate	Avoid contact with eyes or mucus membranes. Stains skin, hair, clothes, jewelry. Strong sulfur odor.
Miconazole nitrate	Antifungal	Shampoo, suspension, spray, flush, rinse, lotion, gel, cream, wipes.	
Mupirocin	Antibacterial	Ointment, cream.	Effective vs. Gram positive bacteria only.
Nitrofurazone	Antibacterial	Solution, ointment, cream, powder	Avoid contact with eyes or mucus membranes.
Nystatin	Antifungal	Ointment, cream, powder	Often mixed into combination products.
Povidone-iodine	Antimicrobial, antifungal, antiviral.	Solution, spray, scrub, shampoo, ointment.	Can stain skin and fabric. Maybe drying. Can cause irritant reactions.
Selenium sulfide	Antifungal (including sporicidal activity), keratolytic, keratoplastic, and degreasing.	Shampoo, lotion.	NOT FOR CATS Maybe drying. Can cause irritant reactions.
Silver sulfadiazine	Antibacterial, aids wound healing.	Cream	Possible sulfonamide reactions when large surface areas are treated.
Terbinafine hydrochloride	Antifungal	Cream, spray, gel	
Three Point Enzyme System	Antibacterial, antifungal, antiviral.	Shampoo, rinse, spray, cream, wipes.	Ingredients include: lactoperoxidase, lysozyme, lactoferrin +/− hydrocortisone.
Triclosan	Antibacterial	Shampoo	Can cause irritant reactions.

Table 20.15 Topical antiseborrheics.

Active ingredient	Properties	Formulation	Comments
Acetic acid/boric acid	Antibacterial, antifungal, ceruminolytic, keratolytic, keratoplastic, astringent.	Shampoo, spray, wipes.	Acetic acid is the main ingredient in vinegar, some products may have a slight vinegar odor.
Benzoyl peroxide	Antimicrobial (especially antibacterial), keratolytic, comedolytic ("follicular flushing"), and degreasing actions.	Shampoo, lotion, cream, gel.	Avoid contact with eyes or mucus membranes. Can be drying to the skin. Can bleach hair and fabrics.
Ethyl lactate	Antibacterial, keratoplastic, antiseborrheic.	Shampoo	
Fatty acids	Soothing, moisturizing, antiseborrheic.	Spray, foam, spot-on.	
Lime sulfur	Antifungal keratolytic, keratoplastic, antiparasitic, and antipruritic.	Concentrate	Avoid contact with eyes or mucus membranes. Stains skin, hair, clothes, jewelry. Strong sulfur odor.
Phytosphingosine hydrochloride	Antiseborrheic	Shampoo, spray, spot-on.	
Salicylic acid	Antiseborrheic, antipruritic, antibacterial (bacteriostatic), keratoplastic, and keratolytic.	Cream, shampoo, ointment.	High concentration products may cause irritation.
Selenium sulfide	Antifungal (including sporicidal activity), keratolytic, keratoplastic, and degreasing.	Shampoo, lotion.	NOT FOR CATS Maybe drying. Can cause irritant reactions.
Sulfur	Keratoplastic and keratolytic.	Shampoo	Often combined with salicylic acid.
Tar, coal	Keratoplastic, keratolytic, vasoconstrictive, antipruritic, anti-inflammatory, and degreasing actions.	Shampoo	Higher concentration products may have carcinogenic effects.

Table 20.16 Topical immunomodulators and retinoids.

Active ingredient	Properties	Formulation	Comments
Adapalene	Anti-inflammatory, keratoplastic.	Cream, gel, lotion, solution.	May cause irritation. Not to be used in pregnant or nursing animals. Prescription only.
Imiquimod	Antiviral, antineoplastic.	Cream	Do not cover after application, avoid sun exposure on treated areas, may cause irritation and/or secondary infections, may cause depigmentation and alopecia. Prescription only.
Pimecrolimus	Anti-inflammatory, immunosuppressive.	Cream	May cause irritation. Prescription only.
Tacrolimus	Anti-inflammatory, immunosuppressive.	Ointment	May cause irritation. Prescription only.
Tazarotene	Anti-inflammatory, keratoplastic.	Cream, gel.	May cause irritation. Not to be used in pregnant or nursing animals. Prescription only.
Tretinoin	Anti-inflammatory, keratoplastic.	Cream, gel.	May cause irritation. Not to be used in pregnant or nursing animals. Prescription only.

Further reading

Koch, S. Torres, S. and Plumb, D. (2013). *Canine and Feline Dermatology Drug Handbook*, 1e. *Ames IA*: Wiley-Blackwell.

Laporte, C., Boothe, D., Cruz-Espindola, C. et al. (2016). Quality assessment of compounded fluconazole capsules and oral suspensions in the United States. *Vet. Dermatol.* 27 (Supplement S1): 6–121.

Mawby, D.I., Whittemore, J.C., Genger, S., and Papich, M.G. (2014). Bioequivalence of orally administered generic, compounded, and innovator-formulated itraconazole in healthy dogs. *J. Vet. Intern. Med.* 28 (1): 72–77.

Papich, M.G., Davidson, G.S., and Fortier, L.A. (2013). Doxycycline concentration over time after storage in a compounded veterinary preparation. *J. Am. Vet. Med. Assoc.* 242 (12): 1674–1678.

Plumb, D. (2015). *Plumb's Veterinary Drug Handbook*, 8e. Ames IA: Wiley-Blackwell.

Renschler, J., Albers, A., Sinclair-Mackling, H., and Wheat, L.J. (2018). Comparison of compounded, generic, and innovator-formulated Itraconazole in dogs and cats. *J. Am. Anim. Hosp. Assoc.* 54 (4): 195–200.

Index

Page locators in **bold** indicate tables. Page locators in *italics* indicate figures. This index uses letter-by-letter alphabetization.

Clinical Atlas of Canine and Feline Dermatology, First Edition. Edited by Kimberly S. Coyner.

Companion website: www.wiley.com/go/coyner/dermatology

Printed in the USA/Agawam, MA
September 16, 2026

910661.203